Geriatric Physical Therapy

Geriatric Physical Therapy

Edited by
ANDREW A. GUCCIONE, Ph.D., P.T.
Director of Clinical Development, Education and Quality Assurance
Physical Therapy Services
Massachusetts General Hospital
Lecturer, Department of Orthopaedic Surgery
Harvard Medical School
Boston, Massachusetts

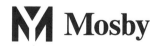 Mosby

St. Louis Baltimore Boston Chicago London Philadelphia Sydney Toronto

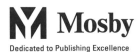
Dedicated to Publishing Excellence

Sponsoring Editor: David K. Marshall
Assistant Editor: Julie Tryboski
Assistant Director, Manuscript Services: Frances M. Perveiler
Production Manager: Nancy C. Baker
Proofroom Manager: Barbara M. Kelly

1 2 3 4 5 6 7 8 9 0 CL/MV 97 96 95 94 93

Library of Congress Cataloging-in-Publication Data

Geriatric physical therapy [edited by]
  Andrew Guccione.
     p.   cm.
    Includes bibliographical references and index.
    ISBN 0-8016-7452-2
    1. Physical therapy for the aged. I. Guccione, Andrew.
    [DNLM: 1. Physical Therapy—in old age. WB 460 G369]
RC953.8.P58G47 1992
615.8′2′0846—dc20
DNLM/DLC   92-49977
for Library of Congress   CIP

Contributors

Dale L. Avers, M.S.Ed., P.T.
Rehabilitation Manager
Lexington Clinic
Lexington, Kentucky

John O. Barr, Ph.D., P.T.
Associate Professor and Director
Program in Physical Therapy
St. Ambrose University
Davenport, Iowa
Research Health Science Specialist
Veterans Administration Medical Center
Iowa City, Iowa

Susan Neufeld Bloom, M.S., P.T.
Geriatric Clinical Consultant
Formerly, Director of Rehabilitation Services
Meridian Healthcare
Baltimore, Maryland

Marybeth Brown, Ph.D., P.T.
Assistant Professor
Program in Physical Therapy
Washington University
St. Louis, Missouri

Julie M. Chandler, M.S., P.T.
Assistant Professor
Graduate Program in Physical Therapy
Duke University
Durham, North Carolina

Charles D. Ciccone, Ph.D., P.T.
Associate Professor
Department of Physical Therapy
Ithaca College
Ithaca, New York

Rebecca L. Craik, Ph.D., P.T.
Associate Professor
Department of Physical Therapy
Beaver College
Glenside, Pennsylvania
Ajunct Associate Professor
Department of Animal Biology
School of Veterinary Medicine
University of Pennsylvania
Philadelphia, Pennsylvania

Jody Delehanty, Ph.D., P.T.
Assistant Professor
Physical Therapy Program
University of Colorado
Denver, Colorado

Marilyn E. DeMont, M.S., P.T.
Director of Professional Development
American Physical Therapy Association
Washington, D.C.

Pamela W. Duncan, Ph.D., P.T.
Associate Professor
Graduate Program in Physical Therapy
Senior Fellow
Center for the Study of Aging and Human Development
Duke University
Durham, North Carolina

Davis L. Gardner, M.A.
Professor
Department of Health Services
College of Allied Health Professions
University of Kentucky
Lexington, Kentucky

Andrew A. Guccione, Ph.D., P.T.
Director of Clinical Development, Education and Quality
  Assurance
Physical Therapy Services
Massachusetts General Hospital
Lecturer, Department of Orthopaedic Surgery
Harvard Medical School
Boston, Massachusetts

Douglas P. Kiel, M.D., M.P.H.
Henry J. Kaiser Family Foundation
Faculty Scholar in General Internal Medicine
Assistant Professor of Medicine
Harvard Medical School
Associate Director of Medical Research
Hebrew Rehabilitation Center for Aged
Research and Training Institute
Boston, Massachusetts

John F. Knarr, M.S., P.T., A.T.C.
Clinical Instructor
Physical Therapy Program
University of Delaware
Newark, Delaware

Wendy Kohrt, Ph.D.
Research Assistant Professor
Department of Medicine
Washington University
St. Louis, Missouri

Carolee Moncur, Ph.D., P.T.
Professor, Division of Physical Therapy
College of Health
Adjunct Associate Professor
Division of Rheumatology
University of Utah School of Medicine
Salt Lake City, Utah

Donald A. Neumann, Ph.D., P.T.
Associate Professor
Program in Physical Therapy
Marquette University
Milwaukee, Wisconsin

Nancy L. Peatman, M.Ed., P.T.
Clinical Associate Professor
Academic Coordinator of Clinical Education
Department of Physical Therapy
Sargent College of Allied Health Professions
Boston University
Boston, Massachusetts

Jean Oulund Peteet, M.P.H., P.T.
Professional Services Director
The Sargent Clinic at Boston University
Adjunct Clinical Assistant Professor
Department of Physical Therapy
Sargent College of Allied Health Professions
Boston University
Boston, Massachusetts

Kenneth E. Perkins, M.S.P.T., P.T., C.O.
Owner and President
Maine Orthotics Lab and Physical Therapy
Gorham, Maine

Elizabeth J. Protas, Ph.D., P.T.
Assistant Dean and Professor
School of Physical Therapy
Texas Woman's University
Houston, Texas

Carol Schunk, Psy.D., P.T.
Regional Director
Medicare and Rehab Specialists
Portland, Oregon

Deborah H. Shefrin, J.D., P.T.
Arnstein and Lehr
Chicago, Illinois

Lynn Snyder-Mackler, Sc.D., P.T., S.C.S.
Assistant Professor
Physical Therapy Program
University of Delaware
Newark, Delaware

Patricia E. Sullivan, Ph.D., P.T.
Associate Professor
MGH Institute of Health Professions
Clinical Consultant
Physical Therapy Services
Massachusetts General Hospital
Boston, Massachusetts

Mary Ann Wharton, M.S., P.T.
Associate Professor
School of Physical Therapy
Slippery Rock University
Slippery Rock, Pennsylvania

Ann K. Williams, Ph.D., P.T.
Associate Professor
School of Physical Therapy
Pacific University
Forest Grove, Oregon

Rita A. Wong, M.S., P.T.
Assistant Professor
Physical Therapy Program
School of Allied Health Professions
University of Connecticut
Storrs, Connecticut

Preface

The overall purpose of this textbook is to provide a comprehensive treatment of geriatric physical therapy for the entry-level student. Practicing clinicians who are new to geriatric physical therapy will find this text helpful as well. Each chapter should help answer the question, How does physical therapy change—if at all—when evaluating and treating the older adult? The intent of this approach was to provide ways of organizing clinical findings and integrating geriatric physical therapy into the context of physical therapy in general. Toward this end, this book was not designed with a multidisciplinary gerontologic perspective written by professionals representing a broad spectrum of disciplines. Instead, contributing authors (with two exceptions) are physical therapists with established expertise in particular areas of physical therapy or a related field.

The text has been organized into five parts. Part I concerns the fundamental process of the art of physical therapy, communication, and four fundamental areas of physical therapy science: clinical epidemiology, exercise physiology, arthrokinesiology, and neuroscience. Part II contains seven chapters related to assessment. Chapter 6 in this part presents a problem-solving model based on the concepts of health status, impairment, functional limitation, and disability as articulated by Nagi. Chapters 7 and 8 detail clinical and formal functional assessments of basic and instrumental activities of daily living in the elderly, and review sensory changes of aging and environments that facilitate independence. Cognitive loss and depression are two impairments known to influence elderly function, and Chapters 9 and 10 on these conditions provide information that is essential to physical therapy evaluation of the geriatric patient. Chapters 11 and 12 promote an understanding of the medical workup and how medical evaluation and pharmacologic treatment interface with physical therapy evaluation and treatment.

Part III contains eight chapters covering the "nuts and bolts" of geriatric physical therapy. These chapters present current research on the scientific basis of specific physical therapy interventions in key areas: endurance training, posture, balance and falls, ambulation, lower extremity orthotics, pain management, wound healing, and patient education. These chapters highlight how physical therapy treatment of the older adult differs from treatment for younger individuals, and in what instances assessment strategies and treatment techniques need to be modified for the geriatric patient. Furthermore, contributing authors have attempted to draw some conclusions about what outcomes can realistically be achieved with an older adult with respect to a particular problem.

The chapters in Part IV consider the social context of geriatric physical therapy: reimbursement issues as well as the ethical and legal issues that surround the daily practice of geriatric physical therapy. Part V presents some of the programmatic aspects of physical therapy services for elders who fall into one of four groups: those who live in nursing homes; those who live in the community and are generally well; those who continue to engage in athletics; and those who are perhaps newest to the ranks of the elderly, older adults with developmental disabilities. Each of these chapters outlines the characteristics of the target population and indicates how physical therapy services might be built around these needs.

The goal of geriatric physical therapy is to provide optimal clinical care to the thousands of individuals we see daily. The authors whose work is presented in this text rose to the challenge of defining the scientific basis of geriatric physical therapy, yet intellect alone does not ensure the best care possible. The best thoughts must be translated into the best clinical actions. It is the hope of all the authors who contributed to this text that the reader will skillfully employ the principles that have been learned to perfect the practice of geriatric physical therapy.

ANDREW A. GUCCIONE, PH.D., P.T.

Acknowledgments

An edited textbook cannot be produced without commitment from numerous individuals. The contributors to this text deserve credit for its quality and thanks for making my task as relatively easy as any editor might wish. The efforts of their support staffs and their colleagues who reviewed draft manuscripts should also be noted. I am particularly grateful to Michael G. Sullivan, Mary Knab, John Hayes Mason, and Ann Jampel for their insights. Peter J. Wagner's work in creating and reconfiguring many of the illustrations is also acknowledged.

David Marshall proposed this project with the promise that he and the staff at Mosby–Year Book would support the book and its editor unfailingly. That promise was kept in full. I am especially indebted to David and also to Julie Tryboski and Fran Perveiler for their efforts. Thanks also to Production Manager Nancy Baker for her help in producing this book.

It is perhaps impossible to write a manuscript on any geriatric topic without pausing to reflect on aging, one's own mortality, and ultimately, a fundamental dimension of the universe: time itself. From a sociological perspective, time is not best measured by subtle deteriorations of physical matter. Rather, a person's own history is better understood as a sequence of interpersonal relationships in particular social contexts. Simply put, our family and friends allow us to mark where we have been, who we are now, and what we shall become. This work is dedicated to my parents, especially the memory of my father, Anthony S. Guccione; to my wife Nancy; and to my children Katie and Nicole.

Andrew A. Guccione, Ph.D., P.T.

Contents

PART I

Foundations of Geriatric Physical Therapy

Implications of an Aging Population for Rehabilitation: Demography, Mortality, and Morbidity in the Elderly

Andrew A. Guccione, Ph.D., P.T.

INTRODUCTION

What are the implications of an increase in the number of older persons in American society, particularly as it affects rehabilitation specialists such as physical therapists? On the one hand, the "graying" of America has been portrayed as a social problem, one that particularly threatens to strip the current health care system of its scarce resources. On the other hand, we are barraged by images of healthy, active elderly, still very much engaged in life and, in fact, a resource to their families and their communities. Is it possible that these two contrasting representations of America's older persons refer to the same set of individuals?

The purpose of this chapter is to review the sociodemographic characteristics of the elderly, then relate these factors to mortality and morbidity in this population. In doing so, we shall find that conflicting portrayals of all older persons as active and healthy or as sick and frail elders are not incorrect, but more appropriately applied to only some segments of an entire population subgroup.

Although physical therapists evaluate and treat individuals, each of us has physical, psychological, and social characteristics by which we can be categorized into groups. Knowing that individuals with certain characteristics—being a particular age or sex—are more likely to experience a particular health problem can assist therapists in anticipating some clinical presentations, placing an individual's progress in perspective, and even sometimes altering outcomes through preventive measures. It is also useful to know the prevalence of a particular condition (i.e., the number of cases of that condition in a population) and its incidence (the number of new cases of a condition in a population over a specified period of time). Taken beyond treatment of a single person, physical therapists can use this information to plan and develop services to meet the needs of an aging society whose members span a continuum across health, infirmity, and death.

DEMOGRAPHY

Definition of the "Elderly"

The first gerontologic question is, How does a particular segment of a population come to be categorized as "old"? The chronologic criterion that is presently used for identifying the old in America is strictly arbitrary and usually has been set at 65 years. Yet the onset of some of the health problems of elders may occur as soon as they enter their early 50s, and as detailed in Chapter 25, "older" athletes may be only in their 40s. As the mean age of the population increases each decade and more individuals live into their ninth decades, we can expect that our notion of who is old will change.

The number of Americans aged 65 and over is growing at an unprecedented rate. In 1988 there were 30.4 million people aged 65 or older,[64] reflecting the major changes in the population structure of the United States in this century. Individuals who had reached their 65th birthday accounted for only 4% of the total population in 1900. In 1940 they were 6.9% of the population, and by 1950, they were equal to 8.2%. Although they represented just less than 10% of the population in 1970, they accounted for approximately 12% of the US population in 1986. This percentage is expected to grow to 12.8% by the year 2000 and over 20% by the year 2040, when the children of the post–World War II baby boom will have grown well into old age.[3, 11] In 1986, 41% of those over 65 years old were actually over 75 years old, and it is predicted that this percentage will increase to 48% by the year 2000. Although the number of elders aged 85 or older currently account for just over 1% of the population, their number will triple by 2040.[3]

One factor that has affected the increase in the proportion of aged in our society is the declining birthrate.[6] With fewer births, the age structure of the population changes from a triangular shape, with a larger number of younger individuals at the base, to a more rectangular distribution of the population by age (Fig 1–1), with a larger number of older individuals at the top. In 1988 the median age of the United States was 32.3 years.[64]

Racial and nonwhite ethnic minorities are currently

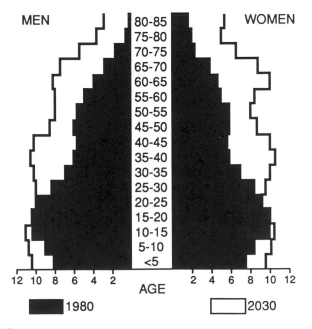

FIG 1–1.
Total population in millions by age group and sex. (Redrawn from Cassel CK, Brody JA: Demography, epidemiology, and aging, in Cassel CK, et al (eds): *Geriatric Medicine*, ed 2. New York, Springer-Verlag, 1990.)

underrepresented among the nation's elders relative to the distribution of these subgroups in the general population. In the overall population, approximately 15% of the United States is nonwhite, and almost 80% of these individuals of all ages are black.[64] Only about 10% of American elders are nonwhite, of which approximately 84% are black.[46] The current racial disparity among the elderly widens in the oldest age group, as there is a slight preponderance of white women among the oldest-old (85 years or older).[3] Hispanic elders, however, have the highest growth rate of any subgroup, and the number of Hispanic elders within the population is expected to quadruple by 2015.[1, 40] More recent immigrations of peoples from Southeast Asia will likely also result in increased representation of these groups among the elderly in the future. Overall, the proportion of nonwhites among all American aged is expected to grow so that over 20% of all elders will be nonwhite by the year 2050.[46] Therefore, the geriatric physical therapist must recognize that "the elderly" of the future will be more racially and culturally diverse than those elderly patients whom are currently served.

Sex Distribution and Marital Status

Because women usually live longer than men, the problems of America's elders are largely the problems of women. In 1986, there were 79 men for every 100 women in the 65-to-74 age-group; this ratio widened to 39 men for every 100 women over the age of 85.[3] Older women have a significant probability of living longer than their mates and, therefore, stand a significant chance of living alone. These women, once widowed, are also likely to remain unmarried. In contrast to the 51.3% women between 65 and 74 years old who are married, over 80% of their male counterparts in the same age-group have spouses. Among those 75 years or older, married men outnumber married women 3:1.[3] Elderly blacks are more likely than elderly whites to be widowed.[44]

Widowhood poses its own set of challenges to the individual.[62] The widow experiences a severe disruption in many of her usual social roles: wife, homemaker, confidant, and member of a couple. This disruption complicates the search for self-validation through the recognition, esteem, and affection of another that were present in marriage.[68]

Living Arrangements

Although over 70% of elders have surviving children, the proportion of elders living alone increases with age[33] (Fig 1–2). Hispanic elders are less likely than whites or blacks to live alone.[72] Little is known about Asian elderly. When

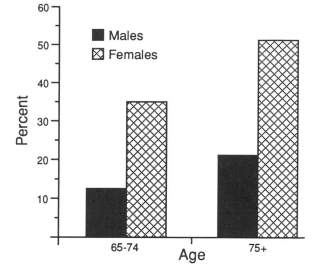

FIG 1–2.
Percentage of community elderly living alone, 1984. (From Kovar MG: Aging in the eighties, age 65 and over and living alone, contacts with family, friends, and neighbors. Preliminary data from the Supplement on Aging to the National Health Interview Survey: US, January–June 1984. *Advance Data From Vital and Health Statistics,* No 116. Hyattsville, Md, Public Health Service, DHHS No (PHS) 86–1250, 1986. Redrawn from Kane RL, Kane RA: Long-term care, in Cassel CK, et al (eds): *Geriatric Medicine,* ed 2. New York, Springer-Verlag, 1990.)

elders need assistance in basic and instrumental activities of daily living (ADL), spouses and children often provide the majority of help. Only a small portion of these services is usually provided by formal care givers.[33] Decline in functional abilities strongly predicts the likelihood that an elder living alone will seek other arrangements.[72] The unavailability of informal social support through family and friends has been implicated as a factor contributing to nursing home placement.[33]

Overall, just under 5% of elders reside in a nursing home. It has been suggested, however, that for every disabled elder in a nursing home there may be as many as three equally disabled elders who are able to continue living in the community with strong social support.[33] Furthermore, an analysis of the proportion of elderly in nursing homes by age reveals that nursing home utilization increases from 2% among those 65 to 74 years old to 20% for those 85 years and older.[33] In general, female nursing home residents outnumber males (Fig 1–3,A), and white nursing home residents are more numerous than nonwhite residents (Fig 1–3,B).[44] Some evidence suggests that elders have as great as a 40% chance of spending at least some time in a nursing home in their lifetimes.[33] Many of these individuals will have short-term admissions and return to their premorbid living arrangements.[44]

Hing found that nursing home placement may be af-

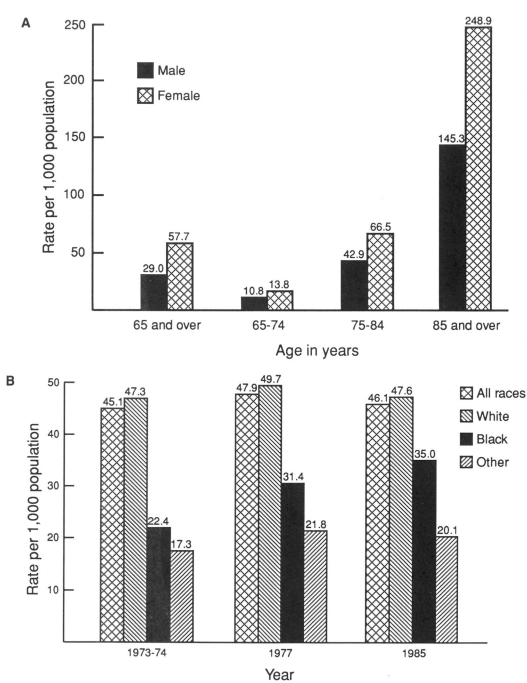

FIG 1–3.
A, number of nursing home residents per 1,000 population 65 years of age or older, by sex and age: United States, 1985. **B,** number of nursing home residents per 1,000 population 65 years of age and over, by race: United States, 1973–1974, 1977, and 1985. (Redrawn from Hing E: Use of nursing homes by the elderly: Preliminary data from the 1985 National Nursing Home Survey. *Advance Data From Vital and Health Statistics, No 135. Hyattsville, Md, Public Health Service, DHHS No (PHS) 87–1250, 1987.)*

fected by functional dependency, cognitive impairment, marital status, and previous living arrangements.[28] Although comparisons made between nursing home usage in 1985 and in 1973–1974 indicated some growth in minority placements, black males and females used nursing homes substantially less than their white counterparts. This underutilization pattern may be due to the presence of extensive informal care-giving networks among blacks even in the face of possibly greater activity limitations. Hing, for example, has noted that black nursing home residents tended to be more cognitively impaired than white residents, although these differences were not significant.[28] This informal care-giving network may be a critical factor that will allow these elders to remain in the community in the future, given the likelihood that black elders will live alone as survivorship among blacks improves. Geriatric physical therapists may need to expand their notion of "family" in their efforts to do patient-"family" teaching beyond the blood relatives of a minority elder.

Family Roles and Relationships

Despite recent changes for younger generations, the degree to which female elders are still bound by society to their traditional homemaking roles should not be underestimated. A disabled male is able to retire from work, his primary socially ordained role, without taking on additional responsibility within the home. In contrast, a disabled woman, regardless of her employment status outside the home, is still expected to continue to do homemaking activities such as housekeeping and grocery shopping, whatever her level of physical function. Women are therefore more likely than men to report disability with respect to social roles.[30] The relative unavailability of assistance with home chores in comparison with other social support services may subtly discriminate against older women, although the level of unmet need in this area is not well documented. These home services can often be the essential element in allowing an elder to remain living independently at home when functional abilities are compromised. Physical therapists will need to join with other health professionals to advocate for easier access to a wider range of services than is currently available in order to facilitate the highest level of independent living for the aged.

Although it is common to promote an image of American elders as abandoned by their children, there is ample evidence that elders do have frequent contact with their families (Fig 1-4). Chappell has reported that most elderly in the United States and Canada live close to at least one child, yet prefer to maintain their independence (Fig 1-5).[7] Several factors that affect the amount of contact between elder and offspring have been cited. Daughters, particularly those who are middle-aged, tend to have more contact than sons. Widowed parents tend to have more contact with their children than their still-married peers, and unmarried children may be in contact with their parents more often than married children. It also appears that working-class children are in greater contact with their parents. The evidence also suggests Hispanics have a greater degree of contact than blacks or whites, whose levels of contact with their parents are similar.[2] There has been little research to explore this issue among Asian families.

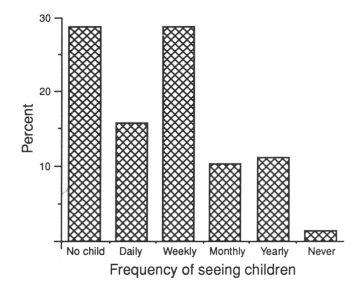

FIG 1-4.
Frequency elderly living alone saw children, 1984. (Redrawn from Kovar MG: Aging in the eighties, age 65 and over and living alone, contacts with family, friends, and neighbors. Preliminary data from the Supplement on Aging to the National Health Interview Survey: US, January–June 1984. *Advance Data From Vital and Health Statistics, No 116.* Hyattsville, Md, Public Health Service, DHHS No (PHS) 86-1250, 1986. From Kane RL, Kane RA: Long-term care, in Cassel CK, et al (eds): *Geriatric Medicine,* ed 2. New York, Springer-Verlag, 1990.)

Elders who do live with family often can find themselves in multigenerational families, growing old with their children.[2, 25] While a sick elder is often the recipient of direct care and emotional support, healthy elders are often a source of financial and emotional support as well.[2] Spouses are the most likely individuals to care for their partners in old age and sickness. When a spouse is unable or unavailable to provide assistance, who does what for an aging parent in need can depend on whether the care giver is a son or a daughter.[7] In general, sons tend to take a "managerial" role. The actual provision of direct care to elders has traditionally been "women's work".[4] It still often falls to daughters, daughters-in-law, and nieces to provide direct care despite the ongoing cultural redefinition of women's (and men's) social roles in the past three decades. Fewer children and increases in the number of women entering the work force have decreased the number of otherwise unemployed women available to take care of family elders.[2, 4] Many of these middle-aged women find themselves caught with multiple and often competing obligations to their own children (some of whom may still be living at home), to their parents, and to themselves. Employed women apparently provide as many hours of direct care to their parents as their nonworking peers, although working women tend to use outside help for personal care and meal preparation for their parents more often than

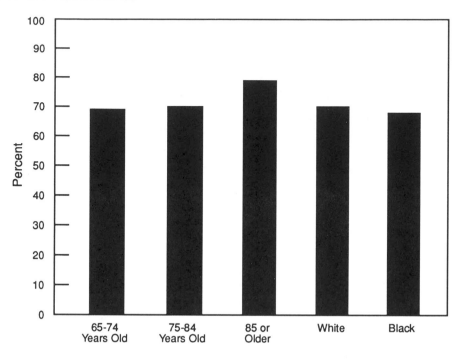

FIG 1-5.
Percentage of elderly people living alone who have children with children nearby. (Data source: National Center for Health Statistics, National Health Interview Survey, Supplement on Aging, 1984. Adapted from Commonwealth Fund Commission on Elderly People Living Alone; *Aging Alone—Profiles and Projections.* Baltimore, The Commonwealth Fund, 1988.

nonworking women.[4] Recommendations by physical therapists that increase the tasks of care giving among family members—for example, assisting with a home exercise program—may be perceived as a substantial burden by these "women-in-the-middle."

The role of grandparent has also changed, especially for women.[2] Increased longevity increases the amount of one's life that might be spent being a grandparent. It is not unusual for an elder to witness a grandchild's movement through the life course from birth up to the grandchild's adulthood. Healthy elders still provide substantial financial and emotional support to their children. Many grandparents find themselves taking on additional baby-sitting and child-rearing responsibilities, particularly as their daughters remain employed outside the home. Therefore, an evaluation of an elder's functional abilities in this social context might need to consider whether there is the dexterity to change a diaper, the strength to lift a toddler, and the stamina to walk young children home from the school bus.

Economic Status

Regarding the elderly as a single group with similar needs is a habit that is easy to acquire. The heterogeneity of the elderly as a group is perhaps best illustrated by considering how financially well-off economically the elderly are. If we treat the aged as a homogeneous group, they overall

appear to be doing better economically than expected. This is due to the entrance of the very youngest of the old, who currently benefit from private and workers' pension programs, into the ranks of the aged. Furthermore, the elderly are not generally as bad off as children, the other population subgroup that is largely dependent on society's resources. In comparison with poverty among children aged 17 years or younger, the elderly have experienced a relatively steady decline in poverty (Fig 1-6).[60] These group figures obscure the realities of poverty among the elderly: poverty increases with age; women are more often in poverty than men; married males and females are better off than their nonmarried peers; widowed females tend to show the highest poverty rate of all; and once poor, elders are likely to remain poor.[60]

In 1987, the poverty line for a single person over 65 was $454 per month and $573 per month for an elderly couple.[60] Using this figure, 12.2% of the American population over 65 were below the poverty line in 1987, whereas an additional 8.1% were classified as near poor (i.e., at 125% of the poverty line).[60] Disaggregating the poverty rate by race demonstrates additional disparities, with about one third of black elders and one quarter of Hispanic elders living in poverty.[57, 64] These figures do not adequately portray the economic disadvantage of 20% of all persons aged 65 or older who are between 100% and 200% of the poverty line. These individuals are in particu-

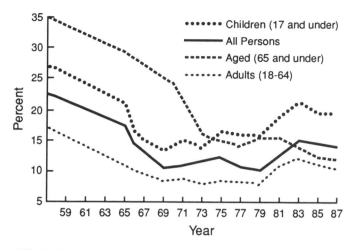

FIG 1–6.
Comparison of trends in official poverty rates among all persons, children, adults, and aged individuals. (Redrawn from US, Bureau of the Census: Money income and poverty status in the United States, 1987. *Current Population Reports* (Series P-60, No 161, August). Washington, DC, Government Printing Office, 1988.)

lar economic jeopardy: too "wealthy" to qualify for means-tested assistance and too poor to provide well for themselves. In 1987, average Social Security benefits were $485 per month for a single elder and $727 for elderly couples.[60] When one considers that Social Security benefits account for 90% or more of the income for over 20% of the elderly population, it becomes apparent that many elders, especially widowed women, live on the edges of poverty.[8]

It is worthwhile to inquire as to why women, even former working women, are especially prone to poverty in old age. Three reasons have been suggested.[69] First, women who did work usually held jobs in occupations and industries dominated by women and characterized by high rates of turnover, lack of unionization and pension coverage, and low wages and fringe benefits. Second, women have tended to have interrupted careers that reduce their overall earnings histories. Because Social Security benefits are calculated on wage histories, average Social Security benefits for women are usually lower than men's. Third, the reduction in benefits that occurs when a woman is widowed may hasten her slide into poverty, as a single income may be insufficient to meet basic needs. Although the market for physical therapy services will continue to increase with the growth of the geriatric population, the capacity of this predominantly female group to purchase physical therapy and other health care services "out of pocket" is likely to be limited. Given their overall economic resources, a substantial proportion of elderly income goes for medical insurance, deductibles, and coinsurance payments. The failure to remove these financial barriers could ultimately prevent access to physical therapy, despite the needs of this population.

MORTALITY

Life Expectancy

In addition to a declining birthrate, the other factor that accounts for the increasing number of elderly is an increasing average life expectancy. Life expectancy can be calculated from two points: at birth and a time closer to death. Taking the first approach, a child born in 1900 would have been expected to live only 49 years on the average, and only 41% of the children born that year would have been expected to reach age 65. By 1974 the average life expectancy of a child born that year had grown to 71.9 years, and 74% of that birth cohort is expected to reach age 65.[61] An American male born in 1990 is expected to live 72.1 years on the average and a female 7 years longer.[64]

Despite recent medical advances in treating geriatric conditions, particularly cardiovascular disease, most of the changes in average life expectancy took place prior to 1955.[61] Since then, only a few years have been added to life expectancy calculations. Furthermore, the major gains in life expectancy in this century have occurred primarily due to advances in postnatal and infant care rather than advances in adult or geriatric health care.[61] The benefits of improved infant care, however, have not been distributed evenly throughout the population with respect to either race or gender. Male black children born in 1990 are expected to live 5 years less than their white counterparts. Although black females born in 1990 are generally expected to live longer than white males, these women will fall short of the life expectancy of white females by 4.6 years on the average.[64]

A slightly different picture of differences in longevity emerges if we consider life expectancy at age 65 rather than at birth. Although women aged 65 in 1985 are expected to live longer than men, whites and blacks at age 65, compared as two groups, have been found to be separated by little more than a year.[9] This finding prompts the question as to why there should be such little difference between elderly blacks and whites when there was a great disparity at birth and through most of adulthood. One of the most intriguing facts to emerge from studies of racial differences in mortality is a phenomenon called "black-white crossover."[71] Simply put, when comparing age-specific death rates, we find higher rates among young or elderly blacks compared with whites the same age and lower rates among very old blacks compared with very old whites (Fig 1–7). Thus, if we include very old black elders in our frame of reference, their lower death rate counterbalances the higher death rate among younger blacks.

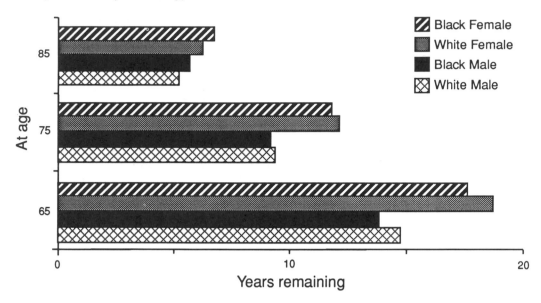

FIG 1–7.
Life expectancy of the elderly in 1984. (Redrawn from Havlik RG, Liu MG, Kovar MG: Health statistics on older persons, United States, 1986. *Vital and Health Statistics Series 3, No 25.* Washington, DC, Public Health Service, DHHS No (PHS) 87–1409, 1987.)

Combining young blacks and old black elders into a single group statistically lowers the overall black mortality rate, even though younger blacks continue to have greater mortality than whites of the same age.[29] Crude generalizations of groups data, which underplay the heterogeneity of the elderly and differences among older persons across age-groups, can be misleading and should therefore be avoided.

Factors other than age itself have been hypothesized to influence death rates among elders. It is not clear, however, that what holds true for the overall population in general or for white elders in particular will hold true in studies of minority elders. In their review of the physical health of middle-aged and aged blacks, Jackson and Perry found that there were no statistically significant differences in death rates between married and nonmarried blacks, despite the expectation that there would be such a difference based on other studies that have shown a direct relationship between survivorship and marital status.[29] They concluded that other factors such as income and education may be more important predictors of the life expectancy of black Americans. Gibson has proposed that risk factors for ill health in old age may be distinctly different for blacks than for whites.[16] Hypotheses about the life expectancy and health of minority elders are difficult to confirm, as there have been very few sources of data with sufficient numbers of minority elders. To reverse long-standing emphasis on studies of white males, the federal government has recently required researchers to state specifically how information on women and minorities will be collected and analyzed as part of the grant application process.

While the racial disparity in average life expectancy has been persistent throughout this century, a percentage analysis reveals that minority gains have been substantial. Although fewer black males reached 65 than their white counterparts in 1977, this represents a 190% increase from 1900, double the increase documented for white males in the same time period. White females reaching their 65th birthday increased 91% from 1900 to 1977. Nonwhite females made an even more remarkable gain of a 230% increase in those reaching age 65 in comparison with their counterparts in 1900.[61]

Causes of Death

Advancing age and sex are the two most important predictors of mortality in the elderly (Fig 1–8). Male death rates at every age are consistently higher than those for women.[5] The three most common causes of death for all elderly are coronary heart disease (CHD), cancer, and stroke.[70] CHD accounts for 31% of all deaths in both men and women over age 65.[5] It is believed that declines in mortality from CHD in the past 30 years have been due to risk factor reduction earlier in the life span.

Almost 20% of deaths in all elders are due to cancers.[5] Once again, however, it becomes important to distinguish between data on elders taken as a single group and data broken down by specific age-groups. Deaths from cancer rise through middle adulthood and decline with old age. Generally speaking, there are fewer deaths attributable to cancer in the elderly overall due to the prolonged survival of individuals with cancer to older ages. This con-

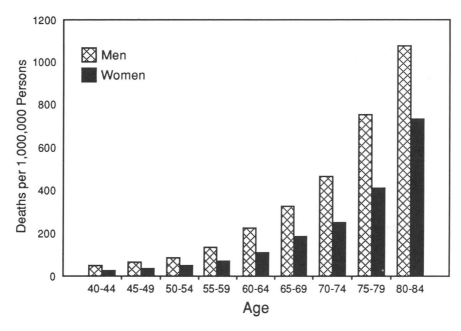

FIG 1–8.
Death rates by age and sex, United States, 1984. (Redrawn from Bush TL, et al: Risk factors for morbidity and mortality in older populations: An epidemiologic approach, in Hazzard WR, et al (ed): *Principles of Geriatric Medicine and Gerontology,* ed 2. New York, McGraw-Hill, 1990.)

trasts with death from cardiovascular causes, which continues to increase rapidly with advancing years.[70] Age-specific cancer death rates, however, show an increase in cancer mortality in each successive age-group.

The death rate from stroke increases exponentially with age and is higher for men than women at every age.[5] Stroke mortality has declined in the United States for most of this century, most likely due to improvements in the detection and treatment of hypertension.

MORBIDITY

Active Life Expectancy

While gains in overall life expectancy are important indicators of a nation's well-being, active life expectancy, that is, the years spent without and with a major infirmity or disabling condition, may provide more meaningful information for health professionals.[35] Using data from the Massachusetts Health Care Panel Study, Katz and colleagues calculated a score on each individual's overall level of independence in bathing, dressing, transfers, and eating. They found that active life expectancy decreased with age, with the largest decrements for those over 79 years old (Fig 1–9). Elders who were 65 to 69 years old could anticipate another 10 years of independent ADL, whereas those elders who were 80 to 84 years old would likely remain independent for only another 4.7 years. Individuals aged 85 or older who were independent in these

four ADL were likely to enjoy an active life expectancy of a mere 2.9 years. Although active life expectancy did not differ in this study between men and women, there were substantial differences between the poor and nonpoor, especially at younger ages. Nonpoor elders aged 65 to 69 had 2.4 additional years of active life expectancy than poor elders. This difference narrowed dramatically to less than 1 year between poor and nonpoor groups for those 75 years or older.[35]

Figure 1–10 encapsulates our current view of the life span. As an individual ages, the likelihood of onset of disease, followed by a period of disability and ultimately death, increases. Rowe and Kahn have proposed that human aging be classified into two categories: usual and successful.[53, 54] Traditionally, geriatric research has focused on the pathologic changes associated with "normal" aging (disease and disability in Fig 1–10), while ignoring the elders who do not exhibit these changes. Thus, "normal" aging has been used erroneously to mean "usual" aging. Although elders who are "successful" agers do not escape the eventuality of disease, disability, and death, they are able to decrease their overall morbidity and delay the onset of disability. Their success has been attributed to "intrinsic" factors such as heredity but also to extrinsic factors such as stress, diet, and exercise. Harris and Feldman have suggested a third category for "high-risk" or "accelerated" aging. Their recommendations for the epidemiologic study of aging are also applicable to health care.[27] Physical therapists can assist the promotion of successful aging by en-

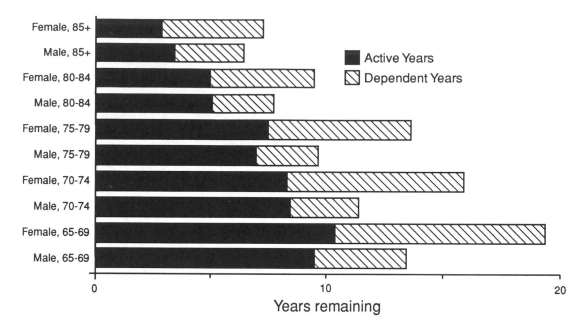

FIG 1-9.
Active versus dependent life expectancy in Massachusetts elderly, 1974. (Redrawn from Katz S, et al: *N Engl J Med* 1983; 309:1218-1224.)

couraging modification of some extrinsic factors, particularly in teenagers and young adults. Among usual agers, physical therapists can concentrate on reducing the disabling effects of disease and stopping a vicious cycle of "disease–disability–new incident disease." The goal of physical therapy for "accelerated" agers would be to maintain their current level of function and prevent further rapid deterioration.

The degree to which disease and disability can be "compressed" and postponed until the last years of life has been a source of great controversy. Fries first proposed that if the average age of onset of significant morbidity increases more rapidly than increases in life expectancy, both the proportion of one's life spent infirm and the overall length of infirmity will be shortened.[13-15] While particular individuals might experience such a compression, the data do not now support Fries' hypothesis for the entire population of this country's elderly.[21] Guralnik and his colleagues compared the prevalence of disability in 531 elders who had received three annual examinations to that of the 8,821 survivors in the same cohort.[23] Their findings indicated that decedents in every age-subgroup group had more disability than survivors. Those dying at the oldest ages had more disability than those dying at younger ages. Thus, if more elders die at older ages, they will likely experience even greater functional deterioration for more years prior to their deaths than if they had died at younger ages.

Opposite to proposing a compression of morbidity, Olshansky and others have argued that there will be an expansion of morbidity as medical technology improves the

likelihood of survival from previously fatal diseases without improving overall quality of life for these individuals.[49] Furthermore, the older individuals live, the more likely they are to experience functional decline. Thus, they appear to have traded death at an earlier age for more years spent with one of the nonfatal diseases of aging and its associated disability prior to death.

Prevalent Chronic Conditions

The proportion of elderly at any age without any chronic conditions is small.[22] Over half of male elders over 80

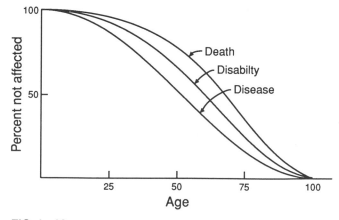

FIG 1-10.
Relationships among disease, disability, and death. (Adapted from Rowe JW: Toward successful aging: Limitations of the morbidity associated with "normal" aging, in Hazzard WR, et al (eds): *Principles of Geriatric Medicine and Gerontology,* ed 2. New York, McGraw-Hill, 1990.)

years and 70% of female elders of similar age have two or more chronic conditions. In 1988, arthritis was the most prevalent self-reported condition of the elderly, followed by high blood pressure, hearing impairments, and heart disease (Fig 1–11). These conditions are even more prevalent among elders who are alone and poor (Fig 1–12).

Functional Limitations

In 1985 the total number of disabled elderly living in the community with any degree of chronic limitations in any basic or instrumental ADL was 5.5 million persons.[42] Limitations in functional activities increase with age. Those elders in the 65- to 74-year-old group are thought to be healthier and generally better off than their counterparts aged 75 years or older, who are often termed the "frail elderly."

In 1984, data were gathered on 11,497 elders through the Supplement on Aging to the National Health Interview Survey.[12] More than three fourths of all these elders experienced no difficulty in self-care activities or walking. Age, however, did have a substantial effect on disability. Whereas 85% of elders between the ages of 65 and 69 experienced no difficulty in self-care activities or walking, only 66% of elders between 80 and 84 and 51% of elders over 85 could report similar levels of well-being. While only 5.7% of elders aged 75 to 79 reported difficulty with four or more self-care activities, this figure almost doubled in the 80- to 84-year-old group and more than tripled in those 85 years or older. Preliminary data from the National Institute on Aging Established Populations for Epidemio-

logic Studies of the Elderly (EPESE) corroborate this finding that physical disability is most prevalent in the oldest-old.[10] The EPESE data also indicate that physical disability is more prevalent for elderly women than men at every age.

It should be noted that while there is substantial evidence that function declines with age, there is also some evidence that some elders are able to maintain a high level of function. In a longitudinal study of physical ability of the oldest-old based on data from the Longitudinal Study on Aging, Harris and associates found that one third of elders over age 80 reported no difficulty in walking one-quarter mile; lifting 10 lb; climbing ten steps without resting; or stooping, crouching, and kneeling.[26]

As in the general population, it is generally agreed that physical disability overall increases with age among blacks.[29] The linearity of this increase has been challenged, as there is mounting evidence that younger blacks, that is, those 74 years old or younger, are more physically disabled than those aged 75 to 79, and that those aged 80 to 84 are more disabled than those 85 and over.[17] There are also important sex differences as well that parallel what is known about the general population. Black women are consistently more disabled in heavy housework than black men. Only black men aged 85 or over are more disabled in light housework than their female counterparts.

Disease and Disability

Several studies have implicated cardiovascular diseases as a cause of disability in the elderly. We know from the

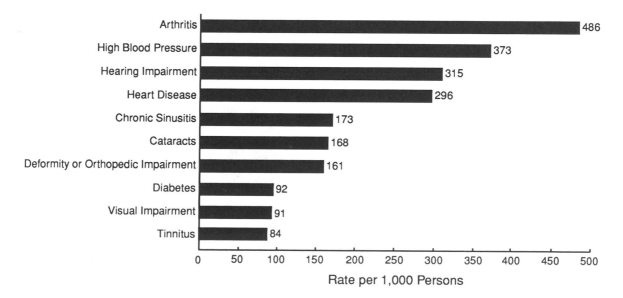

FIG 1–11.
Prevalence of chronic conditions in individuals over age 65 in 1988. (Redrawn from National Center for Health Statistics: Current estimates from the National Health Interview Survey, 1988. *Vital and Health Statistics Series* 10, No 173. Washington, DC, Public Health Service, DHHS Publication No (PHS) 89–1501, 1989.)

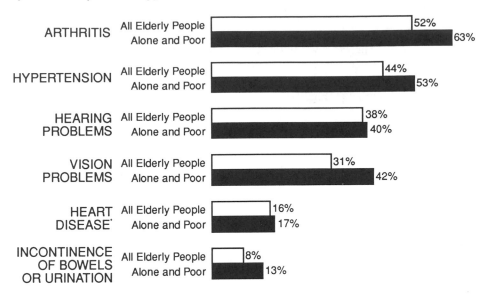

*Includes rheumatic or coronary heart disease, angina, myocardial infarction, and heart attacks.

FIG 1–12.
Percentage of selected chronic conditions among all elderly and elderly who are alone and poor. (Data source: National Center for Health Statistics, National Health Interview Survey, Supplement on Aging, 1984. Adapted from Commonwealth Fund Commission on Elderly People Living Alone: *Aging Alone–Profiles and Projections.* Baltimore, The Commonwealth Fund, 1988.)

Framingham studies, for example, that angina pectoris is related to disability in men and women. Furthermore, long-term and current hypertension, being overweight, and diabetes are associated with disability in women, but long-term hypertension is related to disability in men.[50,51] The demonstration of a relationship between angina and disability in women has been replicated in other studies as well.[47]

The Framingham Heart Study has also provided some insight into the relationships among stroke, mortality, and disability. Kelly-Hayes and colleagues reported on all incident strokes over a 10-year period in 3,920 elders who were free of stroke at the start of the study in 1971.[37] Only 154 patients out of 213 incident cases of stroke survived more than 30 days. Of those who survived more than 30 days, 42 were living in institutions 1 year later. Factors predicting institutionalization were different in women than in men. Age, severity, and education were associated with institutionalization in women, whereas not being married was the only variable that predicted institutionalization in men following a stroke. These findings have been corroborated in a study of 1,274 stroke cases in Australia. In addition to severity and side of paralysis, Shah and colleagues found that age, sex, marital status, and ethnicity were associated with the outcome of rehabilitation.[58]

Kelly-Hayes replicated her previous finding of the high mortality rate of stroke in another analysis of new cases of stroke in a 4½-year period in the early 1980s.[38] Only 67 individuals out of 119 subjects who sustained a

stroke were alive at 1 year. Using baseline data that were available on 46 of these survivors, Kelly-Hayes also analyzed functional recovery. She used the Barthel index to compare the difference in rate of recovery and maintenance of function of those 12 survivors who had been admitted to inpatient rehabilitation programs with the recovery of the 36 individuals who had not been inpatients and found a significant difference in functional levels at baseline. Inpatients were more functionally disabled at admission and made significantly greater improvement in the first 3 months. There were no significant differences between groups at 6 months or a year.

It is still unclear as to how long one can expect functional recovery after a stroke. Do patients reach a plateau of optimal function within 3 to 6 months of their stroke, or do they continue to make slow, progressive gains? Tangeman and associates found improvement in weight shifting, balance, and ADL in 40 individuals who were at least 1 year poststroke following an intensive rehabilitation program.[63] These subjects also demonstrated their new abilities at follow-up 3 months later. Although baseline measures were collected 1 month prior to the start of the study, these investigators were unable to determine if the improvement demonstrated after intensive therapy represented a return to a previous plateau of optimal function or in fact demonstrated additional recovery. They could also not determine whether additional rehabilitation would benefit more severely impaired elders. All subjects could walk independently within the home when they entered the study. This research, however, does indicate that a short trial of therapy may be beneficial to some patients whose functional level has begun to fall or who may not have achieved their optimal functional level during rehabilitation immediately following their strokes.

Hip fractures in the elderly represent an enormous threat to their well-being. Depending on the study, the mortality rate of hip fracture patients may be as high as 25%. Estimates of recovery following a fracture have suggested that anywhere from 25% to 75% of these individuals will not achieve their premorbid level of function.[41] A study of 526 hip fracture patients over a 2-year period found that most recovery of the ability to walk and perform ADL occurred within 6 months. Poor recovery was associated with older age, prefracture dependency, longer hospital stay, dementia, postsurgical delirium in patients without dementia, and lack of contact with a social support network. It has also been shown that depression will negatively affect outcomes in these patients.[45]

Not all diseases affect function globally, as might be expected based on our understanding of the impacts of stroke or hip fracture. Some conditions have effects that are limited to activities that use the afflicted body part. For example, Satariano found that breast cancer, the most prevalent cancer of older women, limited activities that required upper body strength but did not affect other activities.[56] Similarly, in a study of knee osteoarthritis, a commonly afflicted joint in a highly prevalent disease, Guccione and coworkers found that limitations in only those activities that used the lower extremity were more likely among elders with this condition than elders without it.[18]

Few studies have attempted to establish the relationship between disease and disability in nursing home residents. Guccione and colleagues reported the functional status of 126 nursing home residents, of whom 51 had either rheumatoid or osteoarthritis.[19] Controlling for age, residents with arthritis had more pain and were more likely to require assistance dressing, bringing a glass to the mouth, turning a faucet, getting in and out of bed, bending down, and walking. They were also more likely to use a wheelchair daily than other residents without arthritis.

Comorbidity and Function

Guralnik and colleagues have provided ample evidence that an increase in the number of activities with which an elder has difficulty increases linearly with comorbidity, that is, coexistent medical conditions (Fig 1–13).[22] Thus, it is not unusual for physical therapists to find that the most disabled patients are also likely to have a number of medical conditions that complicate not only understanding of the genesis of functional deficit but treatment as well. For example, the individual with a stroke, who also has degenerative changes in the foot and low tolerance for stressful activity secondary to angina with exertion, can present a particular challenge to the geriatric physical therapist's knowledge and skill.

Although there is an emerging body of knowledge on

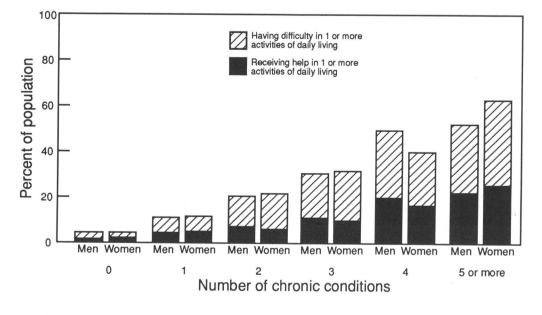

FIG 1–13.
Age-adjusted prevalence of men and women 60 years of age and over having difficulty and receiving help in one or more activities of daily living, by number of chronic conditions: United States, 1984. (Redrawn from Guralnik J, et al: Aging in the eighties: The prevalence of comorbidity and its association with disability. *Advance Data From Vital and Health Statistics,* Hyattsville, Md, Public Health Service, DHHS Publication No (PHS) 89–1250, 1989.)

the effects of disease on function, far less is known about the effects of coexistent disease on function. Elders vary a great deal in the degree to which their chronic comorbidity affects their functional capacities. Based on analyses of data from the 1984 Supplement on Aging, Verbrugge and coworkers concluded that relative to other diseases the most prevalent conditions do not appear to have the highest risks of physical disability in the elderly.[65] This conclusion should not be taken out of the context of its research aim to rank the relative impact of diseases on function. The impacts of prevalent conditions on function in the elderly are still considerable, even if somewhat less than rarer conditions, regardless of the rank order of their impacts. Guccione and colleagues analyzed the independent association of ten different medical comorbidities with disability among 1,769 community-based elders in the Framingham Heart Study cohort.[20] They found that disability in seven functional activities was most associated with stroke, hip fracture, and depression, three of the least prevalent conditions, even after controlling for age, sex, and the presence of any other medical conditions. The likelihood of disability associated with knee osteoarthritis and heart disease, the two most prevalent conditions, was substantial, even though these relationships were not as strong or consistent across all the functional activities as the less prevalent conditions. The combination of their prevalence and the magnitude of risk for disability that these two conditions pose for elders accounts for a larger percentage of disability in community-based elders than is attributable to more disabling, but less prevalent, diseases. Furthermore, even in stroke which has a broad impact on function, disease-related disability may be attributable to different conditions in men and women.[31] Strategies to prevent diseases in younger adults and efforts to retard the effects of disease on function should ultimately alter the trajectory of disability in the elderly in a positive direction.[42]

Psychosocial Factors and Function

Physical therapists must also not forget that factors other than disease can modify disability in the elderly. Mor's finding in a study of 1,737 elders aged 70 to 74 years old that those who did not report exercising regularly or walking a mile were 1½ times as likely to decline functionally over 2 years is especially relevant to physical therapists.[43] Other research provides clues for other interventions involving life-style modifications prior to old age. In an analysis of data from the Alameda County Study, Kaplan found income, smoking, social isolation, and depression associated with trouble climbing stairs and getting outdoors in elders with incident heart trouble, stroke, diabetes, or arthritis.[34] Using the same cohort, Guralnik and

Kaplan compared the function of elders in the top 20% of functioning with that of the remainder elders at follow-up 19 years later.[24] They found several longitudinal predictors of good function: not being black, higher family income, absence of hypertension, absence of arthritis, absence of back pain, being a nonsmoker, having normal weight, and consuming moderate amounts of alcohol. Although being male predicted higher levels of functioning in men, being female did not predict higher levels of functioning in women. This last finding highlights an important statistical problem in geriatric research: any population-based sample of elders is likely to contain more women, who, by virtue of living longer, are also more likely to be disabled. Thus, without controlling statistically for age and sex, any positive effect on functional outcome that might accrue to women at younger ages may be obscured.

One of the most intriguing issues in minority health care is the effects of race on the health status of elders compared with the effects of income.[48, 66] Wallace has suggested that race had effects on the health care of African-American elderly living in St. Louis that were independent of income.[67] Satariano, on the other hand, could not find an independent effect for race in a sample of 906 black and white elders living in an economically depressed area of Alameda County.[55] When Keil and colleagues analyzed data on the elders in the Charleston Heart Study cohort, which included 71 high socioeconomic status (SES) black males, they found that black females had the highest rate of disability (55.8%), followed by white females, black men, and white males.[36] The high SES group of black males had the lowest prevalence of disability. Although further research is necessary to untangle the contributions of race and income to functional well-being in the elderly, it is important to consider the potential impact of these factors on the outcomes of rehabilitation, whether it be for the purposes of research or for clinical practice.

Factors that contribute to good function in the elderly may also differ between men and women. Using data from the Framingham Heart Study, Pinsky and coworkers found that age, alcohol use, smoking, ventricular rate, and education were all significantly related to function 21 years later in men but that only education predicted functional well-being in women.[52] Thus, in analyzing what factors may predispose an elder to functional decline, physical therapists should remember that what is generally known about the elderly may not apply equally to men and women.

Utilization of Services

Functional deficits are important markers for death, further functional decline, and increased utilization of services. In a 2-year follow-up study of 1,791 white elders aged 80 or

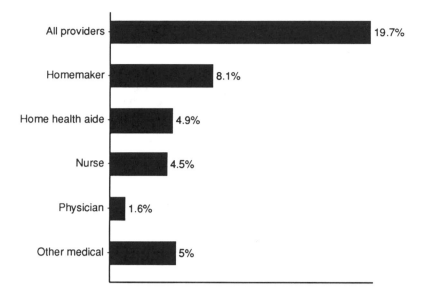

FIG 1–14.
Percentage of persons 65 and older with any functional difficulty using particular services. (Redrawn from Short P, Leon J: Use of home and community services by persons ages 65 and older with functional difficulties. *National Medical Expenditure Survey Research Findings 5.* Rockville, Md, Agency for Health Care Policy and Research, Public Health Service, DHHS Publication No (PHS) 90–3466, 1990.)

older, Harris and colleagues found that those who had received help with any ADL were four times more likely to have died.[26] Among those elders who survived, elders with functional limitations in any ADL were six times as likely to have used a nursing home in the intervening 2 years and two times as likely to have been hospitalized at

least twice or to have had six or more physician visits in the year prior to follow-up.

Although it was estimated that in 1987, 5.6 million noninstitutionalized elders had difficulty in walking or with at least one basic or instrumental ADL, many (3.6 million) received no formal services.[59] Almost 20% of

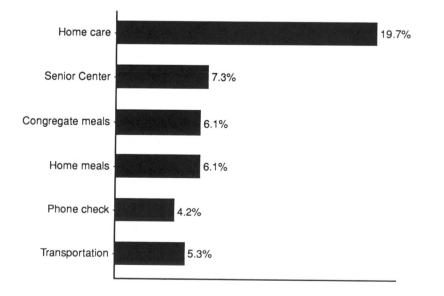

FIG 1–15.
Percentage of persons 65 and older with any functional difficulty receiving service from home care providers. (Redrawn from Short P, Leon J: Use of home and community services by persons ages 65 and older with functional difficulties. *National Medical Expenditure Survey Research Findings 5.* Rockville, Md, Agency for Health Care Policy and Research, Public Health Service, DHHS Publication No (PHS) 90–3466, 1990.)

these services were for professional or homemaking services provided in the home, except meals delivered to the home (Fig 1–14). Adult day care accounted for less than 1%. When an elder received care at home, it was typically provided by a homemaker (Fig 1–15). Functional limitations are strongly associated with the use of formal services. Elderly persons with three or more limitations in ADL are more likely to use home-based services rather than community-based services.

Rehabilitation specialists are quick to assume that offering their services to elders living in the community will delay functional decline and reduce the threat of institutionalization. Unfortunately, there is little evidence to support this assumption. Liang and coworkers provided intensive multidisciplinary care, including physical therapy, to frail elders living in the community and were unable to alter the long-range course of their physical decline.[39]

SUMMARY

Changes in the demographic characteristics of the US population represent a critical challenge to geriatric physical therapists. Elders are expected to live longer than ever before, but the quality of their lives in these added years is still a matter of conjecture. Aging with multiple diseases further aggravates a propensity toward physical decline with advanced age. Function deficits are the expected outcomes of disease; in turn, functional limitations predict increased utilization of services, further morbidity, and death. Future research must establish the ability of physical therapy to delay the onset of disease and disability and to prolong optimal function into old age.

REFERENCES

1. Ailinger RL: Functional capacity of Hispanic elderly immigrants. *J Appl Gerontol* 1989; 8:97–109.
2. Bengston V, Rosenthal C, Burton L: Families and aging: Diversity and heterogeneity, in Binstock RH, George LK (eds.): *Handbook of Aging and the Social Sciences,* ed 3. San Diego, Academic Press, 1990.
3. Brock DB, Guralnik JM, Brody JA: Demography and epidemiology of aging in the United States, in Schneider EL, Rowe JW (eds): *Handbook of the Biology of Aging,* ed 3. San Diego, Academic Press, 1990.
4. Brody EM: "Women in the middle" and family help to older people. *Gerontologist* 1981; 21:471–480.
5. Bush TL, et al: Risk factors for morbidity and mortality in older populations: An epidemiologic approach, in Hazzard WR, et al (eds): *Principles of Geriatric Medicine and Gerontology,* ed 2. New York, McGraw-Hill, 1990.
6. Cassel CK, Brody JA: Demography, epidemiology, and aging, in Cassel CK, et al (eds): *Geriatric Medicine,* ed 2. New York, Springer-Verlag, 1990.
7. Chappell NS: Aging and social care, in Binstock RH, George LK (eds): *Handbook of Aging and the Social Sciences,* ed 3. San Diego, Academic Press, 1990.
8. Clark RL: Income maintenance policies in the United States, in Binstock RH, George LK (eds): *Handbook of Aging and the Social Sciences,* ed 3. San Diego, Academic Press, 1990.
9. Commonwealth Fund Commission on Elderly People Living Alone: *Aging Alone—Profiles and Projections.* Baltimore, The Commonwealth Fund, 1988.
10. Cornoni-Huntley JC, et al: Epidemiology of disability in the oldest-old: Methodologic issues and preliminary findings. *Milbank Mem Fund Q/Health Soc* 1985; 63:350–376.
11. Crystal S: *America's Old Age Crisis.* New York, Basic Books, 1982.
12. Dawson D, Hendershot G, Fulton J: Aging in the eighties. Functional limitations of individuals age 65 and over. *Advance Data From Vital and Health Statistics, No 113.* Hyattsville, Md, Public Health Service, DHHS Publication No (PHS) 87–1250, 1987.
13. Fries JF: Aging, natural death, and the compression of morbidity. *New Engl J Med* 1980; 303:130–135.
14. Fries JF: The compression of morbidity. *Milbank Mem Fund Q/Health Soc* 1983; 61:397–419.
15. Fries JF: The compression of morbidity: Miscellaneous comments about a theme. *Gerontologist* 1984; 24:354–359.
16. Gibson RC: Age-by-race differences in the health and functioning of elderly persons. *J Aging Health* 1991; 3:335–351.
17. Gibson RC, Jackson JS: The health, physical functioning, and informal supports of the black elderly. *Milbank Q* 1987; 65(suppl 2):421–454.
18. Guccione AA, Felson DT, Anderson JJ: Defining arthritis and measuring functional status in elders: Methodological issues in the study of disease and physical disability. *Am J Public Health* 1990; 80:945–949.
19. Guccione AA, Meenan RF, Anderson JJ: Arthritis in nursing home residents: A validation of its prevalence and examination of its impact on institutionalization and functional status. *Arthritis Rheum* 1989; 32:1546–1553.
20. Guccione AA, et al: Disability in the elderly: The risks associated with knee osteoarthritis (OA) vs other diseases. *Arthritis Rheum* 1991; 34(suppl):S34.
21. Guralnik J: Prospects for the compression of morbidity: The challenge posed by increasing disability in the years prior to death. *J Aging Health* 1991; 3:138–154.
22. Guralnik JM, et al: Aging in the eighties: The prevalence of comorbidity and its association with disability. *Advance Data From Vital and Health Statistics, No 170.* Hyattsville, Md, Public Health Service, DHHS Publication No (PHS) 89–1250, 1989.
23. Guralnik JM, et al: Morbidity and disability in older persons in the years prior to death. *Am J Public Health* 1991; 81:443–447.
24. Guralnik JM, Kaplan GA: Predictors of health aging: Prospective evidence from the Alameda County Study. *Am J Public Health* 1989; 79:703–708.
25. Hagestad GO: Problems and promises in the social psychology of intergenerational relations, in Fogel RW, et al (eds):

Aging—Stability and Change in the Family. New York, Academic Press, 1981.

26. Harris T, et al: Longitudinal study of physical ability in the oldest-old. *Am J Public Health* 1989; 79:698–702.

27. Harris TB, Feldman JJ: Implications of health status in analysis of risk in older persons. *J Aging Health* 1991; 3:262–284.

28. Hing E: Use of nursing homes by the elderly: Preliminary data from the 1985 National Nursing Home Survey. *Advance Data From Vital and Health Statistics, No 135.* Hyattsville, Md, Public Health Service, DHHS Publication No (PHS) 87–1250, 1987.

29. Jackson JJ, Perry C: Physical health conditions of middle-aged and aged blacks, in Markides KS (ed): *Aging and Health.* Newbury Park, Sage Publications, 1989.

30. Jette AM, Branch LG: Impairment and disability in the aged. *J Chronic Dis* 1985; 38:59–65.

31. Jette AM et al: The Framingham Disability Study: Physical disability among community-dwelling survivors of stroke. *J Clin Epidemiol* 1988; 41:719–726.

32. Kane RL, Kane RA: Long-term care, in Cassel CK, et al (eds): *Geriatric Medicine,* ed 2. New York, Springer-Verlag, 1990.

33. Kane RL, Ouslander JG, Abrass IB: *Essentials of Clinical Geriatrics,* ed 2. New York, McGraw-Hill, 1989.

34. Kaplan GA: Epidemiologic observations on the compression of morbidity. *J Aging Health* 1991; 3:155–171.

35. Katz S, et al: Active life expectancy. *Engl J Med* 1983; 309:1218–1224.

36. Keil JE, Gazes PC, Sutherland SE, et al: Predictors of physical disability in elderly blacks and whites of the Charleston Heart Study. *J Clin Epidemiol* 1989; 42:521–529.

37. Kelly-Hayes M, et al: Factors influencing survival and need for institutionalization following stroke: The Framingham Study. *Arch Phys Med Rehabil* 1988; 69:415–418.

38. Kelly-Hayes M, et al: Time course of functional recovery after stroke: The Framingham Study. *J Neuro Rehabil* 1989; 3:65–70.

39. Liang MH, et al: Evaluation of a rehabilitation component of home care for homebound elderly. *Am J Prev Med* 1986; 2:30–34.

40. Lopez-Aqueres W, et al: Health needs of the Hispanic elderly. *J Am Geriatr Soc* 1984; 32:191–198.

41. Magaziner J, et al: Predictors of functional recovery one year following hospital discharge for hip fracture: A prospective study. *J Gerontol* 1990; 45:M101–107.

42. Manton KG: Epidemiological, demographic and social correlates of disability among the elderly. *Milbank Q* 1989; 67 (suppl, pt 1):13–58.

43. Mor V, et al: Risk of functional decline among well elders. *J Clin Epidemiol* 1989; 42:895–904.

44. Moritz DJ, Ostfield AM: The epidemiology and demography of aging, in Hazzard WR, et al (eds): *Principles of Geriatric Medicine and Gerontology,* ed 2. New York, McGraw-Hill, 1990.

45. Mossey JM, Knott K, Craik R: The effects of persistent depressive symptoms on hip fracture recovery. *J Gerontol* 1990; 45:M163–168.

46. Myers GC: Demography of aging, in Binstock RH, George LK (eds): *Handbook of Aging and the Social Sciences,* ed 3. San Diego, Academic Press, 1990.

47. Nickel JT, Chirikos TN: Functional disability of elderly patients with long-term coronary heart disease: A sex-stratified analysis. *J Gerontol* 1990; 45:S60–68.

48. Nowlin JB: Geriatric health status: Influence of race and economic status. *J Minority Aging* 1973; 4:(4):93–98.

49. Olshansky SJ, et al: Trading off longer life for worsening health: The expansion of morbidity hypothesis. *J Aging Health* 1991; 3:194–216.

50. Pinsky JL, et al: Framingham Disability Study: Relationship of disability to cardiovascular risk factors among persons free of diagnosed cardiovascular disease. *Am J Epidemiol* 1985; 122:644–656.

51. Pinsky JL, et al: The Framingham Disability Study: Relationship of various coronary heart disease manifestations to disability in older persons living in the community. *Am J Public Health* 1990; 80:1363–1367.

52. Pinsky JL, Leaverton PE, Stokes J: Predictors of good function: The Framingham Study. *J Chronic Dis* 1987; 40 (suppl 1):159S–167S.

53. Rowe JW: Toward successful aging: Limitations of the morbidity associated with "normal" aging, in Hazzard WR, et al (eds): *Principles of Geriatric Medicine and Gerontology,* ed 2. New York, McGraw-Hill, 1990.

54. Rowe JW, Kahn RL: Human aging: Usual and successful. *Science* 1987; 237:143–149.

55. Satariano WA: Race, socioeconomic status, and health: A study of age differences in a depressed area. *Am J Prev Med* 1986; 2:1–5.

56. Satariano WA, et al: Difficulties in physical functioning reported by middle-aged and elderly women with breast cancer: A case-control comparison. *J Gerontol* 1990; 45:M3–11.

57. Schulz JH: *The Economics of Aging,* ed 4. Dover, Auburn House, 1988.

58. Shah S, Vanclay F, Cooper B: Stroke rehabilitation: Australian patient profile and functional outcome. *J Clin Epidemiol* 1991; 44:21–28.

59. Short P, Leon J: Use of home and community services by persons ages 65 and older with functional difficulties. *National Medical Expenditure Survey Research Findings 5.* Rockville, Md, Agency for Health Care Policy and Research, Public Health Service, DHHS Publication No (PHS) 90–3466, 1990.

60. Smeeding TM: Economic status of the elderly, in Binstock RH, George LK (eds): *Handbook of Aging and the Social Sciences,* ed 3. San Diego, Academic Press, 1990.

61. Spence DL, Brown WW: Functional assessment of the aged person, in Granger CV, Gresham GE (eds): *Functional Assessment in Rehabilitation Medicine.* Baltimore, Williams & Wilkins, 1984.

62. Streib GF, Binstock RH: Aging and the social sciences: Changes in the field, in Binstock RH, George LK (eds): *Handbook of Aging and the Social Sciences,* ed 3. San Diego, Academic Press, 1990.

63. Tangeman PT, Banaitis DA, Williams AK: Rehabilitation of chronic stroke patients: Changes in functional performance. *Arch Phys Med Rehabil* 1990; 71:876–880.

64. US Bureau of the Census: *Statistical Abstract of the United States,* ed 110. Washington, DC, 1990.

65. Verbrugge LM, Lepkowski JM, Imanaka Y: Comorbidity and its impact on disability. *Milbank Q* 1989; 67:450–484.

66. Wallace SP: The political economy of health care for elderly blacks. *Int J Health Serv* 1990; 20:665–680.

67. Wallace SP: Race versus class in the health care of African-American elderly. *Social Problems* 1990; 37:517–534.

68. Ward RA: *The Aging Experience,* ed 2. New York, Harper & Row, 1984.

69. Warlick JL: Why is poverty after 65 a woman's problem? *J Gerontol* 1985; 40:751–757.

70. White LR, et al: Geriatric epidemiology. *Annu Rev Gerontol Geriatr* 1986; 6:215–311.

71. Wing JS, et al: The black/white mortality crossover: Investigation in a community-based study. *J Gerontol* 1985; 40:78–84.

72. Worobey JL, Angel RJ: Functional capacity and living arrangements of unmarried elderly persons. *J Gerontol* 1990; [No], 45:S95–101.

Communication, Values, and the Quality of Life

Marilyn E. DeMont, M.S., P.T.
Nancy L. Peatman, M.Ed., P.T.

INTRODUCTION

What we believe about human nature, perceive as valuable in our world, and identify as "quality of life" drive our decisions, our behavior, and our communication. Our personal and professional values guide and direct our behavior and choices based on what we perceive to be "most important" within a situation of conflicting demands. Health care professionals share some common professional values. These professional values must limit and define the parameters of our professional relationships and roles with clients and colleagues. As health care professionals, our role is to do no harm; to develop a trusting relationship based on honesty and truthfulness; to promote independence; to display an "unconditional positive regard"; and to promote a belief in each individual as unique, able, and capable of change.

Professional communication is a learned skill that promotes the establishment of a professional "helping" relationship. These relationships remain within the scope of our physical therapy skills, are directed toward the goals and independence of the client, and focus only on the client. Our professional communication is a tool consciously implemented to facilitate our physical therapy therapeutic interventions.

The purpose of this chapter is to highlight significant components of communication with the elderly, to address the parameters of one's professional role in relation to the elderly, and to identify the issues commonly affecting the quality of life of the elderly.

COMMUNICATION

Communication is commonly defined as the transmission of information or messages between individuals.[18] Communication is a learned, culturally based skill.[4] It is a complex process, conveyed in written, oral, and nonverbal forms. An effective communicator adapts the content of the message and the style of transmission of the message to the needs of the receiver.[18] For example, "That's HOT!"—a simple warning about a hot stove—would be communicated quite differently to a young child, to an adult, to a person with a hearing impairment, or to a person not fluent in the English language.

Similarly, effective communication with the elderly requires adaptation to the common physiologic, psychologic, and social changes that result from the aging process. These changes, when unrecognized in an elderly individual, are common barriers to effective communication. These changes, which can be incorrectly generalized to exist in all elderly persons, can also be barriers to communication. It must be remembered that the aging process produces a slowly progressing, yet individually unique, set of variations in physiologic, psychologic, and social functioning.[4, 6] Thus, effective communication with an elderly individual considers the effects of the aging process on that individual and adapts accordingly.

Effects of Physiologic Changes of Aging on Communication

Hearing

Presbycusis, the form of hearing loss due to age-related physiologic changes of the inner ear, is one of the most widespread sensory deficits associated with aging.[23, 27, 28, 32, 33, 44] The physiologic changes in the inner ear may cause loss of high-frequency sounds and of sound localization; impairment of speech discrimination, especially for the specific sounds of the alphabet *(s, sh, ch, f, g, t, z);* and distortion of received messages.

Auditory impairment is often gradual, with even mild to moderate hearing losses resulting in significant communication and social dysfunction.[1] Elders with inner ear hearing loss have difficulty modulating the volume of their voice, may appear to be "not listening," may show confusion or puzzlement when being addressed, may respond slowly with repeated questions of "What?", and may complain of not "understanding." These behaviors common with inner ear hearing loss must be differentially diagnosed from dementia, depression, or impaired cognitive function.

Outer or middle ear hearing loss, commonly known as *conductive hearing loss,* is not limited to high-frequency sounds. Unlike the sensorineural hearing losses of the inner ear, conductive hearing loss may be corrected by increasing the volume of transmissions with a hearing aid. Table 2–1 details common strategies that facilitate communication with the hearing impaired.[8, 23, 27, 32, 33, 55, 56]

Sight

Visual deficits affect receptive communication in the elder, especially when the visual deficit is only one of many sensory changes restricting communication. Low vision interrupts communication and social interaction for the elder who can no longer perceive nonverbal cues. All structures of the eye develop age-related changes to varying degrees.[6, 27, 28] These changes affect the ability to see in low light or to adapt to darkness or changes in light. Elders may also have difficulty in judging distances, seeing objects that are too close or located in peripheral fields of vision, or accommodating between close and distant objects. Colors, especially blue and green, may be poorly differentiated. Highly reflective surfaces will also challenge an elder.

The maintenance of autonomy and the optimizing of

TABLE 2–1.

Improving Communication With the Hearing Impaired

1. Move closer to the listener for increased ease of hearing and seeing.
2. Face the listener with nonglaring light on the speaker's face.
3. Signal before speaking to gain the listener's attention.
4. Ask the listener what you can do to assist his hearing better.
5. Assist in adjusting eyeglasses or hearing aids.
6. Request permission to decrease background noise and music.
7. Speak at eye level, facing the listener.
8. Do not obscure your mouth or face, as lipreading assists comprehension.
9. Speak at a normal to slightly louder volume but not shouting.
10. Speak at a normal to slightly slower rate and articulate clearly.
11. Watch the movement of the listener's head, which may indicate an ear with better hearing.
12. Be concise, as listening requires great concentration.
13. Identify the topic of conversation and avoid sudden changes.
14. Stress key words by increasing their duration.
15. Pause after key words.
16. Give the listener time to respond.
17. Ask the listener to repeat information to ensure comprehension.
18. Never use "baby talk."
19. Use gestures to supplement speech.
20. Rephrase rather than repeat missed statements.
21. Use a notepad for messages as needed.
22. Choose a voice pitch and sound frequencies within the individual's hearing range whenever possible.

visual reception are the key elements to effective communication with a vision-impaired individual. Table 2–2 suggests strategies for effective communication with a vision-impaired elder.[31]

Speech

Decreased respiratory efficiency and laryngeal function with aging results in a lower-pitched voice, a lower volume, and a shortened controlled expiration rate with speech production. These effects of aging may result in a softer, lower voice with a breathiness, hoarseness, or vocal tremor. Sentences may shorten to accommodate a reduced, controlled expiration rate.[22] Communication with an elder with age-related speech changes is facilitated by a quiet environment, which permits the therapist and the patient to listen attentively. It is often helpful if the therapist watches the elder's lips and asks for clarification or repetition if the elder is not understood.

An increase in time between a stimulus and a response, or *reaction time*, is a manifestation of the gradual slowing of performance that is a normal physiologic process. Increased reaction time is a phenomenon that begins early in life and only becomes prominent with age. Clinically, an increase in reaction time will contribute to a decrease in memory, especially recent memory; a decrease in the speed of processing information; a decrease in vocabu-

lary; and a decrease in the rate of speech.[45] Promoting self-pacing and accommodating your rate of communication to match the elder's reaction time will significantly increase learning.[6]

Facial Expression

Facial expression is another normal age-related change that may affect expressive communication. Campbell notes that sagging cheeks or jowls, which gives a resting appearance of "anger" or "crabbiness" to many elderly men and women, are actually the result of significant loss of fat in the muscle fibers of the face.[6] The assumption of mood or frame of mind from the resting facial expression of an elder could be misleading and impede effective communication.

Sleep Patterns

Age-related changes in sleep patterns begin in the fourth decade. Variability of sleep patterns is evident with an increase in the amount of time spent sleeping, a change in the stages of sleep, and increase in the number of nighttime awakenings.[29] By the sixth decade, deep, or stage 4, sleep is almost gone. With advancing age there is a gradual increase in the total amount of sleep time, in napping, in the amount of nap time, and in wake episodes after sleep onset. After the age of 85 years, going to sleep often takes longer. An elder's mental acuity and overall ability to function are affected by problems of sleeplessness or changes in sleep patterns. Therefore, attention to sleep patterns may help a therapist understand a patient's affect, communication style, and response to treatment.

Strategies for Effective Communication

Communication is an essential component of the role of a health professional. Interpersonal skills are learned skills that focus on the patient, promote trust and confidence, allow the expression of feelings and concerns, efficiently

TABLE 2–2.

Improving Communication With the Visually Impaired

- Avoid startling an elder. Approach slowly and use verbal greetings and touch.
- Avoid positioning an elder in glaring light and adjust levels of light to accommodate the elder's vision. This may be up to three times more light than a younger adult may require.
- Provide Large-print materials with high-contrast colors.
- Use tactile stimulation for cueing.
- Avoid moving personal belongings and discuss any changes in placement of furniture or belongings.
- Wait for the elder's vision to adapt to changes in light.
- Reduce glare on surfaces including floors, bedside tables, and bathroom sinks.

collect information, and effectively impart important information.

There are a variety of facilitative techniques that promote the effective treatment and overall well-being of one's patient or client when used appropriately. Several approaches to assist health professionals in developing the attitudes and interpersonal skills of an effective communicator have been developed.[16, 18, 30, 40] All these strategies are founded on several commonly held professional values. Respect for the individual, the promotion of the patient's autonomy, and the nurturance of a trusting relationship are the guiding principles of all professional relationships. The strategies for improving communication with elders listed in Table 2–3 translate these principles into common actions.[7, 37, 46]

Facilitation of Communication and Socialization

Basic communication and interpersonal skills for the "helping professional" are outside the scope of this text. All health care providers should recognize the use of facilitatory communication skills and the establishment of a professional "helping" relationship as essential vehicles to their provision of care. The essence of our professional interventions and effectiveness is our ability to respond to a human being as a unique, worthwhile individual. The use

of touch, reminiscence, humor, and pets are effective stimuli to interaction and socialization with the elderly.

Touch
Touch has a significant effect in reinforcing our interactions with the elderly. Studies show touch to be a positive motivator that engenders a sense of trust, shows caring, and generally increases the duration of verbal responses from an elder.[20, 21, 53]

Reminiscence
Reminiscence is a useful communication approach that provides validation of the individual's place in the community, increases self-esteem, and assists in the resolution of losses. Reminiscence is a normal coping skill that begins in middle childhood. It is defined as "the act or habit of thinking about or relating past experiences, especially those considered personally most significant."[35] Studies on reminiscence report an increase in communication, life satisfaction, and positive self-image.[3, 39] The use of pictures; music; or topics such as "the depression," "FDR," hometowns, or favorite pastimes are examples that promote the expression of feelings and a sense of self-worth.[38]

Humor
Humor has numerous positive physiologic and psychologic effects on the body. Laughter "stimulates the production of catecholamines and hormones which enhance feelings of well being as well as pain tolerance. It decreases anxiety, increases the flow of endorphins, cardiac and respiratory rates, enhances metabolism and improves muscle tone."[50] Humor and laughter are very effective forms of communication that build trust, defuse anger or frustration, and promote shared experience. Humor is infectious and, similar to other types of communication, can be learned. The use of humor between a therapist and a patient requires three conditions: (1) a relationship that allows for the introduction of playfulness without misinterpretation; (2) a social environment that allows for playfulness without disrupting the serious business; and (3) a joker who provides clues to set the mood and takes the risk that the message will be ignored.[43, 50] It must be remembered that healthy humor is not abusive or diminishing. Instead, healthy humor promotes understanding through positive shared experience.

Pets
Communication can also be fostered by nonhuman means. Pets can play a significant role in combating loneliness and decreasing isolation by increasing verbalization and socialization among the elderly. Pets have been found to be natural "icebreakers" facilitating social interaction. The physical act of petting promotes a mutual relaxation, a therapeutic "caring for a living thing."[13] A pet is a companion,

TABLE 2–3.
Strategies for Improving Communication With Elders

1. Do not stereotype. Do not assume a level of decreased mental function or confusion. Posture, gesture, and facial expressions can be deceiving.
2. Be aware of, and adapt to, any age-related physical limitations that an elder may possess. Consider the sensory deficits in sight, hearing, speech, and reaction time, which may be barriers to communication.
3. Secure the elder's attention by eye contact or a gentle touch.
4. Identify yourself when greeting an elder.
5. Request information from each elder on how best to communicate, e.g., "Should I speak louder?" or "Would you like your glasses?"
6. Ask each individual what form of address is preferred. Do not use generic or pet names such as "Grampa" or "Mama." Each individual has a unique identity.
7. Request permission to adjust the volume of the television or radio or to change the amount or angle of light.
8. Maintain eye contact.
9. Do not pretend to understand an elder's response. Request confirmation or clarification of a message you do not understand.
10. Avoid speaking to elders as if they were children. Do not use a singsong voice or baby talk or give orders.
11. Do not ignore individuals or talk about them in the presence of others as if they were not there.
12. Respect an elder's routines and control of his life. Schedule and keep appointments at mutually agreed-on times.

a "significant other," that provides structure to daily activities, gives and requires attention, and usually instigates a greater degree of physical exercise.

VALUES

Autonomy

Elders are people first and thus are entitled to be treated with respect and dignity and without bias. It is imperative that health care professionals respect and address the individuality of each elder they encounter, regardless of the circumstances in which they encounter them. It is not immediately important whether the elder is living alone or is a resident of a nursing home; whether the person has multiple chronic illnesses or none; or whether the individual is cognitively alert or exhibits signs of dementia. A basic tenet of the geriatric physical therapist is that respect for the elder is the paramount principle underlying all interactions.

The concept of respect implies choice on the part of elders—freedom to actively participate in decision making, to the extent that they are capable of doing so, and to choose what is or what is not done to them, irrespective of their chronologic age.[5] The ability of elders to retain this decision-making power and their enforceable right to make those decisions have been the impetus over the years to enact legislation on informed consent and protection of patient's rights. When these legal requirements are enforced, the elder is in control of the decision rather than subject to the imposition of decisions from external sources.

Societal and cultural beliefs, however, can significantly dilute the autonomy that is an elder's right. It is essential to explore how these influences, whether subtle or overt, affect therapeutic outcomes. For the geriatric physical therapist, it is not enough to be just aware of such factors. Rather, it is necessary that conscious attention be paid to these influences so that the elder client can be valued as a contributor to the health care team.

Ageism

Although awareness of the dangers of stereotyping elders is increasing, most would agree that conscious efforts to educate against negative generalizations need to continue; many elders continue to be stigmatized. Unfortunately, we continue to live in an ageist society. *Ageism* has been variously described as the discriminatory treatment of old people, or a personal revulsion to growing older.[2, 40] It fosters the development of erroneous assumptions about the capabilities, intelligence, and physical skills of elders, based purely on deep-seated beliefs about aging. It supports judgments about a person on the basis of chronologic age and negates the concept of an individual approach to patient care by encouraging premature decisions regarding the elder's status and potential. More important, in an era where collaboration between the health care provider and the client is being espoused, ageism effectively eliminates the elder as the primary decision maker and significantly reduces the value of the elder's contribution on any level.

One example of ageism can be readily seen in the words and language used when referring to elders.[2] For example, the term *old people* connotes a more negative image than the word *elders*. The council of elders in various churches is a positive image, implying a knowledgeable, decision-making group. Perhaps the difference lies in the fact that in many cultures elders are accorded positions of respect and authority. For example, in many native American cultures, elders are viewed in much the same way, commanding the respect of the tribe and dispensing wisdom collected through the years. Yet the uses of many demeaning and derogatory terms, such as *old biddy, fogey,* and *geezer,* continue to flourish in our culture. If we accept the principle that the language we use is reflective of what we are thinking, and that what we think is shaped by our values and beliefs, then the use of negative terminology when referring to the elderly is more than a simple choice of words.[2] Rather, it is the verbalization of deeply held negative values and beliefs. Ageist language is common and is continually reinforced by the mass media. Over time, a term that was once offensive becomes less so, sometimes to the extent that it may become acceptable. The danger is that use, and eventual acceptance, of ageist language may contribute to maintaining the very stereotypes to be dispelled.[2] Although health care workers may consciously state that they do not subscribe to an ageist philosophy, they may in fact undermine their good intentions through the use of language with negative connotations of aging.

Elders themselves can be guilty of ageism, conditioned through experience or observation of societal trends and behavior to expect, and then accept, the words attributed to them as they age. Unfortunately, as Rodin and Langer have shown, continued labeling decreases feelings of self-worth and brings about negative changes in behavior and decrements in perceived control.[44] Real losses occur all around elders by virtue of their life stage, e.g., loss of spouse, loss of friends, and in some cases, loss of home. These changes are adjustments to life that elders are expected to adapt to as their chronologic age increases. However, they may be so conditioned to losing control, as a result of societal influences such as ageism, that they unnecessarily and voluntarily give up additional control over their lives, self-imposing further loss. When examining quality-of-life issues, Ryden states that perceived control factors very strongly in the overall equation.[46] It would seem, then, that fostering an elder's control of decision making improves an individual's quality of life.

Perceived Control vs. Helplessness/Hopelessness

Who controls the decision making for an elder is especially pertinent to quality-of-life issues among our aging population. Perceived control of decision making is actually a very strong contributor to the level of morale of elders, and that morale factors strongly into the overall equation of quality of life experienced by elders.[46] Conversely, loss of control and feelings of helplessness can lead to lack of motivation and withdrawal. Logically, then, fostering an elder's control of decision making should be preserved if we are committed to retaining or improving the quality of life. However, just as ageist language has become accepted in society, so has the expectation that responsibility for decision making slowly, but automatically, shifts away from the elder, presumably to someone who has the best interest of the elder at heart. The presumption is faulty; none of us knows anyone better than we know ourselves. The practice of taking decision-making authority away from elders, however, persists, and the elder is robbed of the opportunity to contribute to the decision and relegated instead to the role of passive recipient of someone else's judgment. Because of the powerful role that control of decision making has in maintaining the morale of elders, it is not surprising that loss of control may precipitate a lack of interest in interacting with people or the environment. These elders may then be characterized as lacking motivation, or as apathetic, listless, and uncommunicative, and engender a sense of helplessness and even hopelessness or despair.[51] Particularly in institutional settings, passive, withdrawn behavior may be unconsciously reinforced by health care professionals who support the notion that the passive residents are the good residents, because they are not disruptive to the flow of work.[51] The likelihood of this occurrence is magnified in situations where the facility is consistently understaffed or where staffing patterns are irregular. Under these circumstances, as might be expected, quality of life for the elder is further threatened, and therapeutic outcomes are seriously hampered.

Loss of control over decision making and its sequelae, as described above, have devastating, but not irreversible, effects on the quality of life of an elder. Research supports the reversible nature of such behavior. Strategies and techniques that address improving perceived control of decision making have been correlated with increased self-reports of happiness, morale, and enthusiasm as well as increased alertness and activity levels noted by others.[51] It would seem logical, then, that any strategy designed to return control of decision making to the elder not only will

help in improving quality of life for that individual but also will benefit all professionals involved in that individual's care. Teitelman and Priddy offer six basic therapeutic strategies that can be used to facilitate such control.[51] Although designed for use in long-term–care settings, their recommendations can be extrapolated to most environments.

1. *Promotion of choice and predictability.* Even small, or what may appear to others as insignificant, choices can have a positive impact on the elder's perception of control and can be readily incorporated on a daily basis. For example, recognizing that elders, like all persons, have preferences for example, what they wear, what food they eat, and when they go to therapy, . . . and allowing them to voice those preferences with the knowledge that their choices will be honored, empowers them and can improve their mental as well as physical well-being. Predictability can be included by keeping the elder informed of overall goals and expectations.

2. *Elimination of helplessness-engendering stereotypes.* Establishing effective, productive relationships with elder clients—respecting and valuing their worth and recognizing their potential contributions and decision-making abilities—is the most useful health care delivery model. Self-awareness, by the health provider, of ageism and the serious consequences of loss of control is paramount. Educating others to its devastating effects is the logical next step.

3. *Promotion of therapeutic attributions and a sense of responsibility.* This strategy involves redirecting the elders' sense of guilt or blame for the cause of their problems and encouraging more personal responsibility for effecting a positive outcome or solution. Self-blame is destructive and has the potential to fuel existing feelings of helplessness/hopelessness, whereas taking a role in identifying/effecting a solution is generally therapeutic.

4. *Provision of success experiences early on in care.* Care needs to be taken, early on, not to overwhelm the elder with demands and tasks that are intimidating. Less-challenging decisions should be attempted first, while the elder's self-confidence is built. Negative results and errors need to be anticipated and minimized by the therapist, while praise and positive reinforcement are maximized.

5. *Modification of an elder's unrealistic goals for care.* The geriatric therapist's overall goal, individualized for each elder, is to simultaneously maintain hope and promote a therapeutic relationship while modifying any unrealistic expectations.

6. *Use of control-enhancing communication skills.* Communication that is respectful and genuine and that values the client's views and feelings can reduce helplessness and improve cooperation in the therapeutic environment.

Culture

Ensuring that elders are in control of their own decisions has a positive influence on outcomes, quality of life, adherence to professional recommendations, and motivation. However, culture is a broad factor that can effectively negate a positive outcome if overlooked. Wood describes ethnicity as "common history and shared culture," while culture itself refers to "socially transmitted beliefs, institutions and behavior patterns that are characteristic of a particular population group."[58] Culture and ethnicity have only recently begun to receive the attention that they deserve in the health care community. However, the potential impact of each of these factors on the eventual outcome of an elder's care must be considered from the outset, if professionals are committed to providing the best possible care.

Ethnicity and culture can impact on elders' views of death, dying, the role of the family in illness, and the importance attached to folk beliefs and medicines as opposed to current technology and medical advances. Ethnic and cultural beliefs can significantly influence the level of respect bestowed on an elder, the dynamics of the family and support system in general, the development of provider-patient relationships, the need for control of decision-making power, and certainly the extent to which an elder will adhere to professional recommendations.[17, 58] In fact, an elder may persist in rejecting professional recommendations despite efforts by the provider to increase elder control of decision making if attention is not given to ethnic and cultural considerations. Wood cautions that elders may believe that their own assessments of their health, "often described in colorful folk medicine causalities," should be regarded by health professionals as seriously as these opinions are taken within the ethnic subculture.[58] Furthermore, dismissal of long-standing, culturally based beliefs is not conducive to establishing a mutually rewarding, therapeutic relationship that is built on trust.

It is not realistic to expect that health care professionals have in-depth knowledge of all subcultures, but it is recommended that sensitivity to cultural issues be encouraged and that empathy be practiced.[58] In the absence of in-depth knowledge of specific cultural beliefs, attention to the nonverbal signals of the elder client, such as body language, facial expression, and eye contact, can provide the health care provider with clues that perhaps further investigation into the cultural background of the client is appropriate. Family members and colleagues also may be able to provide valuable insight into a cultural or ethnic group.

Of course, when providing health care in a region with known cultural influences it is incumbent on the professional to become knowledgeable of local customs and beliefs and to be creative in working to incorporate them into the overall plan of care when possible. For example, in some subcultures, the individual is traditionally a passive recipient of care, dependent on a traditional healer and local customs to effect a change in health. In addition, these individuals may wait to consult with the traditional healer before accepting even minor professional recommendations. This oftentimes further delays the initiation of care. The health professional who unknowingly expects full, active cooperation is likely to be frustrated by these practices but, once informed, can effectively plan a reasonable course of action. The professional must have a healthy respect and appreciation for ethnic and cultural differences among elders and recognize that culture can be a powerful influence on the entire therapeutic process.

Advocacy

One way in which quality-of-life issues in elders can be addressed is to emphasize the concepts of patient advocacy and informed consent. Informed consent may be simplistically misrepresented as meaning only that the elder is part of the decision-making process. While this may be true on a superficial level, this simply does not accurately portray the full requirements. The original intent of informed consent legislation is that health professionals provide the elder with sufficient information about the situation so that the elder can make informed choice.[19] In other words, efforts should allow the elder to be a person who has enough information to actually make the decision and not simply to act as a contributor to the decision-making process.

Historically, however, a paternalistic attitude has been utilized and reinforced in the medical model of health care.[14, 57] In paternalism, decisions regarding what is best for the patient are made by the professionals. Most often this occurs when individuals are truly incapable of making independent decisions because of lack of consciousness or serious cognitive impairment.[57] However, in the case of elders, a paternalistic approach is often taken even when there is no evidence to suggest that either of these conditions is present. Wetle has remarked that paternalistic attitudes employ an ageist assumption that equates old age with incompetence.[57] Unnecessary paternalism perpetuates ageism and fosters dependent, hopeless, and helpless individuals.

On the opposite end of the spectrum from the more familiar practice of paternalism is what Gadow has called *consumerism*.[14] Rather than making all the decisions for the client, the consumerism model finds the health professional providing the elder with factual information and then withdrawing, leaving the decision totally in the hands of the client. While at first glance this model may appear to meet the requirements of patient self-determination, neither it nor paternalism provides a mechanism in which the client is assisted with the decision process itself. One model eliminates the patient from the equation (paternalism), whereas the other eliminates the professional (consumerism).[14]

Advocacy is a third model and one that empowers the elder. It relies heavily on the dynamics of the patient-provider relationship and on the active participation by the professional in assisting the elder to make a decision. As defined by Gadow, the advocacy model is "an effort to help individuals become clear about what they want in a situation, to assist them in discerning and clarifying their values, and to help them in examining options in light of their values."[14]

There are five components to the advocacy model. The first is that of self-determination or *autonomy.* The more information that an elder has, the more able the person will be to choose what course of action is right for a particular circumstance. In the absence of complete information, informed choice is not possible. The second component is that of the *patient-provider relationship.* The provider's role is to enable the client to determine the amount and type of information to be presented.

The third component in this model is one that may be new to many health care professionals but one that is uniquely important to this model: providers need to *share their own values* with the patient. To be able to examine all options freely the client is entitled to know what the provider's feelings and values are. This does not imply an imposition of the provider's values on the patient, nor a coercion to decide in a prescribed way. Rather, it is a sharing perspective that serves to strengthen the patient-provider relationship by affirming that the provider is genuinely concerned with protecting the elder's right to self-determination by providing all the information. Disclosing provider values also has the effect of assisting individuals to *clarify their own values,* the fourth component in the model. It is absolutely essential for the provider to discern what is important to the individual, in terms of quality-of-life issues, in order to provide appropriate information. For example, will a proposed intervention increase or decrease the quality of life that the patient values? Are proposed interventions in keeping with or discordant from strongly held cultural beliefs? This component emphasizes the need for the provider to be able to set aside personal values in deference to letting the patient's values be decisive.[14]

The final component of Gadow's model is the concept of *individuality.* Individuality includes considerations other than values that can be decisive in self-determination. How injury or insult to the body affects a person's perception of self can significantly influence the ability to exercise free choice. The perception of self and body may be so tightly intertwined that behavior after an injury will not be consistent with how the person might have been expected to behave prior to the illness. For example, depression following illness or injury can significantly influence decision making. Decisions made under these circumstances may not be in keeping with usual and customary behavior prior to the incident. In order to protect an elder's right to free choice, it is critical that the health provider be aware of the person's sense of individuality and how it may affect the capacity for self-determination. Most important, the provider needs to be prepared to actively assist the client in exploring these issues.

Gadow's advocacy model conceptualizes the compassionate health care provider as one who not only places the well-being of the elder above all else but also recognizes that the elder is solely responsible for defining the conditions of "personal well-being." In this model, extensive consideration is given to the elder as a unique being—an individual with a history of unique experiences; with values, needs, and desires that do not fade as age increases; and with a right to self-determination in all matters. Using this model, "patient compliance" becomes an obsolete phrase. Compliance, after all, is only an issue if one fails to abide by, obey, or do what someone else has deemed critical. As Ramsden so aptly states, "Failure of patient to comply with treatment may be related to failure of the health care professional to plan a strategy that is in tune with the individual's needs."[41]

ISSUES AFFECTING AN ELDER'S QUALITY OF LIFE

The Role of the Family

Family plays a significant role in the quality of life of the elderly. Families are sources of information, care givers, and major sources of emotional support and socialization.[12] In turn, family members need support to fulfill these critical roles and to meet the needs of aging parents and relatives. Families require information on (1) the normal changes with aging, (2) available community resources, (3) knowledge and skills in the actual physical care of the elder, and (4) communication skills training to deal with physiologic changes and psychologic changes of the aging elder.[9, 34, 42, 47, 48, 54] When an elder becomes impaired, the family members are understandably grieved and often frustrated by the loss. Families require assistance in coping with their feelings, understanding the causes of impairment, and learning communication strategies that promote the elder's well-being and sense of control.[52] Thus, providing care for an elderly patient is usually a team approach that requires professional communication with the elder, the family, and other health care providers. Teaching the elder patient and the family is an important professional skill that directly affects the elder's quality of life.

Grief and Loss

Grief is a natural, emotional response to an actual or impending loss.[10] The loss of physical function; loss of a limb; loss of a job; loss of life roles, and their responsibilities and pleasures; loss of a loved one, especially a spouse; or imminent loss of one's own life—all cause painful suffering. Grieving is a normal reaction for a patient and that patient's family. The grieving process, although recognized to have identifiable symptoms and phases, remains a unique, individual response strongly embedded in social and cultural values and beliefs.[10, 15, 36, 49] Studies indicate that an individual's personality traits are the most powerful predictors of one's style of coping with grief.[15]

Symptoms of Grief

Somatic symptoms are a common response to grief. Tightness of the throat, shortness of breath, choking, frequent sighing, muscle weakness, tremors, an empty feeling in the abdomen, and chills are all common somatic symptoms present with grief. Sensory responses are known to be heightened or erratic. The grief-stricken individual may appear tense, restless, irritable, or hostile. Preoccupation with the image of the deceased or the lost object is common and often the only topic of conversation. Mental distress is often exhibited by disorientation to time, lack of ability to concentrate, restlessness, and a tendency to daydream. Similar to common depression, disturbances in sleeping, eating, and normal activity patterns, including hygiene, are common.

Phases of Grief

A number of models and theories of stages of grieving exist.[10, 15, 25] Each model attempts to delineate the gambit of human emotions associated with loss, including shock, disbelief, sadness, sorrow, anger, disgust, guilt, and relief. Although these models may assist our understanding of the complexity of the grieving process, none are meant to show a linear sequence of emotions or stages. The actual grief process is a total emotional response that is highly individualized.

Grief work does have some commonly recognized phases.[10, 15, 49] Shock, disbelief, and numbness are common initial reactions. Preoccupation with the loss of a person or object, intense pining, restlessness, irritability, intense loneliness, and overall anxiety are often-displayed initial responses. With time, intense grief work may display a wide range of emotional responses, from anger to apathy. The intensity of the grief response is related to the perceived significance of the loss, the bereaved's personality traits and coping methods, and the elder's accepted social and cultural norms. This time of grief work for the bereaved elder patient may be confused with a clinical depression. The apathy, mood swings, and aimlessness common in grief are similar to depression and may be treated like a major depressive episode. Caution is advised in the use of medications that may trigger additional mood swings or produce significant side effects that may actually prolong the grieving process.[49] Finally, a gradual reorganization and balance occur in the emotional and physical well-being of the grieving individual. It is important to recognize that significant new events or anniversary dates may continue to trigger grief reactions or mood swings. Health professionals have an important role in supporting their patients through the grieving process. Verbal and nonverbal support, empathy, respect, and acknowledgment of their individual needs are all part of a comprehensive plan of care.

Fear of Dying

All individuals have fears related to dying and terminal illness. Some of the most common fears are isolation, pain, and dependence.[24, 40] The health care provider has a decided role in supporting the dying patient by providing security, alleviating suffering, and providing as much control for the patient as possible. Continued physical and emotional support diminishes the fears associated with terminal illness and dying.

The fear of isolation is a fear of physical as well as emotional isolation. Family and health care providers confronted with the loss of the patient and their own inability to prevent the inevitable are known to retreat. This retreat is not only from the patient but also from the health care providers' own sense of loss or lack of control. The patient has the desire to be responded to as a living, worthwhile individual up to the time of death. A dying patient, facing the unknown, is supported by knowing that one will not be left alone.

The fear of pain is frequently expressed by dying patients. A decrease of, or freedom from, pain significantly increases an individual's quality of life. A clear commitment by health care providers to alleviate pain is a significant source of comfort for the dying patient.[24]

The dying patient's fear of dependence and of lack of control is compounded by fears of isolation and pain. With the loss of physical and mental functions, the dying patient faces loss of control of aspects of life. The health care providers' role is to empower the dying patient in whatever ways possible by promoting or sustaining an environment that is responsive to that patient's needs. All health care providers would do well by adopting the hospice philosophy of "affirming life and providing support and care" to dying patients so that they may live as fully and as comfortably as possible.[36] In addition, the adoption and promotion of Living Wills and Medical Directives could greatly enhance the dying patient's sense of control.[11]

COMMUNICATING WITH THE TERMINALLY ILL PATIENT

Communicating with a terminally ill patient should be no different than any other patient-therapist interaction. The uniqueness in our response to the patient with a terminal illness comes from our awareness of the significance and finality of death facing the patient and from the enormity of our own perceptions and fears of death and loss. These are complex issues that we face as individuals and as health care providers. The support of other health care providers is advisable when dealing with your own grief and loss for the dying patients. Our helping professional role is not automatic, or easy. It requires significant practice and skill in communication, in the ability to listen, to empathize, and to consistently promote the well-being of an individual from that individual's own perspective. The key to all our professional interactions is the provision of care from the patient's perspective.

Maintaining Hope

Hope for a terminally ill patient may not necessarily be for a cure. Hope for a patient may be to see his next grandchild, to have time to settle the family finances, to have one more Thanksgiving with the family, or to ultimately have a quick and painless death. As illness progresses, patients' hopes may change. Your role is to facilitate the fulfillment of that patient's hope as realistically possible. Open, direct communication is required if the therapist is to learn what is important to the patient. The setting of mutual goals is essential.

Alleviating Suffering

Suffering is not a simple physiologic response. Suffering—the lack of comfort or physical well-being—can be greatly reduced by the alleviation of fears. Patients need the support of knowing that they will not be abandoned or allowed to suffer as they approach death. Although a dying patient's decreasing physical capacity may greatly limit his independence, the role of the health care provider is to maintain that patient's dignity and self-control by promoting the patient's decision making as much as possible.

Saying Good-bye

Saying good-bye to a patient, especially a patient with a terminal illness, can be very difficult. Ned Cassem[26] gives a clear perspective of what one may choose to say and why:

> What we often do because losses hurt so much is we don't say good-bye to anybody. The day comes and we disappear. . . . What should be said is, I want you to know the relationship was meaningful, I'll miss this about you, or I'll find it hard to go down to the corner for a beer, it won't be the same, I'll miss the bluntness that you had in helping me sort out some things, or I'll miss the old bull sessions, or something like that. Because those are the things you value. Now what does that do for the other person? The other person learns that although it's painful to separate it's far more meaningful to have known the person and to have separated than never to have known him at all. He also learns what it is in himself that is valued and treasured.

SUMMARY

Communication is an essential component of the role of the health professional. Communication and interpersonal skills are learned skills, which are driven by some commonly held professional values. Respect for the individual, promotion of the individual's autonomy, and nurturance of a trusting relationship are values that drive the communication approaches and interpersonal skills of health care professionals.

Effective communication with an elder requires adaptation to the common physiologic, psychologic, and social changes associated with the aging process. Changes in hearing, sight, speech, and facial expression alter the elder's communication intake and response. Effective communication with an elder considers the effects of the aging process on that individual and adapts to those physiologic and social changes. Age-related learning, sight, hearing, and speech deficits in an elder require conscious adjustments in the communication approach of the health care provider. Effective communication with an elder may be facilitated through a variety of strategies and approaches including the use of touch, reminiscence, and humor.

An imperative for health care professionals is to respect and address the individuality of each elder they encounter. Ageism remains in our society and continues to foster erroneous assumptions about the capabilities, intelligence, and physical skills of the elder client. Our use of language is a telling example of the insipid influence of ageism. Terms such as *old biddy* and *geezer* continue to thrive in our culture.

Our quality of life is directly related to our ability to control decisions and make choices. Ensuring that elders are in control of their own decisions has a positive influence on therapeutic outcomes, their quality of life, and adherence to professional recommendations. A significant variable when considering anyone's quality of life is the impact of culture and ethnicity. Sensitivity to cultural and ethnicity issues is essential. A model of advocacy embraces the principles of compassionate health care that truly empowers elders.

Grief, death, and dying are significant issues of life for all of us but are particularly prominent for the elderly. Communicating with the terminally ill patient and family is complex. Alleviating suffering, maintaining hope, and saying good-bye can be difficult skills for health care providers to learn. Health care professionals have an important role in supporting their patients. Communication is our tool.

REFERENCES

1. Anand JK, Court I: Hearing loss leading to impaired ability to communicate in residents of homes for the elderly. *Brown Med J* 1989; 298:1429.
2. Barbato C, Feezel J: The language of aging in different age groups. *Gerontologist* 1987; 27:527.
3. Bennett SL, Maas F: The effect of music-based life review on the life satisfaction and ego integrity of elderly people. *Br J Occup Ther* 1988; 51:433–436.
4. Brownlee AT: *Community, Culture, and Care: A Cross-Cultural Guide for Health Workers.* St Louis, CV Mosby, 1978.
5. Buehler D: Informed consent and the elderly. *Crit Care Nurs Clin North Am* 1990; 2:461–471.
6. Campbell JM, Lancaster J: Communicating effectively with older adults. *Fam Community Health* 1988; 11:74–85.
7. Caporael LR, Culbertson GH: Verbal response modes of baby talk and other speech at institutions for the aged. *Lang Communication* 1986; 6:99–112.
8. Cohen G, Faulkner D: Does "elderspeak" work? The effect of intonation and stress on comprehension and recall of spoken discourse in old age. *Lang Communication* 1986; 6:91–98.
9. Cohen PM: A group approach for working with families of the elderly. *Gerontologist* 1983; 23:248–250.
10. Despelder LA, Strickland AL: *The Last Dance: Encountering Death and Dying,* ed 2. Mountain View, Calif, Mayfield, 1987.
11. Emanuel LL, Emanuel EJ: The Medical Directive: A new comprehensive advance care document. *JAMA* 1989; 261:3288–3293.
12. Epstein JL: Communicating with the elderly. *J Market Res Soc* 1983; 25:239–262.
13. Erickson R: Companion animals and the elderly. *Geriatr Nurs* 1985; March-April:92–96.
14. Gadow S: Advocacy: An ethical model for assisting patients with treatment decisions, in Wong CB, Swazey JP (eds): *Dilemmas of Dying: Policies and Procedures for Decisions Not to Treat.* Boston, GK Hall Medical Publishers, 1981.

15. Gallagher DE, Thompson LW, Peterson JA: Psychosocial factors affecting adaptation to bereavement in the elderly. *Int J Aging Hum Dev* 1982; 3:79–95.
16. Gazda GM, Childers WC, Walter RP: *Interpersonal Communication.* Rockville, Md, Aspen, 1982.
17. Gelfand DE, Kutzik AJ (eds): *Ethnicity and Aging: Theory, Research and Policy,* vol 5. New York, Springer, 1979.
18. Gerrard BA, Boniface WJ, Love BH: Interpersonal Skills for Health Professionals. Reston, Va, Reston, 1980.
19. Guccione A: Compliance and patient autonomy: Ethical and legal limits to professional dominance. *Top Geriatr Rehabil* 1988; 3(3):62–84.
20. Hollinger LM: Communicating with the elderly. *Gerontol Nurs* 1986; 12:8–13.
21. Howard DM: The effects of touch in the geriatric population. *Phys Occup Ther Geriatr* 1988; 6:35–50.
22. Jackson MM: Aging and motor speech production, Top Geriatr Rehabil 1986; 1:29–43.
23. Kaplan H: Communication problems for the hearing impaired elderly: What can be done? *Pride Inst J Long Term Home Health Care* 1988; 7:10–22.
24. Kinzel T: Relief of emotional symptoms in elderly patients with cancer. *Geriatrics* 1988; 43:61–65.
25. Kubler-Ross E: *On Death and Dying.* New York, Macmillan, 1970.
26. Langhorne J: *Vital Signs: The Way We Die in America.* Boston, Little, Brown, 1974.
27. Maloney CC: Identifying and treating the client with sensory loss. *Phys Occup Ther Geriatr* 1987; 5:31–46.
28. Mulrow CD, Aguilar C, et al: Association between hearing impairment and the quality of life of elderly individuals. *Am Geriatr Soc* 1990; 38:45–50.
29. Muncy JH: Measures to rid sleeplessness: 10 points to enhance sleep. *Gerontol Nurs* 1986; 12:6–11.
30. Navarro T, Lipkowitz M, Navarra JG: Therapeutic communication: A guide to effective interpersonal skills for health care professionals. Thorofare, NJ, Slack, 1990.
31. Null RL: Low-vision elderly: An environmental rehabilitation approach. *Top Geriatr Rehabil* 1988; 4(1):24–31.
32. Palumbo MV: Hearing Access 2000. Increasing awareness of the hearing impaired. *Gerontol Nurs* 1990; 16:26–31.
33. Patten PC, Piercy FP: Dysfunctional isolation in the elderly: Increasing marital and family closeness through improved communication. *Contemp Fam Ther Int J* 1989; 11:131–147.
34. Pfeiffer E: Some basic principles for working with older patients. *Am Geriatr Soc* 1985; 33:44–47.
35. Pincus A: Reminiscence in aging and its implications for social work practice. *Soc Work* 1970; 15:47–53.
36. Pizzi M: Hospice and the terminally ill geriatric patient. *Phys Occup Ther Geriatr* 1983; 3:45–54.
37. Portnoy EJ: Communication and the elderly patient. *Activ Adapt Aging* 1985; 7:25–30.
38. Price C: Heritage: A program design for reminiscence. *Activ Adapt Aging* 1983; 3:7–52.
39. Priefer BA, Gambert SR: Reminiscence and life review in the elderly. *Psychiatr Med* 1984; 2:91–100.
40. Purtilo R: *Health Professional and Patient Interaction,* ed 4. Philadelphia, WB Saunders, 1990.

41. Ramsden E: Compliance and motivation, *Top Geriatr Rehabil* 1988; 3(3):1–14.

42. Remnet VL: How adult children respond to role transitions in the lives of their aging parents. *Educ Gerontol* 1987; 13:341–355.

43. Robinson VM: *Humor and the Health Professions*. Thorofare, NJ, Slack, 1977.

44. Rodin J, Langer E: Aging labels: The decline of control and the fall of self esteem. *J Soc Issues* 1980; 36:12–29.

45. Ryan EB, Giles H, et al: Psycholinguistic and social psychological components of communication by and with the elderly. *Lang Communication* 1986; 6:1–24.

46. Ryden MB: Morale and perceived control in institutionalized elderly. *Nurs Res* 1984; 33:130–136.

47. Santora G: Communicating better with the elderly: How to break down the barriers. *Nurs Life* 1986; 6:24–27.

48. Shulman MD, Mandel E: Communication training of relatives and friends of institutionalized elderly persons. *Gerontologist* 1988; 28:797–799.

49. Stewart T, Shields CR: Grief in chronic illness: Assessment and management. *Arch Phys Med Rehabil* 1985; 66:447–450.

50. Sullivan JL, Deane DM: Humor and health. *Gerontol Nurs* 1988; 14:20–24.

51. Teitelman J, Priddy J: From psychological theory to practice: Improving frail elders' quality of life through control-enhancing intervention. *Appl Gerontol* 1988; 7:298–315.

52. Thompson RF, Montalvo B: Psychosocial aspects of geriatrics: A six-point orientation scheme for training. *Fam Syst Med* 1989; 7:397–410.

53. Tobin SS, Gustafson JD: What do we do differently with elderly clients? *Gerontol Soc Work* 1987; 10:107–121.

54. Truglio LM, Hayes PM: Carers learn to cope. *Geriatr Nurs* 1986; 7:310–312.

55. Walsh C, Eldredge N: When deaf people become elderly: Counteracting a lifetime of difficulties. *Gerontol Nurs* 1989; 15:27–31.

56. Washburn AD: Hearing disorders and the aged. *Top Geriatr Rehabil* 1986; 1:61–70.

57. Wetle T: Ethical issues in long-term care of the aged, *Geriatr Psychiatry* 1985; 18:63–73.

58. Wood J: Communicating with older adults in health care settings: Cultural and ethnic considerations. *Educ Gerontol* 1989; 15:351–362.

CHAPTER 3

Physiological Change and Adaptation to Exercise in the Older Adult

Elizabeth J. Protas, Ph.D., P.T.

INTRODUCTION

The purpose of this chapter is to discuss the profound physiologic changes that occur as people age. These changes tend to occur in every bodily system. The extent of these physiologic changes has a significant impact on the ability of an individual to function in daily life. Topics to be included in this chapter are issues in normal aging, changes in cardiopulmonary and musculoskeletal function, and the effects of exercise on these changes.

Classification of Aging

Since there are vast differences between a 65-year-old individual and a 100-year-old individual, classifications into smaller age ranges are recognized. These arbitrary divisions represent three ranges of biologic age groups. The young-old are individuals between 65 and 75 years of age. This group often has the least loss of function and impairment. The young-old are the most common subjects of physiologic studies, particularly exercise studies. Individuals between the ages of 75 and 85 fall within the middle-old group. The old-old group is comprised of individuals older than 85.[27] The incidence of disease and disability increases dramatically in the middle-old and old-old groups. Thus, these are the more likely groups with which a physical therapist will work.

Criteria for Normal Aging

A central issue in aging research is, What constitutes normal aging? This is an extremely complex question. Who should be studied to represent normal aging? Should we select healthy individuals who fall within the correct age range? A 90-year-old who is free of significant disease or disability may be unusual and not represent the "average" 90-year-old with a range of health problems. Should we select a group who are conveniently available, for example, at the community health clinic or in the senior citizens housing complex? Selecting available groups may introduce a particular sampling bias into studies. Sampling bias occurs in exercise studies when only the fittest elderly individuals will volunteer for a study that demands physical activity. Subject selection is a particularly important concern in studies dealing with the physiologic changes of normal aging.

Another real research problem in studies dealing with aging is the increasing incidence of undiagnosed and diagnosed pathologies. Failure to rule out latent heart or lung disease in physiologic studies can significantly skew the results of a study. Individuals with heart disease can have reduced cardiovascular capacities not due to aging but due to their disease. Confusion results in the literature from studies that include poorly screened subjects, making the aging literature somewhat difficult to interpret.

Many studies on the physiology of aging have used cross-sectional rather than longitudinal study designs. The obvious advantage of cross-sectional designs is the ease of conducting a study. Comparing individuals within each decade is much easier than following individuals over 10 or so years; however, this may not give the most accurate picture of normal aging. Longitudinal designs, on the other hand, are susceptible to problems such as dropouts due to death and disease that can distort the results.

Theories of Aging

The theories reviewed below concerning why organisms age are diverse and complex and deal with cellular mechanisms of senescence. Many theories attempt to identify a single mechanism for aging; however, aging probably does not have one cause. Even a president of the United States has speculated about aging (Fig 3–1). Aging reflects the accumulated results of reduced cellular function, cell injury, and cell death. Why these changes occur is a key question. Some changes may be interdependent. For example, a change in cell function may result in vulnerability of the cell to injury.

Some theories suggest that aging is related to an aggregation of "insults" from the environment. One theory states that background radiation may produce cellular mutations that accumulate and lead to function failure and death.[12] Since most of us are familiar with the negative, cumulative consequences of radiographic exposure, this theory notes that smaller exposures over a lifetime may cause aging.

There is some research evidence that points to an increasing number of mistakes or "noise" in the system as a cause of aging. This noise can lead to problems in duplicating molecules that are essential to the replication and repair of the cell. For example, if a protein containing an error is involved with protein synthesis, then more "incorrect" proteins can be produced and begin to affect function.[40] Although more altered proteins have been observed with aging, there is little evidence for a change in protein synthesis, but there is evidence for a change in the ability to remove old cells.[17]

There are many processes in cellular synthesis, repair, and degradation that can alter cell function and that may be affected by environmental insults or cellular mistakes. Multiple theories have been formulated from this insight. One theory suggests that the ability to repair ultraviolet damage to DNA may be associated with life span. This may play a part in increased "skin aging" and exposure to the sun. Another proposal implicates an increasing number of cross-linkages in molecular matrixes such as collagen

> "I firmly believe that the aging process would be slowed if it had to move through Congress."

FIG 3–1.
A quote from President George Bush's 1992 State of the Union message before the US Congress.

and elastin with the aging process, although the relationship between greater cross-linking, reduced function, and aging is not clear.[6] From another theoretical perspective, deterioration may be a result of a change in the dynamic balance between cellular synthesis and degradation. Mechanical deterioration often occurs over time and with use. The view of osteoarthritis as a "wear-and-tear" phenomenon of the joints is an example that joint use or "abuse" leads to degeneration. Perhaps the dynamic balance between synthesis and degeneration becomes disproportionate and allows more deterioration to occur.

In contrast to environmental and mistake theories of aging, another approach contends that aging is intrinsic to the organism and is genetically controlled and programmed.[25] Theories in this category are probably easier to understand when we compare different species. In my house, for example, our pets consist of a gerbil, a dog, and a parrot. The gerbil has a life span of 1 to 2 years. The dog has a life span of 12 to 16 years, but the parrot's life span is comparable to humans, about 80 years.

An interesting genetic theory is that changes in the neuroendocrine system are central to aging. It has been proposed that the neurons and hormones that compose the hypothalamus, pituitary, and adrenal glands act as a "Master Timekeeper" for the organism.[14] Degeneration in these systems may result in degeneration in many other bodily systems.

Another genetic theory is a variation of the mistakes theory discussed previously but postulates that mistakes or mutations are intrinsic.[7] Each species is genetically programmed to regulate the exactness of genetic replication. According to this theory, less exact cell replication increases the likelihood of mutations, reduced function, and possibly death. The immune system also has been implicated in the aging process.[63] Aging is associated with reduced immune system function, reduced resistance to infectious disease, and an increase in autoimmune disease.

It has been hypothesized that an accumulation of undesirable substances within the cell interferes with function. These substances are thought to be free radicals, which are very reactive and can cause random damage within the cell.[24] The accumulation of lipofuscin, or the "age pigment," is thought to result from free radical reactions on fatty acids. The effect of these substances within the cell remains unclear.

The free radical theory may be related to the metabolic rate associated with body size. Animals with larger body sizes generally have lower metabolic rates and longer life spans. An hypothesis generated from this theory is that lower metabolic rates produce fewer free radicals and, presumably, less aging damage. If the number of calories a species burns in a lifetime is genetically determined, rapid caloric burning may shorten the life span.[51]

A note of caution must be interjected here about the free radical theory, as there are a number of obvious exceptions to this proposal. First, my pet parrot has a high metabolic rate, low body weight, but an expected life span similar to humans. Second, individuals who are very active and burn more calories should have a shorter life span if the theory is correct; yet adults who exercise regularly have a longer life than sedentary individuals.[42]

The basis of aging may differ for different tissues. For example, bone continuously remodels, whereas nerve cells are stable and exist for a lifetime. Anything that interferes with cell repair and duplication will have a greater impact on the dynamic cells than on more stable cells. On the other hand, damage in the central nervous system has devastating effects, because the damaged cells cannot be replaced.

Another interesting possibility is that individual cells contain mechanisms that produce aging. This idea is supported by evidence that cells grown in culture, without environmental insults, hormonal influences, or immune system changes, grow old and die.[26] From this point of view, aging is an inherent process in the fundamental structure of the organism, the cell, rather than a tissue or system failure.

What the reader should understand is that all of the theories do not fully explain aging and the entire phenomenon that we know as aging is poorly understood. None of the current theories accounts for the changes in senescence. This section should have provided an appreciation of why aging is such a difficult thing to explain and what some of the possibilities are.

CARDIOVASCULAR FUNCTION

Cardiovascular function will be discussed for several different conditions: rest, submaximal exercise, and maximal exercise. This will give a perspective on the range of function performed by this system and the changes that occur under each circumstance. The changes that occur with exercise training will also be discussed in this section. Some areas are fairly well documented with a series of consistent research findings. Other areas are controversial, with studies presenting data both supporting and questioning certain changes. Still other points are poorly understood and need further research. In this section, changes in cardiovascular function and its response to exercise conditioning will be discussed particularly from the point of view of the ability of the system to deliver and utilize oxygen and the possible outcomes of exercise interventions. This information should help the clinician to interpret clinical observations and discuss the effects of exercise programs on the cardiovascular function of elderly individuals.

Oxygen Consumption

Oxygen consumption reflects the abilities of the lungs, the heart, and the tissues. Simply, the lungs deliver oxygen to the blood whereas the heart pumps the blood to the tissues. The peripheral tissues then extract and use the oxygen. Changes occur with aging in the lungs, the heart, and the periphery that alter oxygen consumption. The cardiovascular components of these changes will be discussed in this section, and the pulmonary changes will be discussed in the next section.

The cardiovascular aspects of oxygen consumption are the product of cardiac output and peripheral extraction. The cardiac output is the product of the heart rate (HR) times the stroke volume (SV). The peripheral extraction of oxygen is the difference between the arterial and venous oxygen content or the $a-\bar{v}o_2$ difference. The formula representation of oxygen consumption is:

$$\dot{V}o_2 = (HR \times SV) \times (a-\bar{v}o_2 \text{ diff})$$

The resting oxygen consumption or basal metabolic rate does not change with aging.[48] The resting cardiovascular functions remain the same as in the younger person. The average resting heart rate, for example, continues to be about 75 beats per minute (BPM) for elderly persons.[1, 10]

Between resting and maximal exercise there is a broad range of intensities that is referred to as *submaximal exercise*. Most functional activities require minimal to moderate responses of the cardiovascular system. Therefore, understanding submaximal responses will generally describe what happens to the cardiovascular system during activities of daily living.

The oxygen consumption response to submaximal exercise does not change with aging.[4, 54] Oxygen consumption is linearly related to submaximal exercise intensity. A progressive increase in exercise intensity will be accompanied by a progressive increase in oxygen consumption. Given a similar heart rate in the younger and older adult,

the oxygen consumption will be similar. Submaximal heart rate is also linearly related to exercise intensity. We infer that the stroke volume and arteriovenous oxygen difference would also be the same. Stroke volume increases proportionally to the demands of the exercise until maximal exercise. Similarly, the arteriovenous oxygen difference can increase through a range of values up to a maximal value. Increasing abilities to deliver oxygen during exercise depend on increases in heart rate, stroke volume, and arteriovenous oxygen differences.

If the cardiovascular dynamics are the same during submaximal exercise, the astute reader might ask why it seems harder for the elderly to perform even light exercise. There are several explanations for this. First, the elderly individual may have to perform less external work to reach the same heart rate as the younger person. For example, a brisk walk on a level surface by the 75-year-old may yield a heart rate of 140 BPM, whereas the 25-year-old may have to jog at a medium speed to reach the same heart rate. In addition, the 75-year-old is generally exercising at a higher percentage of that individual's maximum exercise capacity than the 25-year-old. A heart rate of 140 BPM can be 85% of maximum capacity for the 75-year-old but only 75% for the 25-year-old.

If an individual is undergoing an exercise test in which the exercise intensity is progressively increased until the individual can no longer exercise, this is described as the *maximum exercise capacity*. The oxygen consumption and heart rate will progressively increase with each increase in exercise until at some point the oxygen consumption and heart rate level off despite an increase in exercise intensity. This point indicates the maximal ability of the cardiovascular system. The level of oxygen and the heart rate are described as the *maximal oxygen consumption* and the *maximal heart rate*.

The gold standard for defining an individual's ability to exercise is maximum oxygen consumption.[5] A higher maximum oxygen consumption gives the individual a higher ability to exercise. The maximum ability of the body to use oxygen during exercise (maximum oxygen consumption) declines with age.[4, 31] The maximum oxygen consumption averages about 28.5 mL/kg of body weight per minute (mL/kg/min) for a 65-year-old man and is approximately 25.5 mL/kg/min for a 65-year-old woman.[54] This can be compared with average amounts for 25-year-olds of about 43 mL/kg/min for men and 35 mL/kg/min for women. Thus, the decline from the young adult years is substantial. Factors that contribute to this decline are changes in the maximum heart rate, maximum stroke volume, and maximum arteriovenous oxygen difference. Each of these factors will be discussed separately.

The maximum heart rate or the highest heart rate during exercise does decline with age. We frequently use the formula 220 minus a person's age to estimate the predicted maximum heart rate. Although this formula is inaccurate, it indicates a direct relationship between heart rate and age. As an individual ages, the expected maximal exercise heart rate decreases. The maximum heart rate for the 25-year-old is approximately 195 BPM, whereas the healthy 75-year-old can be expected to reach a heart rate of around 165 BPM.[55] The clinical implication of this is that the elderly have a lower exercise capacity and can reach an intense level of exercise at lower pulse rates than a younger person. A pulse rate of 125 in an older person in response to assisted ambulation may indicate considerable cardiovascular stress.

Several studies indicate that the maximum stroke volume during heavy exercise in the elderly is smaller than in the young adult. The maximum stroke volume is also reached at a lower oxygen consumption.[21, 32, 39] These studies examined the changes in stroke volume as exercise intensity progressively increased. Although stroke volumes were similar between young and older subjects during low-intensity work, the stroke volume decreased in the older subjects as the effort approached maximum. Maximum stroke volumes were 10% to 20% smaller for the older subjects compared with the younger exercisers.

The change in maximal stroke volume with age, however, is controversial. Several other studies have reported that the maximum stroke volume increases in elderly subjects to compensate for reduced maximum heart rates.[45, 49] These studies were careful to screen subjects for any sign of heart disease. It is also possible that the subjects in these studies were also more physically fit since they were able to achieve higher maximum oxygen consumptions and had higher cardiac outputs than in the studies where reduced maximum stroke volumes were observed. It has been shown that level of fitness is associated with stroke volume at any age.

Factors that influence the stroke volume are diastolic filling (end-diastolic volume), myocardial contractility (end-systolic volume), perfusion of the myocardium, and peripheral vascular resistance (Fig 3–2). How each of these factors results in the observed changes in stroke volume is still unclear. Decreased end-diastolic volume, myocardial contractility and perfusion, and increased blood pressure can reduce stroke volume.[54] Latent heart disease can result in reduced myocardial contractility and perfusion. This is a good example of contradictory results in the literature that may be related to insufficient screening of subjects for undiagnosed disease. Further research is needed to determine if maximal stroke volume decreases or increases during normal aging.

The changes that occur with maximum cardiac output

as a result of aging are also unclear. If both the maximum heart rate and maximum stroke volume decrease, then the cardiac output will decline. On the other hand, if the maximal heart rate decreases, but the maximal stroke volume displays a compensatory increase, then the cardiac output could remain the same during maximal exercise. What is clear is that the maximum values occur at a lower level of exercise intensity.

The peripheral extraction of oxygen at rest and during submaximal exercise increases somewhat in the elderly.[39] Shephard suggests that this may be a response to a reduction in mechanical efficiency in the elderly.[54] Mechanical efficiency during exercise in the elderly decreases to 21.5%, compared with 23% in the young adult.[4, 55] Increased body weight, joint stiffness, and loss of tissue compliance contribute to increasing the work of exercise.

The maximum arteriovenous oxygen difference may decrease or remain the same as individuals age.[22, 23] Exactly which factors contribute to the differences in results concerning arteriovenous oxygen extraction are not well defined. Losses in muscle mass, reductions in the number of capillaries in muscle tissue, and greater blood flow to the skin may diminish oxygen extraction with aging.[59, 60] Similar changes also happen with disuse and lack of activity in the elderly.[54] This suggests that a decrease in oxygen extraction may be more closely tied to low levels of exercise rather than to aging per se.

A summary of the changes associated with aging in terms of cardiovascular function appears in Table 3–1. While relatively few changes occur at rest and during submaximal exercise, significant declines in maximal oxygen consumption and maximal heart rate occur with maximal exercise. The reduction in maximal heart rate is thought to

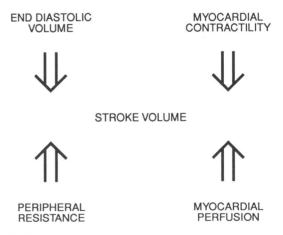

FIG 3–2.
Factors that influence the stroke volume are diastolic filling (end-diastolic volume), myocardial contractility (end-systolic volume), perfusion of the myocardium, and peripheral vascular resistance.

be the single most important factor in relation to a reduced exercise capacity in the elderly.

Effects of Exercise on Cardiovascular Function

Resting and submaximal exercise oxygen consumption levels do not change as a result of an exercise training program in the elderly.[32, 39, 59] There is no change in resting heart rate, stroke volume, or cardiac output. There is, however, some decrease in the submaximal heart rate to a standard level of exercise.[1, 55]

Maximal oxygen consumption increases significantly with exercise training of the young-old.[37] A 12-week exercise training program on cycle ergometers at an intensity of 70% of heart rate reserve (maximum heart rate minus resting heart rate) performed three times per week increased maximum oxygen consumption from 26.6 to 31.9 mL/kg/min in 60-year-old men and women, compared with an increase from 45.6 to 51.1 mL/kg/min in a group of 20-year-olds. The absolute amount of improvement of 5.5 to 6.0 mL/kg/min in 60-year-olds after the exercise training program was similar to that seen in younger people, although the maximal oxygen consumption was lower in the older group.[36]

Seals and his colleagues demonstrated that the amount of improvement is dependent on the intensity of the training.[53] They trained 11 men and women in their 60s for 6 months of low-intensity exercise consisting of 20 to 30 minutes of walking three times per week. The average heart rate reached during the walks was 107 ± 6 BPM. For the next 6 months the subjects engaged in high-intensity training for 30 to 45 minutes initially at 75% of heart rate reserve, working up to 85% of heart rate reserve during the last 8 weeks of training. The exercise training was preceded and followed by appropriate warm-up and cooldown activities. These sessions occurred three times per week. In the final 2 months the average exercise heart rate was 156 ± 6 BPM. There were substantial differences between the intensity and duration of the low- and high-intensity exercise sessions. Although maximum heart rate did not change with exercise training, maximum stroke volume did increase. High-intensity training resulted in an increase in the arteriovenous oxygen difference, whereas low-intensity training did not. Neither low- nor high-intensity training had a significant impact on maximum cardiac output.[53] Few studies have documented an association between increased maximum oxygen consumption, stroke volume, and arteriovenous oxygen difference in older people as a result of exercise training. Although the mechanism for the increase in maximum oxygen consumption in younger people is the increased cardiac output and arteriovenous oxygen difference, this has not been established in the elderly.[60]

Most exercise training studies have examined short-term exercise interventions lasting between 6 weeks and 6 months. Another interesting line of inquiry looks at the effects of longer-term programs of a year to several years. These studies address questions concerning whether exercise reduces or eliminates the decline in exercise capacities among the elderly. A study by Hagberg and colleagues tested the maximum exercise performance in a group of 50-year-old Master's athletes, a group of sedentary 50-year-olds, a group of 25-year-olds who were matched to the Master's athletes, and a group of 25-year-old competitive runners.[23] Although the 50-year-old athletes had almost twice the maximum oxygen consumption of the sedentary 50-year-olds, it was significantly less than the maximum oxygen consumption of the younger groups. This suggests that even a high level of exercise training will not eliminate the decline in maximum exercise capacity associated with aging but that endurance training can produce substantial improvement in exercise capacity. The Master's athletes did have comparable maximal stroke volumes and arteriovenous oxygen differences when compared with the younger groups (Figs 3–3 and 3–4). The maximal cardiac output of the Master's athletes was greater than in the sedentary older group but less than the two younger groups. Finally, both older groups had comparable maximum heart rates that were significantly less than the younger groups. Data such as these point to a decrease in maximum heart rate as the major contributing factor to declining maximum oxygen consumption with aging. Many other cardiovascular changes that occur can be substantially reduced by endurance training.

TABLE 3–1.

Cardiovascular Changes With Aging*

	Due to Aging	After Exercise Training
Resting		
Oxygen consumption	↔	↔
Heart rate	↔	↔
Stroke volume	↔	↔
Arteriovenous oxygen difference	↑	?
Submaximal exercise		
Oxygen consumption	↔	↔
Heart rate	↔	↓
Stroke volume	↔	?
Arteriovenous oxygen difference	↑	?
Maximal exercise		
Oxygen consumption	↓	↑
Heart rate	↓	↔
Stroke volume	↓ or ↑	↑
Arteriovenous oxygen difference	↓ or ↔	↑ or ↔
Cardiac output	↔ (?) or ↑	↔

*↑ = increases; ↓ = decreases; ↔ = no change; ? = insufficient data on elderly subjects.

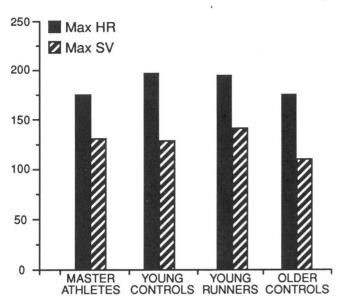

FIG 3–3.
Comparisons of Master's athletes, young and older matched controls, and young competitive athletes on maximum heart rate and stroke volume. Maximum heart rates were significantly different for the older than the younger groups. (Redrawn from Hagberg JM, Allen WK, Seals DR, et al: *J Appl Physiol* 1985; 58:2041–2046.)

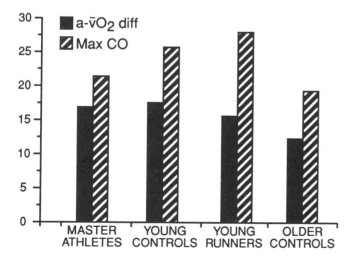

FIG 3–4.
Comparisons of arteriovenous oxygen differences and maximum cardiac output in Master's athletes, young and older matched controls, and young competitive athletes. The arteriovenous difference is significantly less in the older matched controls than the other groups. The cardiac output was highest for the younger groups, but the Master's athletes had higher cardiac outputs than the sedentary older matched controls. (Redrawn from Hagberg JM, Allen WK, Seals DR, et al: *J Appl Physiol* 1985; 58:2041–2046.)

Coronary artery disease (CAD) is the most prevalent disease that affects cardiac function in the elderly and the most common cause of death. CAD has been associated with reduced maximum exercise capacity, decreased maximum oxygen consumption, decreased maximum heart rate, and reduced maximum stroke volume. CAD may affect the contractility and function of the myocardium. Individuals with CAD have reduced exercise reserves and abilities to respond to the benefits of exercise training. Exercise in these instances may increase the risk of myocardial infarction and sudden death. Most of the changes in cardiac function that occur with aging will be exacerbated with CAD, and heart disease is so common among the elderly that it is a significant concern for the clinician.

PULMONARY FUNCTION

A discussion of pulmonary function is different from that of the cardiovascular system in that although there are changes, these changes have less of an impact on the ability of an individual to function unless distinct pulmonary pathology exists. The changes that have been described will be presented along with the ventilatory response of the older person to exercise, and the effect of exercise training on ventilation.

Lung Volumes and Capacities

Prior to considering the effect of aging on pulmonary function, a brief review of the definitions and values of lung volumes and capacities is helpful. The amount of air in the lung is operationally divided into specific volumes as follows:

1. *Tidal volume.* The amount of air breathed in or out during one breath.
2. *Inspiratory reserve volume.* Additional air that can be inspired beyond a tidal inspiration.
3. *Expiratory reserve volume.* The amount of air that can be exhaled beyond a tidal exhalation.
4. *Residual volume.* The amount of air remaining in the lung after a forceful exhalation. This volume will prevent the lung from collapsing even during maximal breathing.

A combination of two or more volumes creates various lung capacities as follows:

1. *Inspiratory capacity.* The amount of air that can be breathed in following a normal exhalation until

maximum lung capacity. This is the combination of tidal volume and inspiratory reserve volume.

2. *Functional residual capacity.* The amount of air remaining in the lung after a normal exhalation—residual volume plus the expiratory reserve volume.

3. *Vital capacity.* The maximal amount of air that can be exhaled after a complete inspiration. The vital capacity is the tidal volume plus the inspiratory and expiratory reserve volumes.

4. *Total lung capacity.* The total volume of air in the lung after maximal inspiration—residual, expiratory reserve, inspiratory reserve, and tidal volume combined.

There is an overall decrease in the functional ability of the lung to move air in and out as people age. The vital capacity averages 2.61 and 3.88 L for 65-year-old women and men, respectively, compared with 3.35 and 5.05 L for 25-year-old women and men.[54] Thus, the vital capacity of the 65-year-old is about 77% the value of the 25-year-old. Since the total lung capacity decreases only slightly throughout life, an increased residual volume compensates for a decreased vital capacity.[30] The percentage of the total lung capacity that is residual volume in the 65-year-old rises to 38.5% for women and 34.5% for men, compared with 29.5% and 25.3% for 25-year-old women and men.[54] These changes are attributed to a loss of elastic recoil in the lung. There is also some evidence that these changes may accelerate after age 65.[52]

Loss of elastic recoil also contributes to a reduction in several dynamic functions of breathing. The percentage of the vital capacity an individual can force out of the lungs in 1 second, the ratio of forced expiratory volume in 1 second to vital capacity, is one of those functions. This ratio is approximately 84% in the 25-year-old but only about 74% to 77% in the elderly. Another important function affected by elastic recoil is the closing volume, which is the lung volume at which small airways begin to close. The percentage of the vital capacity where the closing volume occurs increases as people age. These changes and increased residual volume create more anatomic and physiologic dead space in the elderly. More dead space means that less of the air breathed is contributing to oxygenating the blood.[54]

Changes in the rigidity of the rib cage and declining strength of the respiratory muscles with aging contribute to increase the work of breathing.[65] Loss of efficiency in breathing and greater work of breathing mean that the elderly person must have more ventilation for the same oxygenation than the younger person.[56]

Other changes affect pulmonary gas exchange functions with aging. Fewer small pulmonary blood vessels increase the resistance and reduce distribution of blood flow in the lung. This increases the mean pulmonary arterial pressure, reduces diffusion capacity (the ability of oxygen to diffuse from the alveolar air space into the pulmonary capillary), and contributes to poor ventilation to perfusion matching (having less circulation in aerated portions of the lung). Although these changes reduce arterial oxygen pressure (generally around 95 mm Hg in arterial blood in the young adult), the oxygen saturation (the amount of oxygen held by the hemoglobin in the blood) continues to be about 95% or about the same as in a younger person.[30]

Ventilatory Responses to Exercise

In the healthy adult, lung function does not limit exercise capacity.[50] The impact on exercise performance of the pulmonary function changes that occur with aging are unclear; however, patients with obstructive lung disease have to have a significant loss of the vital capacity before much functional loss is evident.

The ventilatory response of the elderly person to low and moderate exercise is similar to a young adult; however, there is an increase in ventilation as exercise becomes more intense. Some of this has to do with the changes discussed previously. In addition, the older adult is often exercising at a higher percentage of maximal capacity to perform the same exercise as a younger individual. More intense exercise produces a higher blood lactate concentration and greater blood acidosis. The body responds by increasing ventilation to expire more carbon dioxide and reduce the acidosis.[30] Greater pulmonary demands and lower exercise efficiency result. In clinical settings, the older person is often breathing harder and faster during submaximal exercise than the young adult and, as a result, experiences a greater perceived exertion in relation to exercise. The older individual with obstructive lung disease may also experience shortness of breath at relatively low exercise intensities. In the instance of obstructive lung disease, exercise capacity may be limited by the patient's shortness of breath rather than cardiovascular capacity. Shortness of breath may occur sooner during upper extremity activities as a result of a greater ventilatory response than during lower extremity activities. Patients often complain of more difficulty carrying a bag of groceries than walking down the street.

Effects of Exercise Training on Ventilatory Function

An aerobic exercise program that lasts 3 months can significantly change ventilatory function in 60- to 70-year-old individuals.[36] Makrides and her colleagues placed 20- and 60-year-olds on 5-minute cycle ergometry exercise at a heart rate that corresponded to 85% of maximum oxygen consumption, or 160 and 140 BPM, respectively. These

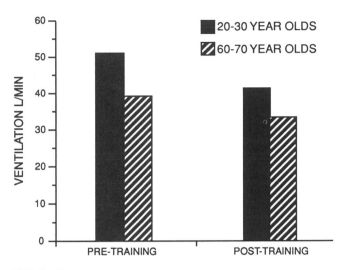

FIG 3–5.
Submaximal minute ventilation for 20- to 30-year-olds compared with 60- to 70-year-olds pretraining and following exercise endurance training. (Redrawn from Makrides L, Heigenhauser GJ, McCartney N, et al: Physical training in young and older healthy subjects, in Sutton JR, Brock RM (eds): *Sports Medicine for the Mature Athlete*. Indianapolis, Benchmark Press, 1986.)

bouts were interspersed with 3-minute bouts at a bike power intensity corresponding to 50% to 60% of maximum oxygen consumption for a 1-hour period three times per week. Ventilation decreased significantly during submaximal exercise as a result of the exercise training (Fig 3–5). A decrease in the carbon dioxide production and the respiratory exchange ratio, a ratio of the carbon dioxide produced to the oxygen consumed, occured with the decreased ventilation.[36] The blood lactate level also declined. These changes suggest that the exercise training has improved the efficiency of the muscle metabolism by producing less of the metabolic by-products in response to exercise. Exercise training also increases the maximal ventilation during exercise (Fig 3–6).[23] These changes will reduce the breathlessness experienced by the elderly, the sense of exertion, and the percentage of maximal ventilation used during exercise.[29] Exercise training improves the effectiveness of ventilation with moderate exercise and enhances the maximal capability. Exercise training may also improve the efficiency of exercise for individuals with obstructive disease. Table 3–2 provides a summary of these changes.

MUSCULOSKELETAL FUNCTION

This is an important area in relation to physical therapy. Significant changes occur in muscle performance and body composition that affect the functional status of the elderly patient. The responses of these changes to exercise train-

ing are similar to those we would expect in younger persons. A common bias is to approach muscle weakness in the 100-lb 90-year-old woman differently than the young athlete after an injury. This section assists the reader in objectively examining that issue.

We will also look at changes that occur in the bony skeleton as people age. These changes have taken on greater importance as people live longer. Fractures resulting from osteoporosis are an unfortunate outcome of this longer life span. As a consequence, hip fractures are encountered more frequently in geriatric rehabilitation. Understanding the dynamics of bone loss and possible preventive interventions are important for the clinician.

Muscle Performance

There is a decline in muscle strength as people age.[33] These changes in strength happen in men and women, a variety of muscle groups, and during different types of muscle contractions.[54,61,62] Strength declines take place beyond the age of 60 and accelerate in individuals 80 years of age or older.[62]

Changes in strength are associated with a decrease in the size of muscles that occurs with aging.[22] There is significant reduction in the cross-sectional area of the muscles in the upper and lower extremity for both men and women.[46,64] There is also a loss of the gross number of muscle fibers and the size of individual muscle fibers when young and older people are compared.[15,35] Reduction in the size of muscle fibers may be attributable to reduced activity and disuse atrophy. An area that is still unclear is what happens to the muscle composition when muscle size decreases? Some studies have suggested that there is a pref-

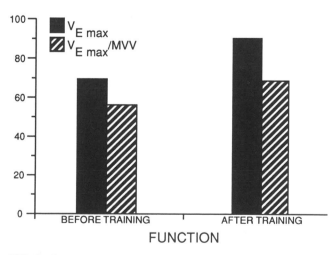

FIG 3–6.
Maximum exercise ventilation and a ratio of maximum exercise ventilation to maximum voluntary ventilation (VE_{max}/MVV) before and after training. (Redrawn from data presented in Hagberg JM, Allen WK, Seals DR, et al: *J Appl Physiol* 1985; 58:2041–2046.)

TABLE 3–2.

Pulmonary Changes With Aging*

	Due to Aging	After Endurance Exercise Training
Volumes and capacities		
Vital capacity	↓	
Total lung volume	↔ or ↓	
Residual volume	↑	
Flow volume	↓	
Dead space/tidal volume ratio	↑	
Submaximal exercise		
Minute ventilation ($\dot{V}_E$)	↑	↓
CO_2 production	↑	↓
Respiratory exchange ratio	↑	↓
Blood lactate	↑	↓
Maximal exercise		
Maximum exercise ventilation ($V_{E_{max}}$)	↓	↑
Maximum voluntary ventilation (MVV)	↓	↑
$V_{E_{max}}$/MVV	↓	↑

* ↑ = increases; ↓ = decreases; ↔ = no change.

erential atrophy of type II or fast twitch muscle fibers that results in greater loss of type II fiber area.[34] Other studies suggest that there is a loss of fiber area in all muscle fibers regardless of the fiber type.[20]

Despite the loss of fiber numbers and size, there does not appear to be a decrease in the enzymes related to energy metabolism in human skeletal muscle.[34] Consequently, the capacity for both aerobic and anaerobic metabolism in skeletal muscle does not seem to decline with aging.[19] Likewise, the number of mitochondria within the muscle appears to remain stable, although there is a decrease in the mitochondrial volume in older individuals.[41]

As every physical therapist should know, there is more to muscle performance than just the assessment of maximum strength through isometric or isotonic torque measures. Muscle groups also should contract during exercise over time, that is, demonstrate endurance, and resist fatigue. Little research addresses these aspects of muscle performance in elderly persons. Makrides et al. employed a 30-second maximal cycling test on an isokinetic ergometer at pedaling frequencies of 60 and 110 rpm to measure the maximum power, total work, and the percent decline in power (fatigue) during 30 seconds of exercise in 20- and 60-year-olds.[36] The 60-year-olds had significantly less maximal power and total work on this test than the younger group; however, the fatigue measure was similar in both groups.

Effects of Exercise Training on Muscle Performance

Isometric and progressive resistive exercise regimes that are of sufficient intensity and take place over 6- to 25-

week durations produce significant increases in strength in elderly people.[2, 13, 15, 44] High-intensity resistances that use 70% to 80% of a one-repetition maximum produce more predictable increases in shorter periods of time, but low to moderate resistances also produce improvements.

Although many strength training studies concentrate on knee extension, a study by Panton and her colleagues demonstrated that strength gains occur in both the upper and lower extremities with resistance exercises aimed at various muscle groups.[43] The strength changes after resistance training are better than a walk/jog exercise program designed to increase general exercise endurance.[43] Significant increases in strength can even occur in frail, institutionalized 80- and 90-year-olds.[13]

Attempts have been made to relate muscle performance to functional ability in the elderly. Neither aerobic nor resistance training improved reaction time or speed of movement in a group of 70-year-olds after 6 months of exercise.[43] In the frail elderly population, quadriceps strength correlates negatively with the time to stand from a chair and to walk 6 m; however, improvements in strength did not improve these functional abilities.[13]

Skeletal Changes

Bone mineral density declines as people age.[47] Women experience an accelerated loss immediately postmenopause; however, bone density declines at the rate of about 1% per year for men and women beyond the age of 60. A 20% loss of cortical bone width in men, and 30% loss in women, occurs in people who survive to be 90.[18] Reduced bone density and thickness increase the risk of fractures in the elderly.[3] One third of women older than 65 will experience vertebral fractures, and one third of 80-year-old women will suffer a hip fracture.[28] Vertebral fractures result in back pain and kyphotic postures. Few elderly people fully recover following a hip fracture, despite extensive rehabilitation. The consequences of reduced skeletal integrity in older people are debilitating and often life threatening.

Exactly why bone loss occurs with aging is still unclear. One explanation deals with the dynamic aspects of bone remodeling. Bone is a tissue that is constantly being broken down and rebuilt. If the balance between bone turnover degenerates, then more bone can be broken down than is replaced, thus leading to bony loss.[54] Low dietary calcium, reduced calcium absorption, and hormonal changes such as reduced postmenopausal estrogen levels have all been implicated in bone loss.[11, 38] Since bone loss begins to occur as early as the 30s for women, physical inactivity and lack of exercise may contribute to bone loss.[16, 47] An increasingly sedentary life-style in older adults has been associated with reduced skeletal mass.[54]

Gender, low body weight, and genetic factors have also been cited.

Effects of Exercise on the Skeletal System

Exercise can decrease bone loss as people age.[8, 9, 38, 57, 58] Both aerobic-type activities such as walking and jogging or strengthening activities that are pursued for at least 9 months to a year will influence bone density.[9, 16] Nelson and her colleagues studied the effects of a supervised year-long walking program and increased dietary calcium on 36 postmenopausal women.[38] The exercise group showed a 0.5% increase in lumbar trabecular bone mineral density, whereas the sedentary group decreased by 7.0%. High dietary calcium, on the other hand, increased femoral neck bone mineral density. The combination of exercise with high dietary calcium did not enhance these results. The authors conclude that exercise and high calcium intake may have different effects at different skeletal sites. Low-dose estrogen supplements also may stabilize bone density.[3] There have been few randomized control group research projects that have looked at the issue of exercise and bone density, and the possible interactions of exercise, dietary calcium, and estrogens. Consequently, the effect of exercise on skeletal integrity remains uncertain.

Table 3–3 is a summary of the musculoskeletal changes that occur with aging and the effects of exercise training. The specific exercise routine needed to produce a specific effect may depend on which musculoskeletal function is targeted. Exercise that increases muscle torque may not increase range of motion. Likewise, exercises that increase bone mineral density at one skeletal site may not improve muscle endurance in that region. We still have much to learn in this arena.

TABLE 3–3.

Musculoskeletal Changes With Aging*

	Due to Aging	After Exercise Training
Muscle		
Torque	↓	↑
Cross-sectional area	↓	↑
Muscle fibers	↓	↔ (?)
Fiber size	↓	↑
Fibertype	↔ (?)	↔
Enzyme activity	↔	↑
Mitochondria	↔	↑
Mitochondrial volume	↓	↑
Skeletal		
Bone mineral density	↓	↑ (?)
Susceptibility to fractures	↑	↓ (?)

*↑ = increases; ↓ = decreases; ↔ = no change; ? = insufficient data on elderly subjects.

SUMMARY

Significant physiologic changes occur in the cardiopulmonary and musculoskeltal systems with aging. Some of these changes reduce function and the quality of life as people age. Many of these changes can be influenced by appropriate exercise interventions. A knowledgeable clinician is in a position to prevent problems as well as rehabilitate problems when they do occur.

REFERENCES

1. Adams GM, DeVries HA: Physiological effects of an exercise training regimen upon women aged 52 to 79. *J Gerontol* 1973; 28:50–55.
2. Agre JC, Pierce LE, Raab DM, et al: Light resistance and stretching exercise in elderly women: Effect upon strength. *Arch Phys Med Rehabil* 1988; 69:273–276.
3. Aloia JF: Estrogens and exercise in prevention and treatment of osteoporosis. *Geriatrics* 1981; 37:81–89.
4. Astrand I: Aerobic work capacity in men and women with special reference to age. *Acta Physiol Scand* 1960; 49(suppl 169):1–92.
5. Astrand PO, Rodahl K: *Textbook of Work Physiology.* New York, McGraw-Hill, 1986.
6. Bjorksten J: Cross linkage and the aging process, in Rothstein M (ed): *Theoretical Aspects of Aging.* New York, Academic Press, 1974, p 43.
7. Burnett M: *Intrinsic Mutagenesis: A Genetic Approach for Aging.* New York, Wiley, 1974.
8. Chow R, Harrison JE, Sturridge W, et al: The effect of exercise on bone mass of osteoporotic patients on fluoride treatment. *Clin Invest Med* 1987; 10:59–65.
9. Dalsky G, Stocke KS, Ehsani AA, et al: Weight bearing exercise training and lumbar bone mineral content in postmenopausal women. *Ann Intern Med* 1988; 108:824–828.
10. DeVries HA, Adams GM: Comparison of exercise responses in old and young men. I. The cardiac effort/total body relationship. *J Gerontol* 1972; 27:344–348.
11. Drinkwater BL, Nilson K, Chestnut CH, et al: Bone mineral content in amenorrheic and eumenorrheic athletes. *N Engl J Med* 1984; 311:277–281.
12. Fialla G: The aging process and carcinogenesis. *N Y Acad Sci* 1958; 71:1124.
13. Fiatarone MA, Marks EC, Ryan ND, et al: High-intensity strength training in nonagenarians. *JAMA* 1990; 263:3029–3034.
14. Finch CE, Landfield PW: Neuroendocrine and autonomic functions in aging mammals, in Finch CE, Schneider EJ (eds): *Handbook of the Biology of Aging,* ed 2. New York, Van Nostrand Reinhold, 1985, p 567.
15. Fontera WR, Meredith CN, O'Reilly KP, et al: Strength conditioning in older men: Skeletal muscle hypertrophy and improved function. *J Appl Physiol* 1988; 64:1038–1044.
16. Gleeson PB, Protas EJ, LeBlanc A, et al: The effect of weight training exercise on the bone density of premenopausal women. *J Bone Miner Res* 1990; 5:153–158.

17. Gracy RE, et al: Impaired protein degradation may account for the accumulation of "abnormal" proteins in aging cells, in Ademan DC, Dekker EE (eds): *Modification of Proteins During Aging.* New York, Alan Liss, 1985, p 1.

18. Gran SM: Bone loss and aging, in Goldman R, Rockstein M (eds): *The Physiology and Pathology of Aging.* New York, Academic Press, 1975, p 215.

19. Green HJ: Characteristics of aging human skeletal muscles, in Sutton JR, Brock RM (eds): *Sports Medicine for the Mature Athlete.* Indianapolis, Benchmark Press, 1986, p 22.

20. Grimby G, Aniansson A, Zetterberg C, et al: Is there a change in relative muscle fiber composition with age? *Clin Physiol* 1984; 4:189–194.

21. Grimby G, Nilsson NJ, Saltin B: Cardiac output during submaximal and maximal exercise in active middle-aged athletes. *J Appl Physiol* 1966; 21:1150–1156.

22. Grimby G, Saltin B: Mini-review. The aging muscle. *Clin Physiol* 1983; 3:209–218.

23. Hagberg JM, Allen WK, Seals DR, et al: A hemodynamic comparison of young and older endurance athletes during exercise. *J Appl Physiol* 1985; 58:2041–2046.

24. Harman D: Aging: A theory based on free radical and radiation chemistry. *J Gerontol* 1956; 11:298–300.

25. Hart RW, Setlow RB: Correlation between DNA excision repair and life span in a number of mammalian species. *Proc Natl Acad Sci U S A* 1974; 71:2169–2173.

26. Hayflick I, Moorhead PS: The serial cultivation of human diploid cell strains. *Exp Cell Res* 1961; 25:585–621.

27. Heikkinen F: Normal aging. Definition, problems, and relation to physical activity, in Orimo H, Simada K, Irika M (eds): *Recent Advances in Gerontology.* Amsterdam, Excerpta Medica, 1979, pp 501–503.

28. Holbrook TL, Grazier K, Kelsey JL, et al: *Frequency of Occurrence, Impact, and Cost of Selected Musculoskeletal Conditions in the United States.* Chicago, American Academy of Orthopedic Surgeons, 1984.

29. Jones NL: The lung of the Master's athletes, in Sutton JR, Beck RM (eds): *Sports Medicine for the Mature Athlete.* Indianapolis, Benchmark Press, 1986, pp 319–328.

30. Jones NL, Overton T, Hammeslindel DM, et al: Effect of age on regional residual volume. *J Appl Physiol* 1978; 44:195–199.

31. Kasch FW, Wallace JP, Van Camp SP: Effects of 18 years of endurance exercise on the physical work capacity of older men. *J Cardiac Rehabil* 1985; 5:308–312.

32. Kilbom A, Astrand I: Physical training and submaximal intensities in women. II. Effect on cardiac output. *Scand J Clin Lab Invest* 1971; 28:163–175.

33. Larsson L, Grimby G, Karlsson J: Muscle strength and speed of movement in relation to age and muscle morphology. *J Appl Physiol* 1979; 46:451–456.

34. Larsson L, Sjödin B, Karlsson J: Histochemical and biochemical changes in human skeletal muscle with age in sedentary males, ages 22–65 years. *Acta Physiol Scand* 1978; 103:31–39.

35. Lexall J, Henriksoon-Larsen K, Winblod B, et al: Distribution of different fiber types in human skeletal muscles. Effects of aging studied in whole muscle cross sections. *Muscle Nerve* 1983; 6:588–595.

36. Makrides L, Heigenhauser GJ, McCartney N, et al: Physical training in young and older healthy subjects, in Sutton JR, Brock RM (eds): *Sports Medicine for the Mature Athlete.* Indianapolis, Benchmark Press, 1986, pp 363–373.

37. Meredith CN, Fontera WR, Fisher EC, et al: Peripheral effects of endurance training in young and old subjects. *J Appl Physiol* 1989; 66:2844–2849.

38. Nelson ME, Fisher EC, Dilmanian FA, et al: A 1-year walking program and increased dietary calcium in postmenopausal women: Effects on bone. *Am J Clin Nutr* 1991; 53:1304–1311.

39. Niminimaa V, Shephard RJ: Training and oxygen conductance in the elderly. I. The respiratory system. II. The cardiovascular system. *J Gerontol* 1978; 33:354–361, 362–367.

40. Orgel LE: The maintenance of the accuracy of protein synthesis and its relevance to aging. *Proc Natl Acad Sci U S A* 1963; 49:517–521.

41. Orlander J, Kiessling KH, Larsson L, et al: Skeletal muscle metabolism and ultra-structure in relation to age in sedentary men. *Acta Physiol Scand* 1978; 104:249–261.

42. Paffenberger RS: Physical activity, all-cause mortality, and longevity of college alumni. *N Engl J Med* 1986; 314:605–613.

43. Panton LB, Graves JE, Pollock ML, et al: Effects of aerobic and resistance training on fractionated reaction time and speed of movement. *J Gerontol* 1990; 45:M26–31.

44. Perkin LC, Kaiser HL: Results of short-term isotonic and isometric exercise programs in persons over sixty. *Phys Ther Rev* 1961; 41:633–635.

45. Port S, Cobb FR, Coleman RE, et al: Effect of age on the response of left ventricular ejection fraction to exercise. *N Engl J Med* 1980; 303:1133–1137.

46. Rice CL, Cunningham DA, Patterson DH, et al: Arm and leg composition determined by computed tomography in young and elderly men. *Clin Physiol* 1989; 9:207–220.

47. Riggs BL, Wahner HM, Melton J, et al: Rates of bone loss in the appendicular and axial skeletons of women. *J Clin Invest* 1986; 77:1487–1491.

48. Robertson JD, Reid DD: Standards for basal metabolism of normal people in Britain. *Lancet* 1952; 1:940–943.

49. Rodeheffer RJ, Gerstenblith G, Becker JL, et al: Exercise cardiac output is maintained with advancing ages in healthy human subjects: Cardiac dilation and increased stroke volume compensate for a diminished heart rate. *Circulation* 1984; 69:203–213.

50. Ross RM: *Interpreting Exercise Tests.* Houston, CSI Software, 1989.

51. Sacher GA, Duffy PH: Genetic relation of life span to metabolic rate for inbred mouse strains and their hybrids. *Fed Proc* 1979; 38:184–188.

52. Schoenberg JB, Beck GJ, Bouhuys A: Growth and decay of pulmonary function in healthy blacks and whites. *Respir Physiol* 1978; 33:367–393.

53. Seals DR, Hagberg JM, Hurley BF, et al: Endurance training in older men and women. I. Cardiovascular responses to exercise. *J Appl Physiol* 1984; 57:1024–1029.

54. Shephard RT: *Physical Activity and Aging.* Rockville, Md, An Aspen Publication, 1987, pp 16–29, 97.

55. Sidney KH, Shephard RJ: Maximum and submaximum exercise tests in men and women in the seventh, eighth, and ninth decades of life. *J Appl Physiol* 1977; 43:280–287.

56. Sidney KH, Shephard RJ: Frequency and intensity of exercise training for elderly subjects. *Med Sci Sports Exerc* 1978; 10:125–131.

57. Sinaki M: Exercise and osteoporosis. *Arch Phys Med Rehabil* 1989; 70:220–229.

58. Smith EL, Reddan W, Smith PE: Physical activity and calcium modalities for bone mineral increase in aged women. *Med Sci Sports Exerc* 1981; 13:60–64.

59. Stamford BA: Effects of chronic institutionalization on the physical working capacity and trainability of geriatric men. *J Gerontol* 1973; 28:441–446.

60. Stamford BA: Exercise and the elderly, in Pandoff KB (ed): *Exercise and Sports Sciences Reviews*. New York, Macmillan, 1988, pp 341–380.

61. Vandervoort AA, Hayes KC, Belanger AY: Strength and endurance of skeletal muscle in the elderly. *Physiother Can* 1986; 38:167–173.

62. Vandervoort AA, Vramer JF, Wharram ER: Eccentric knee strength of elderly females. *J Gerontol* 1990; 45:B125–B128.

63. Walford RL, et al: Immunopathology of aging, in Eisendorfer C (ed): *Ann Rev Gerontol Geriatr* New York, Springer, 1981, p 3.

64. Young A, Stokes M, Crowe M: Size and strength of the quadriceps muscles of old and young women. *Eur J Clin Invest* 1984; 14:282–287.

65. Zadai CC: Pulmonary physiology of aging: The role of rehabilitation. *Top Geriatr Rehabil* 1985; 1:49–57.

Arthrokinesiologic Considerations in the Aged Adult

Donald A. Neumann, Ph.D., P.T.

INTRODUCTION

Arthrokinesiology is the study of the structure, function, and movement of skeletal joints. This term combines the word *kinesiology*, which is the science of movement, with the Greek prefix *arthro*, which means "joint." The purpose of this chapter will be to address specific arthrokinesiologic issues that are unique to the musculoskeletal system of the aged adult. The chapter will focus on the age-related changes in periarticular connective tissue and not the neuromuscular system per se. This chapter assumes that natural age-related changes can occur in joint function even in the absence of disease.

A strict chronologic classification of the "aged" adult will not be given since so much variation exists in the manner that adults actually grow old. *Aged,* however, is not synonymous with *aging,* since technically this process begins immediately after conception. The *aged adult* therefore will refer to the adult whose biologic systems have already matured, and owing to their advanced age, structural and functional joint changes have occurred or are imminent. These changes may be extremely subtle and pose virtually no disability, or they may be extremely profound and result in total disability.

This chapter is organized into three parts. In the first part the principles and terminology unique to communicating concepts of arthrokinesiology will be reviewed. The basic structure and related function of each major joint tissue will then be considered. This brief review will be followed by the main topic of the second part, which covers the specific age-related changes that are known or hypothesized to occur in periarticular connective tissues. Finally, this chapter will describe how age-related changes at the tissue level can cause changes in movement at the joint level.

This chapter should enhance the ability to observe a typical aged adult and relate some movement or postural dysfunction to specific mechanical age-related causes within the joint. This ability should ultimately enhance the therapist's ability to evaluate and treat the specific physical needs of the elderly.

REVIEW OF BASIC PRINCIPLES OF ARTHROKINESIOLOGY

The first part of this chapter will describe the mechanical principles of arthrokinesiology that govern normal joint function. These principles will serve as a foundation for the third part, which will describe changes in joint mobility and stability that may be likely in the aged individual.

Bone and Joint Kinematics

Kinematics, as defined with respect to arthrokinesiology, is the study of the motion within a joint or between bones, without regard to forces or torques that have caused the motion.[84] *Osteokinematics,* therefore, describes the motion of a rotating *bone* about an axis of rotation that is oriented perpendicular to the path of the moving bone. For example, if elbow flexion occurred from the anatomic position, the osteokinematic motion of the forearm would take place in the sagittal plane about a mediolateral (ML) axis (Fig 4–1). When we move our limbs, the distal bone of an articulation may move in relation to a fixed proximal bone (as in Fig 4–1), or the proximal bone may move in relation to a fixed distal bone. An *open kinematic chain* describes the linkage of two bones where the distal bone rotates in relation to a more stable proximal bone. In contrast, a *closed kinematic chain* describes the movement of a proximal bone rotating in relation to a more stable distal bone. Regardless of which bone is performing most or all of the rotation, a given bone's osteokinematic motion is really determined by the mechanical events that have occurred *between* joint surfaces.

Arthrokinematics describes the relative rotary and translatory movements that occur between joint surfaces.[95] Translation, in this context, refers to the *glide* (or slide) of an articular surface where all points along the bone glide in a direction somewhat parallel with each other. For example, glenohumeral abduction may be described as an action of the convex humeral head *rolling* (or rotating) superior and simultaneously gliding inferior on the concave surface of the glenoid fossa. The rotary motion of the humeral head may be likened to a large marble rolling up a slight depression on the glenoid fossa. In order for the marble to remain within the confines of the concave fossa, the rolling marble must simultaneously glide inferior to compensate for any distance the marble may have gained "rolling" up the glenoid surface. In this present example, these "roll and glide" arthrokinematics must occur if full glenohumeral abduction is to be accomplished. Full abduction may be limited in the aged person if the joint's connective tissue resists either the translation or the rotation of the bone. This example will be discussed in greater detail in the final part of this chapter.

Bone and Joint Kinetics

In the scope of arthrokinesiology, *kinetics* describes the joint forces and torques that cause potential motion at a joint.[84] In order to fully understand potential motion about a joint, one must appreciate the difference between a force and a torque. Think of a force as a "push or a pull" that originates from muscle activation, the pull of gravity, the

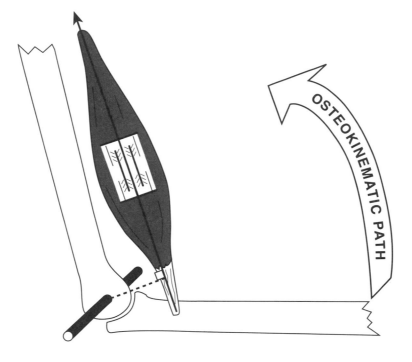

FIG 4–1.
Elbow model showing the osteokinematic motion of flexion in the sagittal plane. The *dark rod* is the axis of rotation, and the muscle's force line is the *dark, thin arrow.*

push from a therapist, or connective tissue's inherent resistance to stretch. Forces cause bones to translate in space and/or rotate in a plane about an axis. In this chapter, *active forces* will refer to forces produced by muscle contraction through active effort. *Passive forces,* on the other hand, will be the forces produced purely by the resistance generated when periarticular structures are stretched. As subsequent discussions will suggest, increased stiffness in "aged" connective tissues may contribute to decreased range of motion in the elderly.

As depicted in Figure 4–1, forces acting on a bone may cause the bone to rotate within a plane about an axis of rotation. This "turning effect" of a bone is called a joint *torque*. This torque, or moment, may be estimated by the product of the force times a given moment arm.[84] In this chapter, an *internal* moment arm (*dashed line* in Fig 4–1) will be defined as the length of a line that extends from the axis of rotation (*dark rod* in Fig 4–1) to the perpendicular intersection of the muscle's force line (*dark, thin arrow* in Fig 4–1). Furthermore, the product of an active muscle force and internal moment arm will be referred to as an *internal torque.* The modifier *internal* is used since the torque was produced by a force *internal* to the musculoskeletal system. The torque effect of a muscle group's contraction is often measured in the clinic by various "isokinetic" testing devices.[84]

In this chapter, an *agonist* muscle will be considered the muscle or muscle group that is primarily responsible

for producing the active forces that direct bone movement. The *antagonist* muscle, in contrast, will be considered the muscle or muscle group that has an action opposite to the agonist muscle.[51] Realize that as the agonist muscle contracts and shortens, the antagonist muscle must elongate while creating a passive force that would not significantly inhibit the intended movement.

In most joint systems, large active muscle forces are required to "drive" the movement or provide joint stability. These forces have been referred to as *myogenic,* since they are produced by action of muscle.[67] Myogenic joint forces most often compress joint surfaces and assist with certain physiologic activities such as joint stability and cartilage nutrition. In the case of disease or weakened articular tissue secondary to advanced age, large myogenic joint forces can cause joint damage, pain, and dysfunction.

To illustrate the concept of a compression force between joint surfaces, consider the model in Figure 4–2, which shows the kinetics about the right hip during single-limb standing.[66] Since the pelvis is assumed to be fixed about the right femur, the model assumes a condition of static equilibrium. The "external" torque caused by body weight is prevented from rotating the pelvis clockwise due to an equivalent counterclockwise torque produced by the hip abductors. Since the external moment arm used by body weight is about twice as long as the internal moment arm used by the hip abductors (D_1 vs. D in Fig 4–2), the hip abductor force must equal twice body weight.[68, 70] As

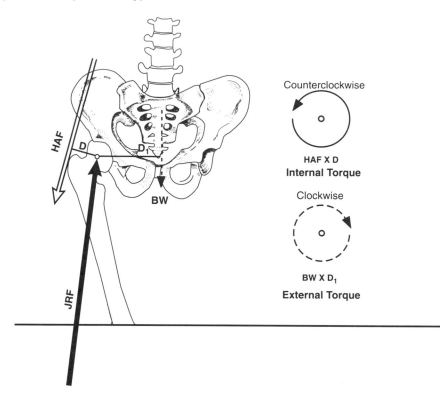

FIG 4-2.
Closed-chain action of the right hip abductor muscle when the pelvis is held stationary about the right femoral head. Assume that the pelvis is only free to rotate *within the frontal plane* about an anteroposterior *(AP)* axis that pierces the right femoral head. The hip abductors must generate an internal torque that stabilizes the pelvis and trunk about the right hip during single-limb support. This stability requires that the internal torque equal the external torque. *HAF* = hip abductor force; *D* = internal moment arm; D_1 = external moment arm; *BW* = body weight; *JRF* = joint reaction force. *Note:* The external moment arm is equal to the length of a line that extends from the axis of rotation to a point of right-angle intersection with body weight's force vector. (Modified from Neumann DA, Cook TM: *Phys Ther* 1985; 65:306.)

Figure 4-2 shows, body weight and hip abductor force produce a combined force that must be matched by an equivalent joint force oriented in an opposite direction. This force, often called a joint reaction force, most often compresses the joint together (*JRF* in Fig 4-2). Normally, in the healthy young joint, this large force is transferred across the joint without problem. In certain pathologic or osteoporotic conditions, however, the joint reaction forces exceed the physiologic tolerance of the weakened bone, and hip fracture may result.

Posture and Positions of Natural Joint Stability

In order to fully appreciate the implications of faulty posture in the aged population, a brief review of the mechanical interactions between joint tissue and the pull of gravity on body segments is required. Consider that a pair of articular surfaces assume a position of maximal congruency at one unique position within a joint's range of motion. This position of natural stability has been referred to as the joint's *close-packed position*.[95] In this position, the ligaments and joint capsule may be relatively elongated and stretched slightly. The resistance to this stretch may be temporally stored as a passive force that may provide an element of transarticular stability.

In the hip and knee joints, the major component of each joint's close-packed position corresponds to positions where stability is required during standing, that is, in hip and knee extension. Ideal standing posture of the lower extremity is shown in Figure 4-3. The alignments of the various body segments position the force line of gravity posterior to the hip and anterior to the knee and ankle.[51] This force line produces a series of external torques that maintain hip and knee extension and bias slight dorsiflexion at the ankle. These hip and knee joint positions stretch various periarticular connective tissues and subsequently produce passive forces that stabilize the joints for standing. In these positions, active muscle forces may be minimized that would reduce energy expenditure as well as levels of myogenic joint force. Gaining useful force

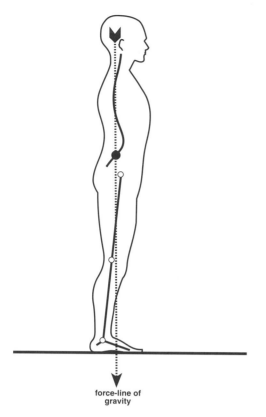

FIG 4–3.
A person with "ideal" standing posture places his force line of gravity *(arrow) posterior* to the mediolateral axis of the hip and anterior to the mediolateral axes of the knee and ankle. Gravity acts to maintain the hip and knee in their close-packed and stable position.

through noncontractile and metabolically "inexpensive" tissues for certain static, low-torque stability functions may have certain physiologic advantages. This discussion will resume in the third part of this chapter with specific clinical significance to the aged person.

AGE-RELATED CHANGES IN JOINT CONNECTIVE TISSUE

Growing old is usually associated with a reduced level of physical activity. In fact, the body's physiologic responses to both are quite similar.[15] Furthermore, as one reaches an advanced age, the chance of being affected by a disease increases. The interaction of these facts requires that three points be considered when studying the arthrokinesiologic aspects of geriatric physical therapy. First, changes in the structure and function of joint connective tissue may occur simply as a natural process of growing old. The manner in which these natural "age-related" changes affect joint function will be the main focus of this chapter. Second,

the type and degree of physical activity one engages in also have a significant influence on the structure and function of connective tissues.[87] The third point to consider is that pathology can affect the joint's connective tissue *at any age* and lead to profound functional limitations and disability. The effects of disease, reduced physical activity, and advanced age often occur simultaneously and may have a combined effect on joint function. Countless other factors, such as genetics, previous postural habits, and earlier injury, also interact and influence an aged person's arthrokinesiologic function. The exact nature of the interaction is very complicated and not fully understood.

This part of the chapter will proceed with a brief review of the structural and functional aspects of the various joint connective tissues. This review will set the stage for an overview of the functional changes that are believed to occur in aged joint tissue.

Periarticular Connective Tissue

Review of Tissue Structure and Function
Periarticular connective tissue (PCT) includes ligament, associated joint capsule, aponeurosis, tendon, intramuscular connective tissue, and skin. All these tissues are physically linked to joints, and therefore their extensibility will influence a joint's range of motion. The predominant histologic components of all PCT are fibroblasts and fibrous proteins, namely, collagen and elastin, extracellular ground matrix, and water. The ground matrix resembles a viscous gel that consists of large branching proteoglycan molecules. These macromolecules, often referred to as glycosaminoglycans, are made of about 95% polysaccharides and 5% protein.[39] The proteoglycan complex and water act as filler and cementing substance for the embedded fibrous protein.

Collagen provides most of the structure and strength to all connective tissues in the body. Twelve different types of collagen have been identified in connective tissue, but subsequent discussion in this chapter will refer to type 1 collagen since this is the main protein in PCT.[14]

Collagen fibers strongly resist stretch and are capable of providing great strength to the tissue in which they reside. The mechanical stability of collagen is maintained through life by a complex mechanism referred to as *intermolecular cross-bridging*. The tropocollagen molecules, the building blocks of the collagen fibril, are strongly linked together at regular parallel intervals. Many fibrils are grouped together to form the collagen fiber and ultimately the collagen fasciculi. Once collagen fibers are formed, their rate of turnover is very slow. The protein should not be considered inert or static. Collagen metabolism can be influenced by physical and chemical stimuli. This can be observed in tissues that are in the process of producing a scar or after periods of decreased physical activity.[72]

Elastin is another protein in most PCT and, as its name implies, provides tissue with a degree of natural elasticity.[39] Connective tissues with high proportions of elastin resist elongation *gradually* as they are stretched. Like any elastic material, this tissue tends to return to its natural length after extensive stretch. The physical alignment and relative proportions of the collagen and elastin within each PCT reflect the tissue's role in limiting, guiding, or stabilizing a joint's motion.

Ligaments are a type of dense connective tissue composed chiefly of thick, longitudinal bands of collagen with relatively few cells and extracellular gel substance. Macroscopically, ligaments resemble thick cords that connect bone to bone and thereby provide structural stability across a joint. Each collagen fiber within a ligament best resists elongation in the direction parallel to the long axis of the fiber. Since the collagen within ligaments is aligned essentially straight and parallel with each other, significant elongation of the ligament itself is restricted by the inherent stiffness in the collagen. The stiffness within the ligament stabilizes and protects a joint against unnatural motion that may injure other joint structures, including muscle. Ligaments often blend in with, and are structurally part of, each joint's *articular capsule*. The collagen fibers within ligaments and capsule may be arranged slightly oblique to the long axis of the ligament or capsule.[92] This arrangement provides resistance to the multidirectional elongations that may arise due to various joint movements.

Collagen fibers provide a limited amount of elasticity to capsular ligaments. This is based on the fact that unstretched collagen fibers are oriented in a wavy or coiled manner. Significant ligamentous resistance to stretch is delayed slightly until the collagen fibers are actually pulled straight. After the stretch is removed, the elastin fibers may aid in recoiling the collagen fibers back to their pre-stretched appearance.[62] As stated earlier, forces that stretch collagen and elastin may be temporally stored and used to perform joint stability functions.

A *tendon* functions to transfer muscle force to bone. The fibrous tissue within the tendon is mostly white collagenous bands of dense connective tissue with limited amounts of elastin. The collagen bundles are thick, tightly packed, and aligned parallel with each other and to the long axis of the tendon. The parallel fiber arrangement allows tendons to resist elongation even in the presence of very high stretching forces.[95] This characteristic high stiffness of the tendon reflects a function of transmitting large muscular forces to bone. Since tendons contain a limited amount of elastin, they elongate slightly due to muscle pull but return to their original length after the removal of the muscle force.

Skeletal muscle is composed chiefly of contractile proteins that are ensheathed in a continuous sheath of *intramuscular connective tissue*. This tissue surrounds each muscle fiber, muscle fasciculi, and external surface of the individual whole muscle. The intramuscular connective tissue ultimately blends with the connective tissue fabric of the tendon and periosteum.[39] The intramuscular connective tissues contain both collagen and elastic fibers.[23] When these tissues are stretched beyond a specific length, the inherent elasticity within these tissues may assist in the production of forces that move and/or stabilize our joints.[43] Internal torques produced about a joint may therefore be the result of *both* active and passive forces.[8, 84] Active forces may be considered *neurogenic* since the nervous system "actively" initiates the coded impulses that cause contractile proteins to shorten and exert a pull on adjacent intramuscular connective tissues. Passive forces generated from stretched muscle, on the other hand, do not require any volitional neural input. These forces may be considered *elastogenic* since they are produced by the forces that are stored within the stretched elastic connective tissue elements of a whole muscle.[69]

Finally, the basic structure of *skin* must be considered since this tissue surrounds all joints and must deform slightly to allow the extremes of a joint's range of motion. The dermis, a deeper skin component, is a form of connective tissue that contains large amounts of collagen.[81] The majority of the thickness of the dermis is a dense, irregular connective tissue that consists of collagen fibers oriented in a wavy and coiled pattern. Elastin fibers are also present in the dermis, but to a much less extent than collagen. As is well known by watching a joint move through full motion, the dermis can be stretched quite a distance before any significant resistance is encountered. The eventual resistance is due to the straightening out of the coiled collagen fibers. When the stretch of the skin is removed, young, healthy skin returns to its original position by the rebound action of the elastic fibers. The wavy and multidirectional physical orientation of all the fibrous elements in the dermis allows the skin to resist forces in many directions.

Review of Mechanical Properties of Connective Tissues

Before proceeding further with the discussion of age-related changes in PCT, a few selected mechanical properties that are relevant to the study of connective tissue need to be reviewed.

Researchers may deform connective tissues in vitro, and the resistance the tissue produces to the deformation may be measured as a force. A deformation-force curve may be plotted that yields information about the tissue's ability to tolerate certain biologic or environmental factors. Ligaments or tendons are often tested for their ability to produce a *tensile force,* that is, a force generated as a resistance to stretch. Hyaline cartilage, on the other hand, is often tested to determine its ability to resist *compression.* Elasticity and viscosity each describe a unique property of a tissue's resistance to deformation.[99] Connective tissues are partially *elastic* and therefore temporally store a component of the force that originally caused their deformation. Like a spring, stretched elastic tissues tend to return to their original prestretched length after the removal of the force. *Viscosity* describes the extent to which a tissue's resistance to deformation is dependent on the *rate* of the deforming force. Viscosity is a time-dependent property, whereas elasticity is not. Realize that most connective tissues demonstrate a *viscoelastic property* since both the rate of deformation *and* instantaneous tissue length determine the amount of resistance the tissue generates when deformed. Usually the greater the amount and rate of deformation, the greater the resistance offered by the tissue.

Connective tissues may be excised from animals of different ages and subjected to various forms of mechanical testing. As an example, Figure 4–4 shows a plot depicting the results of a typical "stress vs. strain" test on an excised tendon of a rabbit.[93] The terms *stress* and *strain* are somewhat analogous to the terms *force* and *deformation,* respectively. For purposes of normalization, the force developed in the deformed tissue is divided by the tissue's cross-sectional

area and thus presented as a pressure measurement called *stress.* The deformation, either in elongation or compression, that is applied to the tissue is often normalized to a percent change in original length and referred to as *strain.* The plot in Figure 4–4 illustrates several mechanical characteristics common to many viscoelastic tissues that are stretched to a point of rupture. This graph shows five regions that each show specific information about mechanical properties of connective tissue. *Region A* shows that at the beginning of the stretch the increase in length in the tendon does not result in a significant increase in stress in the stretched tendon. This region of low resistance is reportedly due to the straightening out of the unloaded coiled collagen fibers.[1] Once the fibers have been stretched out straight, the stress-strain relationship becomes linear due to the parallel arrangement of the fibers *(Region B).* The slope of the stress vs. strain curve in Region B is a measure of the tissue's *stiffness.* Region B is often referred to as the *elastic region,* since at this length removal of the stretch force would result in the tissue recoiling back to its original length. *Region C* shows a property of stretched tissue known as *plasticity.* This is evident by continued elongation of the tissue *without* an increase in resistance from within the tissue. Connective tissue that is stretched to a length where plasticity actually begins may remain permanently deformed. In fact, this is part of the logic used in a therapeutic stretching program in phys-

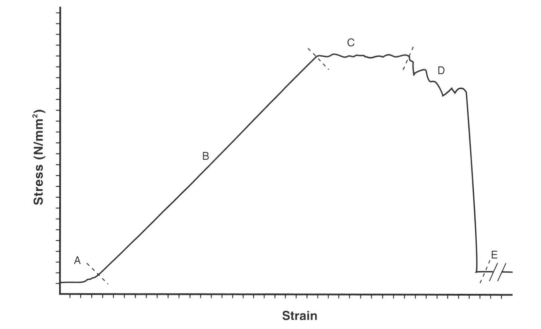

FIG 4–4.
Hypothetical data showing the typical mechanical behavior of an excised tendon that has been stretched to a point of rupture. Tissue *stress* (or force per unit cross-sectional area) has been plotted against a constant *strain* (stretch) rate. *Region A* shows the length where the slack is taken up from the tendon and little, if any, stiffness is recorded. *Region B* shows the length where the tendon shows a linear elastic stiffness. *Region C* depicts the length where the tissue starts to exhibit permanent deformation. *Region D* shows the length at which the tendon actually starts to rupture, and *Region E* shows complete structural failure of the tissue.

ical therapy. *Region D* shows a stretch length that causes actual structural failure within the tendon. In this case, the force of the stretch exceeded the ability of the collagen to transmit the force. Continued elongation of the tissue will eventually cause complete tissue failure, as evident by a complete lack of resistance to increased stretch *(Region E)*. It is important to realize that the characteristics of the plot in Figure 4–4 would most likely vary as a function of tissue age, specific type, and rate of the stretch.

Age-Related Changes in PCT

The mechanical properties of PCT do appear to change with advanced age. The structural and functional changes in the collagen protein probably account for most change; however, the precise physiologic mechanisms are not known or universally agreed.[23, 75, 91] Much of the research literature presented in this chapter regarding the effects of advanced age on human PCT is based on animal research. Human research in this area obviously cannot be conducted with rigid experimental control for variables such as previous physical activity, earlier tissue trauma, nutrition, or breeding. Making direct inferences to human aged tissue based on animal data may be done, however, with caution. Extensive research is needed before definitive descriptions can be given to account for purely age-related changes in the structure of human PCT.

Age-related animal research suggests that ligaments and tendons increase in stiffness and demonstrate a decrease in the maximal length at which rupture occurs.[21] A biochemical analysis of aged tissue usually shows an increase in the relative amount of collagen; an increase in fibril size and aggregation; and a relative decrease in water, elastin, and proteoglycan content.

A mechanism to account for the increase in stiffness in age-related PCT may be the fact that aged collagen shows increased numbers of cross-links between adjacent tropocollagen molecules.[10, 38, 40] Increased rates of cross-linking would increase the mechanical stability of collagen and may explain the increased stiffness in the tissue.[76] This increase in stiffness has been shown in almost all PCT, including the skin.[36]

The unique structure of collagen provides a natural element of stiffness and rigidity to connective tissue. Increased amounts of collagen in PCT may partially explain the increased PCT stiffness shown in aged animals and perhaps humans.[38] Increased collagen content in the endomysium of the rat's intramuscular connective tissue has been shown to correlate with increased stiffness of the whole muscle.[4] Increased numbers of cross-linkages may increase collagen's resistance to degradative enzymes, therefore increasing the relative content of the protein in aged PCT.[63]

Reduced physical activity tends to be a natural part of advanced aging in animals and humans. Understanding the *interactive* effect of advanced age and reduced physical activity on connective tissue stiffness would be very beneficial. Williams and Goldspink[97] monitored the changes in muscle's connective tissue in relatively *young* animals following rigid limb immobilization. They reported marked increases in relative intramuscular collagen as well as stiffness after 4 weeks of immobilization, particularly evident if the muscles were immobilized in a shortened length. The immobilized "young" muscles appeared to show qualitative and quantitative changes similar to what has been observed in aged tissue. These results suggest that physical activity, regardless of age, has a very important influence on muscle stiffness. Further research is needed to understand the precise manner in which physical activity influences the stiffness of aged PCT in general.

Hyaline Cartilage

Review of Tissue Structure and Function

Hyaline cartilage lines the articular ends of bone and protects the joint from damaging transarticular forces. Without this shock-absorbing and lubricating function, normal everyday joint forces would exceed the compression limits of underlying subchondral bone, thus causing fracture.[96] The elastic quality of articular cartilage dissipates high loads as well as decreases the rate of the compression on the joint surfaces.

Hyaline cartilage consists of a small population of chondrocytes widely dispersed in a relatively dense extracellular matrix. The matrix is chiefly composed of water, collagen fibers, and long branching proteoglycan macromolecules.[56, 79] The collagen fibrils within the matrix provide "scaffolding" to the cartilage, lending both shape and tensile strength. The negative electrochemical charges on the proteoglycan side chains cause adjacent chains to repel, adding additional stiffness to the collagen-proteoglycan mesh. The structure of the matrix is further reinforced by the presence of water molecules that bind to and fill the spaces between the hydrophilic proteoglycans.[30] The "crowded" extracellular matrix of articular cartilage may be visualized as a "stuffing" that supports the collagen network. This structure provides healthy articular cartilage the ability to deform repeatedly and re-form following an exceedingly large number of compressions throughout a lifetime. The rate of the deformation of the articular cartilage is controlled somewhat by the action of water slowly oozing through the impedance offered by the matrix. The water under pressure flows toward the relatively unloaded areas of the cartilage. As the joint is unloaded, the water returns to its original location by the swelling pressure produced by the hydrophilic macromolecules within the matrix.[18] The amount of swelling is physically restrained by the tensile properties of the collagen network.

Age-Related Changes in Articular Cartilage

Histologic observation of healthy articular cartilage in the aged adult shows that the density of chondrocytes and the amount of collagen within the extracellar matrix remain essentially unchanged.[31] The water content in the tissue, however, does reduce with advanced age. The hydrophilic proteoglycans have been shown to become shorter in aged tissue and therefore lose their ability to hold water in the matrix.[19] Dehydrated articular cartilage may have a reduced ability to dissipate forces across the joint.

Aged articular cartilage may become more susceptible to mechanical failure. Freeman and Meachim[31] have hypothesized that the loss of physical strength of aged cartilage may be due to fragmentation of the collagen network and/or ruptures of the interfiber bonding. This collagen fragmentation and weakening may, in part, explain the high incidence of localized structural disintegration often observed on the surface of aged articular cartilage. Cartilage lesions, often referred to as *fibrillated* cartilage, can be observed with the naked eye when joints such as the knee and undersurface of the patella are observed in gross dissection. Fibrillated articular tissue may be limited to superficial layers of articular cartilage, or the tissue may show vertical splitting and fragmentation that reach and expose subchondral bone.

The literature tends to support the notion that some amount of fibrillation in articular cartilage is normal and a natural age-related process. Of course, the increased fibrillation may be partially due to the reduced physical activity that often accompanies advanced age. Figure 4–5 shows the results of a random sampling of cadaver knee joints, which clearly indicate that the incidence of fibrillation increases with age.[60] Figure 4–6 shows data that suggests

that other joints including the knee also exhibit natural degeneration with increased age.[42] According to Freeman and Meachim,[31] histologic analysis of fibrillated tissue reveals rupture of the collagen network and an associated weakness in the tissue. Fibrillated cartilage does not tolerate compression and tensile forces nearly as well as intact aged cartilage. Freeman suggests that the collagen structure of aged fibrillated cartilage experiences mechanical fatigue that causes the proteoglycans to "leak out" of the tissue.[30] Decreased proteoglycans within the matrix would diminish the natural dampening effect of cartilage. The cumulative mechanical wear of advanced age may cause, or is strongly associated with, a weakening of articular cartilage.[31]

In summary, some degree of mechanical degeneration of aged human articular cartilage should be considered a normal process. The wear may be from repeated loading of joints over the good part of a lifetime. The ability of even "healthy" articular cartilage to dissipate transarticular forces may diminish in the aged population.

Any discussion of aged articular cartilage should include the point that osteoarthritis is not an imminent consequence of the natural fragmentation of collagen. Fibrillated tissue does not always lead to the disease of osteoarthritis. The link between the hypothesized wear-and-tear theory of fibrillated cartilage and the development of osteoarthritis has not been shown conclusively. Granted, osteoarthritis does occur with greater frequency in the elderly. As a matter of fact, by age 60, more than 60% of the population may have some degree of cartilage abnormality in certain joints.[85] Nevertheless, one cannot assume that the disease of osteoarthritis is purely a mechanical result of aging. If this logic were true, then *all* old persons

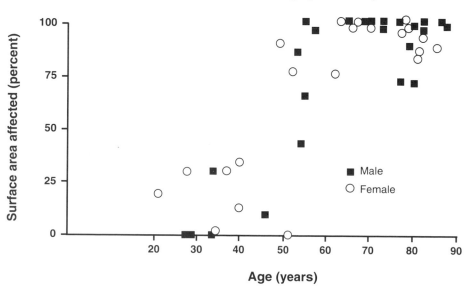

FIG 4–5.
Plot recording the percentage of the surface area of human lateral tibial plateau that showed "overt" fibrillation as a function of age. Data were collected from 47 necropsies. (Redrawn from Meachim G: *J Anat* 1976; 121:97–106.)

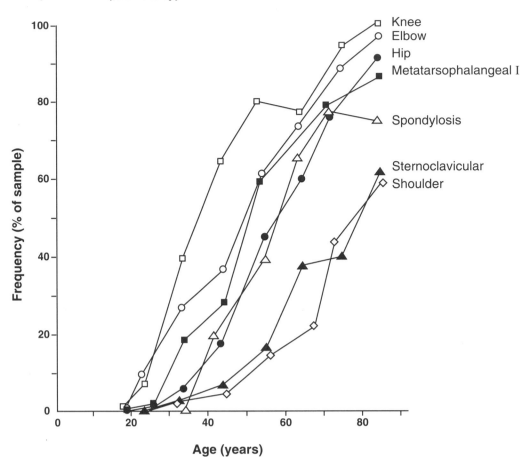

FIG 4–6.
Plot showing the frequency of location of degenerative joint disease as a function of age. The joints were inspected during 1,000 necropsies. (Redrawn from Heine J: *Virchows Arch Pathol Anat Physiol Klin Med* 1926; 260:521–663. Used by permission.)

should develop osteoarthritis, and this is not the case. Genetic, biochemical, traumatic, and morphologic factors may also be interrelated with the effect of aging and development of osteoarthritis.[31]

Due to the relatively high incidence of osteoarthritis in the aged population, the physical therapist should be aware of the basic clinical consequences of the disease.[35] Osteoarthritis often presents with severely degenerated and thinned articular cartilage. The severe collagen weakening and proteoglycan depletion observed in advanced osteoarthritis markedly reduce the cartilage's ability to resist tensile and compressional forces. As a consequence, undampened joint forces may cause a reactive hardening or sclerosis of the unprotected subchondral bone.[74] This reactive response is in accord with the century-old Wolff's law (1892) that bone is laid down in areas of stress and reabsorbed in areas of nonstress. Degenerated cartilage and stiffer subchondral bone are not able to adequately attenuate high transarticular forces. Osteophytes and various remodeling may occur as a further progression of Wolff's law, and the entire morphology and geometry of the joint surfaces may change.[89] Physical therapists need to understand the deleterious consequences of having their patient's arthritic joints subjected to large and repetitive joint forces. Concepts of "joint protection" need to be used with these patients.[66]

Bone

Review of Tissue Structure and Function

Bone contains widely dispersed specialized cells that manufacture and secrete a dense, fibrous extracellular matrix. Compact bone's characteristic rigidity and stiffness are due to the presence of the dense collagen network within the extracellular matrix. This collagen lattice is structurally reinforced by calcium phosphate–based minerals. Bone would be a very soft and pliable material if it were not for the mineralization of the calcium salts on the collagen and matrix material.

The collagen fibers within compact bone possess some degree of elasticity and therefore are well suited to resist tensile forces.[25] Calcium phosphate, in contrast, is very good at resisting compression forces. The interaction of these two materials provides bone with a unique ability to resist forces in multiple directions. The outer cortex shell of bone is very dense to withstand the high forces produced by muscle pull and weight-bearing activities. The inner, more spongy, cancellous bone is porous, which allows bone to flex slightly under a load.

Despite bone's inert appearance, the tissue is physiologically very dynamic and hence possesses a rich blood supply.[55] Osteocytes constantly differentiate into active osteoblasts that produce new bone. Simultaneously, the osteoclasts act as macrophages and reabsorb unneeded or extra bone.[39] The net result of this constant process of syntheses and reabsorption is to change the shape, density, and ultimate weight-bearing ability of bone. This dynamic process allows bone to remodel and heal itself in response to mechanical stress and trauma. Bone, by being a reactive tissue, can alter geometric shape to withstand the force demands imposed by muscle contraction and gravity. The exact mechanism by which bone cells actually sense and alter cellular synthesis in response to mechanical stress is not known for sure. One popular theory suggests that as a bone bends slightly from a mechanical stress, small piezoelectric charges induce an electric field that stimulates osteoblastic activity.[49]

Age-Related Changes in Bone

The precise shape and density of bone are maintained through life by a balance of mechanical and physiologic mechanisms. Mechanical stress stimulates the formation of new bone, whereas the endocrine system functions to ultimately reabsorb bone.[55] Increased internal stress stimulates a net increase in bone density so that the bone can withstand higher forces. As an individual advances in age and becomes less active, a loss of bone mass per unit volume usually occurs. If the bone becomes excessively brittle and prone to fracture, the condition may be classified as *osteoporosis*. This process is characterized by a progressive loss of both fibrous matrix and mineral content[57]; new bone is not made at a rate to replace the natural rate of bone absorption. Decreased bone mass results in a decreased ability of bone to support loads and resist external forces.[20] As an example, consider the relatively common incidence of avulsion fracture of the tibial tuberosity in the aged population. This fracture occurs when the ligamentum patella and tibial tuberosity are pulled free from the shaft of the tibia due to excessive force produced in the quadriceps muscle. The large tensile force developed through the ligamentum patella exceeds the capability of the bone to maintain an intact tibial tuberosity.

The medical impact of osteoporosis in the elderly is significant, particularly evident by the high incidence of fracture of the hip.[100] According to a longitudinal study by Gallagher et al.,[33] the rate of hip fracture doubles each decade after age 50. There are also sex differences. Hip fracture affects 32% of women and 17% of men by age 90.

Physical therapists should note that about 50% of these patients never resume walking after the hip fracture. The mechanical strength of the proximal osteoporotic femur could not withstand the high forces that result from a fall and/or vigorous muscle contraction. Hip fracture in the elderly often results from high torsional forces created about the shaft of the femur during a twisting motion.[32] Interestingly, the aged femur has demonstrated increased stiffness when stressed at high force levels. The femur therefore would lose some ability to "give" under high forces. This may partially account for the fact that older bones fracture at significantly lower force levels than younger bones.[44]

The decline in physical activity and subsequent diminished stress placed on bone are often associated with growing old. Therefore, the loss of bone mass and increased susceptibility to fracture should be considered a normal age-related process. Experiments have shown that males lose about 3% of their cortical bone mass each decade after age 40.[57] Women, on average, lose cortical bone at a similar rate but show an accelerated rate of bone loss following menopause. The postmenopausal loss of bone in women reflects the normal physiologic role of estrogen in the maintenance of cortical bone mass. One should keep in perspective, however, that diminished physical activity from bedrest may have a more significant demineralizing effect on bone than does the decrease in estrogen following menopause.[44] Fortunately, bone loss in postmenopausal women can be minimized somewhat through active dynamic exercise.[83]

ARTHROKINESIOLOGIC IMPLICATIONS OF AGING

Joints in the elderly tend to display a subtle decrease in both angular velocity and displacement.[86] This observation may be made even in the absence of overt pathology such as stroke, arthritis, or Parkinson's disease. The following discussion will suggest reasons why the elderly tend to reduce the speed and amount of extremity movement from primarily an arthrokinesiologic perspective. This discussion will close by analyzing the effects that torques and forces may have on the structure and function of the aged joint system.

Kinematic Considerations of the Joints in the Aged

Reduction in Joint Angular Velocity

Reduced Physical Activity.—Decreased velocity of joint movement in the aged seems to parallel a natural decline in overall physical activity. The exact reason why the elderly slow down is multifaceted and not as obvious as would first appear. Consider that the elderly often assume a more sedentary life-style. This life-style may be chosen due to a combination of personal, family, cultural, or socioeconomic reasons. The decline in physical activity may also be related to actual age-related physiologic changes in the sensorimotor systems, such as decreased muscle strength or decreased vision. Excessive medication, debilitating medical problems or poor nutrition, and a general overcautiousness, coupled with a fear of falling, are additional factors that may contribute to the decreased physical activity.

The elderly often experience major life stresses that may have a subtle effect on their psychologic as well as physiologic ability to engage in physical activity. For example, the elderly woman who has just lost her husband may not feel as comfortable taking evening walks on her own. This decreased daily level of physical stress placed on her cardiovascular system, for example, would reduce her system's aerobic capacity. Eventually, an attempt at any significant physical exertion becomes an uncomfortable experience rather than a rewarding one. The cycle of inactivity, decreased physical fitness, and continued inactivity tends to perpetuate itself in the elderly as well as in the young.

Sensorimotor Changes.—The general responsiveness of the nervous system tends to slow with advanced age. This may partially account for a decline in physical activity and subsequent slowed joint movement. Age-related changes in the nervous system include decreased reaction times; increased rate of loss of brain cells; altered level of neurotransmitter production; and a decreased acuity of the auditory, vestibular, and visual systems.[5, 27, 41, 46, 71, 78, 88] Furthermore, perception of vibration, temperature, touch, proprioception, and pressure stimuli all naturally decline as we reach advanced age.[47, 80, 82, 86] Possibly, the slowed volitional joint movement displayed by many elderly is simply a natural mechanism that provides additional time to adequately interpret and process incoming environmental stimuli. We have all experienced the situation of driving behind a slow-moving automobile with an elderly person at the wheel. The person may not be acting inconsiderately, but rather driving at a "top" speed at which their slowed neuromuscular system can safely process and react to multiple streams of sensory input.

A subtle decline in sensorimotor processing in the elderly is certainly just one of many possible explanations that may account for their reduced level of physical activity. Skeletal muscle fibers atrophy with age, and this atrophy may be more prevalent in the fast twitch muscle fibers.[37] Also, a research study has shown the conduction velocity of motor nerves decreases with advanced age.[28] These factors, coupled with the factors previously mentioned, would theoretically decrease the rate or magnitude of force generated by muscle and partially account for diminished joint angular velocity.[50]

Stiffness in Periarticular Connective Tissue.—Increased PCT stiffness may be another contributor to slowed movement in the aged. Increased levels of resistance to joint motion has been measured directly in the elderly.[99] To discuss the implications of this concept, consider an example where an elderly person demonstrates slowed neck rotation to the left, let us say, in response to the call of his name. The motion of left cervical rotation requires a concentric contraction of the left rotators. These muscles must provide sufficient force to rotate the neck as well as elongate the antagonistic right rotator muscles. Increased intramuscular connective tissue stiffness in the right rotator group, for example, could act as a resistance to the left rotation motion. Since most connective tissues demonstrate viscoelastic properties, the passive resistance generated by the right rotators would be dependent on these muscles' length as well as the rate of their elongation. Attempts at increasing the velocity and subsequent amount of left cervical rotation may increase the resistance offered by the right muscle group's intramuscular connective tissue. Significant resistance offered by these tissues would reduce the productive power output of the intended motion of left rotation. Recall that power output about a joint is the product of internal joint torque times the average angular velocity of the movement.

A Natural Adaptive Mechanism.—Regardless of specific physiologic mechanisms, consider the hypothesis that the slowing of extremity motion in the aged may be, in part, simply a natural biologic process intended to ensure the safety and well-being of the individual. For example, age-related changes in the nervous system may slow extremity movement, which would, in effect, protect painful joints, reduce the likelihood of a fall, or protect an osteoporotic skeletal system from the large forces that are inherent to more rapid motion. This adaptive mechanism may be similar to that of the young child's soft and pliable skeletal system. Their pliable bones are able to bend and therefore give slightly to the potentially damaging forces that occur as the young child learns to interact with the relentless pull of gravity.

Reduction in the Extremes of Joint Range of Motion

The loss of passive range of motion in the elderly is often progressive and subtle, occurring usually at the extremes of a joint's potential movement. This reduced magnitude of joint movement may exist even in the absence of pathology.

In general, the magnitude of passive joint range of motion declines with advancing age.[3, 13, 45, 64, 94] Healthy adult men and women tend to have greatest joint mobility in their 20s, with a gradual decrease thereafter.[12] The loss of range of motion is highly variable across joint and subject; however, joint flexibility is clearly inversely related to age. Bell and Hoshizaki[12] have shown that females tend to lose range of motion at a slower rate than males and that joints of the upper extremity remain more flexible than the joints of the lower extremities.

What factors could account for this rather strong association between advanced age and a progressive decrease in joint range of motion? To consider this question, a few prerequisites for full active range of joint motion should be recognized. First, full range of motion requires that the articular surfaces allow a tracking for movement without undue physical interference. Second, a sufficient motor drive with adequate sensory feedback is needed from the neuromuscular system. Third, the PCT must possess a stiffness level that does not inhibit a joint's full range of motion.

Several factors may impede full active or passive range of motion in the elderly. Age-related changes may occur in the joint from previous injury, occupation, or poor posturing. Subsequent excessive joint wear may predispose osteophyte formation and incongruities at the articular surfaces. These factors, in conjunction with increased viscosity of the synovium, calcification of articular cartilages, and increased fatigability of muscle, could all interfere with full joint motion.

Increased Stiffness in PCT.— Stiffness in PCT certainly needs to be considered as a prime factor in reducing the range of joint motion in the elderly. In all joints, aged or otherwise, the extremes of movement are resisted slightly due to the inherent stiffness provided by the PCT. Wright and Johns have determined from in vivo human experiments that articular capsule and muscle combine to account for about 90% of the total passive stiffness in a healthy joint.[99] The resistance generated by tendon and skin accounted for most of the remaining natural stiffness. Human joints of aged individuals have shown significant increases in passive resistance to movement.[16, 99] This phenomenon may be partially explained by increased stiffness in local joint PCT. As reviewed previously in this chapter, the increased stiffness in the PCT may be due to alterations in the structure of the collagen. Increased stiffness may also result from a reduction in physical activity in the elderly and subsequent lack of natural stretch applied to PCT.[2, 11]

Knowledge of the relative influence of each specific PCT to stiffness in the human aged joint would enhance the planning and implementation of physical therapy programs aimed at maintaining overall joint mobility. Clinical evidence suggests that the intramuscular connective tissues may account for a significant amount of the limitation of joint motion in the aged. James and Parker measured passive ankle dorsiflexion in subjects over 80 years old.[45] Significantly less passive ankle dorsiflexion was available when the knee was in full extension as compared with full flexion. The extended knee evidently placed additional

stretch on the aged and somewhat stiff connective tissue within the multijointed gastrocnemius muscle. The increased stiffness in the muscle was only fully realized when the muscle was stretched over both ankle and knee joints simultaneously.

Another aspect of increased stiffness in intramuscular connective tissues of the aged relates to total metabolic efficiency. The increased resistive "drag" provided by stiff intramuscular connective tissue within antagonist muscle may limit the effectiveness of work output of the agonist muscle. This passive resistance, albeit relatively small when expressed over any particular single joint, may be rather significant when *multiple* joint actions are attempted, particularly at the extremes of motion. The increased muscular effort of the agonists may contribute to general fatigue when the elderly engage in physical activity. Poor nutrition or compromised function of the cardiopulmonary system may further compound the problem.

Age-Related Influences in Joint Mechanics.— Increased stiffness in PCT in the aged may have significant influence on joint arthrokinematics. Consider the motion of active glenohumeral abduction to full range. To achieve this motion, all PCT and muscle that have the potential to produce a glenohumeral *adduction* torque (either through active or passive means) must be elongated. Furthermore, the head of the humerus must descend into the pouch formed by the inferior recess of the inferior aspect of the glenohumeral capsule. The inferior translation of the humeral head is part of the natural arthrokinematic pattern of full abduction.[51, 84, 95] Significant capsular and ligamentous stiffness may interfere with the natural translations that constitute the arthrokinematics of glenohumeral abduction. Increased tissue resistance to any expansion of the capsule, for example, would inhibit the descent of the humeral head. This may cause the head of the humerus to roll superior on the glenoid without the necessary compensatory inferior glide. The head of the humerus may impinge on the supraspinatus tendon or make contact with the coracoacromial arch, thus limiting further abduction. Increased transarticular forces may result, since various muscles may have to generate greater forces in attempts to rotate and/or translate the bones and joint surfaces against the resistance imparted by the stiffer capsule. Abnormal muscle synergies may also result over time, since, as in the above abduction example, the serratus anterior may have to develop greater and longer duration forces to upward rotate the scapula on the thorax in efforts to assist the shoulder abduction.

Practical and Clinical Significance of Decreased Joint Mobility.— The real impact that a limitation of joint motion has on aged individuals depends on which joint is limited, the degree of the limitation, and the overall health and mobility of the person. Consider the following research study. Shoulder abduction range of motion was measured in 1,000 persons who were still relatively mobile and living in their homes.[11] The subjects were considered healthy but did possess a wide range of typical age-associated medical problems. The authors found that over 50% of the subjects over age 75 could not actively abduct their shoulder up to 120 degrees. Also, the mean shoulder abduction range of the 75-year-old group was about 30 degrees less than a group of subjects with an average age of 39 years old. From a practical standpoint, a maximal range of 120 degrees of shoulder abduction should be considered a significant impairment, since many functional activities that require the hand to be brought above the head would be limited.[9] The person who could only actively abduct a shoulder to 110 degrees would, for example, have difficulty returning items to a top shelf in the kitchen. Besides the obvious practical limitations imposed from this lack of mobility, consider other more subtle implications. The elderly person may eventually respond to progressive loss of motion by moving the contents of kitchen cupboards to a lower level. From a practical standpoint, this modification is certainly a sensible one. From an arthrokinesiologic standpoint, however, the modification would reduce the number of abduction efforts attempted each day. The tightness in the shoulder may become self-perpetuating. A simple home exercise program may delay the time when the cupboards have to be modified and therefore allow the natural demands of the functional task to maintain required joint flexibility.

Loss of range of motion in the aged may inform the physical therapist of other aspects of a person's overall health. In the study by Bassey et al., the amount of shoulder motion deficit was positively correlated with an index of subject's health.[11] Of interest was a statistically significant correlation between a 10% loss of mean shoulder abduction for women and the presence of arthritis, lack of (overall) mobility, and incontinence. The therapist must be aware that a reduction in joint motion may be an indirect symptom of some other more significant medical problem. According to the multiple regression equation determined from the data in the Bassey study, the therapist should be alerted to a greater statistical likelihood of systemic health problems if the active shoulder abduction motion in 60-year-old persons is less than about 140 degrees.[11]

A distinction should be made between loss of joint motion associated with a disease process and a loss of motion due to the natural process of growing old. Often this distinction is not clear. An interesting example may be made in this regard by considering the data from Bell and Hoshizaki.[12] These researchers measured the range of motion in several joints and correlated this measurement to subject's sex and age. When considering the 17 joint motions tested, cervical motions showed generally the steepest and most consistent decline with age across both genders. One may speculate that this specific loss of motion may, in part, parallel the natural age-related decline in the acuity of some of the special senses. An important function of the cervical spine is to allow the special senses of vision, hearing, smell, and balance to be placed in a wide range of positions. Even a small decline in the acuity of these afferent systems may reduce the functional demand placed on the cervical joints and theoretically contribute to their loss of passive motion. Research could not be found to substantiate this speculation; however, the logic appears to be sound and worthy of study.

Two final points will be made as a conclusion to this discussion on limitation of joint motion in the elderly. First, it is essential to realize that *not all* elderly individuals lose significant range of motion as they age. Exceptions will always exist, and the reasons for such exceptions should be analyzed as clues to effective treatment principles. The literature does report cases of very athletic aged individuals who have significantly greater range of motion than younger or more sedentary persons.[29] Furthermore, significant increases in range of motion can be gained in the elderly through regular stretching programs.[24, 52, 73] Further research is needed to decipher the complex interaction between aging, mental attitude, and physical activity on the mechanical behavior of PCT in the human. Why certain persons maintain full range of motion and others do not is an important research question in the field of geriatric physical therapy. The importance of such a question will only increase as the active elderly occupy an even greater percentage of living persons in our society.

Finally, consider the idea that an age-related "limitation" in extremity mobility may lend a subtle element of safety to aged persons and, therefore, in this regard may be beneficial. For example, aged persons tend to walk at reduced velocities and with a broader and shorter stride length.[65] As Murray et al. state, this gait pattern seems to favor stability and security during walking.[65] This slowed and cautious gait pattern may reduce stride length as well as the amount of closed-chained ankle dorsiflexion required during the stance phase. The reduced magnitude and/or frequency of heel cord stretch may eventually limit the maximal range of available ankle dorsiflexion. In the larger picture, the small reduction in ankle range of motion may be considered beneficial if the altered gait actually prevents a fall and a subsequent scenario of hip fracture and prolonged bed rest.

Joint Mobility and Influence on Whole Body Posture

As just discussed, in certain conditions, subtle restrictions in joint motion may provide a physiologic benefit to the overall health of the elderly. As a contrast to this argument, consider how a moderate limitation in joint motion may have a potentially negative physiologic effect, particularly in regard to standing posture.

Previously in this chapter, we discussed that in erect standing the body's force line of gravity creates multiple external torques that favor stability of various lower extremity joints (see Fig 4–3). Figure 4–7,A shows this same concept, but now the rotary direction of the *external* torques in the sagittal plane acting about the hip and knee is depicted. The relative lengths of the external moment arms that gravity acts about each joint are also shown. Note that in erect standing the ability to achieve full hip extension places the superincumbent force line of gravity *posterior* to the mediolateral axis at this joint (Fig 4–7,A).

Gravity now acts with an external moment arm that is posterior to the hip and therefore produces an extensor torque. This extensor torque helps maintain the stable position at this joint. Furthermore, full hip extension stretches and elongates the hip's capsular ligaments, which produces transarticular hip forces that may also assist the stability of the extended hip.[95] Any person, elderly or young, who can achieve the hip extension shown in Figure 4–7,A should be able to have an extensor (external) torque at the hip be *produced by gravity*. The extensor torque can be balanced by a passive flexor torque produced by the natural stiffness in the taut iliofemoral ligament. Therefore, in theory, the sagittal plane stability at the hip during stand-

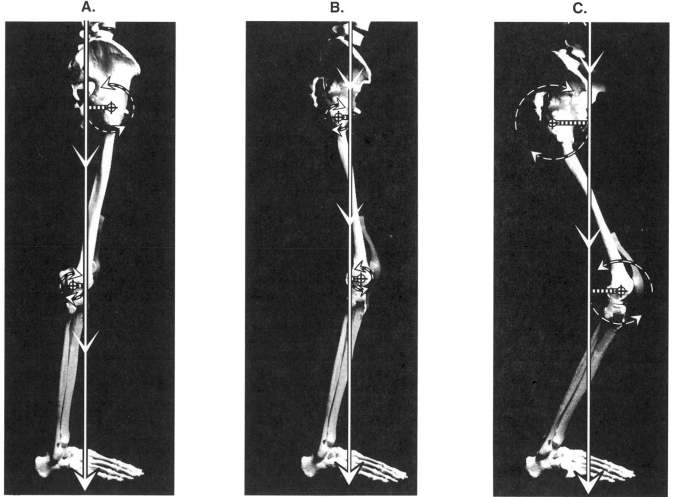

A.   **B.**   **C.**

BW   BW   BW

FIG 4–7.
Model showing the orientation of the force line of gravity (*arrow* labeled *BW,* which refers to body weight) for the major joints of the lower extremity. **A-C** show a progression in severity of hip flexor tightness. Each model demonstrates the mediolateral axis at the hip and knee *(circles with cross hairs),* the associated external moment arms *(hatched line),* and the rotary direction of the external torque in the sagittal plane *(hatched circular arrows).* **A,** ideal standing posture with *hip in full extension.* Body weight acts as an extensor at the hip and knee. **B,** hip with *moderate* hip flexion deformity, that is, lacks full extension. Body weight acts as a flexor at the hip and knee. **C,** hip with *severe* hip flexion deformity. Body weight acts as a very potent flexor at the hip and knee.

ing can be achieved with minimal hip muscle contraction.

In contrast to the relative ease of standing when the hip joint is fully extended, consider the effect of a limitation of hip extension. Assume a situation where an aged person lacks full hip extension and may have a moderate hip flexion deformity caused by PCT tightness (Figure 4–7,B). Lack of full hip extension in the elderly is relatively prevalent[77] and may be predisposed by periods of prolonged sitting. The forward placement of the pelvis-and-trunk shown in Figure 4–7,B would shift the force line of gravity slightly anterior to the hip. The force line of gravity acts now *as a hip flexor,* not as an extensor as shown in Figure 4–7,A. Increased extensor muscle force would be required to maintain the standing position. The subsequent increase in myogenic hip joint force may exacerbate existing hip joint deterioration or possibly increase cartilage wear. Also, as one stands over a hip that is not completely extendable, the joint compression forces[66] may be redirected toward the hip's articular cartilage, which is not naturally suited to disperse forces. Furthermore, the increased metabolic requirements of maintaining low levels of hip extensor muscle contraction may add to general fatigue. This situation may encourage increased sitting, which may perpetuate the cycle of continued or increased PCT tightness.

As Figure 4–7,B shows, PCT tightness at the hip may contribute to a standing posture that incorporates standing over a slightly flexed knee. A knee-flexed posture while standing shifts the force line of gravity to the posterior side of the knee. Gravity now acts as a knee flexor instead of knee extensor as in Figure 4–7,A. Knee extensor force is now required to hold the partially flexed knee from collapsing into full flexion. As with the situation at the hip, increased myogenic joint forces are delivered across the knee, and the metabolic costs of simple standing have undoubtedly increased. Figure 4–7,C shows the biomechanical situation where hip and knee flexor tightness are markedly exaggerated, and as noted, the action of gravity now becomes a very potent hip and knee flexor. This case is quite severe and usually would prohibit functional ambulation.

Kinetic Considerations of the Joints in the Aged

In earlier sections of this chapter, the concepts of joint forces and torques were briefly discussed. This section will focus exclusively on these concepts with continued specific attention on the elderly. Arthrokinesiologic implications that relate to *internal torque* about the joint will be discussed first. The remainder of this section will review a clinical example where aged connective tissue about the joint fails to resist the deforming postures created through *external torques.*

Internal Joint Torque Considerations

Maximal internal torque about a joint is defined as the product of the maximal volitional muscle force times the length of the associated internal moment arm (see Figs 4–1 and 4–2). Aging and various changes in structure and function of connective tissue can alter these variables, and each will be discussed separately.

Reduced Ability to Generate Muscle Force.—Clinically, the elderly patient often shows a reduced "muscular strength" as tested through a dynamometer, isokinetic device, or manual muscle testing. More precisely stated, the maximal internal torque produced about joints tends to decline with advanced age.[6, 7, 58, 90] Assuming that the length of the internal moment arm at any given joint angle remains constant as one reaches an advanced age, the lowered peak internal torque generation must be due to reduced peak muscle force. Skeletal muscle mass declines with advanced age, and this factor alone could account for a significant amount of the loss of force production. The loss of muscle mass may be in part due to simple disuse atrophy secondary to a reduction in physical activity. Other factors that may contribute to the reduced peak muscular force in the aged are a loss in the number of functioning motoneurons,[22] a preferential atrophy of fast twitch (type II) muscle fibers,[37, 54] decreased quality of synapses at the neuromuscular junction,[59] or simply a decreased motivation to produce large forces. Additional factors on sensorimotor changes in the elderly are reviewed elsewhere.

Evidence exists that the natural decline in active muscle force in the elderly may be reduced with exercise programs that increase levels of physical activity.[48] Earlier in this chapter, we discussed evidence that joint range of motion can also be maintained or improved with exercise. Exercise programs that strive to increase or maintain muscle active force production, as well as maintain joint flexibility and angular velocity, are as rational for elderly persons as those designed for the younger persons. Safe levels of stress imposed on bone during properly designed exercise may decelerate osteoporosis, which offers an additional benefit to exercise with the elderly.

Work vs. Power Considerations.—Relating concepts of work and power to this discussion may add a deeper layer of understanding to the physiologic and practical limitations of an aged musculoskeletal system. The *work* that is performed about a joint during concentric muscle contraction is equal to the product of the average internal torque times the degrees (or radians) of joint rotation. The difficulty an elderly person may have in thoroughly cleaning a window, for example, may arise from *both* variables that define work, since both are expected to naturally decline in the elderly. This is why both "strengthening" and range-of-motion exercises are usually recommended for the elderly.

Power is defined as the rate of performing work. In the example above, the *time* required to clean the window becomes a relevant variable. The average power produced about a joint during a task is determined by the product of the average internal torque times the *average velocity* of the joint movement. Decreased velocity of movement, either from increased resistance from antagonist muscle or increased central processing time, would both result in reduced power. When practical, reducing the time element of a task performance reduces some of the limitations im-

posed by the diminished ability of the elderly person to generate significant power. Often, however, the time element of a task cannot be removed, such as the time required to respond with sufficient muscle force to catch oneself from a fall. In this case, the rate of muscle contraction and subsequent speed of joint rotation may be of greater physiologic importance than the amount of peak muscle force.

Change in Length of Internal Moment Arm.—*Joint posture* may be defined as the habitual position of a joint or series of joints. The length and orientation of the inter-

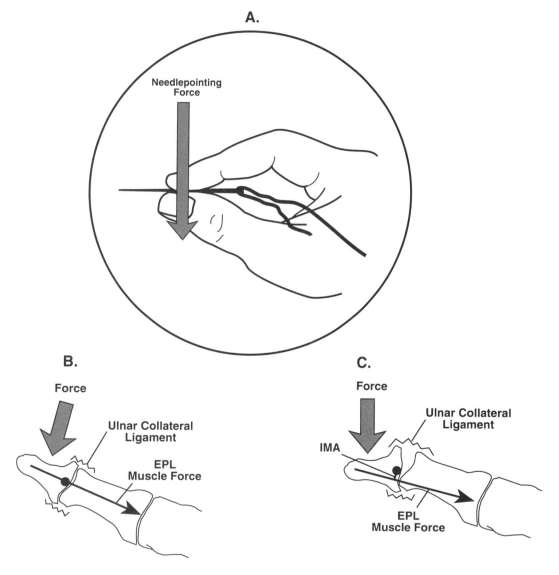

FIG 4–8.
Drawing showing the mechanics involved with thumb interphalangeal *(IP)* deviation deformity secondary to needlepointing activity. **A,** note the "radial" direction of needlepointing force exerted from index finger to the thumb's distal phalanx. **B,** the long-term force causes an excessive and chronic radial deviation torque about the thumb's IP joint. **C,** Throughout the years, the radial deviation torque overstretches the ulnar collateral ligament at the IP joint. The IP deformity created an internal moment arm *(IMA)*, so the extensor pollicis longus *(EPL)* muscle force can now actively radially deviate the IP joint. Axis of rotation for radial deviation torque is shown as a *dark circle.*

nal moment arm may change in the elderly and subsequently alter joint posture. The fact of having lived and worked to old age often provides the time needed for forces to significantly influence the length and therefore effectiveness of the internal moment arm. To illustrate this point, consider the case of a 92-year-old female who has been needlepointing for several hours a day for the last 40 years. She presents with a substantial radial deviation deformity at the interphalangeal (IP) joint of her dominant hand. An analysis of the needlepointing activity in a healthy young hand shows that the index finger produces a radial deviation force that causes the deviation of the IP joint[34] (Fig 4–8,A). Year after year, the chronic tensile forces placed on the IP's ulnar collateral ligament have caused the ligament to elongate beyond its natural length due to the action of a constant external force. The elongated ligament now acts more like a plastic material than an elastic one. The elongated ulnar collateral ligament would offer little resistance to the omnipresent radial deviated (external) torque. What is essential to understand in this particular clinical scenario is that the radial deviated deformity at the IP joint mechanically displaced the tendon of the extensor pollicis longus (compare Fig 4–8,B with 4–8,C). The force line of pull of the thumb extensor now acts with an internal moment arm *that can generate a radial deviation internal torque.* Any active IP extensor muscle activation will now maintain or increase the pathomechanics of the deformity. This self-perpetuating cycle of joint deformity is not limited to the aged population, but this group is particularly susceptible since long periods of time have been available for forces to act on the joints.

The presence of disease may interact with aging and further influence the biomechanics of joint posture. Consider both rheumatoid arthritis and osteoarthritis. Chronic synovitis from rheumatoid arthritis may reduce the ability of the articular capsule to provide resistance to large external torques. A deformity called *ulnar drift* at the metacarpophalangeal joint serves as a prime example of this situation.[17] Also, consider when severe hip osteoarthritis involves a remodeling of the proximal femur such that the distance between the greater trochanter and femoral head diminishes (compare Fig 4–9,A with 4–9,B). The result of this remodeling is a *decrease* in length of the internal moment arm that the hip abductors use to produce frontal plane stability during the stance phase of walking.[66] The hip abductors must therefore produce greater amounts of force during the stance phase in order to offset the loss of length of the internal moment arm. Hip joint forces would therefore increase and possibly stimulate continued bony remodeling with possible continued reduction in internal moment arm length. Once again, a pathomechanical situation is shown to be self-perpetuating. In this case, the del-

eterious effects of the pathomechanics may be alleviated by orthopedic surgery or instruction from physical therapy in the proper use of a cane.[66]

External Joint Torque Considerations

Joint posture is determined by the net effect of all internal and external torques acting about the joint. Recall that *external torque* is the product of a force times the length of the external moment arm (see Fig 4–2). The force component of an external torque may arise from gravity, from a weight applied to a limb, or through some other source that is external to the joint. The external moment arm is the distance from the axis of rotation to the perpendicular intersection with the external force (see Fig 4–2).

Pathomechanics of Senile Kyphosis.— Accentuated kyphosis in the elderly is quite common and may sometimes result in significant disability. This sagittal plane postural asymmetry usually develops gradually over time and is partially responsible for loss of body height in the elderly. Relatively large external (gravitational) torques may develop about the spine of the aged person as a consequence of changes in the mechanics of the connective tissues. To describe the associated pathomechanics, reconsider the ideal standing posture in Figure 4–3, which showed the force line of gravity acting through the center of body mass. Figure 4–10,A illustrates a similar type model of an aged person's spinal column that focuses attention on the cervical and thoracic regions. Note that in ideal standing posture the force line of gravity is directed on the concave side of the normal physiologic curves. This allows the force line to act with an external moment arm that maintains the natural cervical and thoracic curvatures. For purely comparison purposes, assume that a *small* cervical extension torque and *small* thoracic flexion torque are constantly present in the ideal posture of Figure 4–10,A. To limit the rotary extent of these natural cervical and thoracic curvatures, restraining forces must be produced from adjacent tissues. In the thoracic spine, the anterior side of the intervertebral disks are compressed as a result of the natural anterior concavity in the thoracic curve. Since intervertebral disks become more dehydrated and less elastic with advanced age, their effectiveness in resisting compressional forces would diminish.[98] A *small* flexor external torque, *acting over long time periods,* could compress and deform the anterior margins of intervertebral thoracic disks, thereby accentuating the local kyphosis. As the thoracic flexion posture increases, the force line of gravity shifts further anterior, thus increasing the length of the external moment arm and magnitude of the flexed kyphotic posture (Figure 4–10,B).

Sagittal plane X rays of aged adult spines with moder-

A.

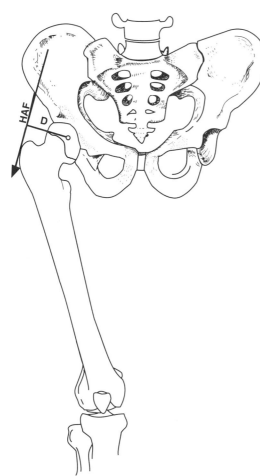

B.

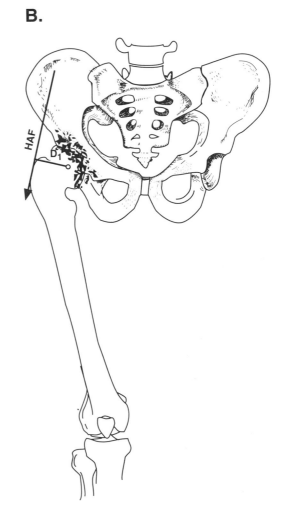

FIG 4–9.
Drawings showing a healthy right hip free of osteoarthritis **(A)** with hip abductor force *(HAF)* and associated internal moment arm *(D)*. Right hip with osteoarthritis is shown **(B)** with diminished internal moment arm *(D₁)* secondary to partial disintegration of femoral head. (From Neumann DA: *Arthritis Care Res* 1989; 2:146–155. Used by permission.)

ate kyphosis often show an anterior translation or shift of the upper thoracic and cervical regions.[61] This anterior shift, observed by comparing Figures 4–10,A and 4–10,B, increases the lengths of the external moment arms, which produces a *moderate* thoracic *and* cervical flexor torque. As a result, increased back extensor muscle force may be needed to hold the person's trunk and head upright. Increased muscle force would increase the magnitude of intervertebral joint forces and possibly predispose arthritic changes, compression fractures, and/or disk injury.[26]

A simple biomechanical principle may be employed to estimate the amount of myogenic joint force transferred across a midthoracic intervertebral segment of a moderately kyphotic spine. Based on an assumption of static equilibrium, the principle states that the sum of the internal and external torques about a joint equals zero.[53, 66] For

sagittal plane rotary equilibrium about a midthoracic region in the spine in Figure 4–10,B, the product of body weight (BW) and the length of the external moment arm (EMA') must equal the product of the muscle force times the length of the internal moment arm (IMA). To estimate the *myogenic* joint force across the *dark circle* indicated in Figure 4–10,B, the extensor muscle force required to maintain the kyphotic spine upright must be estimated. Observe that the length of the external moment arm (EMA') is about twice as long as the associated internal moment arm. The required muscle force therefore can be estimated by multiplying body weight above the chosen axis of rotation times the ratio of EMA':IMA. Assuming BW above the midthoracic vertebra to be 90 lb and moment arm ratio about 2.0, then at least 180 lb of muscle extensor force would be needed to hold the sagittal plane posture of Figure 4–10,B. This force, transferred across a small intervertebral surface area, would result in a relatively large physical pressure that must be supported by adjacent tissue.

Applying this same biomechanical equation to the *ideal* posture shown in Figure 4–10,A, one can estimate an approximate 67% reduction in myogenic joint force at the thoracic spine. This reduction is based on the ideal posture having an external moment arm of only one third the length of that present in the moderately kyphotic posture. This simple mathematical calculation emphasizes the concept that posture and the subsequent length of the ex-

ternal moment arms have a profound effect on forces produced across a joint.

The thoracic posture of Figure 4–10,B may, in extreme cases, progress to that shown in Figure 4–10,C, which was modeled after an actual X ray of a standing elderly person. During standing, this patient showed a small cervical extension torque and a large thoracic flexion torque. Note that despite the large thoracic kyphosis, this particular patient was able to hold her head in enough extension so that the weight of her head assisted in the maintenance of the normal cervical lordosis. However, the

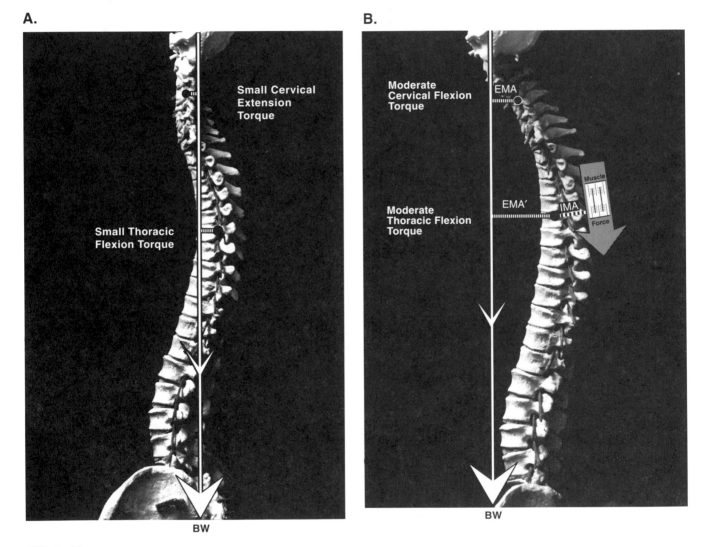

FIG 4–10.

Model showing the orientation of the force line of gravity from body weight *(BW, arrow)* at the cervical and thoracic spine. **A-C** show a progression in severity of kyphosis. Each model demonstrates the mediolateral axis at the midpoint of the thoracic and cervical regions *(dark circles)* and the associated external moment arms *(hatched lines)*. **A,** patient with ideal standing posture and *normal thoracic kyphosis.* Body weight *(BW)* creates a small cervical extension torque and a small thoracic flexion torque. **B,** patient with *moderate thoracic kyphosis.* Body weight *(BW)* creates a moderate cervical and thoracic flexion torque. *EMA'* = external moment arm at thoracic spine midpoint; *EMA* = external moment arm at cervical spine midpoint; *IMA* = internal moment arm for back extensor muscle force.   *(Continued.)*

C.

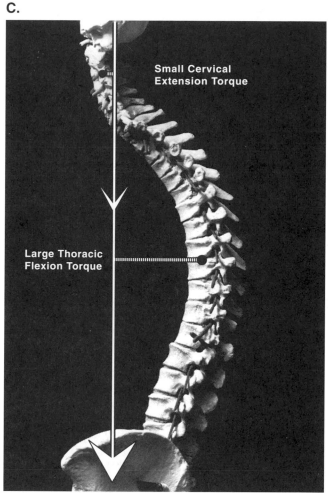

**Small Cervical
Extension Torque**

**Large Thoracic
Flexion Torque**

BW

FIG 4-10 (cont.).
C, patient with *severe thoracic kyphosis.* Body weight *(BW)* causes a small cervical extension torque and a *large* thoracic flexion torque.

main point in Figure 4–10,C to appreciate is the impact that the large external flexor torque would have in the midthoracic region. This large torque will continue as long as the force line of gravity acts with such a large external moment arm length. The increased compression forces produced on the anterior side of the thoracic vertebrae may stimulate bony remodeling with a continued decrease in height of the anterior side of the thoracic bodies. Compression fractures from osteoporosis may augment the kyphosis by increasing the anterior concavity of the middle thoracic spine. This case of severe senile kyphosis should be a reminder of the important role connective tissue has in absorbing the relentless forces of gravity. When aged tissues lose their ability to resist deformation from external forces, gravity wins the ultimate "tug of war" and dominates the clinical course of the posture.

SUMMARY

Arthrokinesiology, or the study of the structure, function, and movement of skeletal joints, is one component of the scientific basis of physical therapy. Age-related changes in joint function can, and do, occur in the elderly, even in the absence of disease. When the effects of disease are coupled with reduced physical activity, the elderly may experience substantial decrements in function. Successful treatment of joint impairments and abnormal posture in the elderly is based on a careful analysis of the pathomechanics of the affected joints.

Acknowledgments

I would like to thank Joan Holcomb, Instructional Media Center, Marquette University, for her ability to draw what I can only visualize. I also extend gratitude to Peter Bland-pied, Ph.D., P.T., for his careful critique of this chapter. Finally, I thank Richard Jensen, Ph.D., P.T., and Marquette University for allowing me the time and resources to continue my intellectual pursuits.

REFERENCES

1. Abrahams M: Mechanical behavior of tendon in vitro. *Med Biol Eng* 1967; 5:433–443.
2. Adrian MJ: Flexibility in the aging adult, in Smith EL, Serfass RC (eds): *Exercise and Aging: The Scientific Basis.* Hillside, NJ, Enslow, 1981.
3. Allander E, et al: Normal range of joint movements in shoulder, hip, wrist and thumb with special reference to side: A comparison between two populations. *Int J Epidemiol* 1974; 3:253–261.
4. Alnaqeeb MA, Al Zaid NS, Goldspink G: Connective tissue changes and physical properties of developing and ageing skeletal muscle. *J Anat* 1984; 139:677–689.
5. Anderson B, Palmore E: Longitudinal evaluation of ocular function, in Palmore E (ed): *Normal Aging II. Reports From the Duke Longitudinal Studies, 1970–1973.* Durham, Duke University Press, 1974.
6. Aniansson A, Hedberg M, Gull-Britt H, et al: Muscle morphology, enzymatic activity, and muscle strength in elderly men: A follow up study. *Muscle Nerve* 1986; 9:585–591.
7. Asmussen E: Aging and exercise, in Horvath J (ed): *Environmental Physiology: Aging, Heat and Altitude.* Amsterdam, Elsevier, 1980.
8. Asmussen E, Bonde-Peterson F: Apparent efficiency and storage of elastic energy: Human muscle during exercise. *Acta Physiol Scand* 1974; 92:537–545.
9. Badley EM, Wagstaff S, Wood PHN: Measures of functional ability (disability) in arthritis in relation to impair-

ment of range of joint movement. *Ann Rheum Dis* 1984;43:563–569.

10. Balazs EA: Intercellular matrix of connective tissue, in Finch C, Schneider EL (eds): *Handbook of the Biology of Aging.* New York, Van Nostrand Reinhold, 1977.

11. Bassey EJ, Morgan K, Dallosso HM, et al: Flexibility of the shoulder joint measured as range of abduction in a large representative sample of men and women over 65 years. *Eur J Appl Physiol* 1989; 58:353–360.

12. Bell RD, Hoshizaki TB: Relationships of age and sex with range of motion of seventeen joint action in humans. *Can J Appl Sport Sci* 1981; 6:202–206.

13. Boone DC, Azen SP: Normal range of motion of joints in male subjects. *J Bone Joint Surg* 1979; 61A:756–759.

14. Bornstein P, Sage H: Structurally distinct collagen types. *Annu Rev Biochem* 1980; 49:957–1003.

15. Bortz WM: Disuse and aging. *JAMA* 1982; 248:1203–1208.

16. Botelho SY, Cander L, Guiti N: Passive and active tension-length diagrams of intact skeletal muscle in normal women of different ages. *J Appl Physiol* 1954; 7:93–95.

17. Brand PW: *Clinical Mechanics of the Hand.* St Louis, CV Mosby, 1985.

18. Brandt KD, Fife RS: Ageing in relation to the pathogenesis of osteoarthritis. *Clin Rheum Dis* 1986; 12:117–130.

19. Buckwalter JA, Kuettner KE, Thonar EJ–M: Age-related changes in articular cartilage proteoglycans: Electromicroscopic studies. *J Orthop Res* 1985; 3:251–257.

20. Burstein AH, Reilly DT, Martens M: Aging of bone tissue, mechanical properties. *J Bone Joint Surg* 1976; 58A:82–86.

21. Butler DL, Grood ES, Noyes FR, et al: Biomechanics of ligaments and tendons, in Hutton RS (ed): *Exercise and Sports Sciences Reviews,* vol 6. Philadelphia, Franklin Press, 1979.

22. Campbell ML, McComas AJ, Petito F: Physiological changes in aging muscle. *J Neurol Neurosurg Psychiatry* 1973; 36:174–182.

23. Caplan A, et al: Skeletal muscle, in Woo SL-Y, Buckwalter JA (eds): *Skeletal Muscle Injury and Repair of the Musculoskeletal Soft Tissues.* Park Ridge, Ill, American Academy of Orthopaedic Surgeons, 1988.

24. Chapman EA, deVries HA, Swezey R: Joint stiffness: Effects of exercise on young and old. *J Gerontol* 1972; 27:218–221.

25. Cochran GVB: *A Primer of Orthopaedic Biomechanics.* New York, Churchill Livingstone, 1982.

26. Cook TM, Neumann DA: The effects of load placement on the EMG activity of the low back muscles during load carry by men and women. *Ergonomics* 1987; 30:1413–1423.

27. Diamond MC, Johnson RE, Protti AM, et al: Plasticity in the 904-day-old male rat cerebral cortex. *Exp Neurol* 1985; 87:309–317.

28. Downie AW, Newell DJ: Sensory nerve conduction in patients with diabetes mellitis and controls. *Neurology* 1961; 11:876–882.

29. Dummer GM, Vaccaro P, Clarke DH: Muscular strength and flexibility of two female Master's Swimmers in the eighth decade of life. *J Orthop Sports Phys Ther* 1985; 6:235–237.

30. Freeman MAR: The fatigue of cartilage in the pathogenesis of osteoarthritis. *Acta Orthop Scand* 1975; 46:323–328.

31. Freeman MAR, Meachim G: Ageing and degeneration, in Freeman MAR (ed): *Adult Articular Cartilage,* ed 2. Kent, England, Pitman Medical Publishing, 1979.

32. Freeman MAR, Todd RD, Pirie CJ: The role of fatigue in the pathogenesis of senile femoral neck fractures. *J Bone Joint Surg* 1974; 56B:698–702.

33. Gallagher JC, Melton LJ, Riggs BL, et al: Epidemiology of fractures of the proximal femur in Rochester, Minnesota. *Clin Orthop* 1980; 150:163–171.

34. Garncarz C, OTR: Personal communication, Sept 23, 1991.

35. Ghosh P: Articular cartilage: What it is, why it fails in osteoarthritis, and what can be done about it. *Arthritis Care Res* 1988; 1:211–221.

36. Grahame R: A method for measuring human skin elasticity in vivo with observations on the effects on age, sex, and pregnancy. *Clin Sci* 1970; 39:223–238.

37. Grimby G, Aniansson A, Zetterberg C, et al: Is there a change in relative muscle fibre composition with age? *Clin Physiol* 1984; 4:189–194.

38. Hall DA: *The Ageing of Connective Tissue.* New York, Academic Press, 1976.

39. Ham AW, Cormack DH: *Histology* ed 8. Philadelphia, JB Lippincott, 1979.

40. Hamlin CR, Kohn RR: Determination of humans' chronological age by a study of a collagen sample. *Exp Gerontol* 1972; 7:377–379.

41. Hayes D, Jerger J: Neurotology of aging: The auditory system, in Albert ML (ed): *Clinical Neurology of Aging.* New York, Oxford University Press, 1984.

42. Heine J: Über die Arthritis deformans. *Virchows Arch Pathol Anat Physiol Klin Med* 1926; 260:521–663.

43. Hill AV: *First and Last Experiments in Muscle Mechanics.* Cambridge, Cambridge University Press, 1970.

44. Hogan DB: Imposed activity restriction for the elderly. *Am Coll R Med Clin Can* 1985; 18:410–412.

45. James B, Parker AW: Active and passive mobility of lower limb joints in elderly men and women. *Am J Phys Med Rehabil* 1989; 68:162–167.

46. Kennedy R, Clemis JD: The geriatric auditory and vestibular systems. *Otolaryngol Clin North Am* 1990; 23:1075–1082.

47. Kokmen E, Bossemeyer RW, Williams WJ: Neurological manifestations of aging. *J Gerontol* 1977; 32:411–419.

48. Kutal I, Parizkova J, Dycka J. Muscle strength and lean body mass in old men of different physical activity. *J Appl Physiol* 1970; 29:168–171.

49. Lanyon LE, Hartman W: Strain related electrical potentials in vitro and in vivo. *Calcif Tissue Res* 1977; 22:315–327.

50. Larsson L: Morphological and functional characteristics of

the ageing skeletal muscle in man. *Acta Physiol Scand [Suppl]* 1978; 457:1–29.

51. Lehmkuhl LD, Smith LK: *Brunnstrom's Clinical Kinesiology*. Philadelphia, FA Davis, 1983.

52. Levarlet-Joye H, Simon M: Study of statics and litheness of aged persons. *J Sports Med* 1983; 23:8–13.

53. Le Veau B: *Williams and Lissner: Biomechanics of Human Motion*, ed 2. Philadelphia, WB Saunders, 1977.

54. Lexell J, Henriksson-Larson B, Winbled B, et al: Distribution of different fiber types in human skeletal muscle: Effects of aging studied in whole muscle cross sections. *Muscle Nerve* 1983; 6:588–595.

55. Martin AD, McCulloch RG: Bone dynamics: Stress, strain, and fracture. *J Sports Sci* 1987; 5:155–163.

56. Mayne R, Buckwalter JA: Collagen types in cartilage, in Kuettner KE, Schieyerbach R, Hascall VC (eds): *Articular Cartilage Biochemistry*. New York, Raven Press, 1986.

57. Mazess RB: On aging bone loss. *Clin Orthop* 1982; 165:239–252.

58. McDonagh MJN, White MJ, Davies CTM: Different effects of ageing on the mechanical properties of human arm and leg muscles. *Gerontology* 1984; 30:49–54.

59. McMartin DN, O'Conner JA: Effect of age on axoplasmic transport of cholinesterase in rat sciatic nerves. *Mech Ageing Dev* 1979; 10:241–248.

60. Meachim G: Cartilage fibrillation on the lateral tibial plateau in Liverpool necropsies. *J Anat* 1976; 121:97–106.

61. Memorial Hospital of Oconomowoc, Radiology Department, May 1991, Oconomowoc, Wi.

62. Minns RJ, Soden PD, Jackson DS: The role of the fibrous components and ground substance in the mechanical properties of biologic tissues. A preliminary investigation. *J Biomech* 1973; 6:153–165.

63. Mohan S, Rahada E: Age related changes in rat muscle collagen. *Gerontology* 1980; 26:61–67.

64. Munns K: Effects of exercise on the range of motion in elderly subjects, in Smith EL, Serfass RC (eds): *Exercise and Ageing: The Scientific Basis*. Hillside, NJ, Enslow Publishers, 1981.

65. Murray MP, Kory RC, Clarkson BH: Walking patterns in healthy old men. *J Gerontol* 1969; 24:169–178.

66. Neumann DA: Biomechanical analysis of selected principles of hip joint protection. *Arthritis Care Res* 1989; 2:146–155.

67. Neumann DA, Cook TM: Effect of load and carry position on the electromyographic activity of the gluteus medius muscle during walking. *Phys Ther* 1985; 65:305–311.

68. Neumann DA, Soderberg GL, Cook TM: Comparison of maximal isometric hip abductor muscle torques between hip sides. *Phys Ther* 1988; 68:496–502.

69. Neumann DA, Soderberg GL, Cook TM: Electromyographic analysis of hip abductor musculature in healthy right-handed persons. *Phys Ther* 1989; 69:431–440.

70. Olson MA, Smidt GL, Johnston RC: The maximal torque generated by the eccentric, isometric, and concentric contractions of the hip abductor muscles. *Phys Ther* 1972; 52:149–157.

71. Peress NS, Kane WC, Aronson SM: Central nervous system findings in a tenth decade autopsy population. *Prog Brain Res* 1973; 40:473–483.

72. Price H: Connective tissue in wound healing, in Kloth LC, McCulloch JM, Feedar JA (eds): *Wound Healing: Alternatives in Management*. Philadelphia, FA Davis, 1990.

73. Raab DM, et al: Light resistance and stretching exercise in elderly women: Effect upon flexibility. *Arch Phys Med Rehabil* 1988; 69:268–272.

74. Radin EL, Paul IL, Tolkoff MJ: Subchondral bone changes in patients with early degenerative joint disease. *Arthritis Rheum* 1970; 13:400–405.

75. Rauterberg J: Age-dependent changes in structure, properties, and biosynthesis of collagen, in Platt D (ed): *Gerontology, 4th International Symposium*. New York, Springer-Verlag, 1989.

76. Rigby BJ: Aging pattern in collagen in vivo and in vitro. *J Soc Cosmet Chem* 1983; 34:439–451.

77. Roach KE, Miles TP: Normal hip and knee active range of motion: The relationship to age. *Phys Ther* 1991; 71:656–665.

78. Rogers J, Bloom FE: Neurotransmitter metabolism and function in the aging central nervous system, in Finch C, Schneider EL (eds): *Handbook of the Biology of Aging*, ed 2. New York, Van Nostrand Reinhold, 1985.

79. Rosenberg LC, Buckwalter JA: Cartilage proteoglycans, in Kuettner KE, Schieyerbach R, Hascall VC (eds): *Articular Cartilage Biochemistry*. New York, Raven Press, 1986.

80. Sabin TD, Venna N: Peripheral nerve disorders in the elderly, in Albert ML (ed): *Clinical Neurology of Aging*. New York, Oxford University Press, 1984.

81. Sams WM, Smith CJ: Alterations in human dermal fibrous conective tissue with age and chronic sun damage, in Montagna W (ed): *Ageing*. Advances in Biology of Skin, vol 6. Oxford, Pergamon Press, 1965.

82. Schmidt RF, Wahren LK, Hagbarth KE: Multiunit neural responses to strong finger vibration. I. Relationship to Age. *Acta Physiol Scand* 1990; 140:1–10.

83. Smith EL, Reddan W, Smith PE: Physical activity and calcium modalities for bone mineral increase in aged women. *Med Sci Sports Exerc* 1981; 13:60–64.

84. Soderberg GL: *Kinesiology: Applications to Pathological Motion*. Baltimore, Williams & Wilkins, 1986.

85. Sokoloff L: *The Biology of Degenerative Joint Disease*. Chicago, University of Chicago Press, 1969.

86. Spirduso WW: Physical fitness, aging, and psychomotor speed: A review. *J Gerontol* 1980; 35:850–865.

87. Staff PH: The effects of physical activity on joints, cartilage, tendons, and ligaments. *Scand J Soc Med Suppl* 1982; 29:59–63.

88. Stelmach GE, Worringjam CJ: Sensorimotor deficits related to postural stability. *Clin Geriatr Med* 1985; 1:679–725.

89. Threlkeld AJ, Currier DP: Osteoarthritis: Effects on synovial tissues. *Phys Ther* 1988; 68:364–370.

90. Vandervoot A, Hayes KC, Belanger AY: Strength and

endurance of skeletal muscle in the elderly. *Physiother Can* 1986; 38:167–173.

91. Verzar F: Ageing of the collagen fibre, in Hall ED (ed): *International Review of Connective Tissue Research,* vol 2. New York, Academic Press, 1964.

92. Viidik A: Biomechanics and functional adaptation of tendons and joint ligaments, in FG Evans (ed): *Studies on the Anatomy and Function of Bones and Joints.* Berlin, Springer, 1966.

93. Viidik A: Functional properties of collagenous tissues. *Int Rev Connect Tissue Res* 1973; 6:127–215.

94. Walker JM, Miles-Elkousy N, Ford G, et al: Active mobility of the extremities in older subjects. *Phys Ther* 1984; 64:919–923.

95. Warwick R, Williams PL (eds): *Gray's Anatomy,* ed 36 (Br). Philadelphia, WB Saunders, 1980.

96. Weightman B, Kempson GE: Load carriage, in Freeman MAR (ed): *Adult Articular Cartilage,* ed 2. Kent, England, Pitman Medical Publishing, 1979.

97. Williams PR, Goldspink G: Connective tissue changes in immobilized muscle. *J Anat* 1984; 138:343–350.

98. Woo SL-Y, Buckwalter JA: *Injury and Repair of the Musculoskeletal Soft Tissues.* Park Ridge, Ill, American Academy of Orthopaedic Surgeons, 1988.

99. Wright V, Johns RJ: Physical factors concerned with the stiffness of normal and diseased joints. *Bull Johns Hopkins Hosp* 1960; 106:215–231.

100. Yano K, Wasnich RD, Vogel JM, et al: Bone mineral measurements among middle-aged and elderly Japanese residents in Hawaii. *Am J Epidemiol* 1984; 119:751–764.

CHAPTER 5

Sensorimotor Changes and Adaptation in the Older Adult

Rebecca L. Craik, Ph.D., P.T.

INTRODUCTION

Age-related decline in sensorimotor performance is a controversial and complex phenomenon. The controversy is focused on the premise that decline in function is due to some subtle underlying pathology rather than the natural processes of aging. Stated in its extreme form, an argument is made that if aging is not responsible for decline in function, then it follows that if disease were controlled, animals and humans would be immortal.[55] As there has been no scientifically validated report of an immortal, totally healthy human or animal, the assumption that disease alone is responsible for functional decline appears invalid. This chapter assumes that aging itself does produce a deterioration of sensorimotor performance, even in otherwise healthy individuals.

The complexity surrounding decline in the quality and quantity of movement is focused on a number of different factors that can contribute to a decline in sensorimotor performance. Declining performance with increased age could be the result of changes intrinsic to the individual, factors extrinsic to the individual, or a combination of both. Some intrinsic factors directly associated with the integrity of the individual's cognitive status and the neuromusculoskeletal system include changes in such variables as neurons, central or peripheral synaptic mechanisms, peripheral nerves, peripheral receptors, muscle, bone, or joints. Other intrinsic factors such as the status of hormones, the cardiovascular system, the respiratory system, and basal metabolism play an indirect but critical role in guaranteeing the integrity of the sensory and muscular systems. Extrinsic factors that can affect the normal function of the neuromusculoskeletal system include death of a spouse, retirement from an occupation, retirement from community involvement, loss of income, change in nutritional status, decline in physical activity level, and inadequate health care. The relationship between age-related decline in the quality or quantity of movement and variables that influence the decline presents a multifactorial problem.

The perfect theory of motor control should offer a framework or model that proposes the interaction within and between intrinsic and extrinsic factors to produce motion. Age-related change in any variable would lead to a predictable change in behavior that could be confirmed by measurement. A variety of motor control theories have been proposed to account for movement, and discussion of these models can be found in two recent publications.[35, 111]

The scope of this chapter will be limited to identifying some of the intrinsic changes that occur in the sensorimotor system including the brain. The assumption will be made that sensation must be intact for the individual to learn and to execute the myriad of motor behaviors produced by the human. Since any model of motor control assumes integrity of the neuromusculoskeletal system, the information presented in this chapter should be relevant regardless of the motor control model assumed.

The purpose of this chapter is to present the kinds of changes that occur in the sensorimotor system of the aging human. A commonly uttered classroom phrase is, "Who cares?" In this case, the question should be more specific: "Why should a physical therapist care about cellular or systems changes associated with aging?" Perhaps the most important reason to care is to emphasize the multiple factors that influence the older person's ability to produce a particular movement in the clinical situation. As more knowledge about performance is gained, it is important to remember the impact of the systems involved in producing the performance. If the nervous system or muscle is incapable, is less capable, or uses different strategies to respond to external stimuli, then clinicians need to be aware of such information to guarantee treatment effectiveness. Age-related changes in function have to be considered as a background to the person who presents in the clinical situation with another primary diagnosis. For example, the older person who had a stroke may recover differently from the younger person who had a stroke because of the age-dependent changes in the sensorimotor system of the older person. This chapter will highlight the changes that occur with aging in the sensorimotor system so that this information can be integrated with the knowledge of various disease processes to provide a more realistic view of clinical expectations for the older person for the clinician and patient.

A variety of research techniques used by individuals in a number of different disciplines will be presented in this chapter. Since individual researchers focus on a specific aspect of aging, there is a need to integrate information collected from a variety of laboratories that have used very different techniques to gather an "impression" of age effects on the whole system—the person. The student who is interested in the impact of aging on sensorimotor changes is therefore faced with a myriad of information from a variety of disciplines that are all relevant to what may have seemed to be a simple question.

Aging is a process that should be considered as spanning development, adulthood, and senescence. While it is difficult to describe any of the processes without consideration of the entire life span, this chapter will focus on the changes seen in the older adult with little emphasis on life span changes.

This chapter assumes a working knowledge of neuroscience, and the reader is encouraged to use a neuroscience textbook as a companion to this chapter. Several figures of normal anatomy have been included to remind the reader of names and locations of some of the nervous system structures referred to in the text.

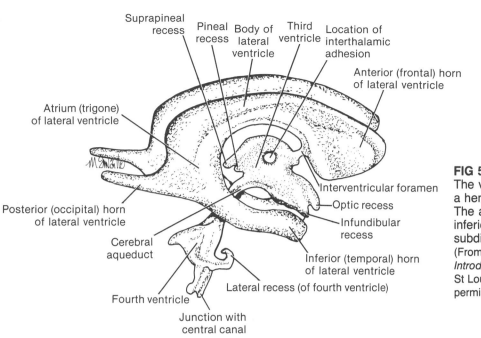

FIG 5–1.
The ventricular system is projected into a hemisected brain to show its location. The anterior horn, body, posterior horn, inferior horn, and atrium are the subdivisions of the lateral ventricles. (From Nolte J: *The Human Brain: An Introduction to Its Functional Anatomy*, ed 2. St Louis, Mosby–Year Book, 1988. Used by permission.)

The chapter is subdivided into five major sections. The first section will focus on neuroanatomic and neurochemical changes that have been reported to occur in the central nervous system (CNS), with primary emphasis on the brain; in the second section, changes in various sensory systems including the visual, auditory, vestibular, and somatosensory systems will be reviewed; the third section will examine the age-related changes reported in the motor unit, including the muscle and its peripheral efferent connections; the fourth section will examine changes in the sensorimotor system and include a discussion of reflex and reaction time testing; and the final section will discuss the possibility of adaptation in the older individual.

BRAIN CHANGES AND NORMAL AGING

One theory associated with the process of aging is that mitotic cells undergo a programmed number of cell doublings until cell division ceases in the senescent cell.[67] Loss of the ability to replicate is, therefore, thought to be a primary mechanism in the aging process. How does this theory apply to the neuron? Neurons are postmitotic cells, that is, cells that do not divide. What causes the loss of neurons and synapses? Is there an indication that the morphology of the aging brain is different from the younger brain? When is the neuron considered an aging cell? Clinically, the assumption has been made that loss of synapses, and therefore loss of neurons, leads to the development of dementia.[78] These are the questions that this section will try to address.

Morphology and Physiology

Neuroanatomic Changes in the CNS
Gross Brain Changes.— An age-related linear decrease in adult brain weight has been well documented, although the rate of decline is controversial.[74] The general trends noted from earlier studies where autopsy materials were used to study brain weight have been confirmed by more recent studies that have used computed tomography (CT), positron emission tomography (PET), or magnetic resonance imaging (MRI) to examine the brain.

Peress et al.,[121] using 7,579 brains from autopsies of subjects from the third to the tenth decade, concluded that both males and females showed a steady linear decline in brain weight and that the decline was in both the supratentorial and infratentorial areas. Miller et al.[105] studied 91 brains from ages 20 to 98 years and found no change until age 50, then a 2% decrease per decade. Other investigators suggest a decrease in brain weight from early adulthood to the tenth decade ranging from 6.6% to 11%.[46] More recent work that has normalized brain weight to body weight and carefully screened for mentally intact individuals continues to support an age-related decline in brain weight and volume.[78]

Changes in gross morphology accompany the change in overall brain weight or volume. The two features examined most frequently are a decline in the physical dimensions of gyri, known as *gyral atrophy,* and ventricular dilation (Fig 5–1). Gyral atrophy describes a decrease in the gray or white matter or both. Significant gyral atrophy is not found throughout the cerebral cortex but appears to be limited to specific regions.[46]

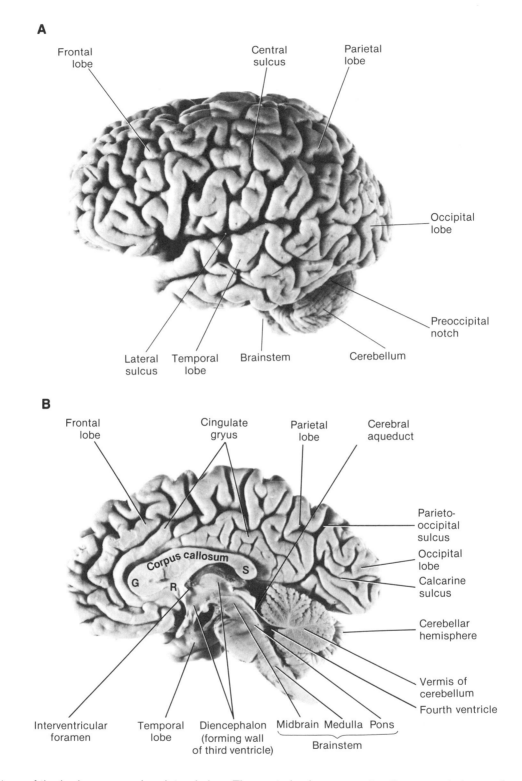

FIG 5–2.
A, major regions of the brain are seen in a lateral view. The central sulcus separates the precentral gyrus from the postcentral gyrus. **B,** regions of the cerebrum, cerebellum, and brain stem shown in a sagittal plane. The portions of the corpus callosum, the major pathway for communication between the left and right hemispheres, are the rostrum *(R)*, splenium *(S)*, and genu *(G)*. (From Nolte J: *The Human Brain: An Introduction to Its Functional Anatomy*, ed 2. St Louis, Mosby–Year Book, 1988. Used by permission.)

In a recent study of healthy men, ranging from 31 to 87 years of age, there was postcentral gyrus atrophy (Brodmann areas 1, 2, 3) in the left parietal lobe and gyral atrophy in association areas (Brodmann areas 5 and 7) of the right parietal lobe in the older subjects[130] (Figs 5–2 and 5–3). There is some significant individual variation in gyral atrophy, and there is also a significant linear correlation in decreasing gyral thickness with increasing age.[50] Some evidence suggests a relationship between a specific area of atrophy and function.[54, 107] For example, enlargement of the left lateral sulcus (fissure of Sylvius), suggesting loss of cortical tissue, has been correlated with decreased intellectual performance.[54] Much additional study using neuropsychologic protocols will be required to define the relationship between mental or functional status and specific areas of cortical atrophy.

Ventricular dilation has also been reported to accompany aging and decreased brain weight.[81] The lateral ventricles have been examined most frequently, and in general, a progressive increase in the size of the ventricles occurs up to the seventh decade, followed by a marked ventricular increase in individuals in the eighth and ninth decade. It is not clear whether an increase in ventricular size is a reliable predictor of impaired intellectual function.

Collectively, decreases in brain weight, gyral thickness, and increase in ventricular size suggest that neurons are lost through the life span. There are an estimated 20 billion neurons in the human brain, and it has been estimated that humans lose approximately 50,000 to 100,000 neurons each day. Age-related changes in the brain weight or brain volume might represent an acceleration of this normal cell loss, or aging might be defined when a critical number of neurons are lost and function is compromised.

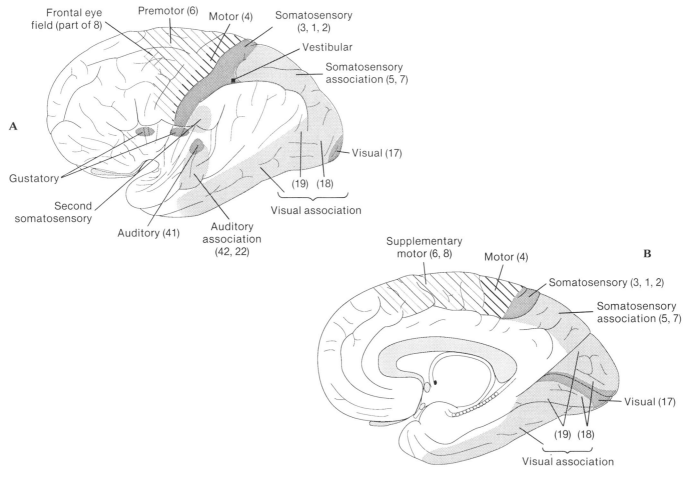

FIG 5–3.
These two diagrams illustrate some of the functional areas of the cerebral cortex and their approximate associations with Brodmann's areas. Brodmann's areas 9 and 10 are not depicted here but are found anterior to the premotor cortex in the frontal lobes and are associated with cognition and other higher functions. (From Nolte J: *The Human Brain: An Introduction to Its Functional Anatomy*, ed 2. St Louis, Mosby–Year Book, 1988. Used by permission.)

If a standard were established for the normal rate of decline of neurons, then a faster rate of decline in brain volume, brain weight, or number of cells might indicate pathology. For example, the demonstration of a significant correlation between a decrease in brain volume and impairment on a dementia rating scale in subjects ranging from the third to the eighth decade might indicate when the decrease in brain volume was pathologic and when it was dependent on age.[73]

Histologic Changes in Brain Anatomy.—The microscopic changes in the anatomy of the brain parallel the gross changes summarized above. Neuronal and glial cell losses have been documented in the aging human cerebrum and brain stem.[69] By the ninth decade, 30% to 50% of cortical neurons are lost in certain areas.[18]

Compiling the results across several studies, all four lobes of the brain show cell loss, with the most severe cell loss in the frontal and temporal lobes.[4, 19, 81] The higher-order association areas, for example, visual association cortex (area 21) and prefrontal cortex (area 10), display greater cell loss than primary motor cortex (area 4) and primary visual association cortex (area 18) (Fig 5–3).

All areas of the hippocampal formation show neuronal cell loss that is age related. Although the precise function of the hippocampal formation is still not understood, it has been associated with learning and memory in the human. No age-related cell loss has been reported in certain portions of the basal ganglia, hypothalamus, or a variety of brain stem nuclei (Fig 5–4). To date, the locus coeruleus (LC) appears to demonstrate the most significant decline in neurons of the brain stem structures that have been examined.[18] LC is found in the brain stem reticular formation at the rostral end of the floor of the fourth ventricle within the pons and midbrain and is rich in neurons containing norepinephrine. Changes in the cerebellum appear confined to the Purkinje neurons; the reduction becomes apparent in the sixth decade.[37] A relationship between loss of Purkinje neurons and age-related changes in motor behavior has not been well established. To summarize, cell loss is more general in the cerebral cortex and hippocampus but highly selective in the basal ganglia, brain stem, and cerebellum.

Prior to cell death, neurons undergo a decrease in the size of the cell body (perikaryon), decreases in number of dendritic spines, and decreases in dendritic length[40, 151]

(Fig 5–5). Some neurons retain the capacity for dendritic growth, which will be discussed in a later section.

In addition to the changes in neurons, there are other changes of the aging brain. The most common changes reported are the presence of lipofuscin, the senile or neuritic plaque, and the neurofibrillary tangle (NFT).

Lipofuscin is a dark, pigmented lipid found in the cytoplasm of aging neurons.[19] The effect of this pigment on cell function is not known at this time. Although there is speculation that an excessive accumulation of lipofuscin may interfere with the function of the neuron, the primary role for lipofuscin at this time is as a hallmark of an aging neuron.[46]

Neuritic (senile) plaques are discrete structures, located outside of the neuron.[46] The plaque is composed of degenerating small axons, some dendrites, astrocytes, and amyloid. Although the senile plaque is found in human disease,[160] it is also reported as a normal age-related change.[109] The plaques have been reported to occur beginning in the fifth decade; to be located primarily deep in the sulci of the neocortex, hippocampus, and amygdala; and to increase in number with increasing age. An increased number of plaques has been related to dementia.[78, 79]

While the neuritic plaque is thought to occur most often in the neocortex, NFTs have been reported to occur in the hippocampal formation and in specific brain stem nuclei in the healthy aging brain.[4] The origin of the NFT is unknown, but it is distinguished in structure and location from the plaque.[159] The NFT appears to occur within the perikaryon and is first identified with silver stain as a darkly stained, thick band that later increases and becomes twisted. The NFT often displaces the nucleus and distorts the cell body. Like the plaque, the NFT is noted to increase in incidence with age, but an even greater incidence, particularly in neocortex, accompanies dementia.

CNS Metabolism and Cerebral Blood Flow

Glucose is the main substrate for cerebral metabolism. The classic view is that cerebral blood flow (CBF) is regulated to meet the requirements of cell metabolism. Various studies have shown the relationship among the rate of cerebral glucose utilization, the need for oxygen to support glucose metabolism, and the integrity of CNS function.[141] Metabolic rates of glucose utilization in the intact human can now be examined using radioactive glucose analogues and PET scans.[126] The assumption that cerebral atherosclerosis

FIG 5–4.   →
A, a coronal (frontal plane) section through the brain. The position of the section in the intact brain is indicated by the *vertical line* in **B** and **C**. The section is through the anterior portion of the diencephalon, so that parts of the thalamus are seen. The caudate, putamen, and globus pallidus are components of the basal ganglia. **D,** is posterior to the coronal section in **A**. The location of the section within the brain is indicated by the *vertical line* in **E** and **F**. Note the position of the hippocampus, which is a portion of the limbic system. (From Nolte J: *The Human Brain: An Introduction to Its Functional Anatomy,* ed 2. St Louis, Mosby–Year Book, 1988. Used by permission.)

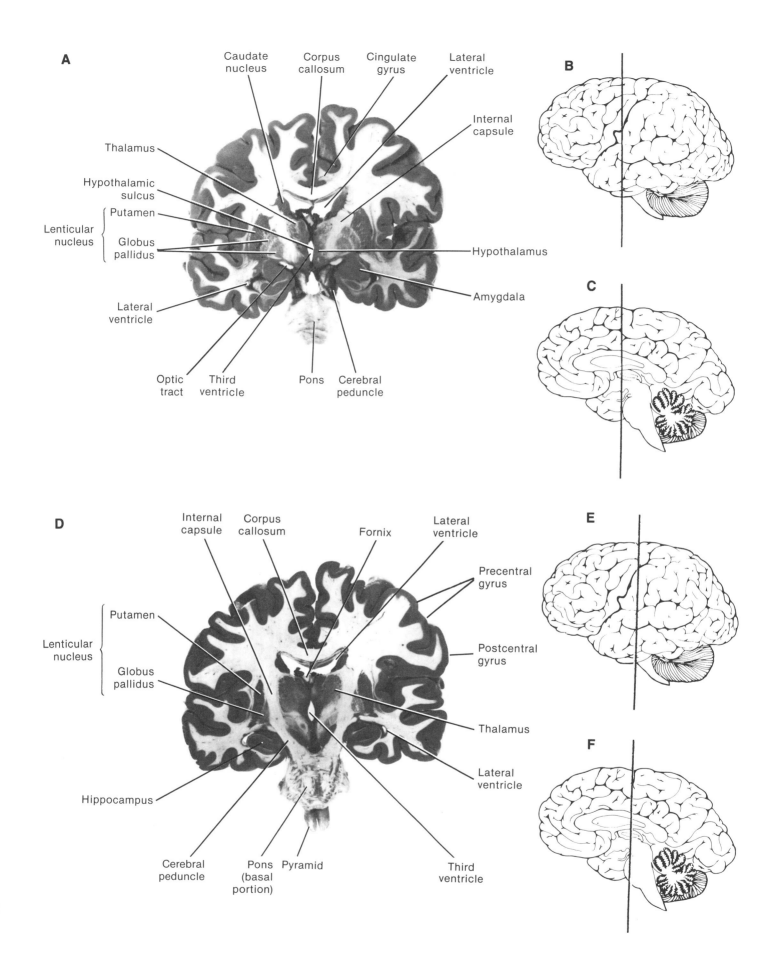

A

Caudate nucleus

Corpus callosum

Cingulate gyrus

Lateral ventricle

Internal capsule

Thalamus

Hypothalamic sulcus

Lenticular nucleus
- Putamen
- Globus pallidus

Lateral ventricle

Hypothalamus

Amygdala

Optic tract

Third ventricle

Pons

Cerebral peduncle

B

C

D

Internal capsule

Corpus callosum

Fornix

Lateral ventricle

Precentral gyrus

Lenticular nucleus
- Putamen
- Globus pallidus

Postcentral gyrus

Thalamus

Lateral ventricle

Hippocampus

Cerebral peduncle

Pons (basal portion)

Pyramid

Third ventricle

E

F

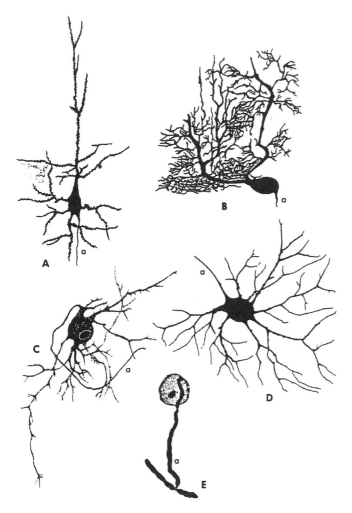

FIG 5–5.
There are a variety of forms of neurons. The neuron in **A** is a pyramidal cell and typical of the cerebral cortex. The bumps on the dendrites are dendritic spines, which appear to enhance synaptic contact area. The axon is labeled *a* in each of the illustrations. The Purkinje cell, the neuron depicted in **B,** may be viewed as the final common pathway leaving the cerebellar cortex. **C,** a sympathetic postganglionic neuron. **D,** an alpha motoneuron; a motor unit consists of this neuron and all the muscle fibers it innervates through its branching axon. The neuron depicted in **E** is a dorsal root ganglion cell. (From Willis WD, Grossman RG: *Medical Neurobiology: Neuroanatomical and Neurophysiological Principles Basic to Clinical Neuroscience*, ed 3. St Louis, Mosby–Year Book, 1988. Used by permission.)

is a natural consequence of the aging process has led to the proposal that poor CBF is the primary mediator of brain aging.[148]

The belief that compromised CBF leads to less oxygen and glucose delivery, which, in turn, compromises neurons and leads to neuronal death, has been challenged. CBF and cerebral metabolic rate of oxygen utilization diminish with normal aging. A rapid decline in CBF and cerebral metabo-lism has been proposed from the first to the third decade of life, whereas a more gradual decline occurs from the third to the tenth decade.[83] The rate of decline in CBF and metabolism are not regarded as important. It has been noted that CBF and metabolism may change at different rates.[74] The age-related rates of decline in blood flow, oxygen need, or glucose utilization by the brain are not profound enough to account for the extent of brain atrophy that accompanies aging. Other reasons for cortical atrophy must be examined to account for changes in the aging neuron.

Summary

A wide variety of changes in brain anatomy and physiology have been described to occur in aging. The extent of such changes is used to distinguish the normal aging brain from a brain with pathology such as senile dementia and Alzheimer's disease (AD). To understand the difference between aging and pathology, relationship among gross morphology, cell integrity, and loss of behavior in persons with AD will be discussed briefly.

AD brains show specific gyral atrophy, NFT, and increased density of neuritic plaques in the association areas of the neocortex and the hippocampal structures. The number of plaques in the neocortex appear to correlate with mental status and functional ability.[14] In a recent review, some of the cellular changes were examined that may lead to the changes in gross morphology and function in the person with AD.[78]

Abnormal phosphorylation or dephosphorylation of proteins within neurons might lead to the early formation of the neurofibrillary tangle. Excessive intracellular NFT may in turn alter other cellular processes. Amyloid beta/A 4-protein precursor (APP) is regulated by many growth factors and is an important protein involved in the regulation of cell growth and neuronal development. Abnormal processing of APP may produce a nonfunctional or cytotoxic protein. Abnormal processing of APP in Alzheimer's disease may lead to an important alteration in the neuron's ability to function. Loss of function of neurons critical to cognitive status may account for marked gyral atrophy, increased density of plaques, and dementia seen in persons with AD.

There is not adequate research to relate the loss of cortical neurons or their connections to decline in cognitive function in the healthy aging human. Neither is there evidence to suggest that decreases in CBF and cerebral metabolism are the primary factors leading to the loss of neurons. Additional research is needed to relate the changes in anatomy and physiology to changes in functional performance. The literature reviewed thus far has pointed out the importance of the combined efforts of basic and clinical research to produce a better understanding of function. The need for standards of normal changes in neuroanatomy that accompany aging is also evident. Without definition of normal, it will remain difficult to define abnormal.

Neurochemical Changes in the CNS With Aging

Morphologic changes in the aging brain just described are accompanied by neurochemical changes. Primary neurotransmitters (NTs) include acetylcholine, dopamine, norepinephrine, serotonin, gamma-aminobutyric acid (GABA), amino acid neurotransmitters, opiod peptides, and other peptide neurotransmitters. Detailed reviews of the age-related changes for the neurotransmitters and the intracellular action of NTs are available.[97, 127] Since most of the research related to NTs and aging was derived from animal models, caution must be exercised in generalizing the research findings to humans. This section will focus only on acetylcholine and dopamine as examples of the kind of research being conducted to relate to changes in neurotransmitters.

Acetylcholine

Acetylcholine (ACh) is essential to the function of the central and peripheral nervous systems and is utilized in both the somatic and autonomic nervous systems. Whole brain assays for the amount of ACh show a small, insignificant decline with aging.[127] There is evidence, however, to suggest a decline in synthesis as well as spontaneous release of ACh with age.[158] Perhaps the overall amount of ACh does not show significant reduction in aging brains because a decreased release of ACh compensates for a decreased synthesis of ACh. Such an assumption suggests that measuring the amount of a particular neurotransmitter from whole brain assays does not provide a true understanding of what is occurring at the cellular level.

Since ACh is found in the hippocampus, and the hippocampus is one of the structures associated with memory and learning, many investigators have tried to establish a link between the presence of ACh and the integrity of short-term memory. For example, animal models that demonstrate a loss of cortical acetylcholine demonstrate a selective memory loss of recent events and information.[11] Other investigators have reported reduced cortical ACh content in the aging human and a profound loss of acetylcholine in specific cortical sites in patients with AD.[58]

Acetylcholinesterase (AChE) is responsible for the inactivation of ACh. Some studies suggest an age-related decline,[101] whereas others suggest no change in AChE with age.[122] A decline in the number of cholinergic receptors has also been reported with age.[127]

A variety of studies using both animals and humans suggest that appropriate pharmacologic or dietary manipulation improves short term memory losses under certain conditions. Rogers and Bloom[127] reviewed a series of experiments in animals and humans that suggested that the AChE inhibitor, physostigmine, or dietary supplements using one of the precursors for acetylcholine, choline or lecithin, showed some promise for delaying or improving senile cognitive deficits. The results are controversial at this time, and additional work is necessary before treatment efficacy is demonstrated.

Dopamine

Although dopamine (DA) is widespread in the CNS, the most frequently studied dopaminergic neurons are those located in the substantia nigra that project to the striatum of the basal ganglia.[127] The dysfunction of these neurons is directly related to Parkinson's disease. DA is also located in the diencephalon and the medulla. Changes in the synthesis, inactivation, catabolism, content, and receptors have all been reported with aging. The synaptic actions of DA are terminated by presynaptic reuptake and by actions of such enzymes as monamine oxidase. Again, the research identifying age-related change to each of the aspects of metabolism and catabolism is incomplete and controversial.

In general, there is consensus that the amount of DA present and the number of receptors in the striatum of the basal ganglia decrease after the fourth decade. On the other hand, the number of receptors increases in persons with Parkinson's disease. Rogers and Bloom[127] explain this disparity by suggesting that the person with Parkinson's disease may still be able to compensate for the decreased amount of neurotransmitter, whereas the aging individual may have lost this compensatory capacity. The administration of L-dopa, a precursor of DA that crosses the blood-brain barrier, has been shown to improve motor function in aged rats and in humans with Parkinson's disease. Much additional research is needed, particularly in regard to the role of DA in motor function of aging human individuals. Mortimer[110] suggested that if the loss of the number of dopaminergic cells in the normal-aged individual was extended to the level of cell count found in persons Parkinson's disease, normal cell counts would approach those of Parkinson's disease at approximately 100 years of age. Thus, he proposed that if more individuals lived to the limit of human age span, the incidence of Parkinson's disease would be greater. This has led to the proposal that Parkinson's disease is an acute and intense aging change,[101, 102] but this view is challenged by other investigators.[131]

Summary

There is evidence to suggest that age-related changes occur in each of the major neurotransmitters, but the precise mechanism that produces a change in NT content is not known. Aging can affect a variety of steps between synthesis of the NT to the final production of a response in the postsynaptic cell. It is difficult to relate the loss of a specific NT to a decline in function in an individual. Loss of function may be related to the synergistic effect of multiple neurotransmitters, or loss of function may reflect an age-related lack of balance between neurotransmitters. At this time the role of neurotransmitters and behavior is still at the descriptive level. Much work needs to be completed before it will be obvious if dietary or pharmacologic supplementation will increase the synthesis or action of a particular neurotransmitter and thereby retard aging or improve function.

Memory and Aging

The integrity of the brain is reflected in the cognitive status of the individual. Since a later chapter in this book will deal with cognition in detail, cognitive state will only be mentioned here as it relates to age-related changes in function and behavior. The description of the morphologic, physiologic, and neurochemical changes in the brain suggests that cognition may change with aging. Early theories of memory proposed that "engrams" for specific memories were contained within a single neuron, whereas other theories placed all aspects of memory and learning within one brain region, the medial temporal lobe. Memory is now viewed as a "multicomponent" process rather than a unitary function.[125] Certain structures are proposed to be associated with a particular aspect of learning and memory. For example, the hippocampal formation and the medial dorsal nucleus of the thalamus are believed to play a critical role in the formation of fact-based, context-dependent memories.[1, 161] The amygdala appears to be important for memory that requires the association of information from different sensory modalities[56] (see Fig 5–4). Other cognitive processes, such as the organization of information in both spatial and temporal contexts, appear dependent on prefrontal cortex.[60]

As expected, all memory functions are not equally susceptible to aging. Studies of normal aging indicate that immediate memory remains intact when tested immediately, but impairment is present when memory for recent events is tested over longer retention intervals.[52] Memory for specific classes of information such as spatial, temporal, or verbal information appears to be differentially compromised during aging.[120] Some patients showing the severe cognitive impairment that accompanies AD display normal motor learning[68] and a relative preservation of very remote memories.[129] The presence or absence of age-related deficits appears to depend on the specific information-processing demands of the tasks. In other words, the results of research to date indicate that memory impairment is task dependent.

In a recent review[39] it was noted that cognitive functioning in older individuals is test dependent. Older individuals do not show significant deterioration when vocabulary and knowledge of the world are tested. Age-related decline is present, however, when the test requires novel combinations and new learning. Such results suggest that memory is not a process that is separate from total cognitive ability. The author argued that instead of trying to correlate anatomic structures with memory loss, investigators should be examining the brain's potential to reconstruct patterns of activity with aging.

A loss of behavior in the presence of age-related changes in the brain has been demonstrated. Additional research needs to be done before mechanisms for specific memory loss are identified and before clinical treatment of memory loss in aging individuals is successful.

SENSORY CHANGES WITH AGING

A generally accepted concept is that sensory integrity declines with aging. The clinician is interested in learning which sensory systems are affected and which part of the system is affected. Are there specific targets of the pathway that are more susceptible to the process of aging? Is there a decrease in the speed with which the nervous system responds to external stimuli in the older individual? If so, where is the change occurring? Are the afferent, central, and efferent systems equally affected by age?

The Visual System

There is a gradual decline in visual acuity prior to the sixth decade, followed by a rapid decline in many patients from 60 to 80 years of age.[2] Visual acuity may decline as much as 80% by the ninth decade. Impairment of visual accommodation has been noted.[17] By age 40 to 55, visual correction is necessary in most people for accurate near vision.

Visual acuity is a measure of visual discrimination of fine details.[32] Since the very center of the macula, the portion of the retina rich in cones, is the portion of the retina used for fine discrimination, a standard eye chart tests the integrity of the cones in the macula and their connection with the visual pathway. Testing for visual acuity with an eye chart assumes that the ability of the eye to resolve the smallest letter demonstrates the eye's ability to resolve larger objects and that contrast is not important.[32] Such assumptions are valid for reading; letters are small, and there is high contrast between the letters on the written page and the background. The need to resolve fine details of high contrast may not be meaningful for other visual tasks such as recognizing a step in a dimly lit hallway or recognizing a larger object such as a face in a crowd of faces. Therefore, traditional acuity testing may describe the person's ability to read but may not test "functional" vision.

Traditionally, changes in visual acuity have been related to a change in the optical portion of the visual system, the structures within the eyeball.[32] The small pupil that occurs with aging, the clouding of the lens, and its inability to change its shape (accommodation) were the primary targets for visual correction in the older individual. Impairment in other aspects of the visual system also accompanies aging so that correction of the optical system in the aging individual may not lead to improved functional vision.

Presentation of a visual stimulus such as a reversing checkerboard pattern to the human eye will reliably evoke consistent electrocortical activity. The visual evoked response (VER) has a characteristic deflection pattern and predictable latency, and results of using this technique have been reviewed.[123] Following maturation, there is a general slowing in the latency of the VER to stimuli with high spatial frequency that appears age related. The slowing has been proposed to occur due to a decrease in the number of axons in the optic nerve and changes in processing in the thalamus and occipital cortex. Although additional research is necessary to correlate the electrical with physical findings, some of the changes in the visual system will be reviewed that may account for the increased latency in the visual pathway.

Age-related changes have been demonstrated beginning at the retina. Photoreceptors demonstrate an age-related loss, as does the function of the ganglion cells within the retina and of their axons which project to the thalamus.[53] The number of neurons in portions of the primary visual cortex (area 17) is significantly reduced with aging.[43] A loss of one half of the cells that process information has been proposed based on the comparison of neuronal density at age 20 to neuronal density at age 80. Therefore, it is obvious that aging affects more than just the optical system.

Other age-related deficits in the visual system have been noted.[32, 136] Aging affects the integrity of the visual fields, dark adaptation, and color vision. There is a differential loss of sensitivity to blue, but there is also some loss of sensitivity over the entire spectrum by the fourth decade. Spatial visual sensitivity decreases in the older adult, especially to low spatial frequencies and slow-moving targets.

The motor integrity of the visual system is not spared during aging. Pupillary responses are diminished, or even absent, and the size of the resting pupil decreases markedly.[96] The corneal touch threshold increases throughout life, although the decline is more rapid after the fifth decade. By the ninth decade, corneal sensitivity is reported to be only one half to two thirds as great as in the second and third decades.[106] The corneal blink reflex may be entirely absent in elderly normal patients.

The ocular motor system also undergoes a progressive loss.[32] Convergence is compromised, ptosis occurs, and there is a symmetric restriction in upward gaze. Smooth pursuit, saccades, and optokinetic nystagmus are each reduced in the elderly.

In summary, corrected visual acuity in the older individual may not lead to enhanced functional vision. There are a variety of changes that occur along the visual sensory and visual motor pathways that lead to a host of age-related changes in the visual system. Careful functional visual screening is essential for elderly persons who are having difficulty maneuvering in the environment.

The Auditory System

Although changes in the auditory system have been demonstrated as early as the fourth decade, functional impairment is not evident typically until the seventh decade.[66] Over one half of all Americans who suffer significant hearing loss are 65 years or older.

Presbycusis, age-related decline in auditory function, is the most common cause of hearing loss in adults.[12] Presbycusis can reflect cellular aging in the peripheral, auditory, and CNS pathways as well as acoustic trauma, cardiovascular disease, and the cumulative effects of ototoxic medications. Presbycusis can occur for at least two distinct reasons; (1) changes in the peripheral sensory organ, the outer, middle, or inner ear; or (2) changes in the central pathway and the auditory portions of the cerebral cortex. The peripheral structures are related more to hearing sensitivity, whereas the central systems are related more to understanding speech, especially under difficult listening conditions.

Age-related changes in hearing include a slowly progressive bilateral hearing loss, affecting high-frequency sensitivity first and later involving loss across the entire frequency spectrum.[66] These changes are related to age-related changes in the cochlea. Word recognition and sentence identification tasks both show an age-related exponential decline, suggesting a decline in perceptual processing of the temporal characteristics of speech.

Results from a recent study reinforce the data just presented where 1,662 men and women were examined between the ages of 60 and 90 years.[57] Pure-tone thresholds increased with age, but the rate of change with age did not differ by gender even though men had poorer threshold sensitivity. Maximum word recognition ability declined more rapidly in men than in women. Hearing aids were being used in only 10% of subjects likely to benefit from these devices.

The relationship between satisfaction with hearing aid

use and the site of lesion was studied in another investigation.[99] As the site of lesion moved from peripheral to central, subject satisfaction with the hearing aid declined. In subjects with purely peripheral, conductive hearing loss, satisfaction with hearing aid use was as high as 84%. In subjects with a change in the CNS, satisfaction declined to less than 15%.

In summary, aging can produce different hearing disorders which interfere with social interaction. Since a primary mode of communication with our patients is verbal, the clinician should be aware of any impairment to the auditory system.

The Vestibular System

Since other chapters in this book will address the functional aspects of the vestibular system, this section will focus on neuroanatomic or physiologic changes and some functional correlates that have been cited for the vestibular system during aging.

The vestibular end organs are responsible for transforming the forces associated with head acceleration into action potentials producing subjective awareness of head position in space (orientation) and motor reflexes for postural and ocular stability.[5] The utricle and saccule sense linear acceleration, and the semicircular canals monitor angular acceleration. At rest, the afferent nerves from these structures maintain a bilateral balanced tonic rate of firing. The tonic activity and its change in level with head movement are used in cortical, brain stem, and spinal centers to elicit the appropriate vestibulo-ocular and vestibulospinal responses.

Presbyastasis is the term to describe age-related disequilibrium when no other pathology is noted.[82] Studies of the vestibular system indicate an age-related 20% decline in hair cells of the saccule and utricle and a 40% reduction in hair cells in the semicircular canals.[75] Age-related changes in the morphology of the vestibular system correspond to changes in vestibular function using caloric testing, douching the auditory canal with warm or cold water and examining ocular responses.[82] Young patients respond with involuntary eye movements of high frequency and large amplitude when warm or cold water is placed in the auditory canal, compared with persons older than 60 years. It is not clear whether these changes reflect a change in the integrity of the labyrinth, a release of CNS modulation, or vascular changes.

Presbyastasis must be distinguished from pathology of the vestibular system in older individuals. Vertigo, nystagmus, and postural imbalance may be symptoms of age-related decline if underlying vestibular pathology is ruled out. The incidence of presbyastasis in the healthy aging population is not available.

The literature suggests that disequilibrium may be attributed to the normal aging of the vestibular system in addition to other factors, which include vestibular pathology, changes in other sensory systems, and changes in the motor system. Differentiating the causes for disequilibrium may lead to more successful treatment intervention.

The Somatosensory System

Anatomic Changes

What indication is there that the morphologic and physiologic changes of the peripheral receptors, afferent pathways, and CNS affect the integrity of the somatosensory sensation? Birren and Schaie[12] cite over 4,000 references on age-related changes in normal human somatosensory function. The problem with many of these studies is that they isolate a single variable for testing such as position sense. It is difficult, therefore, to gain an understanding of how the entire sensorimotor system changes within one individual.

A number of age-related changes in the peripheral nervous system (PNS) have been documented.[128] Morphologic changes in the nerve cells, roots, peripheral nerves, and specialized nerve terminals have been linked with the aging process. Meissner's corpuscles, which detect touch and are limited to hairless skin, decrease in concentration with age[15] (Fig 5–6). In old age, the corpuscles become sparse, irregular in distribution, and highly variable in size and shape. Pacinian corpuscles, responsible for sensing repetitive features of touch such as vibratory stimuli, undergo age-related change in morphology and decrease in density. Merkel cells, which are also touch receptors, do not appear to demonstrate significant age-related change.[135]

In addition to an age-related decline in some of the receptors, there is also an age-related decline in afferent nerve fibers (Table 5–1). A 32% loss of fibers in both the dorsal and ventral roots of T8 and T9 at age 90 years has been reported.[36] The degeneration of the dorsal columns that occurs with aging may reflect the loss of centrally directed axons of the dorsal root ganglion cells. The longer fibers composing the gracile columns are most affected in this process.[112]

The peripheral nerves also show a similar degree of dropout with aging.[116] Age-related loss of fibers in cranial nerves and spinal nerve roots affects thick fibers more than thin fibers.[146] The anatomic site of the nerve may be important since preferential large-fiber loss has been reported in the sciatic, anterior tibial, and sural nerves, for example, but not in the superficial radial nerve.[118, 146]

Aging is also associated with a gradual shortening of the internodal length. The distance between the nodes of Ranvier is normally greater on fibers of larger diameter. Irregularities of internodal length occur in the nerves of older indi-

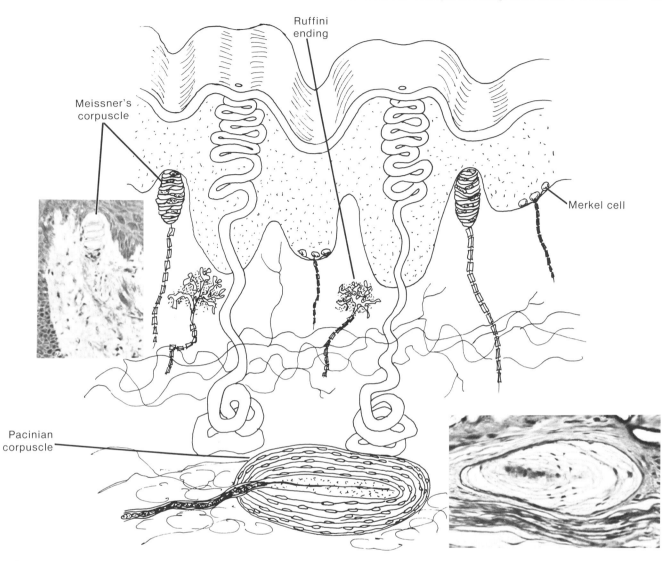

FIG 5-6.
Some of the sensory endings found in hairless (glabrous) skin are illustrated. Note the position of the various mechanoreceptors. Meissner's corpuscles are limited primarily to hairless skin. (From Nolte J: *The Human Brain: An Introduction to Its Functional Anatomy*, ed 2. St Louis, Mosby–Year Book, 1988. Used by permission.)

viduals.[64, 93, 153] Abnormally short internodes for a given axon diameter might result either from segmental demyelination and remyelination or as a result of complete degeneration of fibers followed by regeneration. Since the longer the distance between nodes the faster the saltatory conduction, the shortened internodes contribute to an increased conduction velocity, and therefore, the action potentials may take longer than usual to reach the CNS.

Physiologic Changes
Physiologic age-linked alterations in the PNS have also been documented.[88] While a gradual decline in maximal nerve conduction velocity has been described in some studies,[44, 45] no significant change in normal sensory and

motor conduction velocity is reported in other studies.[104] Table 5–1 lists conduction velocities for peripheral nerve fibers. The collective data on age-related changes in conduction velocity do not suggest that changes are substantial enough to account for the degree of sensory loss reported in older individuals.

The integrity of the sensory pathway from the periphery to various regions within the CNS has been examined using the somatosensory evoked potential (SEP).[42] Peripheral nerve stimulation produces a variety of potentials that can be recorded from the scalp, over the spine, or in the periphery. If recorded from the scalp, the SEP has components that are focally restricted to the somatosensory area contralateral to the stimulated side. Electrical stimulation

TABLE 5-1.

Conduction Velocities, Diameters, and Functions Associated With Various Peripheral Nerve Fibers.*

Roman Numeral Classification	Diameter	Letter Classification	Conduction Velocity	Myelinated	Types of Structures Innervated
Ia	12–20 μm	Not used	70–120 m/sec	Yes	Muscle spindle primary endings
Ib	12–20 μm	Not used	70–120 m/sec	Yes	Golgi tendon organs
Not used	12–20 μm	α	70–120 m/sec	Yes	Efferents to extrafusal muscle fibers
II	6–12 μm	Aα†	30–70 m/sec	Yes	Other encapsulated endings and endings with accessory structures: Meissner's corpuscles, Merkel endings, muscle spindle secondary endings, and so on
Not used	2–10 μm	γ	10–50 m/sec	Yes	Efferents to intrafusal muscle fibers
III	1–6 μm	Aδ	5–30 m/sec	Yes	Some nociceptors; some cold receptors; some hair receptors
Not used	<3 μm	B	3–15 m/sec	Yes	Preganglionic autonomic efferents
IV	<1.5 μm	C	0.5–2 m/sec	No	Most nociceptors; some cold receptors; warmth receptors; some mechanoreceptors; postganglionic autonomic efferents

*From Nolte J: *The Human Brain: An Introduction to Its Functional Anatomy,* ed 2. St Louis, Mosby–Year Book, 1988. Used by permission.
†Some afferents in nonmuscle nerves, particularly joint afferents, range up to 17 μm in diameter. Some investigators refer to these larger fibers, in the 12–17 μm range, as Aα and call those in the 6–12 μm range Aβ. Others refer to all nonmuscle afferents larger than 6 μm as Aα.

is most often used to elicit SEPs, but a mechanical stimulus can also be used. Commonly used peripheral nerves are the median and the peroneal.

SEPs change with maturation and age.[115] Normative data are still being collected, but in general, the latencies appear to increase with increased adult age. The amplitude of the SEP recorded from the scalp appears to decrease with age. Evoked potentials to peroneal nerve stimulation recorded from surface electrodes placed over the spine also show an age-related increase in latency from the lumbar to the cervical region. A delay in central rather than peripheral somatosensory axons is proposed by some investigators as the primary site for the age-related slowing in the SEP.

When sensory detection is studied quantitatively, a progressive impairment with age is noted in many, but not all, peripheral cutaneous modalities. For example, touch-pressure perception approaches a fourfold reduction in males over age 40.[49] The sensory threshold increases the more distal the stimulus application site.[59] Schmidt and colleagues[134, 135] used microneurography to record from median nerve fibers in 12 subjects ranging from 18 to 64 years of age. An age-related decline to flutter and tap (light touch) was reported that appeared due more to changes in the peripheral sensory units rather than conduction along the afferent nerves. Stereognosis, graphesthesia, and double simultaneous stimulation usually remain intact with aging. Although an increase in the thresholds for light touch and pinprick have been reported from laboratory investigations, similar losses are not reported consistently in clinical studies. There are two possibilities that may explain the discrepancy between laboratory and clinical results: (1) the laboratory-reported loss of touch is not a functional loss or (2) clinical testing is not sensitive enough to detect a significant loss. There are no data to support either explanation at this time.

Cutaneous threshold for vibration increases, with lower extremities more affected than upper extremities.[86, 104] Diminished or lost vibratory sensation in the lower extremities has been reported to be present in 10% of individuals at age 60 and in approximately 50% of individuals beyond age 75.[71] Cutaneous pain threshold increases with age.[150] Increased threshold to thermal sensitivity has been reported in laboratory testing, but clinical testing has not indicated an age-related functional decline in thermal modalities with age.

Proprioception has undergone relatively little study in the aging population, and the results are controversial. Perception of passive motion in the metacarpophalangeal and metatarsophalangeal joints was reported to be similar in young and older subjects.[87] Although older subjects detected motion less well at low frequencies of movement, there was not a major decline reported in joint motion sensation. Similarly, impairment of proprioception rarely occurred in a neurologic screening of a sample of subjects ranging from 67 to 87 years of age.[10] On the other hand, passive movement thresholds were reported to be twice as high for the hip, knee, and ankle, with no change in upper extremity perception in subjects over 50 years of age compared with subjects less than 40 years of age.[89] Skinner et al.[140] examined joint position sense of the knee in 29 subjects ranging in age from 20 to 82 years. Both the abilities to reproduce passive knee position and to detect motion were assessed. Joint position sense deteriorated with increasing age as measured by both tests. A more recent study compared the subject's perception of a passively positioned knee angle using a visual analogue scale to the actual angle and reported an age-related decline in position sense.[8] The perception was reported to increase by 40% by applying an elastic bandage around the knee. The research to date on position sense suggests that age-related loss of position sense may be joint specific.

Potvin et al.[124] assessed neurologic status on 61 right-hand dominant men ranging from 20 to 80 years of age. One hundred and thirty-eight tests were used to measure cognition, vision, strength, steadiness, reactions, speed, coordination, fatigue, gait, station, sensation, and tasks of daily living. Tests were excluded if reliability was not demonstrated. Age-related linear decreases were reported for many neurologic functions. The declines over the age span varied from less than 10% to more than 90%, depending on the function. Larger losses of function were observed on the dominant body side.

For the upper and lower extremities, vibratory sensibility showed the greatest decline. The greatest vibratory loss was reported in the toes and ankle. Vibratory loss in the toes and the ankle was also the variable most highly correlated with aging; that is, the oldest subjects demonstrated the poorest ability to detect a vibratory stimulus. Touch of face and upper arm, two-point discrimination, and position sense in upper and lower limbs showed no variance with age. Since the actual testing procedures were not described, it is difficult to compare the results of this study with other research findings. This study serves as a background for additional research since the results address the integrity of the entire sensorimotor system in a large sample of subjects.

Summary

There are a paucity of data that describe age-related changes in somatosensory sensation. The literature is not conclusive because samples remain small, the oldest subjects in some studies are only 65 years of age, different modalities of sensation are not studied in the same population, and protocols differ. Very little attention has been paid to the age-related changes in skin that could also affect the older person's ability to detect a stimulus without directly altering the peripheral receptor or the afferent pathway.[138] Another important deficit in the literature to date is that integrity of one sensation is not studied throughout the body. It is common, for example, to study change in sensation in the knee alone, rather than to report changes in the major joints of the body. This research approach makes it difficult to summarize changes in age-related changes in sensation that occur throughout the body.

Some investigators have used very sophisticated laboratory techniques to document changes in sensation, but the results have not been supported by investigators using standard clinical neurologic screening techniques. Caution must be exercised in generalizing findings about sensory changes reported in one body region to the whole body, or changes reported in one study to the population of healthy older individuals.

The portion of the sensory system primarily responsible for changes in sensation is unclear. Since age-related cutaneous deficits are more often reported in the lower extremities than upper extremities, age-related changes in the afferent pathways are likely to play some role in the sensory changes. The numbers of peripheral receptors decrease, and there is a loss of 5% to 8% of nerve fibers per decade after age 40.[128] Increasing numbers of abnormalities in myelination are reported with increasing age; longer fibers and larger fibers are most affected. A progressive slowing of maximal sensory and motor conduction velocities at a year's rate of 0.12 to 0.16 m/sec has been proposed, and conduction along central afferent pathways to cerebral cortex is prolonged. It appears that the relatively small changes in the conduction velocity along peripheral afferent fibers do not contribute significantly to loss of sensory perception. The loss of peripheral receptors, changes in central afferent pathways, and changes in central processing sites are more likely to be responsible for age-related changes.

The consistent findings across studies are that sensation in the lower extremity appears more affected by aging than the upper extremity and that vibratory sensation is consistently reported to decline with age. Since the integrity of each sensory system is most often tested under static conditions rather than during functional behavior, it is very difficult to predict if seemingly small changes in separate systems will aggregate to produce a profound loss during the execution of a task. Such an assumption needs to be tested under carefully controlled conditions. Additional research must be done before we can interpret the clinical significance of sensory changes with aging on motor performance.

MOTOR UNIT CHANGES WITH AGING

It is difficult to focus on changes in muscle without considering changes in the function of the muscle or the activity level of the individual. This section will focus on the integrity of the aging motor unit (MU); changes in the rate or quality of movement and the effect of physical activity on muscle will be addressed in a subsequent section of this chapter and in other chapters. The MU is defined as the single alpha motoneuron and all the muscle fibers it innervates. It is therefore important to examine changes in the muscle, the neuromuscular junction, and the efferent neuron to completely discuss changes with aging. A commonly reported clinical finding is that older individuals demonstrate decreased strength when compared with younger individuals.[23, 31, 114, 152] *Strength* has been defined operationally in a number of different ways. For the purpose of this chapter, *strength* is defined as some measure of the muscle's force-producing capability such as peak torque, work, or force. What is the reason for a decline in force-producing capability with age? This section will begin by examining changes in the muscle.

Muscle

One of the common changes in aging muscle is reduction in mass, from 25% to 43%, depending on activity level.[94, 137] The decrease in mass is more prominent in lower extremity muscle groups than in upper extremity muscle groups.[63] Consistent with this finding is a reduction in the compound muscle action potentials generated after maximal excitation of the motor nerve and a decrease in strength.[152]

Is the atrophy fiber-type specific? A simple description of the composition of muscle includes the slow twitch, or type I, fibers and the fast twitch, or type II, fibers. There is consensus that both type I and type II fibers demonstrate atrophy with aging in sedentary people.[3, 62, 132] Although there is not consensus that fast twitch fibers (type II) demonstrate more pronounced fiber loss, the majority of studies support this hypothesis. Caution is urged in generalizing the data that support a preferential atrophy of fast twitch fibers in the human; many studies have utilized the vastus lateralis or the biceps brachii. Because all muscles have not been examined, it is possible that different muscles that serve different functions may age differently.[154]

While electrophysiologic[28] and histologic[62] studies support a preferential type II atrophy with aging, results from studies that use histochemistry have produced conflicting data. A common histochemical technique is staining muscle biopsies for actomyosin myofibrillar adenosine triphosphatase (ATPase) because type I and type II fibers contain different ATPases.[21] Larssen et al.[92] reported an age-related decrease in the relative proportion of type II fibers, but other investigators have not confirmed these findings with histochemical techniques.[3, 51] The myosin heavy chain (MHC) composition of a fiber determines its contractile characteristics, and it is MHC that reacts with ATPase stain to yield a muscle fiber type.[41] Recent work suggests that the conflict among investigators using histochemical techniques may be because older fibers are in

transition from one type to another and that the transition is undetected by ATPase stain. For example, examination of MHC within single fibers suggests that older subjects have a higher number of single fibers that contain two forms of MHC,—type I and IIa,—within one fiber than is seen in the younger subjects.[85]

The degree of atrophy does not fully account for the observed loss of strength, suggesting that factors other than simple loss of tissue mass are involved. A wide range of morphologic changes within both type I and type II fibers have been reported. Changes have been reported in mitochondria, sarcoplasmic reticulum, and the transverse tubular system.[65, 149] The physiologic effects of these changes are not known but have been suggested to be coupled with an impaired activation of the myofibrils.[65] Muscle satellite cells, which transform into myoblasts, may also be metabolically less active, and the older muscle may, therefore, not be able to respond to injury as well as the young muscle.

Only modest decreases in high-energy metabolites (adenosine diphosphate [ADP], adenosine triphosphate [ATP], and phosphocreatine) have been reported in the aged muscle.[108] Other enzymes necessary for glycolysis are reduced, however, suggesting a specific disturbance in cytoplasmic glycolysis and gluconeogenesis.[113] Fatty acid patterns appear unchanged in the aged.[147]

Neuromuscular Junction

The neuromuscular junction has been studied, and synaptic failure has been reported to occur more frequently in aged animals.[65, 103] The disturbance in neuromuscular contact is proposed to be related to a marked decrease of protein synthesis in senile motor neurons and the slowing of axoplasmic transport. One theory to account for the muscle changes is a progressive decrease in the trophic factor or trophic (nourishing) function of the nerve cells that results in the random loss of muscle fibers and a decrease in the size of the MU.

Subtle Pathology

Myopathic and neuropathic changes have been reported in aged muscle.[112] Myopathic changes include proliferation of Z-band material, increased numbers of sarcolemmal nuclei, necrosis, and lysosomal accumulations. Neuropathic changes include signs of denervation, and some degree of fiber type grouping. Reinnervation creates an extra burden on the remaining nerve cells, and muscle wasting has been suggested to occur when the pool of viable neurons becomes critically reduced.[152]

Motoneurons

Functioning motoneurons (MUs) appear to decline with age.[144] For example, the number of functioning MUs in both hand and foot muscles has been reported to decline.[22, 28] The remaining MUs become enlarged despite the finding that strength decreases.

Although extensive accurate, quantitative anterior horn cell counts have not been carried out in many human studies, an age-related decline in anterior horn cells is suggested in the available data. A selective loss of small anterior horn cells that subserve the gamma system and small MUs has been noted in the human spinal cord.[80] Axonal counts reveal a significant decrease in both anterior and posterior roots beginning after age 30. By age 89, a 32% reduction in anterior root axons is reported.[48] The reduction includes both large and small myelinated fibers. The remaining axons demonstrate demyelination and remyelination.

Peripheral nerve motor conduction velocities decrease progressively with advancing age.[76] In the ulnar nerve, a reduction of 1 m/sec a decade from age 20 to 55 and 3 m/sec a decade after this age has been reported.[24] However, such slowing may not be as significant as the other age-related changes in the muscle.

Function

What is the relationship between the age-related changes in the neuromuscular system and the muscle's ability to generate force? Other chapters in this book will also describe age-related changes in strength and functional movement changes. However, a brief summary will be offered here to examine mechanisms associated with changes in strength and movement.

Vandervoort et al.[152] reviewed a series of studies that examined isometric muscle torque in groups of young and old adults. The average maximal voluntary contraction (MVC) was at least 20% lower by the seventh decade than in young adults. More advanced age groups show a greater decline, with the suggestion that very old people have only about one half the strength of young adults in their limb muscles. Conclusions from the review were the following: the older the subject, the greater the reduction in strength; the pattern of strength loss is similar for different muscle groups whether they be proximal or distal or located in the upper or lower limbs; and the percentage decrement in old age is similar for males and females.

Is the decline of strength attributed to the declining muscle mass? Kallman et al.[77] conducted a study on 847 healthy volunteers, aged 20 to 100 years. Grip strength was strongly correlated with muscle mass but more strongly correlated with age. Therefore, it appears that factors in addition to decreased muscle mass might account for the age-related decline in ability to generate maximum isometric tension. Osteoarthritis, activity level, and motivation, for example, may each contribute to an age-related decline in force-generating ability. Decreased size and possibly decreased percentage of fast twitch fibers may lead to a loss of strength. Decline in the number of functioning MUs and motoneuron changes are also factors to be considered as contributing to reduced muscle function.

A prolonged patellar reflex time has been noted in healthy older males.[90] Since reflex latency appears relatively unchanged, the delay has been related to the motor time component (the time required to activate the muscle). A prolongation of contraction time, latency, twitch tension rate, and relaxation time have all been noted. Decline in muscle strength has been suggested to represent a circular deterioration: impairment of neural stimulation leads to less powerful muscle contraction, which leads in turn to muscular degeneration, whereas lack of feedback from muscular contraction leads to neural degeneration. Results and theories such as these support the notion that it is not possible to understand muscle function without consideration of the nervous system.

Summary

The best established and functionally more significant changes that have appeared in the literature include the following: a reduced static and dynamic ability to produce torque; atrophy of type I and II myofibers, with a suggested greater type II atrophy; a loss of alpha motoneurons; and a reduced oxidative capacity of exercising muscle. Although myopathic and neuropathic changes have been reported, they appear modest, and no consistent pattern across muscles has been observed. Changes suggestive of denervation are the most common reported pathology, but it is difficult to determine whether these are age linked or secondary to other diseases such as diabetes, nerve root compression, or disuse. All the cited changes suggest aged muscle may have a reduced capacity to respond to injury. While the decline in muscle strength is strongly correlated to muscle mass, other factors also interact to produce the loss of strength seen with aging. Additional research must be completed before the reported anatomic and physiologic changes can be related to a decline in functional performance. Careful study of the strength of a number of muscles within an individual and careful control of physical activity and the presence of subtle disease are necessary before the effect of age on muscle function is understood.

SENSORIMOTOR CHANGES WITH AGING

Paucity of movement is a common observation in old animals and humans.[142, 143] The limited movement becomes hesitant and slow. Even when the speed of movement is retained, the initiation of movement is delayed. Sensorimotor integrity has been examined using a variety of protocols including the study of reflexes, the time it takes the subject to respond to and execute a task, and functional performance. Since other chapters in this book will address age-related decline in functional activities, this section will focus on studies that have been designed to determine why movement time changes, rather than describing the decline in coordinated movement patterns that accompanies aging.

Reflex Testing

Reflex testing is performed to assess the integrity of the sensorimotor pathways without the influence of cognitive processing. The latency of a reflex response can, therefore, be used to assess the integrity of the simplest sensorimotor connection. Investigators who postulate that the Achilles tendon tap elicits a monosynaptic response in the agonist MUs purport to study the simplest sensorimotor connection.

The reflex change most commonly noted with aging is diminution or absence of the Achilles tendon response, which has been reported to occur in 10% of older subjects.[71] Other investigators note only small increases in the latency of the Achilles and patellar tendon reflexes. These latter findings are consistent with the research findings suggesting a small but unremarkable decline in conduction velocity in sensory and motor nerves.[10, 29] Comparison between the latency associated with the Achilles tendon reflex and the latency in a known polysynaptic reflex response reveals the same small age-related increase in latency, rather than a longer latency for the polysynaptic response.[20] Such results suggest that the Achilles tendon reflex may be more than a monosynaptic response[26] or that central synapses are preserved in the polysynaptic pathway. If the latter hypothesis is correct, the increased latency in both monosynaptic and polysynaptic reflexes can be attributed to changes in conduction velocity of the afferent and efferent pathways. The lack of significant changes in the integrity of reflexes with aging suggests that other factors must be examined to account for older individuals' slow movement.

Central Efferent Pathways

Magnetic and electrical stimulation of the motor cortex through the scalp are two recently developed noninvasive techniques used to study the integrity of motor pathways in the human.[16] Motor evoked potentials (MEPs) are recorded from a muscle contralateral to the stimulated motor cortex. Conduction times can be recorded within the CNS by recording over the spinal cord at the level of the relevant motoneurons. For example, conduction time can be recorded between the cortex and the L4-5 level of the spinal cord, and the MEPs can be recorded from the tibialis anterior. Although data indicating age-related changes in MEPs in the sixth through tenth decades are still unavailable, the MEP technique is mentioned here because preliminary data on age-related changes are exciting. Results from subjects ranging from 19 to 50 years of age indicate a trend for decline in central conduction time with age.

Reaction Time

Changes in the peripheral systems have been cited which might account for some slowing in stimulus encoding and execution of movement. Are there changes in central decision, comparison, and response selection as well? In other words, what role does cognition play in producing a slowed movement? Aspects of cognitive processing have been studied using reaction time with the assumption that the time it takes to perform a response reflects the stages of processing involved. *Reaction time* (RT) is defined as the time required to initiate a movement following stimulus presentation. In a simple RT test, the subject knows that a single response is required for the stimulus. Simple RTs have been shown to increase with age.[145] Birren et al.[13] summarized the results from a variety of studies and reported a 20% increase in RT in 60-year-old subjects compared with 20-year-old subjects. However, several investigators have suggested that physically active older subjects have faster RTs than sedentary older individuals.[30, 142]

Measurement of RT includes the time for electromechanical transduction from muscle activity to movement. Some investigators have used electromyography (EMG) activity to separate premotor time (PMT) and motor time (MT). PMT is defined as the time between stimulus onset to the onset of EMG activity, and MT is defined as the time from the onset of EMG activity to the initiation of the movement. By subdividing reaction times, the assumption is that insight can be gained into the extent to which muscular factors slow performance.

The effect of age on PMT and MT appears dependent on the task involved.[157] Although both PMT and MT are affected by aging, different tasks demonstrate more slowing in PMT or MT. For example, when the subject is merely required to move the hand, the PMT seems particularly affected by age.[156] When the subject is required to move the arm against resistance,[139] or to jump,[117] the main slowing is in the MT, which includes the time needed for the muscle contraction. While movements against resistance may increase pain or fatigue, and therefore require new compensatory strategies, the results of this research suggest that as age increases, there is a progressively slower buildup of muscular contraction when action is required. This change is particularly evident when substantial force has to be exerted either to overcome resistance or to produce a very rapid movement. In a recent review of the effect of exercise on improving PMT and MT, the authors conclude that substantial training does not significantly improve the time necessary to complete a task and suggest that slowness of movement reflects a change in the neural pathways that does not appear to improve significantly with increased physical activity.[119]

A two-choice RT test requires choice between two responses instead of one response in simple RT. The two-choice RT is, therefore, a more complex task. As movement complexity increases, the RT increases in the older adults.[95, 145] Older individuals are more sensitive to small changes in movement complexity than younger individuals and also experience more difficulty when tasks demand both accuracy and speed. Choice of accuracy over speed can lead to problems when a whole body response is required quickly to prevent a fall, for example.

To summarize, premotor and movement times are significantly related to chronologic age. Premotor time is slower in older individuals regardless of the task. Motor time appears to depend on the amount of muscle activity required to produce the task; that is, the higher the required muscle force, the longer the motor time. In both speed of reaction and movement, fastest responses are reported for subjects in their second decade. Consistency of response is greatest in the third decade. Beyond age 60, the variability in premotor and movement times increases greatly compared with the younger subjects' performance.[157] More complicated tasks are more sensitive in indicating age-related decline. Collectively, the results indicate the importance of the CNS when considering the effects of age on sensorimotor capacity.

Posture and Motion

The focus thus far has been on involuntary and voluntary movement of the moving limb. Does aging affect trunk and interlimb coordination? For example, is the ability to produce preparatory postural adjustments prior to the onset of voluntary movement altered with increased age? Older subjects have been reported to fail to produce the normal postural adjustments prior to performing a voluntary movement.[72, 145] For example, when asked to perform a unilateral knee flexion during standing, the lack of necessary postural adjustments in trunk and contralateral limb musculature leads to a loss of balance.[98] Loss of balance is increased when the subjects are asked to make the movements more rapidly. Such data suggest a change in coordination of movement and posture that is age related.

Functional Movement

There is a gap in understanding between laboratory studies of human movement and outcome studies that report an older person's ability to perform activities of daily living (ADL). While laboratory studies attempt to describe the quality of movement and mechanisms that may be interacting to produce the movement, outcome studies focus on the person's ability to complete a task successfully without regard to the quality of the movement. The Potvin study[124] cited previously emphasizes this gap in knowledge.

In Potvin's study, neurologic status was assessed in 61 men ranging in age from 20 to 80 years. In addition to examining sensory status, tests of sensorimotor status and ADL were examined. Simple reaction times for the upper and lower extremities showed significant age-related effects. In examining movement using quasi-laboratory conditions, the greatest age-related declines in function in the upper extremity were in hand-force steadiness and speed of hand-arm movements. The most difficult task imposed using the lower extremities was standing on one leg and maintaining balance with the eyes closed. Although the RT demonstrated age-related effects, the declines were far less than those reported for hand-force control and one-legged standing when an age-related decline of at least 50% was reported for these two tasks. Average loss of function for ten ADL tasks was 30%. The ADL tasks most age sensitive were putting on a shirt and cutting with a knife.

Therefore, while well-controlled laboratory studies provide insight into the mechanisms responsible for age-related decline in movement, the results may not reflect the severity of deterioration in functional movement. When subjects are observed functioning under more natural conditions, additional factors may increase the complexity of the task and result in more significant declines in function.

Neural Noise Theory

A number of reviews have attempted to correlate slower performance in older age with the slowing that accompanies other age-related conditions such as diffuse brain damage, cardiac insufficiency, hypertension, and Parkinson's disease.[70, 100] For example, in both aged individuals and patients with Parkinson's disease, tapping rate is decreased 20% to 30%, and tracking is decreased 40% to

50%.[110] Slowing in these conditions and in old age has been suggested to be related in some way to loss of cells or synapses, lower oxygen levels in the brain, and/or neurotransmitter changes. While the correlation between Parkinson's disease and impaired movement time is well established, the mechanisms responsible for the slowness of movement are not clear. Several investigators have proposed that slowness of movement in the healthy elderly reflects central problems such as disorders in the basal ganglia and the extrapyramidal system.[7, 101] There is not, however, substantial evidence to identify a single central mechanism that accounts for the age-dependent slowness of movement.

Since this chapter has suggested age-related change at virtually every level of the neuraxis, it is expected that changes throughout the various systems collectively contribute to the problem of slow movement encountered in the older individual. There is sufficient indication to support the assumption that slowness of movement is task dependent and that disability is more obvious when the task is new or complex or imposes a time constraint. The literature reviewed indicates that age affects the speed of limb movement and coordination among body parts to produce motion without identifying the mechanism responsible for the age-related slowing.

While the literature cited thus far indicates age-related changes throughout the CNS, PNS, and muscle, there is not one region or aspect of movement generation that appears to be the primary reason for the age-related decline in function. In his neural noise theory, Welford[157] suggests that age-related decline in the quality and quantity of movement is the result of the composite changes within the nervous and muscular systems. The electrical activity within the nervous or muscular system from the individual at rest displays a significant amount of background activity. This background activity, or noise, reflects ongoing activity but is not related to any particular process. True signals that may be carrying important information from sense organs or other parts of the nervous system have to be distinguished from this background or random electrical activity. Age-related deterioration in the visual, somatosensory, or vestibular system may produce a signal detection problem. To detect a stimulus correctly with any given level of accuracy, or to decide among several action plans, a longer sampling period may be necessary in the older individual. Slowing of performance with age may, therefore, result at least in part from a decrease in signal-to-noise ratio, leading to increases of time taken by older people to accomplish a task, which may become more obvious when the response is required in a short amount of time. Interacting with this factor is the tendency by older people to adopt higher criteria for responding and to spend more time monitoring their actions. The propositions for the neural noise theory remain to be tested.

Summary

There are adequate data to suggest that aging results in a decline in the speed of movement and the quality of movement. It is obvious that aging alters the function of a variety of mechanisms within the human body. It is not obvious that one particular component is responsible for the slowing of movement seen in older subjects, nor is the mechanism that leads to the beginning of age-related decline obvious. It is critical to recognize that changes, in addition to the changes reported here, in nervous and muscular tissue influence motor performance. As stated in the introduction, both intrinsic and extrinsic factors influence the production of movement. Therefore, if the effect of aging on motor performance is to be understood, attention must be spent integrating the changes in the sensorimotor system with changes in other variables including hormonal status, cardiorespiratory function, nutritional state, environmental variables, and activity level.

ADAPTATION

The dictionary defines *plasticity* as the capacity to change. However, the term has come to have very specific meaning in the scientific literature. Neuroscientists use the term *plasticity* to explain structural or physiologic change in the CNS; plasticity is demonstrated, for example, by morphologic evidence that suggests an altered neural organization or by a change in the efficiency of a synapse. Therefore, plasticity can be defined as a response of neurons to perturbations in their local environment.[33] Plasticity is viewed as an "adaptive" response to a perturbation. While the changes may be the nervous system's attempt to adapt, it is not clear whether the changes in neural networks correlate with functional adaptation.

The term *mutability*, rather than *plasticity*, is often used to describe the muscle fiber's ability to change in response to a new demand. The clinician does not, therefore, observe plasticity or mutability; the clinician observes the consequences of plasticity, which may result in the sparing of function, substitution of function, or recovery of some lost function. Despite the lack of correlation between cellular and functional changes, it is important to know if the nerve and muscle possess the ability to respond to perturbation in the aged individual.

Plasticity

Perturbation of a neuron may be in the chemical composition of the neuron's immediate surroundings, in its afferent supply, in its targets, or in its neighboring neurons and glia. The plastic responses to such perturbations may include alteration in dendritic or axonal morphology, synapses, receptors, or metabolism.[33]

Dendrites account for as much as 95% of the receptor surface, which allows for contact with other neurons.[133] Dendrites are important in the neuron's ability to receive and process information. Most studies of the aged nervous system have focused on the cerebral cortex, hippocampus, and olfactory bulb. There is little information about the cerebellum, brain stem, and spinal cord. Therefore, any evidence presented here cannot be generalized to changes in the entire nervous system. As stated earlier, there is a loss of synapses, dendritic branches, and dendritic spines with age. There is also evidence in the human that there is an age-related increase in the number of dendritic branches and dendritic spines in the aging brain.[25, 38] The presence of increased dendritic growth of remaining neurons, coupled with the loss of other neurons, suggests that the dendritic growth is a compensatory response to the death of neighboring neurons. The mechanism to account for the proliferation of dendrites is speculative. One theory is that the glial cells, particularly the astrocytes, in the CNS and the Schwann cells in the PNS serve as sources of a trophic factor.[6] Another possibility in the CNS is that norepinephrine serves as a trophic (nourishing) system.[61] The relationship between the structural changes in the dendrites and changes in neurochemistry has not been established at this time.

New synapses (synaptogenesis) have been demonstrated to form in the adult brain.[38] In the CNS, partial denervation results in sprouting by the remaining fibers. Sprouting continues to be demonstrated in the aging animal brain, but the rate and magnitude of sprouting appear to decline. It is assumed that sprouting can occur in the aging human brain and can be adaptive or maladaptive. The return or maintenance of function depends on which connections are formed. The relationship between sprouting and functional ability in the human has also not been established.

The factors that accelerate the plastic changes include the environment and diet. There is little evidence in the human to suggest a cause-and-effect relationship among these factors. Research in aged animals suggests that dendritic spine density increases with an enriched environment.[34] There is some evidence, although it is controversial, to suggest that dietary supplements that include the precursors for acetylcholine may delay memory loss in older human subjects.[38] Although the research on human plasticity is scant, there are early indications that plasticity is possible in the aging human and that the clinician may be able to optimize performance.

Mutability

The possibility of preventing age-related changes in the MU is theoretically greater than for age-related changes in other tissues. This assumption is justified because of the well-documented ability of the muscle to respond to physiologic stimulation by improving its functional capacity and by correcting certain types of structural and chemical damage. In response to appropriate stimuli, muscle fibers can enlarge severalfold, as well as increase oxidative capacity. Are age-related functional changes in part a result of disuse? Can activity prevent and/or reverse these regressive changes? Aging is associated with an evolving reduction of physical activity, and deconditioning occurs fairly rapidly.[9] Other chapters will address the literature that suggests that the older individual is capable of regaining strength.

Larsson[91] studied the effect of physical training on vastus medialis morphology in 18 sedentary males ranging in age from 22 to 65 years. Subjects were involved in a 60- to 80-minute strength training program two times per week for 15 weeks. Muscle biopsies were taken, and strength measurements were performed before and after the training period. Maximal isometric and dynamic torque were evaluated using an isokinetic device. Age-related muscle fiber atrophy seen before training diminished after the training period because of an increase in fiber size in older subjects, and the increase in fiber size was more marked in the older subjects. Increased torque was noted in all subjects, but the training effect was more marked in older subjects. Such data suggest that older muscle is mutable, but the oldest subject was only 65 years of age.

Knee extension and elbow flexion have also been studied in young and elderly subjects.[84] The 7 sedentary, young subjects were an average of 28 years, and the 26 older subjects were an average of 69 years of age. The older subjects were subdivided into four groups: sedentary individuals, swimmers, runners, and strength-trained subjects. The older physically active subjects had trained an average of 15 years, three times per week. Maximal isometric torque for knee extension was 44% lower and for elbow flexion was 32% lower in the sedentary elders compared with the young subjects. Speed of movement was 20% and 26% slower in the knee and arm movement, respectively, in the sedentary elders compared with the young subjects. Cross-sectional area for the vastus lateralis and biceps brachii was reduced, and a preferential type II atrophy was demonstrated for the vastus lateralis and the biceps brachii. The only active older group that did not show age-related decline were the strength-trained older men. The strength-trained older men demonstrated no significant difference on any of the variables tested when compared with the sedentary young subjects. This study suggests that muscle mutability may be retained in certain muscles in some older individuals through age 69 and that retention may be dependent on strength training rather than general conditioning. The relationship between muscle fiber types and the quality or quantity of functional performance was not addressed in this study. Since the sample size for this study was small and the older subjects were less than 70 years of age, additional work is necessary to generalize these findings.

In his review of the literature of how physiologic systems change with exercise, Buskirk[27] concludes that a general adaptation occurs with exercise. Although the adaptation is age dependent, he suggests that regular exercise retards the downward trends in systems of the body that are commonly associated with aging. The two studies just cited support the hypothesis that muscle retains mutability with age. Changes in this retention need to be studied within active and sedentary individuals over time.

SUMMARY

This chapter has reviewed topically a wealth of literature on age-related declines in the nervous and muscular systems reported to accompany aging. While the majority of investigators agree that reported nervous system or muscle changes are a natural part of the aging process, there is no consensus about the rate of age-related change within or across systems, nor is there consensus about what factors are primary in accelerating or retarding the aging process. Many investigations have selected a particular region of the brain, a specific sensation, or a particular body region for study. It is important to recognize this limitation and not generalize findings from one body region to the whole body. Since most studies using humans as subjects have been cross-sectional studies, it is not possible to state with certainty that similar findings will be found with prospective studies.

Where possible, studies were cited that attempted to correlate the age-related degeneration with function, but no consensus has, as yet, been established concerning the relationship between the age-related changes within the nervous or muscular systems and the age-related decline in movement ability. The precise reasons or factors associated with the age-related decline in function are not evident. Regardless of the motor control model, the age-related changes in the nervous system or muscle present a complex interaction that requires additional research.

Investigators who use humans must carefully screen the subjects for subtle pathology and include a large sample of subjects over age 70. Ideally, studies should include a variety of hypotheses to encompass many systems so that knowledge is gained about how sensory, cognitive, and muscular performance change within one individual. Protocols should include functional tasks rather than being limited to conduction velocities, reflex times, or reaction times to simple, well-practiced tasks, and they should be prospective.

This chapter on the sensorimotor system may lead initially to readers' concern for their own age-related decline in function, as it has for the author. The more recent and exciting research on plasticity, mutability, and the effects of exercise should buoy reader spirit, however. Additional work will have to be done before it is known whether the proposed plasticity of the nervous system is functional and can be altered by extrinsic factors. It is encouraging to suppose that the quality and quantity of movement may be prolonged with exercise.

Functional change in the aging neuromuscular system as measured by the physical therapist should occur in conjunction with anatomic, physiologic, and neurochemical changes in the sensorimotor system. The reader must recognize that care and treatment of the aging individual require an interdisciplinary knowledge and a multidisciplinary team, however, to fully understand the variables that affect a person's aging process or recovery from a disability superimposed on the aging system.

Acknowledgments

I would like to acknowledge the technical assistance of Kimberly Gallo and the creative assistance of Carol Oatis, Ph.D., P.T., and Mark Haskins, Ph.D., V.M.D. This effort was supported in part by NIH Grant NS22283, University of Pennsylvania.

REFERENCES

1. Aggleton JP, Mishkin M: Visual recognition impairment following medial thalamic lesions in monkeys. *Neuropsychologia* 1983; 21:189–197.
2. Anderson B, Palmore E: Longitudinal evaluation of ocular function, in Palmore E (ed): *Normal Aging II, Reports From the Duke Longitudinal Studies, 1970–1973. Durham, Duke University Press, 1974.*
3. Aniansson A, Grimby G, Hedberg M, et al: Muscle morphology, enzyme activity and muscle strength in elderly men and women. *Clin Physiol* 1981; 1:73–86.
4. Ball MJ: Histopathology of cellular changes in Alzheimer's disease, in Nandy K (ed): *Senile Dementia: A Biomedical Approach.* New York, Elsevier, 1978.
5. Baloh RW: Neurotology of aging: Vestibular system, in Albert ML (ed): *Clinical Neurology of Aging.* New York, Oxford University Press, 1984.
6. Banker GA: Trophic interactions between astroglial cells and hippocampal neurons in culture. *Science* 1980; 209:809–810.
7. Barbeau A: Aging and the extrapyramidal system. *J Am Geriatr Soc* 1973; 21:145–149.
8. Barrett DS, Cobb AG, Bently G: Joint proprioception in normal, osteoarthritic and replaced knees. *J Bone Joint Surg* 1991; 73B:53–56.

9. Bassey EJ: Age, inactivity and some physiological responses to exercise. *J Gerontol* 1978; 24:66–77.

10. Benassi G, D'Alessandro R, Gallassi R, et al: Neurological examination in subjects over 65 years: An epidemiological survey. *Neuroepidemiology* 1990; 9:27–38.

11. Beninger RJ, Wirsching BA, Jhamandas K, et al: Animal studies of brain acetylcholine and memory. *Arch Gerontol Geriatr Suppl* 1989; 1:71–89.

12. Birren JE, Schaie KW (eds): *Handbook of the Psychology of Aging.* New York, Van Nostrand Reinhold, 1977.

13. Birren JE, Woods AM, Williams MV: Speed of behavior as an indicator of age changes and the integrity of the nervous system, in Hoffmeister F, Miller C (eds): *Brain Function in Old Age.* New York, Springer-Verlag, 1979.

14. Blessed G, Tomlinson BE, Rotn M: The association between quantitative measures of dementia and of senile change in the cerebral grey matter of elderly subjects. *Br J Psychiatry* 1968; 114:797–811.

15. Bolton CF, Winkelmann RK, Dyck PJ: A quantitative study of Meissner's corpuscles in man. *Neurology* 1966; 16:1–9.

16. Booth KR, Streletz LJ, Raab VE, et al: Motor evoked potentials and central motor conduction: Studies of transcranial magnetic stimulation with recording from the leg. *Electroencephalogr Clin Neurophysiol* 1991; 81:57–62.

17. Botwinick J: *Aging and Behavior.* New York, Springer, 1978.

18. Brody H: The effects of age upon the main nucleus of inferior olive in the human. *J Comp Neurol* 1975; 155:61–66.

19. Brody H, Vijayashanker N: Anatomical changes in the nervous system, in Finch CE, Hayflick L (eds): *Handbook of the Biology of Aging.* New York, Van Nostrand Reinhold, 1977.

20. Brooke JD, Singh R, Wilson MK, et al: Aging human segmented oligosynaptic reflexes for control of leg movement. *Neurobiol Aging* 1989; 10:721–725.

21. Brooke MH, Kaiser KK: Muscle fiber types: How many and what king? *Arch Neurol* 1970; 23:369–379.

22. Brown WF: A method for estimating the number of motor units in thenar muscles and the changes in motor unit count with ageing. *J Neurol Neurosurg Psychiatry* 1972; 35:845–853.

23. Bruce RA: Exercise, functional capacity, and aging—Another viewpoint. *Med Sci Sports Exerc* 1984; 16:8–13.

24. Buchtal F, Rosenfalck A: Evoked action potentials and conduction velocity in human sensory nerves. *Brain Res* 1966; 3:1.

25. Buell SJ, Coleman PD: Quantitative evidence for selective dendritic growth in normal human aging but not in senile dementia. *Brain Res* 1981; 214:23–42.

26. Burke D: Spasticity as an adaptation to pyramidal tract injury. *Adv Neurol* 1988; 47:401–423.

27. Buskirk ER: Health maintenance and longevity: Exercise, in Finch C, Schneider EL (eds): *Handbook of the Biology of Aging,* ed 2. New York, Van Nostrand Reinhold, 1985.

28. Campbell MJ, McComas AJ, Petito F: Physiological changes in aging muscles. *J Neurol Neurosurg Psychiatry* 1974; 37:131–141.

29. Carel RS, Korcyzn AD, Hochberg Y: Age and sex dependency of the Achilles tendon reflex. *Am J Med Sci* 1979; 278:57–63.

30. Clarkson PM: The effect of age and activity level on simple and choice fractionated response time. *Eur J Appl Physiol* 1978; 40:17–25.

31. Clarkson PM, Kroll W, Melchionda AM: Age, isometric strength, rate of tension development and fiber type composition. *J Gerontol* 1981; 36:648–653.

32. Cohen MM, Lessell S: The neuro-ophthalmology of aging, in Albert ML (ed): *Clinical Neurology of Aging.* New York, Oxford University Press, 1984.

33. Coleman PD, Flood DG: Is dendritic proliferation of surviving neurons a compensatory response to loss of neighbors in the aging brain? in Finger S, et al (eds): *Brain Injury and Recovery: Theoretical and Controversial Issues.* New York, Plenum Press, 1988.

34. Connor JR, Diamond MC, Johnson RE: Aging and environmental influences on two types of dendritic spines in the rat occipital cortex. *Exp Neurol* 1980; 79:371–379.

35. Contemporary management of motor control problems, in Lister ML (ed): *Proceedings of the II Step Conference.* Alexandria, Va, Foundation for Physical Therapy, 1991.

36. Corbin KB, Gardner ED: Decrease in number of myelinated fibers in human spinal roots with age. *Anat Rec* 1937; 68:63–74.

37. Corsellis JA: Some observations on the Purkinje cell population and on brain volume in human aging, in Terry RD, Gershon S (eds): *Neurobiology of Aging.* Aging, vol 3. New York, Raven Press, 1976.

38. Cotman CW, Holets VR: Structural changes at synapses with age: Plasticity and regeneration, in Finch C, Schneider EL (eds): *Handbook of the Biology of Aging,* ed 2. New York, Van Nostrand Reinhold, 1985.

39. Craik F: Changes in memory with normal aging: A functional view, in Wurtman RJ, et al (eds): *Alzheimer's Disease.* Advances in Neurology, vol 51. New York, Raven Press, 1990.

40. Cupp CJ, Uemura E: Age-related changes in prefrontal cortex of Macca mulatta: Quantitative analysis of dendritic branching patterns. *Exp Neurol* 1980; 69:143–163.

41. Danieli-Betto D, Zerbato E, Betto R: Type 1, 2a, and 2b myosin heavy chain electrophoretic analysis of rat muscle fibers. *Biochem Biophys Res Commun* 1986; 138:981–987.

42. Desmedt JE, Brunko E: Functional organization of far-field and cortical components of somatosensory evoked potentials in normal adults, in Desmedt JE (ed): *Progress in Clinical Neurophysiology,* vol 7. Basel, Karger, 1980.

43. Devaney KO, Johnson HA: Neuron loss in the aging visual cortex of man. *J Gerontol* 1980; 35:836–841.

44. Dorfman LJ, Bosley TM: Age related changes in peripheral central nerve conduction in man. *Neurology* 1979; 29:38–44.

45. Downie AW, Newell DJ: Sensory nerve conduction in

patients with diabetes mellitus and controls. *Neurology* 1961; 11:876–882.

46. Duara R, London D, Rapoport St, et al: Changes in structure and energy metabolism of the aging brain, in Finch C, Schneider EL (eds): *Handbook of the Biology of Aging,* ed 2. New York, Van Nostrand Reinhold, 1985.

47. Duara R, Margolin RA, Robertson-Tchabo EA, et al: Cerebral glucose utilization, as measured with positron emission tomography in 21 resting healthy men between the ages of 21 and 83 years. *Brain* 1983; 106:761–775.

48. Dyck PJ: Pathologic alterations of the peripheral nervous system of man, in Dyck PJ, et al (eds): *Peripheral Neuropathy,* vol 1. Philadelphia, WB Saunders, 1975.

49. Dyck PJ, Schultz PW, O'Brien PC: Quantitation of touch-pressure sensation. *Arch Neurol* 1972; 26:465.

50. Earnest MP, Heaton RK, Wilkinson WE, et al.: Cortical atrophy, ventricular enlargement and intellectual impairment in the aged. *J Neurol* 1979; 29:1138–1143.

51. Essen-Gustavsson B, Borges O: Histochemical and metabolic characteristics of human skeletal muscle in relation to age. *Acta Physiol Scand* 1986; 126:107–114.

52. Ferris SH, Crook T, Clark M, et al: Facial recognition memory deficits in normal aging and senile dementia. *J Gerontol* 1980; 35:707–714.

53. Fozard JL, Wolf E, Bell B, et al: Visual perception and communication, in Birren JE, Schaie KW (eds): *Handbook of the Psychology of Aging.* New York, Van Nostrand Reinhold, 1977.

54. Freedman M, Knoefel J, Naeser M, et al: Computerized axial tomography in aging, in Albert ML (ed): *Clinical Neurology of Aging.* New York, Oxford University Press, 1984.

55. Fries JF: Aging, natural death and the compression of morbidity. *N Engl J Med* 1980; 303:130–135.

56. Gaffan D, Harrison S: Amygdalectomy and disconnection in visual learning for auditory secondary reinforcement by monkeys. *J Neurosci* 1987; 7:2285–2292.

57. Gates GA, Cooper JC, Kannel WB, et al: Hearing in the elderly: The Framingham cohort, 1983–1985. Part 1. Basic audiometric test results. *Ear Hear* 1990; 11:247–256.

58. Geula C, Mesulam MM: Cortical cholinergic fibers in aging and Alzheimer's disease: A morphometric study. *J Neurosci* 1989; 33:469–481.

59. Goldberg JM, Lindblom U: Standardized method of determining vibratory perception thresholds for diagnosis and screening in neurological investigation, *J Neurol Neurosurg Psychiatry* 1979; 42:793–803.

60. Goldman-Rakic PS: Circuitry of the prefrontal cortex and regulation of behavior by representational memory, in Mountcastle B, et al (eds): *Handbook of Physiology.* Baltimore, Williams & Wilkins, 1987.

61. Goldman-Rakic P, Brown RM: Regional changes of monoamines in cerebral cortex and subcortical structures of aging rhesus monkeys. *J Neurosci* 1981; 6:177–187.

62. Grimby G, Aniansson A, Zetterberg C, et al: Is there a change in relative muscle fibre composition with age? *Clin Physiol* 1984; 4:189–194.

63. Grimby G, Saltin B: The ageing muscle. *Clin Physiol* 1983; 3:209–218.

64. Gutmann E, Gutmann L, Medawar PB, et al: The rate of regeneration of nerve. *J Exp Biol* 1942; 19:14–44.

65. Gutmann E, Hanzlikova V: Fast and slow motor units in aging. *J Gerontol* 1976; 22:280–300.

66. Hayes D, Jerger J: Neurotology of aging: The auditory system, in Albert ML (ed): *Clinical Neurology of Aging.* New York, Oxford University Press, 1984.

67. Hayflick L: The cellular basis for biological aging, in Finch CE, Hayflick L (eds): *Handbook of the Biology of Aging.* New York, Van Nostrand Reinhold, 1977.

68. Heindel WC, Salmon DP, Shults CW, et al: Neurophysiological evidence for multiple implicit memory systems: A comparison of Alzheimer's, Huntington's and Parkinson's disease patients. *J Neurosci* 1989; 9:582–587.

69. Henderson G, Tomlinson BE, Gibson P: Cell counts in human cerebral cortex in normal adults throughout life using an image analyzing computer. *J Neurol Sci* 1980; 46:113–136.

70. Hicks L, Birren J: Aging, brain damage, and psychomotor slowing. *Psychol Bull* 1970; 74:377–396.

71. Hobson W, Pemberton J: The health of the elderly at home. London, Butterworth, 1955.

72. Horak FB, Shupert CL, Mirka A: Components of postural dyscontrol in the elderly. *Neurobiol Aging* 1989; 10:727–738.

73. Itoh M, Hatazawa J, Yamaura H, et al: Age related brain atrophy and mental deterioration—A study with computerized tomography. *Br J Radiol* 1981; 54:384–390.

74. Itoh M, Hatazawa J, Yamaura H, et al: Stability of cerebral blood flow and oxygen metabolism during normal aging. *J Gerontol* 1990; 36:43–48.

75. Johnsson L, Hawkins J: Sensory and neural degeneration with aging, as seen in microdissections of the inner ear. *Ann Otol Rhinol Laryngol* 1972; 81:179–183.

76. Kaeser HE: Nerve conduction velocity measurements, in Vinken PJ, Bruyn AW (eds): *Handbook of Clinical Neurology,* vol 7. Amsterdam, North Holland, 1970.

77. Kallman DA, Ratco CC, Tobin JP: The role of muscle loss in the age-related decline of grip strength: Cross sectional and longitudinal perspectives. *J Gerontol* 1990; 45:M82–88.

78. Katzman R, Saitoh T: Advances in Alzheimer's disease. *FASEB J* 1991; 5:278–286.

79. Katzman R, Terry R: *The Neurology of Aging.* Philadelphia, FA Davis, 1983.

80. Kawamura YI, Okazaki H, O'Brien PC, et al: Effect of age on glucose utilization and responsiveness to insulin in forearm muscle. *J Am Geriatr Soc* 1977; 28:304–307.

81. Kemper T: Neuroanatomical and neuropathological changes in normal aging and dementia, in Albert ML (ed): *Clinical Neurology of Aging.* New York, Oxford University Press, 1984.

82. Kennedy R, Clemis JD: The geriatric auditory and vestibular systems. *Otolaryngol Clin North Am* 1990; 23:1075–1082.

83. Kety SS: Human cerebral blood flow and oxygen consumption as related to aging. *J Chron Dis* 1956; 3:478–486.

84. Klitgaard H, Mantoni M, Schiffino S, et al: Function, morphology and protein expression of ageing skeletal muscle: A cross-sectional study of elderly men with different training backgrounds. *Acta Physiol Scand* 1990; 140:41–54.

85. Klitgaard H, Zhou M, Schiaffino S, et al: Ageing alters the myosin heavy chain composition of single fibres from human skeletal muscle. *Acta Physiol Scand* 1990; 140:55–62.

86. Kokmen E, Bossemeyer RW, Williams WJ: Neurological manifestations of aging. *J Gerontol* 1977; 32:411–419.

87. Kokmen E, Bossemeyer RW, Williams WJ: Quantitative evaluation of joint motion perception in an aging population. *J Gerontol* 1978; 33:62.

88. La Fratta CW, Canestrari RE: A comparison of sensory and motor nerve conduction velocities as related to age. *Arch Phys Med Rehabil* 1966; 47:286–290.

89. Laidlaw RW, Hamilton MA: A study of thresholds in perception of passive movement among normal control subjects. *Bull Neurol Inst* 1937; 6:268–340.

90. Larsson L: Physical training effects on muscle morphology in sedentary males at different ages. *Med Sci Sports Exerc* 1982; 14:203–206.

91. Larsson L, Grimby G, Karlsson J: Muscle strength and speed of movement in relation to age and muscle morphology. *J Appl Physiol* 1979; 46:451–456.

92. Larsson L, Sjodin B, Karlsson K: Histochemical and biochemical changes in human skeletal muscle with age in sedentary males, age 22–65 years. *Acta Physiol Scand* 1978, 103:31–39.

93. Lascelles RG, Thomas PK: Changes due to age in internodal length in the sural nerve of man. *J Neurol Neurosurg Psychiatry* 1966; 29:40–44.

94. Lexell J, Henriksson-Larsen B, Winbled B, et al: Distribution of different fiber types in human skeletal muscle: Effects of aging studied in whole muscle cross sections. *Muscle Nerve* 1983; 6:588–595.

95. Light KE, Spirduso WW: Effects of adult aging on the movement complexity factor of response programming. *J Gerontol* 1990; 45:107–109.

96. Lowenfeld IE: Pupillary changes related to age, in Thompson HS (ed): *Topics in Neuro-Ophthalmology*. Baltimore, Williams & Wilkins, 1979.

97. Magnoni MS, Govoni S, Battaini F, et al: The aging brain: Protein phosphorylation as a target of changes in neuronal function. *Life Sci* 1991; 48:373–385.

98. Mankovskii N, Mints YA, Lysenyuk UP: Regulation of the preparatory period for complex voluntary movement in old and extreme old age. *Hum Physiol* 1980; 6:46–50.

99. McCandless G, Parkin J: Hearing aid performance relative to site of lesion. *Otolaryngol Head Neck Surg* 1979; 87:871–875.

100. McFarland RA: Experimental evidence of the relationship between ageing and oxygen want: In search of a theory of ageing. *Ergonomics* 1963; 6:339–366.

101. McGeer PL, McGeer EG: Enzymes associated with the metabolism of catecholamines, acetylcholine and GABA in human controls and patients with Parkinson's disease and Huntington's chorea. *J Neurochem* 1976; 26:65–70.

102. McGeer PL, McGeer EG, Suzuki JS: Aging and extrapyramidal function. *Arch Neurol* 1977; 34:33–35.

103. McMartin DN, O'Conner JA: Effect of age on axoplasmic transport of cholinesterase in rat sciatic nerves. *Mech Ageing Dev* 1979; 10:241–248.

104. Merchut MP, Toleikis SC: Aging and quantitative sensory thresholds. *Electromyogr Clin Neurophysiol* 1990; 30:293–297.

105. Miller AKH, Alston RL, Corsellis JAN: Variations with age in the volumes of grey and white matter in the cerebral hemispheres of man: Measurements with an image analyzer. *Neuropathol Appl Neurobiol* 1980; 6:119–132.

106. Millodot M: The influence of age on the sensitivity of the cornea. *Invest Ophthalmol Vis Sci* 1977; 16:240–242.

107. Milner B, Petrides M: Behavioural effects of frontal-lobe lesions in man. *Trends Neurosci* 1984; 7:403–407.

108. Moller P, Bergstrom J, Furst P, et al: Effect of aging on energy-rich phosphagens in human skeletal muscles. *Clin Sci* 1980; 58:553–555.

109. Morimatsu M, Hirai S, Muramatsu A: Senile degenerative brain lesions and dementia. *J Am Geriatr Soc* 1975; 23:390–406.

110. Mortimer JA: Comparison of extrapyramidal motor function in normal aging and Parkinson's disease, in Mortimer JA, et al (eds): *Advances in Neurogerontology: The Aging Motor System*. New York, Praeger, 1982.

111. *Movement Science*. Alexandria, Va, American Physical Therapy Association, 1991.

112. Mufson EJ, Stein DG: Degeneration in the spinal cord of old rats. *Exp Neurol* 1980; 70:179–186.

113. Munsat TL: Aging of the neuromuscular system, in Albert ML (ed): *Clinical Neurology of Aging*. New York, Oxford University Press, 1984.

114. Murray MP, Gardner GM, Mollinger LA, et al: Age related differences in knee muscle strength in normal women. *Phys Ther* 1980; 60:412–419.

115. Noel P, Desmedt JE: Cerebral and far-field somatosensory evoked potentials in neurological disorders involving the cervical spinal cord, brainstem, thalamus, and cortex, in Desmedt J (ed): *Progress in Clinical Neurophysiology*, vol 7. Basel, Karger, 1980.

116. Ochoa J, Mair WPG: The normal sural nerve in man: II. Changes in the axons and Schwann cells due to aging. *Acta Neuropathol* (Berl) 1969; 13:217–239.

117. Onishi N: Changes of the jumping reaction time in relation to age. *J Sci Labour* 1966; 42:5–16.

118. O'Sullivan DJ, Swallow M: The fibre size and content of the radial and sural nerve. *J Neurol Neurosurg Psychiatry* 1968; 31:464–470.

119. Panton LB, Graves JE, Pollock ML: Effects of aerobic

and resistance training on fractionated reaction time and speed of movement. *J Gerontol* 1990; 45:M26–31.

120. Park DC, Puglisi JT, Sovacool M: Memory for pictures, words, and spatial location in older adults: Evidence for pictorial superiority. *J Gerontol* 1983; 38:582–588.

121. Peress NS, Kane WC, Aronson SM: Central nervous system findings in a tenth decade autopsy population. *Prog Brain Res* 1973; 40:473–483.

122. Perry EK: The cholinergic system in old age and Alzheimer's disease. *Age Ageing* 1980; 9:108.

123. Polich J, Starr A: Evoked potentials in aging, in Albert ML (ed): *Clinical Neurology of Aging*. New York, Oxford University Press, 1984.

124. Potvin AR, Syndulko K, Tourtellote WW, et al: Human neurologic function and the aging process. *J Am Geriatr Soc* 1980; 28:1–9.

125. Rapp PR, Amaral DG: Evidence for task-dependent memory dysfunction in the aged monkey. *J Neurosci* 1989; 9:3566–3576.

126. Reivich M, Kuhl D, Wolf A, et al: The [18F] fluorodeoxyglucose method for the measurement of local cerebral glucose utilization in man. *Circ Res* 1979; 44:127–137.

127. Rogers J, Bloom FE: Neurotransmitter metabolism and function in the aging central nervous system, in Finch C, Schneider EL (eds): *Handbook of the Biology of Aging*, ed 2. New York, Van Nostrand Reinhold, 1985.

128. Sabin TD, Venna N: Peripheral nerve disorders in the elderly, in Albert ML (ed): *Clinical Neurology of Aging*. New York, Oxford University Press, 1984.

129. Sagar HJ, Cohn NJ, Sullivan EV, et al: Remote memory function in Alzheimer's disease and Parkinson's disease. *Brain* 1988; 111:185–206.

130. Sandor T, Albert M, Stafford T, et al: Symmetrical and asymmetrical changes in brain tissue with age as measured on CT scans. *Neurobiol Aging* 1990; 11:21–27.

131. Sawle GV, Colebatch JG, Shah A, et al: Striatal function in normal aging: Implications for Parkinson's disease. *Ann Neurol* 1990; 28:799–804.

132. Scelsi R, Marchetti C, Poggi D: Histochemical and ultrastructural aspects of M. vastus lateralis in sedentary old people (age 65–89 years). *Acta Neuropathol* (Berl) 1980; 51:99–105.

133. Schade JP, Baxter CF: Changes during growth in the volume and surface area of cortical neurons in the rabbit. *Exp Neurol* 1960; 2:158–178.

134. Schmidt RF, Wahren LK: Multiunit neural responses to strong finger pulp vibration. II. Comparison with tactile sensory thresholds. *Acta Physiol Scand* 1990; 140:11–16.

135. Schmidt RF, Wahren LK, Hagbarth KE: Multiunit neural responses to strong finger pulp vibration. I. Relationship to age. *Acta Physiol Scand* 1990; 140:1–10.

136. Sekuler R, Hutman LP, Owsley CJ: Human aging and spatial vision. *Science* 1980; 209:1255–1256.

137. Serratrice G, Roux H, Aquaron R: Proximal muscular weakness in elderly subjects. *J Neurol Sci* 1968; 1:275–299.

138. Silverberg N, Silverberg L: Aging and the skin. *Postgrad Med* 1989; 86:131–136.

139. Singleton WT: The change of movement timing with age. *Br J Psychol* 1954; 45:166–172.

140. Skinner HB, Barrack RL, Cook SD: Age-related decline in proprioception. *Clin Orthop Rel Res* 1984; 184:208–211.

141. Sokoloff L, Reivich M, Kennedy C, et al: The 14C deoxyglucose method for the measurement of local cerebral glucose utilization: Theory, procedure, and normal values in the conscious and anesthetized albino rat. *J Neurochem* 1977; 28:879–916.

142. Spirduso WW: Physical fitness, aging, and psychomotor speed: A review. *J Gerontol* 1980; 35:850–865.

143. Spirduso WW: Exercise and the aging brain. *Res Q Exerc Sport* 1983; 54:208–218.

144. Stalberg E, Fawcett P: Macro EMG in healthy subjects of different ages. *J Neurol Neurosurg Psychiatry* 1982; 45:870–878.

145. Stelmach GE, Worringham CJ: Sensorimotor deficits related to postural stability. *Clin Geriatr Med* 1985; 1:679–725.

146. Takahashi J: A clinicopathologic study of the peripheral nervous system of the aged: Sciatic nerve and autonomic nervous system. *J Am Geriatr Soc* 1966; 21:123–133.

147. Thomas TR, Londeree BR, Gerhardt KO, et al: Fatty acid pattern and cholesterol in skeletal muscle of men aged 22–73. *Mech Ageing Dev* 1978; 8:429–434.

148. Thompson LW: Cerebral blood flow, EEG and behavior in aging, in Terry RD, Gershon S (eds): *Neurobiology of Aging*, vol 3. New York, Raven Press, 1976.

149. Tomanga M: Histochemical and ultrastructural changes in senile human skeletal muscle. *J Am Geriatr Soc* 1977; 25:125–131.

150. Tucker MA, Andrew MF, Ogle SS, et al: Age-associated change in pain threshold measured by transcutaneous neuronal electrical stimulation. *Age Ageing* 1989; 18:241–246.

151. Uemura E, Hartmann HA: RNA content and volume of nerve cell bodies in human brain II. Subiculum in aging normal patients. *Exp Neurol* 1979; 65:107–117.

152. Vandervoort A, Hayes KC, Belanger AY: Strength and endurance of skeletal muscle in the elderly. *Physiother Can* 1986; 38:167–173.

153. Vizoso AD: The relationship between internodal length and growth in human nerves. *J Anat* 1950; 84:342–353.

154. Walters TJ, Sweeney HL, Farrar RP: Aging does not affect contractile properties of type IIb FDL muscle in Fischer 344 rats. *Am J Physiol* 1990; 258:C1031–1035.

155. Weiss AD: Sensory functions, in Birren JE (ed): *Handbook of Aging, and the Individual*. Chicago, University of Chicago Press, 1959.

156. Weiss AD: The locus of reaction time change with set, motivation, and age. *J Gerontol* 1965; 20:60–64.

157. Welford AT: Between bodily changes and performance: Some possible reasons for slowing with age. *Exp Aging Res* 1984; 10:73–88.

158. White P, Hiley C, Goodhart M, et al: Neocortical cholinergic neurons in elderly people. *Lancet* 1977; 1:668–670.

159. Wisniewski HM, Soiser D: Neurofibrillary pathology: Cur-

rent status and research perspectives. *Mech Ageing Dev* 1979; 9:119–142.

160. Wisniewski HM, Terry RD: Morphology of the aging brain, human and animal, in Ford DH (ed): *Neurobiological Aspects of Maturation and Aging.* Progress in Brain Research, vol 40. Amsterdam, Elsevier, 1973.

161. Zola-Morgan S, Squire LR, Amaral DG: Lesions of the hippocampal formation but not lesions of the fornix or the mammillary nuclei produce long-lasting memory impairments in monkeys. *J Neurosci* 1989; 9:898–913.

Principles and Concepts of Assessment

Health Status: A Conceptual Framework and Terminology for Assessment

Andrew A. Guccione, Ph.D., P.T.

INTRODUCTION

Many different concepts are required to capture the broad dimensions of an elder's inevitable experience with disease and illness. Terms such as *health status, well-being, quality of life,* and *functional status* have all been used at various times to describe a facet of the human condition of individuals as they age.[18] Physical therapists direct a substantial proportion of their attention toward understanding the relationships among disease, health, and function, especially how the processes of normal aging and medical morbidity interact to alter a person's physical ability to do even the simplest activities of daily living (ADL) and fulfill the role obligations associated with living independently as an adult.

The preceding chapters have reviewed in great detail the multiple changes that occur with aging or result from certain medical problems that an elder is likely to face. When evaluating an individual geriatric patient, who may present clinically with almost any combination of these changes, a therapist may feel overwhelmed by all the abnormal results noted on the initial assessment. One of the greatest challenges of geriatric physical therapy is to collect complete and only pertinent data and to categorize these clinical findings in a way that helps the therapist to understand what the patient's problems are; how they have come about; and what, if anything at all, could be done by a physical therapist to remedy the patient's situation. This chapter has three purposes. The first purpose is to present a model of health status that can be used by physical therapists to categorize the data they might collect during an initial evaluation. Second, we will explore how the parts of the model interconnect and may be used to assist the physical therapist to understand the patient's problems in functional terms that also suggest what a physical therapist might do to maintain or improve the patient's condition. Finally, this chapter will review the major elements of setting up a treatment program and outline some other factors that are relevant to designing a physical therapy plan of care that is tailored to the specific needs of an older individual.

THE CONCEPT OF HEALTH STATUS

Definition of Health

The World Health Organization (WHO) defined *health* as a state of complete physical, psychologic, and social well-being, and not merely the absence of disease or infirmity.[24] According to this definition, "health" is best understood as an end point and pertains to the psychologic and social domains of human existence—not just the physical state of the human being. In contrast to "complete health"

as an end point, there is health that most physical therapists recognize: an objective state between wellness and death. *Illness,* in comparison with "objective" health, refers to the internal subjective experience of the individual who is aware that personal well-being has been jeopardized and how that person perceives and responds to that experience.

Sociologist Saad Nagi constructed a model of health status that furthers our understanding of the relationship between health and functional status, especially in the elderly.[12–15] In this model, health status is parceled out into four distinct components that evolve sequentially as an individual loses well-being: disease or pathology, impairments, functional limitations, and disability (Fig 6–1). Each of these terms will be discussed below. Taken together, these concepts describe the essential elements of a model that will be discussed and expanded below to serve as an overall framework for physical therapy evaluation and treatment.

Disease

In Nagi's model the term *disease* refers to an ongoing pathologic state that is delineated by a particular cluster of signs and symptoms and is recognized externally by either the individual or a practitioner as abnormal. Nagi's concept of disease is rooted in the principle of homeostasis: the human organism responds to an active pathologic state by mobilizing its resources to respond to a threat and to return to its normal state.[15] Disease may be the result of infection, trauma, metabolic imbalance, degenerative processes, or other etiologies. Whatever the cause, Nagi's concept of disease emphasizes two features: (1) an active threat to the organism's normal state and (2) an active response internally by the organism to that threat, which may be aided externally by therapeutic interventions.

The term *disease* in Nagi's model does not cover all the conditions of many elders and other individuals that necessitate the services of a physical therapist. There are also numerous medical conditions that affect an individual's ability to function but are not related to a *single* active pathology. Congestive heart failure (CHF), for example, is a medical syndrome, that is, a recognized cluster of signs and symptoms. Although CHF evolves from active pathologies over time, it is the coexistence of these pathologies over the same period of time that may explain CHF in the elderly.[5] Osteoarthritis, which is neither active nor pro-

Disease ⟶ Impairment ⟶ Functional Limitations ⟶ Disability

FIG 6–1.
Schematic representation of the four components of health status and the process of disablement in the model developed by Nagi.

gressive in all cases, may also be a medical condition that is best understood as a cluster of pathologic processes, not a single disease.[4] A physical therapists's caseload may also include individuals whose medical diagnoses indicate fixed lesions, which identify previous insults to a body part or organ and sites of dysfunction but are not presently associated with any active processes. A patient seen following a stroke is a common example of an individual with a fixed neuroanatomic lesion that is no longer associated with any ongoing pathologic process. Therefore, Nagi's original model can be developed further to include threats to health, other than disease, that can lead to impairment (Fig 6–2).

Impairment

The second term in Nagi's model is *impairment*. Impairments, many of which evolve as the consequence of disease, pathologic processes, or lesions and also contribute to an elder's illness, can be defined as alterations in anatomic, physiologic, or psychologic structures or functions that are the results of underlying changes in the elder's normal state. Physical impairments, such as pain and decreased range of motion in the shoulder, may be the overt manifestations (or symptoms and signs) of either temporary or permanent disease or pathologic processes. This will not be true, however, for every geriatric patient. The genesis of some impairments can often be unclear. Poor posture, for example, is neither a disease nor a pathologic state, yet the resultant muscle shortening and capsular tightness may present as major impairments in a clinical examination. Thus, not all elderly patients are patients because they have a disease. Some elders are treated by physical therapists because their impairments are sufficient cause for concern. Our efforts with geriatric patients are directed primarily at impairments of the cardiopulmonary, musculoskeletal, and neuromuscular systems. Other systems will be intense concerns in certain subgroups of patients, for example, the integumentary system in frail and immobile nursing home residents.

Physical therapists are recognized experts in the measurement of impairments through the application of test procedures such as goniometry and manual muscle testing. Given that much of physical therapy is directed toward remediating or minimizing impairments, some additional elaborations on the concept of impairment are particularly useful in geriatric physical therapy. Schenkman and Butler have proposed that impairments can be classified in two ways.[21, 22] Some impairments are the direct effects of a disease, syndrome, or lesion and are relatively confined to a single system. For example, they note that weakness can be classified as a neuromuscular impairment that is a direct effect of a peripheral motor neuropathy in the lower extremity. There may also be impairments in other systems that can be regarded as indirect effects of the underlying problem. For example, attempts to ambulate a patient with a peripheral motor neuropathy may put unnecessary strain on joints and ligaments that may be detected on clinical examination as musculoskeletal impairments. The combination of weakness and ligamentous strain may lead to a composite effect, the impairment of pain.

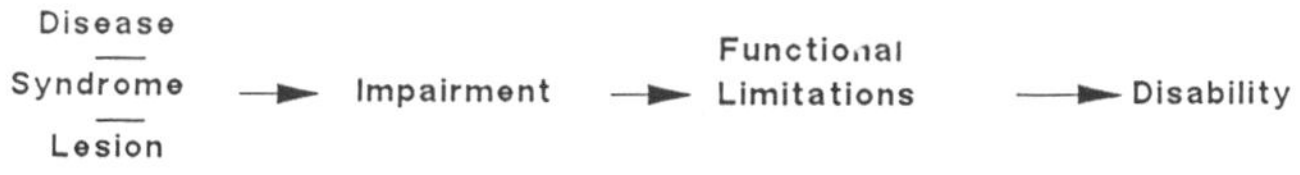

Although Schenkman and Butler expanded the concept of impairment around individuals with neurologic dysfunction, categorizing clinical signs and symptoms into impairments that are direct, indirect, or composite effects can help to bring together the data of the medical history and the findings of the clinical examination into a cohesive relationship. For example, consider a 79-year-old female with severe peripheral vascular disease (PVD). Upon clinical examination, the physical therapist notes that this individual has lost sensation below the right knee. Sensory loss is an impairment that would be classified as a direct effect of PVD. As the individual is ambulating less and cannot sense full ankle range of motion (ROM), loss of ROM may be an indirect effect of the patient's PVD on the musculoskeletal system. The combination of the direct impairment—sensory loss below the knee—and the indirect impairment—decreased ROM in the ankle—may help to explain another clinical finding, poor balance, which can be understood as a composite effect of other impairments. Piecing clinical data together in this fashion allows the therapist to uncover the interrelationships among a patient's PVD, loss of sensation, limited ROM, and balance deficits. Without a framework that sorts the patient's clinical data into relevant categories, the therapist might never comprehend how the patient's problems came to be, and thus how the physical therapist might solve them. Treatment consisting of balance activities alone would be inappropriate, as the therapist must also address the loss in ROM as well as teach the patient to compensate for the sensory loss in order to remediate this patient's impairments.

Disease
——
Syndrome —▶ Impairment —▶ Functional Limitations —▶ Disability
——
Lesion

FIG 6–2.
Expansion of the Nagi model to include conditions other than disease or active pathology that may result in impairments.

Functional Limitations

While most of us anticipate that our body systems will deteriorate with time as we age, an inability to do for one's self from day to day perhaps most clearly identifies when elders are losing their health. Nagi proposed that functional limitations were the results of impairments and consisted of an individual's inability to perform the tasks and roles that constitute usual activities for that individual, for example, reaching for something on an overhead shelf or being able to dress without assistance. As measures of behaviors, and not anatomic or physiologic conditions, limitations in functional status should not be confused with diseases or impairments that encompass aberrations in specific organs or present clinically as the patient's signs and symptoms.

Functional limitations occur in distinct categories of tasks and activities: physical, psychologic, and social. *Physical function,* the intended primary outcome of most physical therapy interventions, covers an individual's sensorimotor performance in the execution of particular tasks and activities. Walking, stair climbing, housekeeping, shopping, and cooking are all examples of physical functional activities. Tasks concerned with fundamental daily activities are further classified as "basic" ADL. The more complex tasks associated with independent community living, for example, using public transportation or grocery shopping, are categorized as "instrumental" ADL, sometimes noted as "IADL." Successful performance of complex physical functional activities, such as personal hygiene and housekeeping, typically requires integration of cognitive and affective abilities as well as physical ones.

Psychologic function has two components: mental and affective. *Mental function* covers a range of cognitive activities such as telling time and performing money calculations that are essential to living independently as an adult. Attention, concentration, memory, and judgment are all elements of mental function. An elder's emotional state or effectiveness in coping with the stresses attributable to disease and other components of the aging process represents the patient's affective function. *Affective function* broadly refers to both the everyday "hassles" of daily existence that are part of every elder's experience as well as the more traumatic events such as death of a spouse. Self-esteem, anxiety, depression, and coping are indicators of affective functioning.

Social function encompasses an individual's social activities such as church attendance or family gatherings as well as performance of social roles and obligations. Grandparenting and being employed outside the home are two examples of social role functioning relevant to an elderly individual and therefore are potential problems to be considered in the physical therapist's initial evaluation. Although physical therapists are chiefly concerned with physical functional activities, individuals typically conceive their personal identities in terms of specific social roles: worker, father, grandmother, wife, community volunteer. All of these roles demand a certain degree of physical abil-

ity. Many opportunities for social interaction for retired elders occur around volunteer and leisure activities, even if it means only the manual dexterity required to dial a telephone. Therefore, the positive effects of physical therapy with the elderly may not be strictly limited to improvement in physical functional status. Improved social functioning may accompany changes in physical ability as well.

Although every geriatric patient can be expected to carry at least two medical diagnoses, each of which will manifest itself in particular impairments of the cardiopulmonary, musculoskeletal, or neuromuscular systems, impairment does not always entail functional limitation. One cannot assume that an individual will be unable to perform the tasks and roles of usual daily living by virtue of having an impairment alone. For example, an elder with osteoarthritis (disease) may exhibit loss of range of motion (impairment) and experience great difficulty in bathing (function). Another individual with equal loss of ROM may use a method for taking a bath without any difficulty, perhaps by using available joint motion to the best advantage or by using assistive devices. Sometimes patients will overcome multiple, and even permanent, impairments by the sheer force of their motivation. In the first case, a decrease in difficulty while bathing following remediation of the joint impairment would usually be accepted as clinical evidence of a causal relationship between impairment and functional loss.

The degree to which any of these limitations in physical functional activities may be linked to impairments has not been fully determined through research. The few studies that have been reported in the literature support a relationship between impairments and functional status. Bergstrom et al., have studied a group of 79-year-old men and women.[2,3] They found that lower extremity joint complaints were more common than upper extremity complaints. Among those elders who had upper extremity complaints, ROM was most restricted in the wrists or shoulders. Hip motion was limited in 84% of the individuals who had lower extremity complaints. When elders with symptoms and joint complaints were compared with elders without such problems, significant differences were found in the ability to use public transportation and climb stairs. Elders with musculoskeletal impairments were also more likely to use ambulation aids. Badley and coworkers conducted a study of 95 patients with arthritis whose mean age was 61.[1] If an individual could not flex the knee more than 70 degrees, they noted that their subjects had difficulty walking to a toilet, transferring to a toilet, getting in and out of a bath, and walking up and down stairs. In a panel of elders in Massachusetts, Jette and colleagues found that musculoskeletal impairments in the hand influenced limitations in basic ADL over a 5-year period.[10] Progression of impairment in the lower extremity had similar significant impact on the progression of deficits in IADL.

Functional assessment, which will be covered elsewhere in this text, allows the therapist to determine if the manner in which tasks and activities are done represents an important quantitative or qualitative deviation from the way in which most people of similar age would perform them. In the absence of norms for elderly functional performance, the therapist must bring previous experience with adults, who are similar to the patient, to bear on this judgment, rather than compare functionally limited elders with healthier and younger adults. Furthermore, even if the therapist concludes that the patient's performance is other than "normal," this does not imply that an elder cannot meet socially imposed expectations of what it means to be independent or that an elder is permanently disabled.

Disability

Nagi reserved the term *disability* for patterns of behavior that emerged over long periods of time during which an individual experienced functional limitations to such a degree that they could not be overcome to create some semblance of "normal" overall role and task performance. The elder who is fully able to use a shower mitt, a tub chair, Velcro-adapted clothing, and elastic shoelaces cannot accurately be described as "disabled," even though functional performance is extremely limited without the use of assisted devices. Although each of the terms that have been presented so far involves some consensus about what is "normal," the concept of a "disability" is socially constructed. The term *disabled* connotes a particular status in society. Labeling a person as disabled requires a judgment, usually by a professional, that an individual's behaviors are somehow inadequate based on the professional's understanding of the expectations that the activity should be accomplished in ways that are typical for an elder's age and sex as well as cultural and social environment.

The evidence suggests that functional limitations in a geriatric population change over time, and not all elders exhibit functional decline.[11] If we follow any cohort of elders over time, there will be more functional limitations overall within the group, but some individuals will actually improve and others will maintain their functional level. Restricting the use of the term *disabled* to describe only long-term overall functional decline in geriatric populations encourages us to understand a particular elder's functional limitations in a dynamic context subject to change, particularly after therapeutic intervention. Disability depends on both the capacities of the individual and the expectations that are imposed on the individual by those in the immediate social environment, most often the patient's

family and care givers. Physical therapists who apply a health status perspective to the assessment of patients draw on a broad appreciation of an elder as a person living in a particular social context as well as having individual characteristics. Changing the expectations of a social context— for example, explaining to family members what level of assistance is appropriate to an elder following stroke—may help to diminish disability as much as supplying the patient with assistive devices or increasing the physical ability to use them.

Granger notes that while the pathways from disease to disability are thought to be unidirectional, disability may itself initiate further functional limitations and impairments and foster disease.[6] Perhaps no clearer example of disability in the elderly exists than the cardiac "cripple" whose rehabilitation has not encouraged resumption of a level of activity that is "normal" for that person. Lack of activity may result in further impairment in both the cardiopulmonary and musculoskeletal systems, which may further put the individual at risk of recurrent cardiac episodes.

Handicap

Nagi did not include the concept of handicap in his model. A *handicap* can be defined as the social disadvantage attached to having a disease, impairment, functional limitation, or disability. In itself, it is not the product of any one of the concepts in the Nagi model but rather a reaction to disablement by the society in which an individual lives. It is quite possible that a person has serious disease, multiple impairments, and functional limitations and is unable to perform most age- and sex-appropriate activities yet is still valued as an individual within a social group. People are handicapped when their place in the human community is denied. As advocates for those whom society would cast off because of their physical condition, physical therapists are deeply concerned with eliminating social attitudes that cause some persons to be handicapped.

THE RELATIONSHIP BETWEEN IMPAIRMENT AND FUNCTIONAL STATUS

Nagi's model describes the major concepts of a diagnostic process that is potentially useful to physical therapists to plan and direct treatment.[8] Although additional research is necessary to elaborate the relationship between impairments and function suggested by the research cited above, the domain of the physical therapist's expertise is found in our ability to identify cardiopulmonary, musculoskeletal, and neuromuscular impairments that may underlie physical functional limitations. To provide physical therapy interventions that will achieve the goal of restoring or improving function, the physical therapist must know more than the patient's signs and symptoms, which are expressions of the individual's disease and impairments. The clinician must also attempt to discern which impairments affect the patient's ability to function. Physical therapy is a complex clinical art and science, but the primary question of the discipline is simple and has two parts: What is the patient's current functional level? and Which impairments contribute to the patient's functional limitations? (See Figure 6–3.) When the therapist's attention turns toward treatment planning, the key question is, Of the impairments that are related to the patient's functional limitations, which ones can also be remedied by physical therapy treatment? Or if the patient's impairments cannot be remedied, How can the patient compensate for them? In the next section, the process of diagnosis in physical therapy will be reviewed using the terminology of health status and the process of disablement presented above.

APPROACHES TO CLINICAL DIAGNOSIS

Physical therapists engage in the diagnostic process every time they assess a patient, cluster findings, interpret data, and label patient problems.[8, 16, 20] Sackett, et al. point to four different approaches that are used by practitioners to arrive at a clinical diagnosis.[19]

One approach to clinical diagnosis uses a *decision tree* to progress the initial evaluation along one of a large number of potential paths.[23] A patient's response to each inquiry or clinical assessment procedure automatically determines the next inquiry to be carried out. The major disadvantage of this approach is that all contingencies have to be worked out explicitly in advance. If a patient's response or clinical presentation has not been included on the tree, then the next step of the evaluation remains unknown. Working out all the possible responses that could be exhibited by an older adult to the number of clinical assessments that are relevant to geriatric physical therapy is a daunting challenge. Furthermore, as the profession of physical therapy seeks to establish its scientific credibility, each step of the decision tree must be validated empirically.

Impairment ➔ Functional Limitations

Impairment	Functional Limitations
Cardiopulmonary	Physical
Musculoskeletal	Psychological
Neuromuscular	Social

FIG 6–3.
The primary goal of a physical therapy evaluation is to determine the relationship between a patient's impairments and functional limitations.

A second strategy for clinical diagnosis is the *complete history and physical,* which has also been termed the *strategy of exhaustion:* "the painstaking invariant search for, but paying no immediate attention to, all medical facts about the patient followed by sifting through the data for the diagnosis"[19] Generally, this is the method of the novice and is abandoned with experience. Sackett and his colleagues have commented that all medical students should be taught both (1) how to do both a complete history and physical and (2) once they have mastered its components, never to do one. A similar admonition may be appropriate for physical therapy students and clinicians, especially those with an interest in caring for the elderly. Students and clinicians must have mastery of all the components of a complete history and physical examination. Performing every assessment and clinical test that a practitioner knows as an initial evaluation is, however, time-consuming, fiscally irresponsible, and likely to yield an uninterpretable catalog of abnormal findings. This does not mean that only cursory and quick clinical examinations of the elderly are indicated. On the contrary, optimal clinical examination may require in-depth evaluations of certain aspects of a patient's clinical presentation in order to understand the factors contributing to the patient's functional deficits. The salient point is that evaluation will be limited to only those aspects.

A third approach to clinical diagnosis is called *pattern recognition,* which can be defined as the "instantaneous realization that the patient's presentation conforms to a previously learned picture." Two examples of patterns relevant to physical therapy are the upper extremity position of the adult with spastic hemiplegia and the bilateral swelling and ulnar deviation of the metacarpals of an individual with rheumatoid arthritis. These patterns represent something immediately identifiable to the experienced therapist that has been learned over time. It has been suggested that pattern recognition is increasingly used as a diagnostic strategy as clinical experience grows.[19]

Unfortunately, pattern recognition is a reflexive approach to categorizing a patient's problems that is not always a reflective process as well. The drawback of pattern recognition is that it can place too much reliance on the therapist's previous experience and lead to a narrow set of premature conclusions. If, for example, we are evaluating someone with shortened bilateral step length in a shuffling pattern, previous clinical experience might suggest that this is a neuromuscular abnormality. On the other hand, previous exposure to patients with rheumatic diseases, who may exhibit the same nonspecific gait abnormalities, may lead to concerns about metatarsalgia. Neither conclusion would be correct without further corroborating evidence.

Experienced clinicians can develop a tendency to see

patterns and assign a diagnostic interpretation to the patient's signs and symptoms prematurely. There is, however, great value to pattern recognition as part of a clinical diagnostic strategy, especially at the start of the diagnostic process. By suggesting that a patient's clinical presentation might conform to some previously encountered pattern, the therapist is able to limit the search for corroborating evidence to substantiate the clinical impression.

The fourth diagnostic method is called the *hypothetico-deductive strategy,* which is defined as the formulation of a short list of potential diagnoses or actions from the earliest clues about the patient, followed by performance of clinical tests that will best reduce the length of the list. This method corrects for the flaw in pattern recognition by not structuring the search for corroborating evidence too narrowly. Neither does it open the search too widely, requiring the therapist to consider every abnormal clinical finding that might be identified through a "complete" history and physical, especially one performed on a geriatric patient. In the next section, the essential steps of the hypothetico-deductive method will be presented as a schema for evaluation and treatment planning.

SCHEMA FOR EVALUATION AND TREATMENT PLANNING

Evaluation

Prior to meeting the patient, a physical therapist should organize the diagnostic approach. Owing to the legal and reimbursement requirements currently imposed on physical therapists, many elders enter physical therapy with a medical referral that may contain a few useful facts about the patient's medical history or the reason for the referral. In these circumstances the first question to ask oneself is, Given the facts about the patient that are available prior to the evaluation, what impairments or functional limitations have been identified? In the event that the referral is incomplete or is not required, the therapist may still hypothesize that certain impairments or functional limitations may exist by virtue of the individual's age, sex, or diagnosis using epidemiologic information and previous clinical experience. For example, suppose that a referral has indicated that the patient to be evaluated has Parkinson's disease, that she is 74 years old, and that she lives alone. The diagnosis of Parkinson's disease suggests the possibility of the following impairments: loss of motor control and abnormal tone, ROM deficits, faulty posture, and decreased endurance for functional activities. Using epidemiologic research about what functional limitations are likely for females living alone, questions about independence in IADL would be appropriate to include in the evaluation. Social isolation, for example, may lead to depression,

which could further aggravate a person's functional difficulties.

After organizing one's thoughts around whatever information about the patient is available, the therapist begins the clinical encounter. If the overall goal is to optimize patient function, then the first step is to ascertain the patient's current level of function. Whenever the patient's communication ability is intact, the initial interview begins by allowing patients to identify what they see as the primary functional limitations that have prompted the need for physical therapy. In their formulation of a hypothetico-deductive strategy for clinical diagnosis, Rothstein and Echternach emphasize the value of listening as patients identify their problems and allowing the individuals to express the desired goal of treatment in their own terms.[17] By talking with the patient the therapist begins to develop not only a professional rapport but also an understanding of the patient's appreciation of the situation. Listening to the patient also permits the therapist to address an ethical dimension of practice. Allowing the patient to identify the goals of treatment is one way to ensure that a person's autonomy has been respected.[7] This is especially pertinent to care provided to older individuals who may find their ability to control their own personal destinies compromised by professional judgments made "in their best interests."

When the patient is unable to communicate effectively, the therapist may turn to proxy information. The therapist may hypothesize about a patient's functional deficits based on previous experience with similar patients. The patient's family and friends may also be able to give some insight as to what the patient would regard as the goal of treatment.

The next two questions to pose in the initial evaluation of the patient are, What impairments could contribute to the patient's functional limitations? and What gross or specific tests would best identify these physical impairments? Proposing that some impairments underlie the functional deficit limits the actual patient testing to just a few alternatives. The tests and measurements that we do as part of an initial evaluation should only be those necessary to confirm or reject a hypothesis about what impairments might lead to specific limitations. A therapist may choose a gross test, for example, a "break" test for strength, to reject a kind of impairment as a contributing factor to the patient's functional deficit. Specific tests can be used to clarify and confirm the exact relationship between the impairment and the limitation. Confirmed impairments may then be stated in the form of a prioritized problem list.

Patients can have multiple impairments, many of which can be identified by a physical therapist and could be treated using physical therapy procedures. Those impairments that are identified during patient assessment but that are not associated with any current or potential functional limitations are excluded from treatment planning. These impairments may, however, be monitored during treatment for any subsequent changes that inhibit a patient's potential for independent function.

Two kinds of clinical data should be integrated into the clinical plan. First, there are a number of factors identified in the literature and reviewed elsewhere in this text that may influence the trajectory of a patient from disease to disability that need to be taken into account (Fig 6–4,A). Specifically, these include a patient's age, sex, education, and income. With respect to the geriatric patient in particular, the therapist must also consider other medical conditions, overall health habits, cognitive ability, mood, and the patient's physical and psychosocial envi-

ronments. Additional information that would assist in setting goals and designing treatment and information from other disciplines can also be very helpful. Data on the individual's current medical conditions and medications, for example, are extremely helpful.

The range of an elder's needs can be very broad, and often a therapist may not know exactly whom to turn to for additional information or help. Health care can be conceived of as a continuum of services (Fig 6–4,B). At one end are medical and nursing care to deal with the patient's disease and illness. At the other end of the continuum is social care by social service professionals to facilitate a patient's re-entry into the community. Although there will always be some overlap, each of these professionals has a

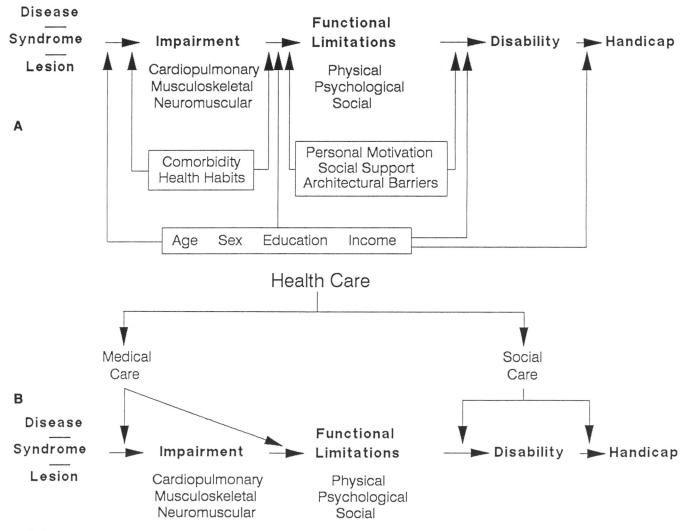

FIG 6–4.
A, personal factors that can affect the trajectory of disability. **B,** professional services in the continuum of health care services and their points of impact on the trajectory of disability. **C,** expansion of the Nagi model to account for the influence of health care services and personal factors on the process of disablement. (Part **C** from Guccione AA: Physical therapy diagnosis and the relationship between impairments and function. *Phys Ther* 1991; 71:499–504. Used by permission of the American Physical Therapy Association.)   *(Continued.)*

C

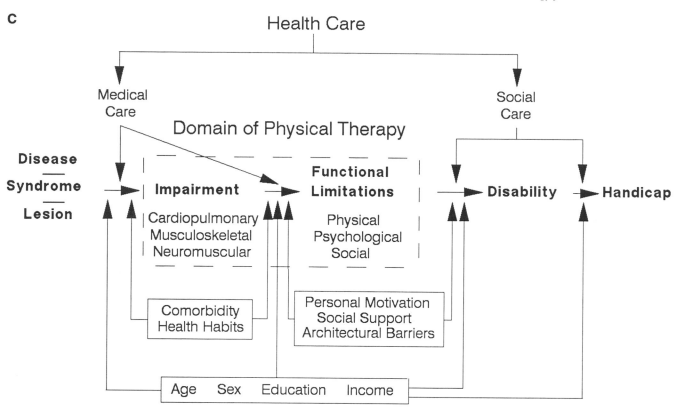

FIG 6–4 (cont.).

primary relationship with the patient in the professional's domain of expertise. Superimposing the continuum of health care onto the patient's clinical needs may provide some clues as to which other practitioners should be consulted (Fig 6–4,C).

The relationship between impairment and function forms the tentative basis for a system of classification for physical therapy diagnosis.[8] Although imprecise, it is useful to say that decreased range of motion of the right shoulder results in dependence in dressing, or to suggest that decreased strength of the left quad leads to dependence in stair climbing. Therapists with additional skill in evaluation can further elaborate the nature of the impairment.[9, 20] Physical therapy treatment will end when the stated functional goals are achieved. Therefore, the functional outcomes of treatment should be stated in behavioral terms.

Treatment Planning

The change in impairment anticipated at discharge should also be described. This helps to identify how much change in impairment will be needed in order for the patient to accomplish the functional activity. The schema for evaluation presented above suggests that physical therapy procedures are aimed directly at remediating impairments that underlie functional limitations, rather than merely addressing the limitation itself. Although physical therapists sometimes apply therapeutic exercise in the position of function—for example, standing balance exercises—or try to simulate the environment in which the functional activity is performed—for example, a staircase—the functional activity alone should not be mistaken for the therapeutic modality. The physical therapist's treatment is still directed at remediating underlying impairment, particularly in the early phases of treatment. As the patient progresses, that is, is less impaired, emphasis will shift to practicing the activity under the therapist's supervision and integrating the task into the patient's daily routine. This general approach of treating impairments first, rather than the functional deficit, has two exceptions. The first exception is the instance in which the therapist determines that the patient has all the requisite physical capacity to perform the task but lacks the knowledge to perform the activity safely and efficiently. A therapeutic strategy to teach only the functional skill directly to the patient would be indicated here. A common example is to teach an individual how to use a cane to reduce weight bearing on an osteoarthritic hip in the absence of any loss of hip range or strength.

The second instance in which a therapist might determine to teach and practice the functional activity rather than change underlying impairments is encountered when the impairments themselves cannot be changed for a certain period of time or are, in fact, permanent. A patient whose lower extremity is immobilized in a cast can be taught to ambulate safely with an assistive device. When the cast is removed, impairments underlying any inability to walk independently may then be addressed. It is particularly helpful for the therapist working with geriatric patients to appreciate that there are some impairments that are not going to change, no matter how much therapy is attempted. This will diminish unnecessary treatment. This does not mean, however, that the patient should automatically be discharged from therapy. Physical therapists can teach patients how to compensate for their permanent impairments. Teaching a nonambulatory elder how to use a wheelchair independently may produce a substantial improvement in the quality of that person's life.

When it is decided that an individual's impairments are amenable to physical therapy, the therapist should establish a schedule for evaluating the effectiveness of the treatment plan. If the patient achieves the desired change in impairment and does not also achieve the functional goal, this is an indication that the therapist has incorrectly hypothesized the relationship between the patient's impairments and functional status.[18] Although a host of physical therapy procedures might be used to remediate an impairment, only those that are most likely to promote the outcome in a cost-effective manner are included in treatment.

SUMMARY

Health status has four components that form a framework for geriatric assessment: disease, impairment, functional limitation, and disability. Handicap results from the negative valuation of a disability by the society in which the disabled individual lives. Physical therapists have particular expertise in the clinical analysis of the relationship between impairments and functional limitations and in the application of therapeutic procedures to remediate impairments. The overall goal of physical therapy for geriatric patients is to maintain or improve their functional status. This goal can be achieved by changing the impairments that underlie the functional limitation or by teaching the patient to compensate for those impairments that cannot be changed.

REFERENCES

1. Badley, EM, Wagstaff S, Wood PHN: Measures of functional ability (disability) in arthritis in relation to impairment of range of joint movement. *Ann Rheum Dis* 1984; 43:563–569.

2. Bergstrom G, et al: Prevalence of symptoms and signs of joint impairment at age 79. *Scand J Rehabil Med* 1985; 173–182.
3. Bergstrom G, et al: Functional consequences of joint impairment at age 79. *Scand J Rehabil Med* 1985; 17.183–190.
4. Ettinger WH, Davis MA: Osteoarthritis, Hazzard WR, et al (eds): *Principles of Geriatric Medicine and Gerontology,* ed 2. New York, McGraw-Hill, 1990.
5. Gerstenblith G, Lakatta EG: Disorders of the heart, Hazzard WR et al (eds): *Principles of Geriatric Medicine and Gerontology,* ed 2. New York, McGraw-Hill, 1990.
6. Granger CV: A conceptual model for functional assessment, in Granger CV, Gresham GE (eds): *Functional Assessment in Rehabilitation Medicine.* Baltimore, Williams & Wilkins, 1984.
7. Guccione AA: Compliance and patient autonomy: Ethical and legal limits to professional dominance. *Top Geriatr Rehab* 1988; 3(3):62–73.
8. Guccione AA: Physical therapy diagnosis and the relationship between impairments and function. *Phys Ther* 1991; 71:499–504.
9. Harris BA, Dyrek DA: A model of orthopaedic dysfunction for clinical decision making in physical therapy practice. *Phys Ther* 1989; 69:548–553.
10. Jette AM, Branch LG, Berlin J: Musculoskeletal impairments and physical disablement among the aged. *J Gerontol* 1990; 45:M203–208.
11. Manton KG: A longitudinal study of functional change and mortality in the United States. *J Gerontol* 1988; 43:S153–161.
12. Nagi SZ: Some conceptual issues in disability and rehabilitation, in Sussman MB (ed): *Sociology and Rehabilitation.* Washington, DC, American Sociological Association, 1965.
13. Nagi SZ: *Disability and Rehabilitation.* Columbus, Ohio State University Press, 1969.
14. Nagi SZ: An epidemiology of disability among adults in the United States. *Milbank Mem Fund Q/Health Soc* 1976; 54:439–467.
15. Nagi S: Disability concepts revisited: Implication for prevention, in Pope AM, Tarlov AR (eds): *Disability in America: Toward a National Agenda for Prevention.* Washington, DC, National Academy Press, 1991.
16. Rose SJ: Musing on diagnosis. *Phys Ther* 1988; 68:1665.
17. Rothstein JM, Echternach JL: Hypothesis-oriented algorithm for clinicians: A method of evaluation and treatment planning. *Phys Ther* 1986; 66:1388–1394.
18. Rubenstein LV, et al: Health status assessment for elderly patients. Report of the Society of General Internal Medicine Task Force on Health Assessment. *J Am Geriatr Soc* 1988; 37:562–569.
19. Sackett DL, Haynes RB, Tugwell P: *Clinical epidemiology: A Basic Science for Clinical Medicine.* Boston, Little, Brown, 1985.
20. Sahrmann SA. Diagnosis by the physical therapist—prerequisite for treatment. *Phys Ther* 1988; 68:1703–1706.

21. Schenkman M, Butler RB: A model for multisystem evaluation, interpretation, and treatment of individuals with neurologic dysfunction. *Phys Ther* 1989; 69:538.

22. Schenkman M, Butler RB: A model for multisystem evaluation and treatment of individuals with Parkinson's disease. *Phys Ther* 1989; 69:932–943.

23. Watts NT: Clinical decision analysis. *Phys Ther* 1989; 69:569–576.

24. World Health Organization: The first ten years of the World Health Organization. Geneva, World Health Organization, 1958.

Functional Assessment of the Elderly

Andrew A. Guccione, Ph.D., P.T.

INTRODUCTION

There can be little dissension that the ultimate goal of all physical therapy interventions with the elderly is to restore or maintain the highest level of function possible for the individual. Whenever physical therapists take on this challenge, they assist elders in maintaining their identities as competent adults. Very young children begin to define themselves, in part, through their independence and mastery over the physical environment, and their pleasure in these achievements is self-evident. Disease and illness threaten more than an older person's physical health. By altering the ability to function, disease and its effects curtail the customary activities that a person identifies as essential to meaningful living. Therefore, functional assessment, in its broadest sense, is particular to the individual and a measure of those activities by which an individual judges the quality of life.

The four purposes of this chapter are to review what is currently known about the physical functional status of the elderly, describe the elements that may be included in a physical functional assessment, discuss some of the methodologic aspects of administering a functional assessment, and describe a few of the formal functional assessment instruments that have been used in geriatric clinical practice and research.

As has been described in Chapter 6 and elsewhere in this text, the data of a functional assessment alone cannot determine the treatment plan. The physical therapist must review functional limitations in light of other clinical findings that identify the patient's impairments. The therapist then hypothesizes which impairments contribute to the patient's functional deficits and will be the focus of physical therapy intervention. Two patients may have the same limitation in transferring from bed to chair, yet require entirely different treatment programs. If the first individual lacked sufficient knee strength to come to a standing position, then the treatment program would incorporate strengthening exercises to remedy the impairment and improve the patient's function. If the other patient lacked sufficient range of motion (ROM) at the hip due to flexion contractures to allow full upright standing, then the treatment would focus on increasing ROM at the hip to improve function. Each individual may achieve a similar level of functional independence, yet neither would have received the exact same treatment to achieve the same outcome.

PHYSICAL FUNCTIONAL LIMITATIONS IN THE ELDERLY

As elaborated in Chapter 6, physical, psychologic, and social function are all dimensions of function that are included in the measurement of a person's overall health status.[32] Physical therapists are most often concerned with evaluating physical functional limitations and remediating the impairments that underlie them. Physical functional activities, the focus of this chapter, can be subdivided into five areas: mobility, which includes transfers and ambulation; basic self-care and personal hygiene activities of daily living (ADL); more complex activities essential to an adult's living in the community known as instrumental ADL (IADL); work; and recreation. Epidemiologic studies of functional limitations in the elderly provide a group context into which a physical therapist can place an individual patient's level of function.[6] In general, we know that the ability to function independently declines with age and that this decline is influenced by a host of biologic, psychologic, and social factors. There are several major sources of epidemiologic data on function in the elderly.[34] These include the Supplement on Aging (SOA) to the 1984 National Health Interview Survey,[8] the 1985 National Nursing Home Survey (NNHS),[18] the 1987 National Medical Expenditure Survey (NMES),[25] the 1982 and 1984 National Long Term Care Surveys (NLTCSs),[26] and the Establishment of Populations for the Epidemiologic Study of the Elderly (EPESE) project begun in 1982.[5]

Community-Dwelling Elders

The SOA data indicate that as few as 19% of the 26.4 million noninstitutionalized persons over age 65 in 1984 had difficulty walking (Fig 7–1).[17] Sex-specific rates of difficulty in walking, however, were different. Just over 20% of women over age 65 had difficulty walking, whereas only 15.5% of their male counterparts did. Slightly over 77% of those surveyed in the SOA reported no difficulty in any of basic ADL, which is not surprising in a noninstitutionalized population. Difficulty in bathing and getting outside were reported by 10% of these elders, whereas 6% experienced difficulty in dressing. Almost one quarter of these elders had trouble with a single home management task, heavy home chores (Fig 7–2). Nearly 27% had difficulty with at least one of six IADL: preparing meals, shopping, managing money, using the telephone, doing heavy home chores, and performing light housework. Male elders reported less difficulty in almost all these tasks than female elders did.

Despite the fact that advancing age increases the risk of functional limitations, there are still a substantial number of old-old who remain physically independent. Harris and her colleagues examined physical ability in 80-year-olds who participated in a longitudinal follow-up to the SOA.[16] Using four items from Nagi's measure of work disability, they found that 67% of all white persons aged 80 or older had no difficulty lifting 10 lb; 57% had no difficulty climbing up ten steps; 49% had no difficulty walk-

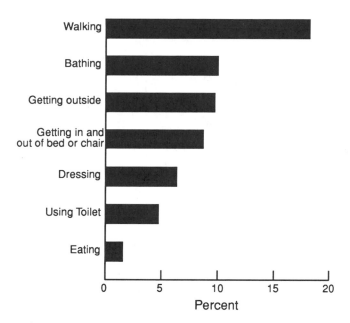

FIG 7–1.
Percentage of the noninstitutionalized population 65 years of age or over who have difficulty with activities of daily living, by type of activity: United States, 1984. (Redrawn from Havlik RJ, et al: Health statistics on older persons, United States, 1986. *Vital and Health Statistics, Series 3, No 25.* Hyattsville, Md, Public Health Service, DHHS No (PHS) 87– 1409, 1987.)

ing a quarter of a mile; and 47% had no difficulty with stooping, crouching, or kneeling (Fig 7–3). The order in which the activities became more difficult was the same for men as for women. Women, however, reported more difficulty with each of these tasks than men.

Given that any sample of elderly will most likely contain a larger proportion of older, and therefore more functionally disabled, women than men, a difference in the rates of functional limitations between men and women is not unexpected. The differential rates of functional limitations in IADL between men and women are also partially explained by a gender bias in the items of many surveys. Among present-day elders, many men do not perform housekeeping and other similar activities. Therefore, men may not report having any difficulty at all performing these tasks as they did not perform them at the time of the interview. Neither have male elders generally ever performed these tasks, a reflection of society's arbitrary notion of what is "proper" for a man or a woman. A similar finding was obtained in the EPESE study of elders with low back pain.[23] Although elderly women with low back pain reported modestly higher rates of limitations in basic ADL than men, the rate of limitation in doing household chores for women was more than double the rate for men.

Besides underscoring the gender bias of some items that might be included in a functional assessment, differences in functional status between men and women remind us that function is also a sociological phenomenon. Functional assessment does not only measure the individual's abilities to perform tasks that are personally meaningful to the individual. Functional assessment also depends on social expectations of what is "normal" functioning for an adult. In some social groups, a man might never be expected to do housecleaning, nor would anyone anticipate that a woman would shovel snow, because performing these activities runs counter to what a man or a woman "should" do. It is therefore necessary that the overall ap-

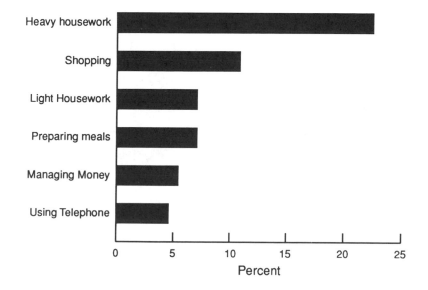

FIG 7–2.
Percentage of the noninstitutionalized population 65 years of age or over who have difficulty with instrumental activities of daily living, by type of activity: United States, 1984. (Redrawn from Havlik RJ, et al: Health statistics on older persons, United States, 1986. *Vital and Health Statistics, Series 3, No 25.* Hyattsville, Md, Public Health Service, DHHS No (PHS) 87–1409, 1987.

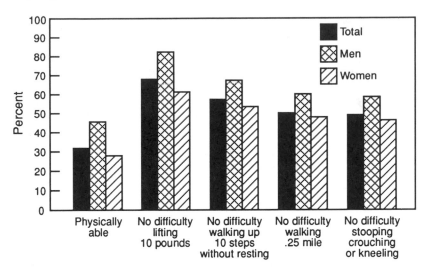

FIG 7-3.
Physical ability of noninstitutionalized white persons, age 80 or older. (Redrawn from Harris T, et al: Longitudinal study of physical ability in the oldest-old. *Am J Public Health* 1989, 79:698-702.)

proach to functional assessment of an elder include items that take into account what is "normal" in that person's social sphere.

A judgment about whether an elder's functional level is normal also draws heavily on cultural and ethnic attitudes. If there is a certain expectation in the family that debilitation is a normal occurrence in old age and that elders are entitled to have even the simplest ADL done for them, there is little likelihood that the goal of independence in all ADL will be achieved. Therefore, physical therapists working with elders from specific groups should have an understanding of different cultural and ethnic expectations of independent function.

Institutionalized Elders

There is a substantial difference in functional limitations between elders still living in the community and those who reside in a nursing home. Inability to perform simple self-care activities typically places an elder at risk for admission to a nursing home. Data from the NNHS that compare nursing home residents to their noninstitutionalized peers clearly indicate the disparity in functional levels between these two groups of elders. While over 90% of elders in nursing homes required assistance in bathing, only 6% of community-dwelling elders needed help in this activity. Similarly, just over 40% of nursing home residents needed assistance to eat, whereas only 1.1% of their peers outside the nursing home were similarly limited (Table 7-1).

Data on the differences in functional limitations between community-dwelling and institutionalized elders provide direction for physical therapists planning a functional assessment for an individual patient. The relation-

ship between ADL and IADL is generally hierarchical; that is, limitations in ADL usually predict limitations in IADL.[3, 33] For example, we know that most elders living in the community are generally independent in all ADL and may experience limitations in a few IADL. Thus, a home-care physical therapist working with a patient recently returning home from an acute care hospital following a hip fracture would first explore the individual's ability in basic ADL such as transfers, ambulation, and toileting. If deficits were found, independence in these activities would serve as the first goals of treatment. If the patient was independent in basic ADL upon initial evaluation, or became independent through the physical therapist's intervention, the therapist would then examine the elder's lim-

TABLE 7-1.

Percentage of Persons 65 Years of Age and Over, By Whether Nursing Home Resident or Noninstitutionalized and Type of Dependency in Selected ADL: United States, 1984 and 1985

Type of Dependency	Nursing Home Residents, 1985 (%)	Noninstitutionalized Population*† 1984 (%)
Requires assistance in		
Bathing	91.2	6.0
Dressing	77.7	4.3
Using toilet room	63.3	2.2
Transferring‡	62.7	2.8
Eating	40.4	1.1

*From Dawson D, Hendershot G, Fulton J: Aging in the eighties. Functional limitations of individuals age 65 years and over. *Advance Data From Vital and Health Statistics, No 133.* DHHS Publication No (PHS) 87-1250, Hyattsville, Md, Public Health Service, April 30, 1987.
†Percentage of the noninstitutionalized elderly dependent in activities of daily living is a measure of those who *received* help rather than those needing it.
‡*Transferring* refers to getting in or out of a bed or chair.

itations in performing IADL, which supports a person's ability to live independently in the community.

Physical therapists should be wary, however, of assuming too quickly that there is a need for institutionalization merely on the broad epidemiologic evidence supporting a relationship between limitations in basic ADL and the ability to remain living in the community. Epidemiologic data summarize various facts about a group, but a particular fact need not apply to every member of that group. Furthermore, despite the fact that most elders living in the community generally function at a higher level than their institutionalized peers, many elders with functional limitations do manage to remain outside of institutions with formal services or through the efforts of families and friends. Physical therapists play an important role in identifying an elder's needs for formal care givers such as homemakers and home health aides and in teaching families how to manage an elderly patient's limitations well enough so that the individual may continue to reside in the community.

At least two other factors also influence whether an elder limited in the most basic ADL continues to live in the community. First, there are not enough nursing home beds in some areas to accommodate the need of the community for such placements. Thus, an elder might benefit from admission to a nursing home but will continue to live at home. Second, even if nursing home beds are available, some elders lack the appropriate insurance coverage or the financial means to claim them. These individuals will therefore remain in the community, sometimes under the most distressing circumstances. Therapists working in the community should anticipate that elders who are disabled enough to require human assistance around the clock will constitute at least a small portion of their caseloads from time to time.

COMPONENTS OF PHYSICAL FUNCTIONAL ASSESSMENT

Functional assessment data can be useful to physical therapists in several ways.[22] On the individual level, a functional assessment can be used as a quick screen to identify the need for more extensive evaluation by a physical therapist or other practitioners. If an elder who has functional deficits becomes a patient, these data determine the overall goals of physical therapy treatment. Such goals serve as indicators of a patient's progress and validate the success (or failure) of the therapist's intervention. Finally, organizing and analyzing functional data by types of patients or patients' problems can provide valuable documentation of the needs of a group for treatment, the benefits of a particular treatment approach, or the success of an innovative program.

Mobility

A primary concern of physical therapists in performing a physical functional assessment of an elderly individual is to identify any functional limitations in mobility: ambulation on level surfaces within the home, stair climbing, negotiating uneven terrain, and walking for longer distances in the community.

Basic Activities of Daily Living (ADL)

Basic ADL include all the fundamental tasks and activities necessary for survival, hygiene, and self-care within the home. A typical ADL battery, which may be administered by a physical therapist alone or cooperatively with other health professionals, covers eating, bathing, grooming, dressing, bed mobility, and transfers. Incontinence and the ability to use a bathroom are especially important elements in the assessment of physical function in some older individuals. The ability of an elder in three aspects of toileting may each require exploration: to get to the bathroom in an appropriate period of time, to move safely on and off the receptacle, and to perform self-hygiene tasks.

Instrumental Activities of Daily Living (IADL)

An evaluation of IADL addresses multiple areas that are essential to living independently as an adult: cooking, shopping, washing, housekeeping, and ability to use public transportation or drive a car. For some individuals, it may also be appropriate to investigate the ability to perform home chores such as shoveling snow or yardwork.

Work

One measure of adult competence is employment. Previously, it has been assumed that elders did not need to or want to work. Changes in federal regulations during the 1980s raised the minimum age at which individuals may receive full Social Security benefits and also removed a mandatory retirement age for most occupations.[21] Therefore, elders who want to, or need to, remain in the work force may do so if they are physically able to perform the tasks of their employment. The ability to work may be investigated in two ways. One approach is to consider the conditions of work itself: whether an individual is working the anticipated number of hours each week, whether the requirements of the job have been modified in any respect to allow the individual to work, and whether the quantity or quality of work done has met the anticipated standard of performance. Another approach to assessing work is to examine the ability to perform ten particular physical tasks, first described by Nagi,[29] that are associated with work disability: (1) walking up ten steps without resting; (2) walking a quarter of a mile; (3) sitting for 2 hours; (4) standing for 2 hours; (5) stooping, crouching, or kneeling; (6) reaching up overhead; (7) reaching out to shake hands; (8) grasping with fingers; (9) lifting or carrying 10 lb; and 10) lifting or carrying 25 lb. Using these data on "advanced" mobility, one can infer what an elderly individual's capacity to work would be.

Recreation

Recreational activities are no less important than work to maintain a sense of well-being. Clearly more older men and women today are maintaining interests in recreational sports that they developed earlier in life. Other elders can be identified who are just discovering the pleasures of physical exertion. Functional assessment of recreational activities, however, is not limited only to sports. Many elders enjoy dancing and gardening, which require a relatively high degree of balance, flexibility, and strength. Even sedentary activities, such as stamp collecting or playing chess, require a certain degree of physical ability in the hand and upper extremity and therefore may be functional measures of the outcomes of treatment for some patients.

METHODOLOGIC ISSUES

There are three methodologic issues that are germane to the discussion of functional status measurement: reliability, validity, and clinical utility.[2, 4, 12, 13, 27, 31] It is sometimes erroneously assumed that measurement issues are relevant only if a clinician uses a formal instrument to assess function. This is simply not the case. All physical therapy assessments involve measurements that provide data used by the physical therapist to render an evaluation of the patient's condition. The certainty of that professional judgment is a function of the quality of the data. It is important to know if apparent improvement in a patient's level of function is a real change in performance or merely a variation in measurement due to the nature of the test or the skill of the tester in administering the test. These are issues of reliability. It is also important to know if the therapist *actually* gathered the information that was intended to be gathered, and what inferences about the patient's status or prognosis are appropriate based on the data. These are the central questions of the validity of a measurement.

Reliability

There are several forms of reliability, each of which is pertinent to judging the value of the information derived from a particular test. The first kind of reliability is termed *internal consistency* and is a measure of how well items on a test, which purportedly measure the same thing, yield similar results.[31] Internal consistency is important in judging the value of assessment instruments that use a battery of multiple items to cover a component of function such as basic ADL, IADL, or mobility. Internal consistency is an indicator of how well the items within a segment "hang together" and measure the same kind of thing. If a battery contains too many questions all measuring the same thing, it may be possible to drop some items and evaluate a patient more efficiently.

Two other kinds of reliability indicate how much variability in test scores is due to the tester. The first of these, *intra-rater reliability* attests to the degree to which a measurement will change when the same tester administers the test on two separate occasions even though no real change has occurred. This form of reliability is often taken as an indicator of the stability of a test between administrations. *Inter-rater reliability* indicates the agreement of test results when two or more testors measure the same thing. Both of these forms of reliability are critical to clinical practice, especially in geriatric physical therapy where multiple care givers may repeat measurements on the same patient over a period of time and use these data to determine a patient's progress or deterioration.

Validity

There are several kinds of validity that are pertinent to functional assessment.[31] The first is *face validity,* which requires the judgment that the assessment appears on the face of it to be a test of what is to be measured. For example, an IADL test should measure activities such as cooking, grocery shopping, and housekeeping in some way. If the test consisted of only sociodemographic data and goniometric measurements, we would conclude that this test lacked face validity as a measure of IADL.

Content validation establishes the degree to which test measures adequately sample a domain of activities. For example, a formal measure of recreational activity might only mention two of the more strenuous sports — hiking and kayaking, list only running and jogging under cardiovascular training activities, and omit more sedentary pastimes altogether. Such an instrument would not have adequately sampled the multitude of activities that constitute "recreation," especially for older adults. Therefore, we would conclude that this instrument lacked content validity.

Although *construct validity* often involves statistical approaches that are far beyond the scope of this text, it is a critical dimension of functional assessment. Construct validation answers the question, Does a test yield measurements that represent the underlying concept of what we want to measure? All the questions posed to a patient during an initial evaluation and all the measurements taken during assessment do not fall into the same category. Some formal functional assessment instruments were developed before there was much concern about the psychometric properties of physical therapy tests and measures. These instruments tend to combine disease severity, impairment, and functional limitations under a single category of "function." Several even combine scores on various subsections of the test to give an overall "functional" score. While a single number appears to be a useful and reliable summary of the patient's status, it can be difficult to determine exactly what construct has been measured by this sort of score. Although these scores may be reliable, their validity is a separate question. Physical therapists should use them thoughtfully, as they may often reflect more than a person's functional status.

Sometimes the results of a test can be compared with a "gold standard," which is accepted as an unimpeachable measure of whatever is being tested. This comparison demonstrates that the test has concurrent validity. For example, the results obtained from a formal ADL instrument that uses a patient's self-report might be shown to be similar to the results obtained from having the patient actually perform the activities listed in the instrument. We might then compare the patient's self-report to that of another individual who knows the patient well. We might also demonstrate that elders who are judged as being independent by this self-report measure also have few impairments in ROM, strength, and balance.

Physical therapists are also responsible to establish the likelihood of achieving goals as part of the process of physical therapy evaluation. Often, we base these judgments on a combination of the patient's clinical presentation and our prior clinical experience. What we lack as often is a clear understanding of the predictive validity of our measurements, which allows us to know that a certain score on a test at the initiation of treatment predicts the outcome of intervention. Knowing the predictive validity of a baseline functional assessment would greatly facilitate the formulation of achievable treatment goals and increase the efficiency of discharge planning from the beginning of treatment.

Clinical Utility

The ultimate value of any clinical data is their usefulness to the task at hand. Reliable and valid data are necessary but not sufficient conditions for test results to have clinical utility. If a test or instrument has clinical utility, all necessary data will be gathered completely and in the shortest period of time. Too many questions and too many compli-

cated steps increase respondent burden. If an elder becomes annoyed, fatigued, or distracted by the evaluation, the therapist may have hindered the development of professional rapport with the patient, an important factor in the success of any rehabilitation program.

Is it necessary to use a formal, structured instrument to conduct a functional assessment? It is doubtful that any instrument will contain all the activities that would constitute a complete evaluation of any one person's function. Therefore, a therapist may wish to combine a formal instrument with unstructured assessment and open-ended questions as part of the overall evaluation. This will ensure that there are similar baseline data with known reliability and validity on all patients as well as data that capture information unique to the individual.

Given that some formal instruments may not be well suited to particular clinical needs, it is tempting to "mix and match" from several instruments. Extrapolating items from a variety of instruments may provide the kind of data desired, but it may be at the expense of reliability and validity. Further methodologic problems may arise when instruments are not administered in the format for which they were developed and tested. Users may prefer or need to gather data in some instances by using trained interviewers. This requires that explicit instructions for the interviewers have been developed to ensure comparability of results.

MODES OF ASSESSMENT

There are three primary methods to measuring functional status. An individual's level of physical function may be collected by self-report, gathered by an interviewer, or observed by asking the subject to perform a function under a specific set of conditions. Therapists are most familiar with direct observation of the activity. The major advantage of this approach is that the professional judgment of functional status is based on clear-cut objective evidence of the ability to perform the task.[15] Physical performance measures are also not limited by language barriers.[14] If the therapist and the patient do not speak the same language, the therapist may act out the activity and signal that the patient should do the same. Direct observation also has some disadvantages. This method assumes that the controlled environment of a structured situation in the clinic is reasonably similar to the environment in which a person functions. An individual may not be able to transfer out of a chair in the clinic but may be totally independent in transferring using any chair in that person's home. Physical performance measures are also time-consuming for the therapist and therefore costly.

While direct observation may have stood as the gold

standard for some time, self-report approaches have become well accepted in research. Self-report is now considered the most feasible and cost-effective means of gathering standardized functional status data on large numbers of individuals.[27] One further consideration in using a self-report mode of assessment is whether to use a trained interviewer to administer the instrument or to allow the respondent to read and answer a questionnaire. There appears to be little difference in the quality of the data obtained by self-report or face-to-face interviewer.[28] It may be the case in the elderly, however, that visual loss or shorter attention spans recommend the use of trained interviewers.

PARAMETERS OF MEASUREMENT

Independence

The concept of functional independence may be conceived in several ways. These include dependence or the degree of assistance needed to perform a task, how much pain accompanies the task, the amount of time it takes to perform the activity, or whether an individual uses an assistive device or aid to perform the task. The amount of difficulty an individual has when attempting to perform functional activities is another way to operationalize independence. The concept of difficulty is composite of several criteria to assess how functional activities are performed and summarizes the degree of effort expended in performing the task. It involves elements of how long the activity takes, how much discomfort the individual experiences, and to what degree assistive devices are required.

In order to collect the appropriate information on an elder's functional status, the therapist must consider the way in which functional limitations are identified and the kind of data needed. Merely using an assistive device and performing an activity with difficulty are appropriate criterion levels of disability for some clinical or research purposes, but each parameter alone may not identify the same individuals as limited. The difficulty of an activity may be diminished, in fact, by using an adaptive device. The need for human assistance may be a more meaningful criterion of dysfunction when the data will be used to plan an elder's need for services or to make public policy decisions.

Therapists must also consider what constitutes a clinically meaningful change in function. If an individual's behavior may be graded only as "independent or dependent," then the scoring system may not be sensitive to real changes that indicate a patient's progress. For example, progression from being totally nonambulatory to requiring only moderate assistance to ambulate can represent substantial improvement in function. However, if the patient can only be rated as "independent/dependent," then treatment might erroneously be judged ineffective. Careful consideration of the precision of descriptors is essential to capture subtle yet noticeable improvements in a patient's condition.

Capacity vs. Performance

Some self-report instruments phrase questions as "Could you. . .?" whereas another may query the same activity by asking "Do you . . .?" These are not equivalent forms of the same question and do not yield the same information. The first way of phrasing a question taps into an elder's beliefs about personal abilities, which may be based only partially on empirical evidence. The second approach establishes whether the individual does the activity. Thus, an elder might respond to a question about stair climbing in the following way: "I could climb the stairs to the second floor of my home (if I had to), but I do not climb the stairs (because it hurts my knee and I don't want to)." Observation of performance can inform us as to what an elder can do but will not let us know what an elder will do any better than asking the person directly. Thus, there may be some disparity between what elders regard as their capabilities and what they may habitually perform at home or under specific conditions in the clinic. Therapists must recognize that even if an elder has the capacity to perform the activity but will not do it, treatment to achieve a higher level of function may be inappropriate.

Time Frames

The time frames of particular items vary from questionnaire to questionnaire. The period of inquiry may be for the same day, the past week, or even the past month. Therapists must decide in advance what is the appropriate time period in which to sample behavior, given the fluctuating nature of many geriatric problems.

SELECTED INSTRUMENTS FOR GERIATRIC FUNCTIONAL ASSESSMENT

A considerable number of functional assessment instruments with particular relevance to geriatric physical therapy have been presented in the literature. Comprehensive reviews of these instruments have been published elsewhere.[1, 12, 13, 27] A few of these instruments are reviewed below. They were selected on the basis of being representative of the current state of the art in geriatric functional assessment as well as their predominance in geriatric clinical practice and research.

Katz Index of Activities of Daily Living

Katz's index is the prototypic instrument for measuring basic ADL in geriatric patients.[19, 20] The index covers activities in six categories: bathing, dressing, toileting, transfers, continence, and feeding. Unfortunately, this instrument does not address ambulation and other components of mobility, which are particularly pertinent to physical therapy. Although designed for use among institutionalized elders, the theoretical foundation of the Katz index is actually taken from a developmental model of children. According to this model, feeding is designated as the "lowest" and most easily acquired function, whereas bathing represents the developmentally "highest" level of function. Each item on the Katz is rated according to the degree of assistance needed to do the task. Responses in each category of activity are then dichotomized as independent or dependent, according to predetermined criteria. The pattern of responses is then converted to a cumulative letter grade from A through G, which denotes a particular pattern of dependency in the hierarchy of function. For example, an "A" means independent in all six functional categories; a "C" indicates independent in bathing, dressing, and one other function; and a "G" denotes dependence in all activities. The psychometric properties of the Katz are sufficient to justify its widespread use in both clinical care and research.

Functional Independence Measure

The Functional Independence Measure (FIM) is an 18-item measure of physical, psychologic, and social function that is part of the Uniform Data System for Medical Rehabilitation.[10, 11] The FIM uses the level of assistance an individual needs to grade functional status from total independence to total assistance. A person may be regarded as independent if a device is used, but this is recorded separately from "complete" independence. The instrument lists six self-care activities: feeding, grooming, bathing, upper body dressing, lower body dressing, and toileting. Bowel and bladder control, aspects of which some may consider as impairments rather than function, are categorized separately. Mobility is tested only through three items on transfers. Under the category of locomotion, walking and using a wheelchair are listed equivalently, whereas stairs are considered separately. The FIM also includes two items on communication and three on social cognition.

The FIM measures what the individual does, not what that person could do under certain circumstances. The inter-rater reliability of the FIM has been established at an acceptable level of psychometric performance. The face and content validity of the FIM as well as its ability to capture change in a patient's level of function have also

been determined. A trained clinician must administer the FIM, as the response for each item requires a professional judgment.

OARS Multidimensional Functional Assessment Questionnaire

The Older American Resources and Services (OARS) was one of the first formal approaches developed explicitly to assess the function of elders in multiple domains.[7, 9] The OARS, which was developed and tested at the Duke Center for the Study of Aging and Human Development, is composed of an instrument to assess functional activities (the Multidimensional Functional Assessment Questionnaire [MFAQ]) and a questionnaire to identify the resources that an elder uses. The MFAQ is designed to be administered by a trained interviewer. In order to ensure the reliability and validity of the responses given to the interviewer, the MFAQ begins with an assessment of the elder's cognitive function. The Services Assessment Questionnaire (SAQ) records both an elder's use of services and the perceived need for services. A total of 24 generic services are covered, for example, nursing and homemaker services, legal and protective aid, and recreation.

The items on the MFAQ cover basic and instrumental ADL, social interaction and resources, economic resources, physical health, and mental health. After reviewing the responses, the interviewer rates the elder in each of the five dimensions using a six-point scale. The scale's end points are "excellent functioning" and "total or complete impaired function." The MFAQ's reliability and validity have been established and meet acceptable levels of psychometric performance. It has also been shown that the MFAQ is sensitive enough to detect gross changes over time and can discriminate among elders who live independently in the community, require adult day care, or are institutionalized.

Philadelphia Geriatric Center Multilevel Assessment Instrument

The Multilevel Assessment Instrument (MAI) is based on Lawton's conceptual model of adult behavior, which is hierarchically organized by the complexity of the behavior.[24] There are five behavioral domains represented in the MAI: physical health, cognition, self-care, and instrumental ADL; time use (employment, hobbies, recreation); social interaction; personal adjustment (morale, psychiatric symptoms); and perceived environment (housing, neighborhood, personal security). The items on ADL investigate the perceived ability of an individual (i.e., "Can you . . . ?") rather than actual performance of the task (i.e., "Do you . . . ?"). Limitations are graded by the degree of human assistance required rather than the quality of the performance. As discussed elsewhere in this text, the psychologic dimension of health status is composed of mental and affective function. The MAI is an excellent example of an instrument that differentiates cognition, morale, and psychiatric symptoms.

The MAI is available in full, midlength, and short forms. The MAI in all its forms had extensive testing of its reliability and validity. In general, the MAI has demonstrated acceptable psychometric characteristics, particularly in its long form. The instrument was designed to be administered by an interviewer and can be completed in under an hour.

Minimum Data Sheet for Nursing Home Resident Assessment and Care Screening

The Omnibus Budget Reconciliation Act of 1987 (OBRA '87) mandated a number of changes in nursing home regulations, which were meant to guarantee quality of care for nursing home residents. One mechanism to monitor care to all Medicare or Medicaid nursing homes developed subsequent to the enactment of OBRA '87, was the Resident Assessment Instrument (RAI).[30] The RAI has two parts: the Minimum Data Set (MDS) and Resident Assessment Protocols (RAPs). The MDS is used to assess the patterns of a patient's function in multiple dimensions: cognitive, communication/hearing, vision, physical functioning and structural problems, continence in the last 14 days, psychosocial well-being, mood and behavior, and activity pursuit. The MDS is also used to collect basic demographic data, disease diagnoses, health conditions, oral/nutritional status, oral/dental status, skin condition, medication use, and special treatment and procedures, an area that specifically lists physical therapy.

Following the initial admission of the patient to a facility, the MDS must be completed by the 14th calendar day of residency but may be updated through the 21st day. After this initial administration, the resident must be reassessed using the full MDS annually. A subset of MDS items must also be assessed on each resident every 3 months. If there is a significant change that appears to be permanent, a resident should be assessed using the MDS within 14 days after the change has occurred, in addition to any quarterly or yearly reassessments. The law requires that each assessment be conducted or coordinated by a registered nurse, who may choose to assign parts of the assessment to other health professionals, including physical therapists.

When physical therapists are part of an MDS assessment team, they will most likely be involved with the MDS section on physical functioning and structural problems. This section considers seven different areas: bed mobility, transfers, locomotion, dressing, eating, toilet use, personal hygiene; bathing; body control problems (e.g., contractures, amputations, hemiplegia, balance); mobility appliances and devices; the need to have tasks broken down into component parts; rehabilitation potential; and change in ADL in the last 90 days. The first six of these items are coded according to the degree of human assistance a resident needed to perform the task and the type of support provided by staff, if assistance was required. The time frame for assessment on each ADL is the 7 days prior to the assessment.

After the MDS is completed, the data are reviewed to determine if the patient has any of the 18 common problems identified by the RAPs. The RAPs address the following clinical problems: delirium, cognitive loss/dementia, visual function, communication, ADL function/rehabilitation potential, urinary incontinence and indwelling catheter, psychosocial well-being, mood state, behavior problem, activities, falls, nutritional status, feeding tubes, dehydration/fluid maintenance, dental care, pressure ulcers, psychotropic drug use, and physical restraints. The RAP review will determine the plan of care for each patient.

Specific data on the reliability, validity, and sensitivity of the MDS have not been published. The MDS was developed with extensive field testing to ensure its clinical utility. Further research clinical use will be necessary to determine if its developers succeeded in producing a clinically relevant and psychometrically sound instrument.

SUMMARY

The purpose of geriatric physical therapy intervention is to improve or maintain the functional status of the individual. Previous studies of the functional status of elders have indicated that age alone is a risk factor for functional decline. When normal aging is coupled with the effects of disease, an elder may experience a severe deterioration in quality of life. A functional assessment is therefore an essential component of the physical therapist's evaluation. Regardless of whether the functional assessment is conducted with a formal structured instrument, an unstructured interview, or direct observation of performance, the results must be reliable, valid, and clinically useful.

REFERENCES

1. Applegate WB, Blass JP, Williams TF: Instruments for the functional assessment of older patients. *N Engl J Med* 1990; 322:1207–1214.
2. Arnold SB: The measurement of quality of life in the frail elderly, in JE Birren, et al (eds): *The Concept and Mea-*

surement of Quality of Life in the Frail Elderly. San Diego, Academic Press, 1991.

3. Åsberg KH, Sonn U: The cumulative structure of personal and instrumental ADL. *Scand J Rehabil Med* 1989; 21:171–177.

4. Bombardier C, Tugwell P: Methodological considerations in functional assessment. *J Rheumatol Suppl* 14(suppl 15):6–10.

5. Cornoni-Huntley JC, et al: Epidemiology of disability in the oldest-old: Methodologic issues and preliminary findings. *Milbank Mem Fund Q/Health Soc* 1985; 63:350–376.

6. Dawson D, Hendershot G, Fulton J: Aging in the eighties. Functional limitations of individuals age 65 years and over. *Advance Data From Vital and Health Statistics, No 133*. Hyattsville, Md, Public Health Service, DHHS Publication No (PHS) 87–1250, 1987.

7. Fillenbaum GG, Smyer MA: The development, validity and reliability of the OARS Multidimensional Functional Assessment Questionnaire. *J Gerontol* 1981; 36:428–434.

8. Fitti JE, Kovar MG: The Supplement on Aging to the 1984 National Health Interview Survey. *Vital and Health Statistics, Series 1, No 21*. Washington, DC, Public Health Service, DHHS Publication No (PHS) 87–1323, 1987.

9. George LK, Fillenbaum GG: OARS methodology: A decade of experience in geriatric assessment. *J Am Geriatr Soc* 1985; 33:607–615.

10. Granger CV, et al: Advances in functional assessment for medical rehabilitation. *Top Geriatr Rehabil* 1986; 1(3):59–74.

11. Granger CV, et al: Functional assessment scales: A study of persons with multiple sclerosis. *Arch Phys Med Rehabil* 1990; 71:870–875.

12. Guccione AA, Jette AM: Assessing limitations in physical function in patients with arthritis. *Arthritis Care Res* 1988; 1:170–176.

13. Guccione AA, Jette AM: Multidimensional assessment of functional limitations in patients with arthritis. *Arthritis Care Res* 1990; 3:44–52.

14. Guralnik JM, et al: Physical performance measures in aging research. *J Gerontol* 1989; 44:M141–146.

15. Harris BA, et al: Validity of self-report measures of functional disability. *Top Geriatr Rehabil* 1986; 1(3):31–41.

16. Harris T, et al: Longitudinal study of physical ability in the oldest-old. *Am J Public Health* 1989; 79:698–702.

17. Havlik RJ, et al: Health statistics on older persons, United States, 1986. *Vital and Health Statistics, Series 3, No 25*. Hyattsville, Md, Public Health Service, DHHS Publication No (PHS) 87–1409, 1987.

18. Hing E: Use of nursing homes by the elderly: Preliminary data from the 1985 National Nursing Home Survey. *Advance Data From Vital and Health Statistics, No 135*. Hyattsville, Md, Public Health Service, DHHS Publication No (PHS) 87–1250, 1987.

19. Katz S, et al: Studies of illness in the aged. The Index of ADL: A standardized measure of biological and psychosocial function. *JAMA* 1963; 185:914–919.

20. Katz S, et al: Progress in the development of the index of ADL. *Gerontologist* 1970; 10:20–30.

21. Kovar MG, LaCroix AZ: Aging in the eighties: Ability to perform work-related activities. Data from the Supplement on Aging to the National Health Interview Survey, United States, 1984. *Advance Data From Vital and Health Statistics, No 136*. Hyattsville, Md, Public Health Service, DHHS Publication No (PHS) 87–1250, 1987.

22. Lachs MS, et al: A simple procedure for general screening for functional disability in elderly patients. *Ann Intern Med* 1990; 112:699–706.

23. Lavsky-Shulan M, et al: Prevalence and functional correlates of low back pain in the elderly: The Iowa 65+ Rural Health Study. *J Am Geriatr Soc* 1985; 33:23–28.

24. Lawton MP, et al: A research and service oriented multi-level assessment instrument. *J Gerontol* 1989; 37:91–99.

25. Leon J, Lair T: Functional status of the non-institutionalized elderly: Estimates of ADL and IADL difficulties. *National Medical Expenditure Survey Research Findings 4. Agency for Health Care Policy and Research*. Rockville, Md, Public Health Service, DHHS Publication No (PHS) 90–3462, 1990.

26. Manton KG: A longitudinal study of functional change and mortality in the United States. *J Gerontol* 1988; 43:S153–161.

27. McDowell I, Newell C: *Measuring Health: A Guide to Rating Scales and Questionnaires*. Oxford, Oxford University Press, 1987.

28. Morris WW, Boutelle S: Multidimensional functional assessment in two modes. *Gerontologist* 1985; 25:638–643.

29. Nagi SZ: An epidemiology of disability among adults in the United States. *Milbank Mem Fund Q/Health Soc* 1976; 54:439–467.

30. *Resident Assessment Instrument (RAI) Training Manual and Resource Guide*. Washington, DC, American Health Care Association, 1990.

31. Rothstein JM: Measurement and clinical practice: Theory and application, in Rothstein JM (ed): *Measurement in Physical Therapy*. New York, Churchill Livingstone, 1985.

32. Rubenstein LV, et al: Health status assessment for elderly patients. Report of the Society of General Internal Medicine Task Force on Health Assessment. *J Am Geriatr Soc* 1988; 37:562–569.

33. Sonn U, Åsberg KH: Assessment of activities of daily living in the elderly. A study of a population of 76 year olds in Gothenburg, Sweden. *Scand J Rehabil Med* 1991; 23:193–202.

34. Wiener JM, et al: Measuring activities of daily living: Comparisons across national surveys. *J Gerontol* 1990; 45:S229–237.

Environmental Design: Accommodating Sensory Changes in the Elderly

Mary Ann Wharton, M.S., P.T.

INTRODUCTION

The ability to function in the everyday environment is essential to older individuals. Maintaining independence, however, may be compromised by sensory changes that individuals experience over their life span. Changes in vision, hearing, taste, smell, and touch may deprive older persons of necessary sensory cues to perceive the environment and may influence both their behavior and the behavior of others toward them. The ability of physical therapists to recognize the relationship between sensory changes and environmental interaction, to recommend adaptations to accommodate those changes, and to teach intervention strategies will promote continued independent functioning of older individuals.

Most individuals will experience gradual sensory loss with age. Such changes are normal and irreversible and may not even be uniform within the same individual. For example, visual loss may occur primarily in one eye, or an individual may have poor vision but excellent hearing. Moreover, loss of the different senses may be experienced at different ages. Hearing loss generally accelerates after age 40, vision and smell after 50, and taste after 55.[63] The important point is that the sensory declines experienced with aging are highly individualized, with some elderly people experiencing relatively minor declines and maintaining optimal functional ability and other individuals experiencing significant declines with resultant increased functional dependency. Typically, the declines occur gradually and may be unnoticed until elderly individuals are no longer capable of independent functioning within the environment.

Throughout life, individuals rely on sensory cues to perceive and interpret information from their surroundings. As sensory declines occur with aging, older persons may misinterpret cues from the environment or may experience sensory deprivation. The consequences may be loss of independence by older individuals. Therefore, individuals may need higher thresholds of stimulation to continue to function in the environment. As individuals experience loss in functional ability, they may also become increasingly reliant on sensory cues from the environment. An interdependence develops between the senses and the environment: one relies on one's senses to perceive and derive pleasure from the environment, and one relies on the environment to promote and support functional ability as age-related sensory declines are experienced.

As physical therapists interact with the elderly, it is critical to recognize the importance of the balance between sensory perception and ability to function effectively in the environment. They need to evaluate elderly individuals for sensory changes and to recommend appropriate interventions and modifications to enhance optimal functional performance in an environment without creating dependence.

SENSORY CHANGES: RELATIONSHIP TO FUNCTIONAL ABILITY WITHIN THE ENVIRONMENT

Vision

Vision is important in identifying environmental cues and distinguishing environmental hazards. As people age, changes in vision and visual perception may lead to misinterpretation of visual cues and result in functional dependence.

Physiologically, this decline in vision can result from age-related changes in the structures of the eye and in external ocular structures. Neuronal changes, perceptual changes, and pathology also contribute to vision and visual perceptual changes in the elderly. The ability to function in the environment, in spite of changes in vision and visual perception, is dependent on the ability to adapt to visual impairment, including decreasing visual efficiency and low vision. Older individuals must adapt to such problems as decreasing visual field, changes in visual acuity, increasing needs for illumination balanced by needs to reduce glare, delayed dark-light adaptation, increasing needs for contrast, decreasing power of accommodation, and changes in color vision and depth perception.

Visual Field

A decrease in both peripheral and upper visual fields accelerates with aging. Decreased pupil size, resulting in admittance of less light to the peripheral retina, may be responsible for early changes. Later changes may result from decreased retinal metabolism. Mechanical causes are due to relaxation of the upper eyelid and loss of retrobulbar fat, which results in the eyes sinking more deeply into the orbits. As a result, upper gaze can be compromised by as much as 20 degrees in a 70-year-old.[62, 63]

Within the environment, this decrease in upper visual field may cause older individuals to miss cues above head level. Common examples of cues found above head level may include traffic and street signs, "Exit" signs in public buildings, hanging light fixtures, and environmental hazards such as hanging tree limbs.[63]

Lateral field or peripheral vision deficits, described as the inability to detect motion, form, or color on either side of the head while looking straight ahead, are particularly significant for elderly persons. For safety in the environment, older persons must be able to detect people or objects in the lateral field, and elderly drivers must possess adequate lateral awareness.[16]

Visual Acuity

There is a general decline in visual acuity with age, although this decline is not universal or inevitable. Factors responsible for decreased visual acuity include increased thickness of the lens, which affects the amount of light allowed to reach the retina, and the loss of elasticity of the lens. These changes result in decreased ability to see clearly and particularly affect near objects. Additionally, changes in the iris and pupil may decrease acuity. As one ages, the iris loses its ability to change width, and pupil size remains small in both dim and bright light. One specific consequence is decreased night vision.[16, 62, 63]

Visual aids can be beneficial in improving visual acuity for the elderly. Corrective lenses can enhance vision when worn properly, especially in the early stages of vision loss. Hand-held magnifiers are adequate for use over short periods, for example, when reading a telephone book. Table stand magnifiers are beneficial when reading books or newspapers, as they cause less eye fatigue by maintaining a constant distance between the object being magnified and the magnifier. Illuminated magnifiers that hang from the neck are useful when sewing or performing craft work. Other low-vision aids can be obtained at low-vision clinics.[53]

In addition to visual aids, certain modifications to environmental stimuli can enhance visual functioning for older persons. Use of large print is suggested for signs and labels, including medication schedules, telephone lists, and home programs. Large-print books and newspapers are also available, as are other large-print devices such as measuring tapes and rulers, measuring cups and spoons, cookbooks, wristwatches, phone dialers, and games. Local agencies for the blind are helpful in identifying such resources.[7, 36, 53, 63]

Illumination

Within the environment, declining visual acuity necessitates a stronger stimulus or light source. This is primarily related to senile miosis (an age-related decrease in pupillary size), changes in the refractory media, and a reduction in retinal cones and rods. As a result of these changes, it has been estimated that older individuals require as much as two to three times more light than younger individuals. Wall-mounted light fixtures and peripheral lighting from floor lamps are superior to a central ceiling source because they do not foster formation of shadows on critical corner and furniture areas. Background lighting should not be as bright as that in the area on which attention is directed. Lighting that focuses directly on the task, rather than overhead lighting, is recommended to meet the needs of older individuals for reading, task performance, and other close work. Small, high-intensity lamps with three-way switches are helpful in achieving the proper ratio of background-to-task lighting.[7, 16, 43, 53, 63]

Glare

When increasing illumination, care must be exercised to avoid excessive and intensive illumination, which can create a hazard for older persons in the form of glare. Glare results from diffuse light scattering on the retina as it passes through mildly opaque refractive media, inhibiting clear vision. A primary cause of glare sensitivity is the increasing opacity of the lens, which diffuses the incoming light. Degenerative changes that take place in the cornea also contribute to glare.[61, 63]

Direct glare occurs when light reaches the eye directly from its source. An example of direct glare is uncontrolled natural light that enters a darkened room through a window. Another example of direct glare would be excessive light from exposed light bulbs. Indirect glare can be the result of light reflecting off another surface. Examples include light reflecting off highly polished surfaces including waxed floors, plastic-covered furniture, polished silverware, or stainless steel assistive devices, including grab bars and walkers.[7, 63]

Glare can be lessened by modifying light sources. Diffuse, soft lighting is preferable to single light sources. Lamp shades should be used to soften the light. Glare from windows can be minimized by use of sheer curtains, venetian blinds, tinted-glass windows, or drapes. Wall-mounted valance or cove lighting that conceals the light source is also recommended. Fluorescent fixtures can be used to reduce glare, but they must be checked to ensure that they do not create another hazard for elderly individuals in the form of flickering.

Another method of controlling glare is to reduce the number of reflective surfaces. Positioning light sources to avoid reflection from shiny surfaces, such as waxed floors, is helpful. Use of carpeting, wallpaper, flat paints, and paneling is preferable to use of high-gloss paints. Glass, plastic, and glossy furniture should be avoided or covered with textured surfaces to minimize the effects of glare. Gleaming metal fixtures can be replaced with wood or plastic fixtures. Assistive devices, including grab bars and walkers, should not be constructed of shiny materials.

Care should be taken to control the sources of glare in public areas. For example, mall directories and bus signs should be covered with nonglare materials rather than highly reflective plastics. Grocery stores and drugstores should refrain from displaying products wrapped in plastic. Name tags, street signs, and publicity for older individuals should be prepared on dull surfaces to minimize glare.

Outdoor areas are also vulnerable to glare, especially

with bright sunlight or with wet, shiny surfaces on rainy or snowy days. Sunscreens and adequate shade from trees are recommended to limit glare from direct sunlight. If it is not possible to provide adequate control for glare, older individuals should be encouraged to use sunglasses, visors, brimmed hats, or umbrellas. Glare that occurs at dusk can be particularly troublesome for older individuals as poorly illuminated objects are contrasted against a bright, post-sunset sky. Night glare that occurs from oncoming headlights can also be hazardous. Use of well-lit routes and divided highways can minimize this hazard for older individuals.[7, 21, 44, 53, 63]

Dark Adaptation

Dark adaptation, or the ability of the eye to become more visually sensitive after remaining in darkness for a period of time, is delayed in older persons. One reason for this visual change is the smaller, miotic pupil, which limits the amount of light reaching the periphery of the retina. It is this area of the retina that contains the rods, which are sensitive to low light intensities. Another reason for delayed dark adaptation in the elderly is the metabolic changes in the retina. The oxygen supply to the rod-dense area of the retina diminishes as a result of vascular changes, which, in turn, affects the efficiency of the rods to respond to low levels of illumination. As a result of these changes, older persons will have difficulty adapting to darkness and to abrupt and extreme changes in light.[62, 63]

Use of a night-light is recommended to assist in overcoming the decreased ability for the eyes to adapt to the dark. A red bulb is suggested since it reduces the time required for adaptation to the dark and permits older individuals to see well enough to function. It is also recommended that older individuals carry a pocket flashlight to aid in transition to dimly lit environments. Improving lighting at the point of entry to an area, through pull cords or light switches near the entrance to a room, is also recommended. Automatic timers or keeping a light on at all times in dimly lit areas can prevent older individuals from having to enter a darkened room.[27, 34, 38]

Accommodation

Accommodation, the ability of the eye to focus images on the retina independent of object distances, is impaired with aging. Functionally, this results in the inability to focus clearly over a range of distances. The decrease in this ability, referred to as *presbyopia,* occurs gradually and affects near vision first.

Loss of accommodation is the result of several factors. Both the cornea and lens lose transparency with aging. In addition, the lens thickens, flattens, and yellows and becomes rigid. The ciliary muscle weakens and relaxes. As a result, the lens gradually loses its ability to change shape and focus at varying distances. Difficulty is encountered by older individuals when attempting to read small print or detail unless the material is held at a distance. Reading glasses are initially indicated. Later, bifocals are needed to compensate for the inability of the lens to change shape and focus on objects of varying distances.[62, 63]

Color

The ability to perceive, differentiate, and distinguish colors declines with aging as a result of changes in retinal cones, the retinal bipolar and ganglion cells, the visual pathways that terminate in the occipital cortex, and the lens. As the lens thickens and yellows with age, it becomes less sensitive to colors having shorter wavelengths. Cool colors—blues, greens, and violets—are particularly impaired since they have the shorter wavelengths. Warm colors with longer wavelengths, including the reds, oranges, and yellows, are easier to differentiate and should therefore be used as focal points against sharply contrasting backgrounds. In addition to loss of color discrimination at the blue end of the color spectrum, there is a loss of sensitivity over the entire spectrum. As a result, light pastel colors may be difficult to distinguish. Monotones also provide difficulty for older individuals, as may dark shades, which tend to blend into shadows. As a result, older persons may have trouble negotiating around dark furniture or in areas where dark floor surfaces and dark walls or doorways come together. Optimal lighting may be needed to minimize this hazard.

Both warm and cool colors can be included in a color scheme when designing living situations for the elderly. The goal with the use of color is to use contrast to assist elderly individuals in distinguishing objects from their backgrounds. It is also important that the use of color be aesthetically pleasing.[7, 16, 21, 62, 63]

Contrast

The ability to discriminate between degrees of brightness appears to decrease in 60- to 70+-year-olds. Typically, older individuals have difficulty seeing objects that have low contrast, especially with a bright background. This decreased ability to discriminate between degrees of brightness appears to be the result of an increase in light scatter secondary to age-related eye changes. Elderly persons require greater than two times as much light to see low-contrasting objects with the same degree of clarity as younger people.[16, 62]

Use of sharp contrast will enhance the visual performance of older individuals. Bright detail on dark backgrounds is easier to distinguish than low-contrast or dark detail on light background. Recommendations would include white lettering on the telephone dial of a black telephone or white lettering on a black background for reference dials on appliances. Use of warm colors—reds, oranges, and yellows—is recommended to highlight important visual targets such as handrails, steps, intersections, and traffic signs. Floors and rugs should contrast with woodwork and walls. To enhance eating, plates should contrast with tablecloths or tabletops. Colored rims on dishes and glasses can provide sufficient contrast to avoid spills. The table covering should also contrast with the floor to enhance the reference point of older individuals and help prevent falls.[24, 63]

Depth Perception

Related to loss of color discrimination is change in depth perception, or the ability to estimate the relative distance and relief of objects. Lack of color contrast results in a flat visual effect, or decreased depth perception and inability to judge distances. As a result of the inability to judge distances, older persons may have difficulty estimating the height of curbs and steps and may have difficulty with activities of daily living that require distance judgment, including feeding tasks.

Related to depth perception is the ability to discriminate figure-ground. It is difficult for older individuals to recognize a simple visual figure when it is embedded in a complex figure background. Specific implications for the elderly are in selection of floor coverings. When a pattern is present on a floor surface, it may create a hazard as older individuals perceive it as one object or several objects. The avoidance of patterns is therefore recommended for floor surfaces, particularly in hallways or living areas.[7, 62, 63]

Hearing

Hearing provides a primary link that allows individuals to identify with the environment and communicate effectively. Age-related hearing loss can lead to decreased awareness of environmental cues, poor communication skills, and ultimately, social isolation. With aging, there are both physiologic and functional changes in the auditory system. Both the peripheral auditory system, which includes the structures of the ear itself, and the central nervous system, which integrates and gives meaning to sound, are affected. Age-related hearing loss can be attributed to three factors: conductive loss, sensorineural loss, and combined conductive and sensorineural loss. Changes that typically occur with aging and are detrimental to the older individual's ability to function independently in the environment include high-tone hearing loss, decreased speech discrimination, and difficulty detecting and appropriately filtering background noise.

Conductive Hearing Loss

Conductive hearing loss results from dysfunction of the external ear, the middle ear, or both. Factors responsible for this type of hearing loss include impacted cerumen, perforation of the tympanic membrane, serum or pus in the middle ear, and otosclerosis. Conductive hearing loss occurs when sound transmission to the inner ear is lost because the intensity of the signal is not sufficient. Even though the signal is weakened, sound received by the inner ear can still be analyzed since the inner ear itself is not affected. Therefore, increasing the intensity of the signal through louder speech or through mechanical amplification, such as a hearing aid, may help restore the ability to hear.

With a conductive loss, some impairment will occur in the ability to hear sounds of all frequencies. The specific pattern is dependent on the etiology of the hearing loss. An appropriate intervention when speaking to older individuals with a conductive hearing loss is to increase the speaker's volume to enable the elderly to hear the signal more clearly and to understand the speech. For individuals with profound hearing loss, an appropriate strategy may be to speak directly into the individual's ear. Devices such as timers, alarm clocks, smoke detectors, and doorbells can be modified or changed so that the signal is within the hearing range of older persons.[7, 21, 33, 36, 37, 62, 63]

Sensorineural Hearing Loss

Sensorineural hearing loss occurs when there is a dysfunction in conversion of sound waves to electrical signals by the inner ear or dysfunction in transmission of nerve impulses to the brain. Age-related sensorineural hearing loss is referred to as *presbycusis*. *Sensory* presbycusis is due to a loss of hair cells at the basal end of the organ of Corti and results in loss of high-frequency hearing. *Neural* presbycusis is due to degenerative changes in nerve fibers of the cochlea. It leads to loss in speech discrimination but not in pure-tone thresholds. As a result, the person continues to hear tone but cannot understand what is heard. Amplifications may be of little benefit, since these devices can amplify unintelligible sounds. *Metabolic* presbycusis results from atrophy of blood vessels in the wall of the cochlea. It is most likely the result of arteriosclerotic vascular changes. It results in a relatively uniform reduction in pure-tone sensitivities for all frequencies and is accompanied by recruitment, which is a rapid increase in loudness as the sound intensity increases. *Mechanical* presbycusis is the result of atrophic changes in the structures involved with vibration of the cochlear partition. The result is increasing hearing loss from low to high frequencies. The ability to understand speech is affected. High-pitched consonants such as *s, t, f,* and *g* are increasingly difficult to understand, especially in the presence of background noise, which masks the weak consonant sounds, or with rapid articulation.[27, 33, 37]

Older individuals with a sensorineural hearing loss may have significant difficulty maintaining independent function in the environment. In addition to difficulty in hearing and/or understanding speech, these individuals may have great difficulty hearing and interpreting key signals from the environment. Recommendations to assist these individuals incorporate strategies to address the hearing loss. Lower frequency and pitch of signals from television, stereo systems, or radio can be achieved by adjusting the treble and bass to compensate for loss of high frequency, that is, by tuning the bass up and the treble down. Use of microphones by speakers and entertainers will also cut out some of the high-frequency sound, making it easier for individuals to hear. Devices that have high-frequency sound, such as smoke alarms, telephones, and doorbells, should also have a visual cue, such as a flashing light.

For individuals with presbycusis, a hearing aid may be of limited benefit, since this device may only amplify a distorted signal. Some assistive listening devices, such as pocket amplifiers with external earphones, microphones, and earphones may be beneficial. As with profound conductive loss, speaking directly into the individual's ear may be of benefit for the person without a device.

Environmental background noise that competes with the older person's ability to hear can be minimized by use of acoustic materials such as drapes, upholstered furniture, and carpets, which absorb noise. Insulating sheet rock should be installed in noisy areas such as kitchens or maintenance rooms. Exterior noise can be minimized by tight window seals.

In institutions and public buildings, noise from telepages, radios, televisions, dishwashers, and air conditioners should be eliminated where possible. Background music should be eliminated, since it contributes to the older individual's inability to hear. Fluorescent lighting should be used with discretion, since the buzzing sound that is produced may also interfere with hearing.[7, 21, 51, 62, 63]

Taste and Smell

Taste and smell intertwine to provide additional links with the environment. These senses allow individuals to appreciate foods and pleasant odors in the environment, such as fresh-baked bread, the smell of newly cut grass, and roses. They also allow detection of unpleasant odors that can serve as warning to environmental hazards. Examples include unsafe drink and foods, fire, and noxious gases. Research on age-related changes in these senses is limited and often contradictory, but there is evidence that they are diminished. This decline in taste and smell can impact on the older individual's behavior, safety in the environment, and nutrition.

Taste

Although there is no agreement on the cause, it is known that the number of taste buds decreases with age. By age 60, most people have lost approximately half of their taste buds. This loss further accelerates after age 70. This loss of functioning taste buds, combined with neuron reduction in taste centers, may account for changes in taste with aging. Other age-related changes that affect taste may include changes in the elasticity of the mouth and lips, decreased saliva flow, changes in oral secretions, increased incidence of gingivitis and periodontitis, and tongue fissures. Smoking and illness may also contribute to the decline of taste sensitivity.

Regardless of cause, age-related changes in taste acuity are thought to be small. Taste buds located in the front of the tongue that are responsible for sweet and salty tastes are the first to atrophy. Stronger stimuli are needed to appreciate these tastes, and older people may use excessive amounts of salt or may prefer sweets. This can pose problems for older individuals suffering from hypertension or diabetes. Taste buds located on the posterior surface of the tongue that are responsible for bitter tastes and allow rejection of bitter toxins are lost later. Additionally, older persons may experience an increased sensitivity to bitterness, with the resultant complaint that food tastes bitter or sour.

Recommendations to enhance the taste experience include suggestions to compensate with other senses. Since smell is so closely intertwined with taste, older individuals can be encouraged to stimulate smell with the aroma of cooking foods. Meals should be prepared using a variety of aromas, temperatures, and textures. Oral hygiene should be encouraged prior to eating to rid the mouth of unpleasant tastes. Spices, herbs, flavor extracts, and sugar and salt substitutes can be used to enhance the flavor of foods.

When dealing with canned foods, older persons should be taught to feel for any bulges in the can and to discard any suspicious cans. Stored foods should be dated and checked for spoilage. Defrosted foods should be used promptly, since thawing and refreezing affects flavor and texture.[37, 62, 63]

Smell

Research on olfactory sensitivity and smell is contradictory, but sensation appears to decline as a result of age, as well as a result of other factors associated with age. These factors may include continuous exposure to odor, leading to decreased acuity, or exposure to environmental pollutants or smoking. Structural causes may include fiber loss in the olfactory bulb, with a loss of approximately three fourths of the olfactory fibers by age 80 or 90. Alterations in nasal anatomy and physiology may also occur secondary to diseases of the respiratory system.

A critical function of the sense of smell is to warn individuals of environmental dangers, including smoke or gas fumes. For elderly persons who experience a decline in the ability to smell and are living alone, it is critical that environmental adaptations be considered. One recommendation is to use smoke detectors with loud buzzers. Since declining sensitivity to odor may limit the individual's ability to detect mercaptans (foul-smelling additives) used to warn of natural gas leaks, safety-spring caps for gas jets of a stove are also recommended. If the sensory loss is profound, switching from gas to electrical appliances may be indicated.

Social interaction of older persons may be affected by a declining sense of smell. Individuals may not be able to detect body odor, so particular attention must be given to bathing patterns. Perfumes may be overutilized, making the scent overpowering and offensive to others.

For the institutionalized elderly person, unpleasant odors from cleaning equipment, sanitizing sprays, and substances designed to mask offensive odors abound. Pleasant odors associated with positive life experiences are often overlooked. Absence of "good" smells adversely affects the quality of life for these individuals. Opportunities should be created to stimulate positive life experiences with pleasant smells. Kitchens can be vented to allow the aroma of cooking food to permeate residential hallways and dining areas. Flowers with fragrant scents can be placed in living areas to enhance the older person's sensory experience.[7, 21, 37, 62]

Touch

The sense of touch is a complicated human response that involves many separate processes, including touch, temperature, pain, and vibration sensitivity, kinesthesia, and stereognosis. Sensory input is subdivided into touch and tactile systems. Touch is used for awareness and protective responses. It can be determined culturally and is often lacking in the older person's environment, contributing to the individual's diminished sensorium. Tactile input is utilized to interact with the environment and allows individuals to perceive multiple characteristics of an object.[7] For example, a surface may feel smooth or rough, soft or hard, warm or cold.

Little conclusive research has been done on the sense of touch. However, evidence suggests that touch decreases with age and varies from individual to individual. Many of the losses in somatesthetic sensitivity are the result of dis-

eases that occur with greater frequency in the elderly, rather than a result of aging per se. Increased thresholds for touch, especially textures, temperature, and kinesthesia, have implications for the older individual's ability to obtain needed sensory input from the environment.

Tactile Sensitivity

Degenerative changes in Meissner's corpuscles may result in decreased sensitivity of the skin on the palm of the hand and sole of the foot but not of hairy skin. The resultant decrease in touch acuity can affect the ability of older individuals to localize stimuli. As a result, older individuals may have problems differentiating or manipulating small objects, including buttons and coins. The decrease in speed of reaction to tactile stimulation can cause harm to older persons, as they take longer to become aware of harmful or noxious stimuli such as temperature extremes, chemical irritants, or simple pressure from a stone in a shoe.[62]

Introducing texture into the environment can be valuable in assisting independent function of older individuals, especially if there is impairment in other senses. Wall hangings, carpet, and textured upholstery on furniture can enhance tactile input and add warmth. Use of texture on handrails or doorknobs can give environmental cues and enhance safety. Tactile deprivation can be minimized by the use of soft blankets and sheets and textured clothing.[7, 21]

Thermal Sensitivity

Changes in vascular circulation and loss of subcutaneous tissue in older individuals may result in changes in thermal sensitivity and impaired ability to cope with extreme environmental temperatures. One consequence is that older persons may feel cold and uncomfortable, even on a day that seems warm to a younger person. Air conditioning may not be tolerated, especially in the institutional environment.

Additionally, extremes in hot temperatures, for example, from hot bathwater or a heating pad, may not be readily detected by older individuals. As a consequence, individuals may suffer a burn from the inability to react quickly to the temperature extreme.[7, 21]

GENERAL PRINCIPLES OF DESIGN

Environmental design principles that accommodate age-related changes in sensation can enhance independent functioning of elderly individuals. The ideal environment will vary according to the needs of individuals but should be supportive of sensory changes while promoting satisfaction, safety, and security. Design that accommodates sensory changes occurring with age should enhance the ability of individuals to function at the maximum level of competence. Overutilization and underutilization of sensory cues should be avoided, since both create dependence and result in a mismatch between the individual and the environment.[7, 61]

When an environment places excessive demands on an individual's ability to function, the phenomenon is known as *environmental press*.[7] As this demanding physical environment fails to support aging individuals, safety, self-image, and interactions with others may be adversely affected, and stress may result.[35] In this circumstance of high environmental demand, individuals with the least capabilities will likely exhibit maladaptive behavior. Simple environmental changes, such as increased lighting, easily identifiable landmarks for cuing, or decreased background noise, may foster meaningful changes in behavior and interaction within the environment.[7]

Recommending too many changes in sensory stimuli within the environment may lead to sensory distortion, resultant overload, and decreased environmental press. This excessive decrease in environmental press may result in lack of challenge for some individuals, leading to marginal performance and dependent behavior. The optimal environment for the elderly is one that provides a measure of challenge and, at the same time, provides the necessary supports for the individual.[35]

Numerous environmental checklists can be found in the literature that address physical barriers in the home and institution.[9, 54, 55] However, special consideration must also be given to accommodating sensory changes. Each area of the physical environment in which older persons function must be addressed, keeping in mind this interdependence of sensory loss, functional ability, and reliance on the environment for support. In addition to recommendations cited previously in this text, several areas deserve further emphasis. These include comments on personal/living space, long-term–care residencies, physical therapy departments, stairs, escalators, and driving.

Personal/Living Space

Since the home is the hub of most activity for older individuals, creating an environment to support sensory loss and enhance maximum functional independence is critical. Incorporating the previously outlined design principles that accommodate losses in vision, hearing, taste, smell, and touch will not only facilitate independence but may also minimize the occurrence of accidents leading to death or disability. Examples include use of enhanced lighting and provision of contrast in personal living space to deter falls that result from decreased vision, and use of smoke detectors with visual cues to decrease vulnerability to death from fires in older individuals with decreased ability to hear and smell.[61]

Long-term–Care Residencies

Long-term–care residencies designed using traditional concepts derived from the medical model may fail to meet the needs of today's frail elderly population who suffer from multiple chronic conditions. In order to enhance the quality of life for these older individuals, architects and administrators are challenged to incorporate design principles that create environments to support age-related changes and enhance functional performance of individuals with sensory losses.

Appropriate lighting can support greater independence and enhance the safety of older individuals with visual deficits. While direct, incandescent lighting adds warmth, it may not provide adequate illumination and may also create light pools and shadows. Therefore, direct lighting is not recommended for use in corridors. It is, however, appropriate as supplemental task lighting. Desk lamps and table lamps by chairs should be provided for reading and close work. Indirect fluorescent lighting is recommended for use in corridors, since this type of lighting provides adequate, even illumination and minimizes glare. Warm white bulbs are recommended because they give a softer tint. Care should be taken to minimize flickering, which can be a hazard for the elderly. A regular schedule for checking ballasts on fluorescent lights and replacing worn-out bulbs can minimize this problem.[11]

Long-term–care facility design should be attentive to choices in materials for window coverings, ceilings, wall coverings, and floors. Window treatments should be chosen to minimize the effect of glare, since this is often a problem in residential facilities. Curtains or blinds can be used for this purpose. Draperies should be considered since they not only minimize glare but also serve to absorb extraneous background noise and assist in lowering energy costs.[5, 11, 43]

Ceilings and wall coverings in residential facilities should be chosen to support sensory deficits of elderly residents. Ceilings should be covered with acoustic tile specially designed to absorb noise and extraneous sounds that interfere with speech discrimination. Use of these materials is particularly recommended in corridors, dining rooms, and other areas where background noise is prevalent. Wall coverings can be chosen to serve multiple purposes. Color can be used for resident orientation and cuing. Choosing paint or fabric of different colors for various areas within the facility can provide meaning, especially for confused or demented residents. Use of contrast on door frames can serve as added landmarks and assist residents in locating their personal room. Color contrast between walls and floors can provide valuable sensory information to minimize falls in ambulatory individuals. Textured wall coverings that are soft to touch have the added benefit of providing tactile cues for older individuals deprived of touch and for visually impaired residents. Repetitive, random, and vivid patterns that create visual illusions and unstable figure-ground relationships should be avoided.[5, 11, 43, 45]

Floor coverings should be selected to enhance the mobility of older residents. Vinyl or linoleum is often chosen since it is easy to clean and provides little resistance for wheelchair mobility. One problem with this surface is that it is a major source of glare. This can be controlled to an extent with use of nonglare wax. An alternative to vinyl is the use of carpet, which has traditionally been avoided because of stains and odor. Newer design, including solution-dyed fibers and liquid-barrier backing, has minimized these problems. One study recommends the use of carpeting to enhance walking in elderly hospital inpatients. This study determined that gait speed and step length were significantly greater on carpeted than on vinyl surfaces.[59] Mobility of wheelchair-bound elderly need not be hampered by use of carpeting, since low-looped pile, that is very tightly woven, can minimize friction.[5, 11]

Furniture selected for residential facilities should be functional and, at the same time, supportive of sensory changes. Use of fabric upholstery can provide tactile cues and eliminate problems of glare created by vinyl upholstery. Choosing color that contrasts with flooring can serve as a valuable visual cue for residents with visual deficits. Repetitive and illusionary patterns should be avoided.[11]

Particular consideration should be given to design of resident rooms in long-term–care facilities. Beds and chairs should be comfortable and stable and support functional ability of residents. Adequate illumination should be provided, with provisions included for task lighting. Glare should be controlled through use of appropriate window treatments, floor surfaces, and furniture choices. Color and contrast should be considered when selecting wall coverings, and even furniture coverings. For example, bedspreads should be chosen to contrast with floor coverings so that a visually impaired resident will be able to safely transfer on and off the bed.

Special considerations for personal bathrooms and central bathing areas focus on features to enhance resident safety. One important consideration is to control glare, which is a particular problem with vinyl flooring, porcelain sinks, bathtubs, toilets, chrome towel bars, and grab bars. Suggestions to minimize glare include use of colored fixtures that can additionally provide contrast with floor and wall coverings. These are aesthetically pleasing and can serve as an important safety feature for older individu-

als with visual deficits, who may experience difficulty in judgment when the toilet, bathtub, or grab bar is of the same color as the floor.[11]

Communal dining areas can pose several design challenges in residential facilities. In addition to the usual problems with lighting and control of glare, there is the added problem of noise control. Since dining areas are frequently located adjacent to the kitchen, background noise from dishwashers and food processors can contribute to difficulty with hearing-impaired residents and can cause further social isolation of these individuals. Use of good insulating materials or locating dining areas away from kitchens is recommended to minimize this problem. Further reduction in background noise can be attained through use of tablecloths and placement of paper pads between cups and saucers.[5, 11]

Physical Therapy Departments

If the elderly are to receive maximum benefit from physical therapy intervention, it is crucial that design principles incorporating recommendations to accommodate for sensory loss with aging be utilized when building new facilities or renovating existing space. Concepts previously discussed that accommodate sensory changes must be implemented. These include controlling light sources; minimizing glare; and choosing appropriate ceilings, wall coverings, and floor coverings. Specific recommendations for physical therapy departments include choosing walkers and other assistive devices that are constructed of nonshiny materials in an effort to control glare. Some equipment, such as parallel bars, some whirlpools, and various other modalities, is, by design, constructed of shiny material. When using this equipment, the effect of glare should be minimized by controlling light sources.

When choosing mat tables and treatment tables, the overall design of the physical therapy department should be considered. These surfaces should be covered with material that provides contrast to floor coverings, so that elderly clients are afforded a specific visual cue that will enhance safety in transfers.

One significant problem in most physical therapy departments is background noise. Suggestions to minimize this noise include confining whirlpool areas to separate rooms that are insulated with acoustic material. Another recommendation is to provide individual treatment booths rather than sectioning treatment areas with curtains. Not only will this afford privacy for older individuals; it will also serve as a means of limiting background noise. And background music from radios and use of intercom devices should be discouraged, since they serve as further distractors for the elderly with hearing loss.

Finally, use of texture is encouraged to enhance tactile

sensation. When possible, linens should be used on mats and treatment tables rather than paper coverings. These should also contrast with floor coverings to enhance visual perception. Carpeting should be considered as floor coverings to enhance ambulation, absorb sound, and minimize glare.

Stairs

Stairs are one area within the environment not previously discussed that require special consideration, since they are frequent sites of accidents leading to injury, hospitalization, and even death. Safe negotiation of stairs requires integration of visual and kinesthetic tests of the conditions of the stairs. This is particularly critical for descent, which is generally more hazardous than ascent. Successful stair negotiation requires that individuals make a transition from free-form movement on level surfaces to the highly circumscribed foot placement that is required on stairs. Visual feedback is used initially in order to judge the position of the stair treads and maximize accuracy of foot placement. Looking at the steps then allows the user to scan the flight of steps for hazards, including broken treads, irregularities, or other obstacles. Once the visual test is accomplished, individuals rely on kinesthetic tests to obtain a feel of the treads and ensure accurate foot placement. In elderly individuals, visual distractions drawing the user's attention away from the stairs as well as visual deceptions built into the design of the stairs were identified as two leading causes of stair accidents. Furthermore, the most critical piece of visual information for successful descent of steps was identified as a singular and unambiguous indication of the edge of each step. Optical illusions created by patterned carpeting overpower the ability of individuals to detect tread edges and create a significant hazard. Similar hazards are created by three-dimensional textures, including shag carpeting, since these textures cause treads to appear to merge into a continuous surface.[2]

Other environmental considerations on stairs include use of adequate lighting to enhance visual feedback. Light switches should be located at both the top and bottom of the flight of steps. Night-lights should also be located near the first and last steps to provide cuing during darkness. Glare reflecting from floor surfaces should be minimized by the use of nonglare surfaces, including appropriate types of carpeting. Light from windows located near stairs should be controlled with window coverings. Glare derived directly from light sources should be minimized by positioning and by avoiding exposed lightbulbs. Kinesthetic feedback may be enhanced by use of carpeting; however, the addition of ribbed vinyl or rubber stair nosing of a contrasting color should be considered to aid in reducing the risk of falls by enhancing detection of the edge of the step. Stairs without carpeting can be marked by a strip of paint or tape in a contrasting color.[44, 55]

Escalators

Escalators have been identified as a hazardous environment for the elderly since their use may result in accidents involving falls. It is thought that the repeated optical image that is a critical design feature of escalators may induce visual depth illusion resulting in disorientation. More research is needed to determine whether the illusion adversely affects postural stability of older individuals more than younger people. However, it is theorized that the higher proportion of falls on escalators for older people may be a result of age-related declines in vision and a suspected relationship to postural stability. Older individuals should be alerted to the potential hazards of escalator use, and individuals with vision and visual perceptual deficits should be encouraged to avoid use of escalators. Additionally, these individuals should be cautioned to avoid similar surfaces such as carpeting or linoleum that employ the use of repeated patterns.[13]

Driving

Since driving is a privilege that enhances independent functioning in the environment, it is important to consider the impact that age-related sensory changes might have on this skill. Vision is a critical sensory modality that undergoes changes with age. Older drivers must learn to give careful consideration to this system in relationship to specific skills needed for driving. Declining visual field is one factor that must be given such consideration. Older individuals must be aware of pedestrians or vehicles in the lateral field, and those individuals experiencing declines in peripheral vision must be taught to compensate by turning their heads or by using car mirrors. Similarly, drivers experiencing loss in the upper visual field must be alerted to the need to look upward to avoid missing overhead road signs and traffic signals.[16]

Depth perception is also known to decline with age and is additionally affected by increased susceptibility to glare, loss of visual acuity, dark adaptation, changing needs for illumination and contrast, and altered color perception. Older drivers need the ability to judge distances between their vehicle and other moving or stationary objects. This is critical for judging distances from oncoming cars, maintaining appropriate distances, safely passing other vehicles, merging onto a highway, or braking before reaching an intersection.[16] Older drivers who experience difficulty with depth perception and are unable to compensate for this loss should be strongly cautioned to avoid driving.

Since older individuals have problems with dark adaptation, they may experience difficulty with changes in illumination coming from oncoming headlights or streetlights. As a result, night driving may pose a safety hazard, and older individuals may need to confine driving to daylight hours.[27] Additionally, older drivers may be limited in night driving by glare intolerance. They should be instructed to compensate for this by avoiding looking at oncoming headlights, traveling on divided highways, or traveling on well-lit roads.[52] Vehicle design modifications introduced on 1986 models have proved beneficial for older drivers experiencing decreased night vision and difficulty with glare. These include changes in headlights, rear lights, and directional signals that can be seen on the side of the vehicle. They also include design concepts that result in reduction in windshield and dashboard glare and installation of rear window defrosters and wipers.[57]

The impact of diminished color discrimination on driving is questionable. However, it has been suggested that it may take some older drivers twice as long as younger drivers to detect the flash of a brake light since red colors may appear dimmer as individuals age.[16] The high-mounted rear brake light introduced in 1986 vehicle models may serve as an accommodation for older drivers.[57]

In addition to visual loss, older drivers may experience difficulty because of age-related changes in hearing. Specifically, they may be unable to hear horns from other motorists warning of oncoming hazards, or they may be unable to localize the source of such signals. Vehicle malfunction warnings, such as brake sensors, may also go undetected with diminished hearing. Older drivers can compensate for this loss by adhering to a strict vehicle maintenance schedule.

The final deterrents to safe driving for older individuals that must be given consideration are hazards specific to the road environment itself, for example, poorly placed and poorly designed road signs. Signs should be of sufficient size and should provide adequate color contrast to be seen by older drivers. Traffic lights pose another difficulty. Hazards pertaining to traffic light changes at intersections occur when older drivers react slowly to light changes from green to red. It has been suggested that older drivers would benefit if engineering slowed the speed at which a traffic light changes to 10% under the current recommended speed of change. Since night drivers rely on median and roadside delineator lines as visual cues, increasing the width of these markers from 4 to 8 in. has also been speculated to be of benefit to older night drivers. Older drivers with visual deficits may have difficulty on two-lane highways and older highways that have closely placed on- and off-ramps. Newer highway design that includes four-lane highways with wide separation and better

delineation of on- and off-ramps should prove valuable for older drivers.[57] Finally, because older individuals are thought to have difficulty with visual depth illusion created by repeated optical patterns, repetitive patterns occurring in bridges, tunnels, and expressways may pose hazards.[13] Some older drivers should avoid these environments in order to foster safe driving.

TEACHING/CONSULTING STRATEGIES

Physical therapists working with the elderly are challenged to incorporate teaching strategies to accommodate sensory loss into treatment programs. Their unique knowledge of sensory changes that accompany aging, coupled with knowledge of appropriate interventions, will maximize the rehabilitation experience and afford the elderly an opportunity to utilize newly acquired skills in an environment that maintains reasonable control over functional ability and enhances quality of life.

Simply indicating which changes accompany normal aging may encourage older individuals to seek appropriate interventions and avoid the resignation that often accompanies a sense of helplessness at thoughts of "growing old." The physical therapist should encourage use of adaptive equipment to compensate for specific sensory loss. For example, individuals with visual loss should be supported in use of glasses and other low-vision aids, and persons with hearing loss should be encouraged to use hearing aids or other amplification devices that have been prescribed. Additionally, therapists should instruct the elderly in environmental modifications that are unique to their individual needs.

Specific teaching strategies incorporate instruction in techniques to strengthen the sensory stimulus. Examples might include adjustments to volume and tone of radios and televisions for hearing-impaired individuals or use of large-print books for the visually impaired. Another technique is to teach older individuals to compensate with other senses. For example, individuals with a diminished sense of smell can be taught to inspect food visually for signs of spoilage. The final strategy is to teach the elderly to modify behavior. One example is to teach older individuals with the visual problem of dark adaptation to pause when entering a darkened room from a bright, outdoor environment.[21, 63]

Because of their knowledge of age-related sensory changes and environmental modifications, physical therapists should assume active roles as consultants. Providing information to architects and designers will foster safe access of facilities by older individuals. This is particularly important in public buildings, including churches, hospitals, outpatient clinics, and senior centers. Additionally, independence of individuals in retirement complexes, senior housing, and long-term–care facilities can be enhanced when design principles are incorporated. Therapists should assist in plans for construction of new facilities and renovation of existing facilities. Also, they should take an active role in purchase of supplies for existing facilities. Quality of life for older residents can be maximized by selecting such items as furniture, wall and floor coverings, and window treatments that enhance, rather than impede, functional performance. Finally, physical therapists can encourage development of appropriate products to meet the needs of older individuals with sensory loss by serving as consultants to companies that design and manufacture these devices.[6, 24]

SUMMARY

It is important for physical therapists who work with the elderly to recognize sensory changes that occur with aging and to understand the affects that these changes have on the ability of older individuals to function in the environment. Knowledge of adaptations within the environment to accommodate and support losses that occur in vision, hearing, taste, smell, and touch can maximize the rehabilitation experience for the elderly and promote optimal functional independence.

Physical therapists should be able to apply this information concerning sensory losses and environmental adaptations to general principles of design in order to create meaningful environments for older persons. Consideration should be given to all aspects of the environment in which older individuals function. These include personal living space and long-term–care residencies. Specific attention should be given to architectural barriers found in physical therapy departments and on stairs and escalators. Since driving is a skill that allows access to other activities of daily living, special consideration must also be given to this function.

Finally, the roles of physical therapists as teacher and as consultant should be emphasized. Physical therapists have unique knowledge of the needs of the elderly, and they should be encouraged to share this knowledge with architects, designers, administrators, and others who deal with facilities and products used by older individuals.

REFERENCES

1. Anderson RG, Meyerhoff WL: Otologic disorders, in Calkins E, Davis PJ, Ford AB (ed): *The Practice of Geriatrics.* Philadelphia, WB Saunders, 1986.
2. Archae JC: Environmental factors associated with stair accidents by the elderly. *Clin Geriatr Med* 1985; 1:555–569.
3. Barrowclough F: Design for geriatric care. *Nurs Times* 1976; 72:1330–1331.
4. Brennan PL, Moos RH, Lemke S: Preferences of older adults and experts for physical and architectural features of group living facilities. *Gerontologist* 1988; 28:84–90.
5. Brown WJ: Planning considerations for resident-oriented long-term care settings. *Contemp Longterm Care* 1987; 10:53–55.
6. Christenson MA: The therapist as geriatric environmental consultant. *Top Geriatr Rehabil* 1987; 3:79–83.
7. Christenson MA: Adaptations of the physical environment to compensate for sensory changes. *Phys Occup Ther Geriatr* 1990; 8:3–30.
8. Christenson MA: Chair design and selection for older adults. *Phys Occup Ther Geriatr* 1990; 8:67–85.
9. Christenson MA: Designing for the older person by addressing environmental attributes. *Phys Occup Ther Geriatr* 1990; 8:31–48.
10. Christenson MA: Enhancing independence in the home setting. *Phys Occup Ther Geriatr* 1990; 8:49–65.
11. Christenson MA, Gieneart D: Redesigning the long-term care facility. *Phys Occup Ther Geriatr* 1990; 8:87–111.
12. Cohen JJ, et al: Establishing criteria for community ambulation. *Top Geriatr Rehabil* 1987; 3:71–77.
13. Cohn TE, Lasley DJ: Visual depth illusion and falls in the elderly. *Clin Geriatr Med* 1985; 1:601–620.
14. Cooper BA: A model for implementing color contrast in the environment of the elderly. *Am J Occup Ther* 1985; 39:253–258.
15. Fernie GR: CAD/CAM approaches to the development of seating and mobility aids for the elderly. *Can J Public Health* 1986; 77(suppl 1):114–118.
16. Fox MD: Elderly drivers' perceptions of their driving abilities compared to their functional visual perception skills and their actual driving performance. *Phys Occup Ther Geriatr* 1988; 7:13–49.
17. Fozard JL: Vision and hearing in aging, in Birren JE, Schaie KW (ed): *Handbook of the Psychology of Aging.* San Diego, Academic Press, 1990.
18. Goodwin S: Not so grand design. *Nurs Times* 1986; 82:26.
19. Gray G: Design of new building for the elderly. *J R Soc Health* 1989; 109:18–20.
20. Grisso JA, Mezey MD: Preventing dependence and injury: An approach to sensory changes, in LaVizzo-Mouvey R, et al (ed): *Practicing Prevention for the Elderly.* Philadelphia, Hanley and Belfus, 1989.
21. Hayter J: Modifying the environment to help older persons. *Nurs Health Care* 1983; 4:265–269.
22. Hiatt LG: Is poor lighting dimming the sight of nursing home patients? *Nurs Homes* 1980; 29:32–41.
23. Hiatt LG: The color and use of color in environments for older people. *Nurs Homes* 1981; 30:18–22.
24. Hiatt LG: Roles for gerontologists, the future of aging and technology. *Generations* 1986; 11:5–8.
25. Horwitz J: Residents' response to retirement community architecture. *Contemp Longterm Care* 1987; 10:92–93.
26. Howard DM: The effects of touch in the geriatric population. *Phys Occup Ther Geriatr* 1988; 6:35–50.

27. Kee CC: Sensory impairment: Factor X in providing nursing care to the older adult. *J Community Health Nurs* 1990; 7:45–52.

28. Kiernat JM: Environmental aspects affecting health, in Maguire GH (ed): *Care of the Elderly: A Health Team Approach.* Boston, Little, Brown, 1985.

29. Kiernat JM: Promoting independence and autonomy through environmental approaches. *Top Geriatr Rehabil* 1987; 3:1–6.

30. Kollarits CR: The aging eye, in Calkins E, Davis PJ, Ford AB (eds): *The Practice of Geriatrics.* Philadelphia, WB Saunders, 1986.

31. Kosnik W, et al: Visual changes in daily life throughout adulthood. *J Gerontol* 1988; 43:63–70.

32. LaBuda DR: Bringing gerontologists and technologists together. *Generations* 1986; 11:8–10.

33. Leibowitz HW, Shupert CL: Spatial orientation mechanisms and their implications for falls. *Clin Geriatr Med* 1985; 1:571–580.

34. Liang MH, et al: Rehabilitation management of homebound elderly with locomotor disability. *Clin Geriatr Med* 1988; 4:431–439.

35. Maguire GH: The changing realm of the senses, in Lewis CB (ed): *Aging: The Health Care Challenge,* ed 2. Philadelphia, FA Davis, 1990.

36. Maloney CC: Identifying and treating the client with sensory loss. *Phys Occup Ther Geriatr* 1987; 5:31–46.

37. Matteson MA: Age-related changes in the special senses, in Matteson MA, McConnell ES: *Gerontological Nursing: Concepts and Practice.* Philadelphia, WB Saunders, 1988.

38. McConnell ES: Nursing diagnoses related to physiological alterations, in Matteson MA, McConnell ES: *Gerontological Nursing: Concepts and Practice.* Philadelphia, WB Saunders, 1988.

39. McGilloway FA: A chair is a chair, or is it? *Nurs Mirror* 1980; 151:34–35.

40. Meltzer DW: Ophthalmic aspects, in Steinberg FU (ed): *Care of the Geriatric Patient in the Tradition of EU Cowdry,* ed 6. St Louis, CV Mosby, 1983.

41. Null RL: Low-vision elderly: An environmental rehabilitation approach. *Top Geriatr Rehabil* 1988; 4:24–31.

42. Owen DH: Maintaining posture and avoiding tripping. *Clin Geriatr Med* 1985; 1:581–599.

43. Parsons HM: Residential design for the aging (for example, the bedroom), *Hum Factors* 1981; 23:39–58.

44. Pease JA: Carpeting, new advances in technology provide more functional homelike environments. *Generations* 1986; 11:41–44.

45. Rapelje DH, Schiff MR: Homes for the aged—improving their interiors. *Dimens Health Serv* 1984; 61:22–24.

46. Raphael CC: An architect's viewpoint. *Top Geriatr Rehabil* 1987; 3:19–25.

47. Rouse DJ: Technology transfer, aerospace technology put to earthly use for elders, *Generations* 1986; 11:15–17.

48. Schwartz S: Chronic care: Improving the quality of design. *Dimens Health Serv* 1982; 59:10–13.

49. Senturia BH, Goldstein R, Hersperger WS: Otorhinolaryngologic aspects of geriatric care, in Steinberg FU (ed): *Care of the Geriatric Patient in the Tradition of EU Cowdry,* ed 6. St Louis, CV Mosby, 1983.

50. Stelmach GE, Worringham CJ: Sensorimotor deficits related to postural stability. *Clin Geriatr Med* 1985; 1:679–694.

51. Stone R, Sonnenschein MA: Can you hear me? Technology for coping with hearing loss. *Generations* 1986; 11:39–40.

52. Sullivan N: Vision in the elderly. Part 2, Coping with declining visual function. *J Gerontol Nurs* 1983; 9:231–235.

53. Sullivan N: Vision in the elderly. Part 1, Declining visual function in old age. *J Gerontol Nurs* 1983; 9:228–231.

54. Tiedskaar R: Geriatric falls, in Gambert SR (ed): *Contemporary Geriatric Medicine,* vol 2. New York, Plenum, 1986.

55. Tiedskaar R: Fall prevention in the home. *Top Geriatr Rehabil* 1987; 3:57–64.

56. Walker JM, et al: Walking velocities of older pedestrians at controlled crossings. *Top Geriatr Rehabil* 1987; 3:65–70.

57. Waller JA: The older driver, can technology decrease the risks? *Generations* 1986; 11:36–37.

58. Wells TJ: Major clinical problems in gerontologic nursing, in Calkins E, Davis PJ, Ford AB (eds): *The Practice of Geriatrics.* Philadelphia, WB Saunders, 1986.

59. Willmott M: The effects of a vinyl floor surface upon walking in elderly hospital in patients. *Age Ageing* 1986; 15:119–120.

60. Wolfson LI, et al: Gait and balance in the elderly: Two functional capacities that link sensory and motor ability to falls. *Clin Geriatr Med* 1985; 1:649–659.

61. Yerxa EJ, Baum S: Environmental theories and the older person. *Top Geriatr Rehabil* 1987; 3:7–18.

62. Yurick AG, et al: *The Aged Person and the Nursing Process.* ed 2. Norwalk, Conn, Appleton-Century-Crofts, 1984.

63. Zegeer LJ: The effects of sensory changes in older persons. *J Neurosci Nurs* 1986; 18:325–332.

Cognitive Impairment

Carol Schunk, Psy.D., P.T.

INTRODUCTION

Decline in cognitive ability from a higher previous level of function brings multiple problems that influence rehabilitation of the older individual. While therapists may focus on physical disability, it is impossible to reach treatment goals without an awareness of the normal cognitive changes with aging and the changes that occur with a specific illness. Consideration of the mental condition will influence the therapeutic plan and result in setting appropriate goals and achieving a successful outcome.

Definition

The terms *confusion, dementia,* and *senility* are commonly used to describe mental function of the elderly. Although many people consider "getting old" to be the reason for mental decline, actual changes attributed to normal aging are minimal. Cognitive changes that are severe enough to interfere with function are part of a cluster of dementing illness and not old age. *Dementia* comes from Latin and means "pathological condition of the mind."[24] *Senility* is a term often used with mental deterioration in the elderly. However, it is not a diagnostic term and is not based on specific organic causes.[21] Chronic encephalopathy, characterized by global intellectual deterioration severe enough to interfere with social and personal activities, is also commonly referred to as dementia. Properly used, dementia is characterized by persistent observed cognitive changes resulting from an illness. The key terms are *acquired* and *persistent*. *Acquired* implies abilities that were once within the behavioral domain of the individual and are now dysfunctional. *Persistence* differentiates dementia from delirium, which produces a fluctuating state.

Prevalence

As some of the dementing illnesses progress slowly, early detection is difficult with the person retaining the social skills and the ability to compensate for deficits. An individual may be quite functional within the structure of the family home with familiar objects and routines. Not until they are out of their natural environment, such as in a new grocery store, will symptoms be noticeable. A spouse may unconsciously begin to help the affected mate, therefore prolonging the identification of dementia. Because of the lack of a solid data base and problems with accurate diagnosis, in the United States prevalence is only estimated. Based on European studies, the prevalence of dementia is between 10% and 20% of all elders, depending on the sample and the criteria of dementia that were used. Although published data on the United States are minimal, approximately 15% of the population over 65 is cognitively impaired.[21] Risk for deterioration increases with advancing age, ranging from 3% of those 65 to 74 years old, 18.7% of those 75 to 84 years old, and over 47% of those aged 85 or more.[6] The prevalence in nursing home residents over age 65 has been estimated as high as 50%.[23] Of those with an organic mental disorder, an estimated 10% to 20% of these elders have reversible or partly reversible conditions.

CHANGES ASSOCIATED WITH NORMAL AGING

Predictable changes in patterns of some cognitive functions are common with normal aging. The health care practitioner should be able to differentiate between normal and abnormal patterns in order to plan the appropriate treatment approach. Often the therapist may be in the initial position to detect the onset of dementia symptoms as related to the individual's ability to participate in therapy. With normal aging, there may be some change in functional activity. There is also a cognitive component to performance of many physical activities of daily living (ADL). Consequently, if a cognitive decline is not correctly identified, change in physical activity may be misinterpreted. If cognitive deficits are also present, early identification provides an advantage in developing strategy to assist with daily activity and maintaining independence. Given that approximately 20% of dementia is reversible, this differentiation is important.[26]

Memory and Learning

Memory loss is the cognitive component most often associated with aging. This has undoubtedly contributed to the perception that the elderly cannot remember basic information and have severe lapses in memory, one of the many myths of growing old. While lapses in memory may occur as one ages, the ability to recall with cues is common. In healthy individuals, these kinds of memory problems usually do not interfere with social or personal activities.

The most prominent structural theory of memory describes three distinct types.[10] *Sensory memory* is the initial momentary memory in which there is brief registration of the physical characteristics of stimulus such as pain with an injection. *Short-term* or *primary memory* is a brief repository for conscious processing of small amounts of information. Recognition of a streetlight changing from green to red is a result of primary memory. Both of these types are relatively unaffected by aging. Changes that have been documented are of little practical importance, given normal demands.[10]

Long-term or *secondary memory* is the level where

documentation of age-related decline is most prominent. Providing for unlimited long-term retention of the information, secondary memory is responsible for analysis and organization of information for storage plus future retrieval.[10] Recall seems to be the primary activity affected by aging, with free recall being more involved than cured recall and recognition—the "Why did I come into this room?" phenomenon. Older individuals may not recall why they walked into the kitchen until the memory is cued by the sight of the phone and the recollection that they intended to make a call. While reduction in effectiveness is gradual, the most notable transition of decline is between 50 and 70 years. There are multiple reasons plus the contribution of intervening variables that influence poor performance with secondary memory tasks. In some memory theories, a tertiary level dealing with remote memory has been described. Research in this area is minimal but does not substantiate the common belief that older individuals are superior in remembering the past but inferior in remembering the present.

The memory factor associated with the normal older person has been termed *benign senescent forgetfulness* (BSF). Early stages of a mental disorder may often be mistaken for BSF. However, functional decline that is evident as the mental disorder progresses is unique to dementia and not present with BSF. Therefore, physical therapists may have a crucial role in diffferentiating between BSF and other mental disorders. Identified as a slowly progressive, mild impairment of cognitive functioning, BSF is not severe enough to interfere with daily activities. While still under investigation, BSF is currently being viewed as a variant of aging occurring in one third of individuals over 85.[16]

Another common, but inaccurate, belief is that the capacity to learn new information declines with age. While there is some evidence that there are age-related changes in learning, problems inherent to the research limits interpretation. These include comparisons across studies and multiple factors that contribute to cognitive changes, including response time, interference of prior material, and retrieval. Also complicating the research are isolating factors such as learning new motor skills, sensory changes, cognitive reorganization of material between stimulus and response, dividing attention between several tasks simultaneously, and highly speeded tasks. Despite these variables, the capacity for cognitive reserve has been demonstrated in the older person. While more limited than a younger person's the ability exists to improve performance.[2]

Intelligence

Age-related deterioration in intelligence is difficult to study given the cohort effects, generational bias of tools,

and selective attrition. While consistent longitudinal studies over many decades can eliminate some of these variables, there still exist factors particular to one generation that are difficult to factor out. The measurement tools are not sensitive to the variety of educational and cultural conditions that influenced the current older person. Actual documented declines are minimal and do not affect daily functioning. The Wechsler Adult Intelligence Scale (WAIS) is the most common tool for measuring intelligence. WAIS studies show peak in verbal and performance scores by age 18 to 30, with stability until mid-50s to early 60s.[10] Based on data from the Seattle Longitudinal Study, Hertzog and Schaie determined 55 to 70 years as the transition time from stability to decline in general intelligence.[11] While decline in performance on many cognitive tests is evident, in the older person substantial decline is generally limited to those over 75. Performance skills that are time related and influenced by decrease in reaction time tend to change more drastically than verbal skills. This phenomenon is known as the *classic aging pattern* and is the basis for age-graded intelligence quotient (IQ) scores.

The difference between *fluid* and *crystal* intelligence is also relevant to understanding cognitive dysfunction in the elderly. Fluid intelligence involves the capacity to use unique kinds of thinking to solve unfamiliar problems and is believed to decline with age. Crystalized knowledge, acquired through education and acculturation, remains stable through age 70. Creativity is often researched as a component of intelligence, with the assumption that declines are universal. Clinically, this can be interpreted as meaning, "If you haven't done it, forget it." While some studies suggest that creativity peaks by about 35 years,[10] there are enough exceptions to encourage our patients to take on new challenges and to personally keep us all inspired. Additional factors that must be considered are the lack of reinforcement for creativity in old age and environmental issues, which geriatric clinicians can positively influence.

Personality

Stereotypic beliefs about personality development such as theories about stages of personality and an aged personality profile are generally inaccurate. The best available evidence suggests that personality types remain fairly stable throughout life.[10] Therefore, those who are characterized by an internal locus of control or believing they have the ability to control the events in their lives will continue to react accordingly as they age. Those who experience a severe mid- to late-life crisis tend to react similarly to the way they reacted to situations throughout life. Activity also follows this model: those elders who were active stay active. In his research on the trait theory of personality, Hartke concluded that "consistency in personality is more the rule than change in personality as one ages."[10] The change that does occur is promoted as a continuation of individuality of the person. Traits that have been predominant will continue to be influential as one ages. Clinically, this means patients who display a negative outlook about therapy have probably always had a negative attitude in a variety of situations.

The area that does warrant additional exploration is personality changes as related to illness. Evidence is minimal that specific changes do occur, but research itself is lacking. The distinction between the influence of aging or the illness process on personality is inconclusive, making any generalizations to aging inappropriate.[10]

DIFFERENTIAL DIAGNOSIS

Diagnostic Criteria

The third revised edition of the *Diagnostic and Statistical Manual (DSM* III-R) of the American Psychiatric Association provides a universal reference of diagnostic criteria for cognitive disorders. When there is no reference to etiology, the cognitive disorder is classified as a mental symptom. Delirium, intoxication, withdrawal, and dementia are the most common mental symptoms. A *mental disorder* designates a mental symptom for which etiology is known or presumed and is characterized by a "psychological or behavioral abnormality associated with transient or permanent dysfunction of the brain."[1] Therefore, a patient is correctly diagnosed as having a mental disorder by the presence of an organic mental syndrome plus the presence of an organic factor etiologically related to the decline in mental function.

Delirium and dementia, one of the six groups of organic mental syndromes, characterize patients as having global cognitive impairment as opposed to select dysfunction. Differential diagnosis between delirium and dementia

is often difficult, as one may be superimposed on the other. Specific features are described in Table 9–1.[24] Dementia cannot be accurately diagnosed in the presence of delirium; to have coexisting diagnosis, it would be necessary for the dementia to have been identified prior to symptoms of delirium.

There is no specific course or pattern for mental symptoms. When associated with a specific episode of a neurologic disease, onset may be sudden but remain stable. This may be in contrast to a gradual onset with a progressive course of involvement, such as found in patients with dementia of the Alzheimer type. In some cases, onset may be gradual, such as an organic brain tumor. In this case, symptoms may subside with treatment.

Dementia

As described in the *DSM,* III-R, the essential feature of dementia is impairment in short- and long-term memory, associated with decline in abstract thinking, judgment, and other disturbances of higher cortical function. These factors must be severe enough to interfere significantly with work, social activities, or relationships with others. Memory is the most classic feature, with retaining new tasks showing greater decline than remembering remote material. As the case progresses, both recent and remote memory may be affected, with the person reaching the stage where recognition of familiar people is impaired. Disorientation may be missed early on, as the individual will attempt to compensate for the loss. Disorganized thinking is apparent in the inability to follow directions or tolerate changes in routine.[1]

Making an accurate diagnosis of dementia requires that the practitioner understand the normal process of cognitive changes with aging. Although research on cognitive changes associated with normal aging is not definitive, a diagnosis of dementia is applicable only when there is de-

TABLE 9–1.

Differential Diagnosis of Delirium and Dementia*

Feature	Delirium	Dementia
Onset	Rapid	Usually insidious
Sensorium	Clouded	Often clear
Orientation	Impaired	Variable
Short-term memory	Impaired	Impaired
Perception	Commonly impaired	Less commonly impaired
Sleep-wakefulness cycle	Disrupted	Normal
Physical findings	Focal neurologic signs and autonomic dysfunction noted often	Higher cortical neurologic dysfunction
Course	Fluctuating	Steady
Reversibility	Reversible in most cases	80% of cases irreversible; 20% of cases arrestable

*From Tobias CR, Lippman S, and Pary R: *Postgraduate Med* 1989; 86:101. Used by permission.

monstrable evidence of memory impairment and other features to the degree where there is interference with social or occupational function. Dementia is characterized as a decline in intellectual functioning from a previous level; therefore, knowing a person's baseline cognitive ability is essential.

Unfortunately, clinical assessment of premorbid cognitive function is not always possible and is complicated in the elderly when family input is unavailable. Consideration of educational, occupational, and socioeconomic level can provide information in determining a previous level, but often the clinician will have to piece together a picture of the individual's prior status. Irreversible dementia disorders cluster into several categories, with primary neuronal degeneration of the Alzheimer type and multi-infarct dementia being the most common.

Alzheimer's Disease

Primary degenerative dementia of the Alzheimer type (DAT), accounting for 60% of those with dementia, is the category of organic mental disorder for individuals with Alzheimer's disease. A definitive diagnosis is made postmorbidly through autopsy, as standard diagnostic criteria have not been found. McKhann and colleagues published clinical criteria that have been widely adopted for the probable diagnosis of Alzheimer's disease.[14] Their criteria include typical insidious onset of progressive dementia, not caused by any other disease known to produce memory loss and cognitive decline. Often the diagnosis is one of exclusion based on results of a medical and family history; neurologic, psychiatric, and clinical examination; neuropsychologic tests; and laboratory studies. Classification by subtypes is possible with the identification of the presence of delirium, delusions, or depression; contribution of family history; rapid or slow progression; and early or late onset.

Diagnosis is difficult in the early stages, as the individual may present very well socially with no physical appearance of a problem. Forgetfulness is often the first characteristic expressed subjectively by the individual and not evident on clinical assessment. Memory impairment as demonstrated by difficulty with acquisition of new information is the first obvious symptom. The actual loss in the process of memory involves poor encoding and retrieval, and poor recognition recall. The course of the disease is usually divided into stages, with the middle stage being identified by cognitive deficits that are quite obvious, such as intellectual decline and language disturbance. Premorbid personality and behavior changes occur along with the cognitive decline, presenting a very difficult situation for the family members. Awareness of the cognitive decline is often accompanied by depression. In the late stage the person is incapable of self-care, often becoming mute and inattentive. Research shows that physicians often overlook dementia of this type even in patients with whom they are familiar.[5]

Behavioral problems are also evident in the clinical presentation, although there are minimal empirical data to support the clinic observations of behavioral problems associated with the cognitive deficits of persons with DAT. Fifty-five families having a member with irreversible dementia, including 60% with DAT, were surveyed by Teri and colleagues to identify the "biggest problem" of patient care. In a list of 22 behaviors, over half the care givers described 4 problems: memory disturbance, catastrophic reactions, suspiciousness, and making accusations. Clarification of the associated behavioral problems and associated cognitive and functional factors was also investigated. Results showed the most common patient problems were cognitively oriented memory loss (84%), confusion (82%), and disorientation (64%). The next most common problems reported by over 20% of the participants were related to activity and emotional distress, decreased activity, loss of interest, tension, apathy, depression, and bodily preoccupation. Despite these results, there was no support for a relationship between overall cognitive impairment and behavioral problems in patients with comparable cognitive impairments. The association between rate of decline and various health and behavioral factors was studied to determine the influence on deterioration. While the results indicated that there was an association between some factors and rate of decline, the progression of the disease is variable.[21]

Multi-infarct Dementia

The *DSM* III-R classifies multi-infarct dementia as an organic mental disorder with the essential feature being cerebrovascular disease. The cognitive disorder is the result of the additive effects of small and large infarcts producing a loss of brain tissue. Deterioration is select, with some functions left completely intact. While the location of the infarction is relevant, predicting the exact course of the mental dysfunction based on site is often misleading. This may be in part because multiple strokes have occurred, obstructing a clear attribution of the deficit to a particular lesion. Common disturbances include problems with memory, abstract thinking, judgment, impulse control, and personality. Three forms of multi-infarct are most common: large vessel disease, strokes, and multiple microcerebral infarcts.[5] While the clinical presentation may resemble some features of Alzheimer's disease, the signs of abrupt onset, step-by-step deterioration, fluctuating course, and emotional lability are specific to multi-infarct dementia.[1]

Reversible Dementia

Dementia was once regarded as a permanent, irreversible, and progressive disorder. It is now known that many cases of dementia are not related to an irreversible pathology of the central nervous system. It is estimated that 10% to 30% of those presenting with dementia symptoms can be treated to correct a metabolic or structural condition, also resulting in restoration of intellectual function.[16] Without investigating the potential medical causes of dementia, a true diagnosis cannot be made. Several of the conditions that can mask the diagnosis of a reversible dementia include drug complications; infectious diseases; nutritional, psychiatric, and metabolic disorders; and trauma. Change in cognitive status secondary to drugs is possibly the most common cause of reversible dementia. The complication may be a result of drug-drug interaction either from self-medicating or inattentiveness by the physician on the drug combinations being prescribed. Given the multiple medical problems of the elderly, there may be several physicians involved in the person's care, each being unaware of the medications prescribed by the other. Psychosocial factors such as depression, social isolation, anxiety, grief, or communication disorders can also be manifested by a decrease in cognitive function. Without exploration of other factors, a misdiagnosis of irreversible dementia is possible.

Data are limited in documenting a relationship between increased incident of dementia and psychosocial factors such as bereavement, isolation, relocation, stress, or life-style changes.[25] However, once dementia is documented, there is evidence that environmental and psychosocial variables do have an impact on severity and progression. Factors may include inadequate stimulation, diet, and medical care.

Pseudodementia

Pseudodementia is the term used when dementialike behavior is actually the result of a major depressive episode. Characteristics of depression, sometimes estimated as affecting 25% of the older population to some degree, include psychomotor retardation, flattened affect, and disinterest in events around them. Patients presenting in this fashion could be labeled as having a decline in mental ability simply because they do not have the interest in answering questions intended to establish a cognitive level. Also termed *dementia syndrome of depression,* the presenting symptoms of memory impairment—decline in intellectual function and poor performance on mental status examinations—can be diagnostically confusing. Since the two conditions can coexist, there is a contemporary trend not to use the term *pseudodementia,* which may imply that the individual must be either depressed or demented but not both.[9]

Although persons with dementia or depression may present similarly, observation of behavioral characteristics is revealing. While depressed patients may respond to testing in a slow, labored manner, they are aware of content and provide accurate responses.[24] Those with true dementia will be unable to produce the correct response even when pressed for an answer. Dysphoria is a distinguishing characteristic in depression, as evident in profound sadness, apathy, and feelings of helplessness and hopelessness. Social contact and activity are lessened with low self-esteem and an increase of self-blame.

A study by Pearson and colleagues examined the relationship between depressive diagnosis and cognitive and functional limitations in DAT patients.[17] They found that depression did affect functional status beyond the effects of cognitive impairment. Therefore, if depression is an overlying condition, functional status may improve with successful treatment of the depressive episode. A trial of antidepressants may provide information for a clear diagnosis. If the mood improves as the depression is resolved, cognitive function will return to predepressive level. Should the individual continue to display characteristics of decline in mental ability, then investigation for dementia would be initiated.

Given change in functional status, involvement of the physical therapist is appropriate. The focus will not only be on physical training but on monitoring the cognitive orientation to therapy. As improvement in functional activities requires aspects of cognition such as attention and memory, the therapist may be the primary practitioner to note decline or improvement in mental function.

Anxiety

Given the number of stressful situational changes that occur as one ages, anxiety-type behavior may be more common than in the younger years. Early stage dementia can be a cause of anxiety as the person becomes aware of his deteriorating mental capacity. If related to organic causes, a diagnosis of organic anxiety syndrome may be appropriate.[1] Common diseases in the older person that may be the etiologic cause of an anxiety syndrome include pulmonary embolus, chronic obstructive pulmonary disease, and alcohol withdrawal. According to the American Psychiatric Association, the primary diagnostic criterion is prominent, recurrent panic attacks or generalized anxiety with evidence of specific organic factors related to the disturbance. Anxiety disorders have a similar symptomatic picture but without similar etiology. In the elderly, situational factors such as relocation may precipitate an anxiety disorder.

Coping Behavior

Given multiple changes in later life, the older individual's ability to cope may influence behavior. Coping styles are closely related to personality styles, developed throughout life, as one confronts challenges and changes. Stress is often the by-product of factors and situations occurring later in life. Although the stresses may occur more frequently, there is no indication that the ability to cope with stressful events declines with age. Economic, health, and social resources may be minimized with old age and therefore compromise the ability to deal with stressful life events. However, if all is constant, the notion of declining ability to cope in later life has not been validated.

Given pain as a major stress for many older persons, Keefe and Williams were prompted to do a comparison study of coping strategies for different age-groups.[12] Results showed that chronic pain patients of different ages tend to rely on similar coping strategies to deal with pain and rate the effectiveness of their pain in a similar fashion. Those who used catastrophizing or an emotional nonparticipatory reaction had higher levels of pain and psychologic distress, whereas those who indicated a high ability to deal with the pain reported lower levels of pain and depression. Given the lack of differences in coping strategies, a study by Middaugh et al. concluded that there is no reason why older persons would not be good candidates for chronic pain programs, as they were able to benefit as much as younger patients.[15] Subjects showed decrease in level of pain and ability to enhance functional activity regardless of age.

ASSESSMENT

There are no neurodiagnostic procedures or electrophysiologic techniques that unequivocally confirm the presence of primary degenerative dementia. Therefore, diagnosis is often made on clinical grounds.[25] Given the number of individuals with possible cognitive deficits in long-term–care facilities, there is a need for a rapid bedside assessment tool. One commonly used instrument is the Pfeiffer Short Portable Mental Status Questionnaire, which contains ten questions and can be used to screen for moderate to severe cognitive impairment.[19] The Mini Mental Status Exam (MMSE) seems to be the most accepted of the brief standardized tests, providing the most information in the greatest number of domains.[7, 13] In addition, the MMSE provides specific norms for older adults.[3] Viewed as a screening tool rather than a diagnostic tool, a score of less than 24 out of the 30 possible points indicates cognitive impairment, warranting evaluation by a physician. Since there are various parts of the examination, the total score may identify a cognitive deficit but does not provide information on the specific area of loss. Individualized scores of the examination sections provide a better picture of the nature of the decline. The first part measures orientation. Serial sevens, if done correctly, suggests that cognitive function is good. However, the task when failed is nonspecific, given the factors such as education or poor calculation skills that can influence the outcome. The recent memory or recall section is essential in assessment for dementia, especially in relation to functional activities. Odenheimer suggests that the one cognitive domain neglected is "executive control" or "intention," which measures stick-to-itiveness, goal setting, and flexibility.[16] Since functional independence depends on the ability to move from one task to another, this can be assessed by asking the patient to copy a figure that alternates in form or listing items in a grocery store for 1 minute.

The MMSE and the Blessed Orientation-Memory-Test (BOMC)[4] are both bedside tools that have excellent test-retest reliability. They are utilized for identifying cognitive disabilities and in describing changes in mental status over time. Other advantages are the simplicity and clarity of the instruments, which are important given the minimal training of the care givers in the nursing homes.[26] Criticisms of these tools include limited ability to provide specific neurobehavioral descriptions as compared with more extensive tests; and neglect of nonverbal functions, making them nonmultidimensional.[26] Therefore, they have been reported to be vulnerable to high false-negative rates. Given these problems, the tests' wide utilization is based on the tests' ability to discriminate between different diagnostic subgroups, related to severity and course of dementia and reliability when applied in nursing home settings.

Comparing the BOMC and the MMSE, Zillmer et al. found that the MMSE may be more useful since it identifies more than one mental process, as compared with the BOMC.[26] The study emphasized that brief mental status examination should be confined "to measuring limited dimensions of mental processes." Results of the study concluded that the BOMC and MMSE are appropriate tools if "primarily interpreted as measures of memory, attention and limited (i.e., highly stereotyped) linguistic facility." They counseled against broader interpretation.

THERAPEUTIC MANAGEMENT

While the treatment goal of maximizing functional independence is consistent with goals of patients without dementia, there are special considerations when treating an older person with a cognitive disability. Rehabilitation potential for individuals with cognitive dysfunction was considered to be minimal according to the early literature.[23] The features of dementia that most influence the rehabilitation process are memory decline and the difficulty or inability to learn new material. Since therapy is viewed as a teaching process, these features of dementia may be perceived as major obstacles to successful outcome. In addition, physical therapy reimbursement for persons with a dementing disease is often questioned based on the perceived inability to follow a treatment plan. Research now demonstrates that the presence and severity of cognitive status should not eliminate a patient from rehabilitation.[23] Therapists must modify treatment methods and goals in relation to the limitations of the cognitive disability, but therapy should not be denied based on mental dysfunction. Reassessment of progress in relation to treatment goals may be necessary on a more frequent basis, given the inconsistent pattern of mental deterioration.

The initial step in planning a therapeutic program is to determine the exact nature of the cognitive dysfunction. The screening tools discussed can be utilized for a global picture of the condition. If available, a neuropsychologic assessment with consultation by a psychologist will provide additional information to delineate the deficit. The attempt is to clearly define specifics of the memory loss or other disability. Then the treatment can be modified, such as using one-step consistent commands or providing cues. The approach to teaching is to avoid criticism; use consistent, simple commands; give sensory cues: demonstrate; and allow the person to rest.[13] Learning should be approached in a simple, repetitive manner, often requiring cooperation from the family or nursing staff for consistency in the approach and directions for the individual.

The patient's physical disability may be part of the same disease that has caused the cognitive impairment, such as a cerebrovascular accident. In other cases the two components are separate, such as the patient with Alzheimer's disease who suffers a hip fracture. In either case the therapy assessment and treatment program must be modified to accommodate the mental dysfunction. A physical therapy evaluation technique like manual muscle testing may not be valid with an individual who is inconsistent in following directions. Modification to accommodate the mental limitation may result in a generalized assessment of strength documented as "voluntary motion noted in extremities; unable to grade specifically secondary to inconsistency following directions." Muscle testing procedures are not familiar tasks to most people, which therefore necessitates learning that can be difficult for a person with dementia. While strength can be assessed and reported, the approach is modified in relation to the limitations of the mental symptoms.

The orthopedic patient with DAT and a lower extremity fracture presents an example of alteration of the treatment program. A physician's order for gait training, partial weight bearing with a walker, is appropriate given the physical problem. However, modification is necessary with dementia symptoms. Given the limitations of memory caused by dementia, the patient will probably not be able to understand and remember the weight-bearing status nor conceptualize the mechanics of using the walker. Therefore, the physician must be consulted to change the status to either full– or non–weight-bearing status. If the dementia is severe enough, gait training may be postponed until the patient is able to walk without the use of an assistive device that can be too complicated to comprehend. Exercise for those with a cognitive deficit may be modified with the focus on following the therapist's demonstration rather than the expectation of an independent program. Likewise self-range of motion for a cognitively impaired person with hemiparesis is better accomplished through function rather than attempting to teach a new activity. Skills and activities that occurred daily prior to the onset of the mental decline such as eating, walking, or dressing can usually be relearned with a higher degree of success than introduction of a new skill.

Manipulation of the patient's environment is often more successful than attempting to teach the person techniques to compensate for cognitive loss. Items and surroundings that are familiar minimize the impact of memory deficit, allowing the person to perform routine daily activities by rote without having to problem solve. The emphasis on the environment includes safety as a valid factor in the therapeutic program. Failure to recognize and react to hazards becomes a major consideration in the person's ability to remain in an unsupervised situation. Since confusion is often an issue, protection of the patient is part of the treatment program.

Because control of the environment seems to help with the person's confusion, many facilities have developed dementia units that emphasize a structured low-key environment with consistent staffing.[8] The focus is on safety, specially trained staff, admission criteria, physical design, and activity schedules.[18] Management is facilitated by reinforcing the environment with constant reminders to orient them to time, the place, and care-giver identity. Glickstein and Bottorf have presented suggestions for modifying the home, hospital, or day-treatment area with the goal of function at the highest level of independence.[8]

The health professional must assess not only the patient's environment but also available support systems and family situation in order to implement an individual plan of care.[8] Education and training for the care giver are essential, as management of the patient is heavily dependent on the family support and coping resources. Those without an understanding of the limitations of the patient may have unrealistic goals that are translated into demands on the patients, resulting in failure and frustration. The patient should be engaged in activities that can be performed successfully without failure. Identification of community support groups for the care giver is also part of the treatment plan, offering an opportunity for education and emotional assistance.

CASE STUDY

JD was an 84-year-old male living at home with his 72-year-old companion. Also living in the home was the patient's 17-year-old nephew and the nephew's pregnant 16-year-old girlfriend. According to the family, JD had been fine until he fell, fracturing his left hip. Following a total hip replacement, JD was placed in a nursing home for rehabilitation. Physician's orders were for physical therapy; transfer and gait training; partial weight bearing on the left. Upon initial evaluation the therapist found the patient to be very confused. He was unable to identify family members and was not orientated to time or place, with minimal awareness of the restrictions of his injury. Consultation with the family revealed that JD was fine prior to the fall, with some signs of "getting old" but much more aware than presently displayed. The therapist modified the treatment program to accommodate the cognitive status, including utilization of an adductor cushion to prevent dislocation and allowing no weight bearing until the patient could follow partial–weight-bearing limitations. The therapist considered postsurgical confusion as a possible reason for the cognitive dysfunction. When the mental function only slightly improved in the next few days, the therapist scheduled an interview with the individuals living with JD in his home.

As an introduction for the family, the therapist explained that she was interested in JD's ability to perform daily activities prior to the accident. She told them that "just getting old" is usually not the reason for individuals to change the way they function, that most people who experience normal aging have minimal changes in their memory, personality, or intelligence. With questioning, those interviewed recalled that JD had become more forgetful about 2 years ago. He began to get lost while driving, only to be returned by a neighbor in the small farming community. The animals were neglected, as JD either fed them five times a day or not for several days. When he forgot repeatedly to milk the cow, the nephew moved in to help out with the chores. In the last 6 months the family reported that they had to answer the phone, as people outside the family were unable to understand JD when he talked. JD had also become very suspicious of the neighbors, accusing them of taking his fence down. Following the interview, the therapist conducted an MMSE. JD scored 15 out of 30, with low scores on the orientation and memory portion. Given the presenting cognitive function,

history as revealed by the family, and MMSE score, JD was referred to a psychologist for testing to rule out dementia of the Alzheimer type.

To maximize the therapy sessions, JD's treatment program was modified to accommodate the cognitive dysfunction. The physician was consulted regarding the difficulty of maintaining partial–weight-bearing status and agreed to allow the patient to bear weight to tolerance if a wheeled walker were used. This allowed the patient to transfer with a modified standing pivot method and to begin gait training. The family was involved in therapy, as JD continued to respond to instructions when a familiar person was present. They also were instructed in simple exercises that they encouraged JD to do whenever they visited. This modification in the treatment plan compensated for JD's inability to comply with an independent exercise program. As the family was very vested in JD's returning to his prior living situation, a home assessment was conducted with suggestions on safety, precautions for danger when wandering, and cues to minimize the effects of the memory loss. Family concerns were also addressed by explaining Alzheimer's disease, which had been confirmed by the consultant, and the effects on the living situation and the family members. With an extended therapy period due to the dementia, JD reached treatment goals of independent ambulation and transfers. He returned home with supervision as a safety precaution.

SUMMARY

With the elderly population the probability of cognitive dysfunction increases with age. While affecting only a small percentage of the population under 80 years, cognitive dysfunction must be considered by therapists when treating the older individual. Dementia is the most common mental dysfunction, with a varied symptomatic picture, depending on the type. With healthy aging, there are some changes in memory, intelligence, and personality. However, such variations do not interfere with daily relationships or function. Knowledge of normal aging as related to mental function allows the practitioner to recognize abnormal changes and plan an appropriate therapy program.

Memory impairment is the primary feature of dementia. Some forms of dementia are reversible. Therefore, etiology must be investigated to make treatment recommendations if appropriate. Dementia of the Alzheimer type is the most common of the irreversible categories, with multi-infarct dementia also often diagnosed in the elderly. Depression may mimic dementia, although it is now thought that the two conditions can coexist. Pseudodementia is often-used terminology when dementialike symptoms are eliminated with successful treatment of depression. Assessment of cognitive status can be accomplished by several brief standardized examinations. Since there are no procedures that definitively confirm dementia, clinical symptoms are often used for diagnosis. While the brief tools can be used to screen, referral to a psychologist or physician may be appropriate for a more comprehensive assessment.

While the focus is the same—maximizing the individual's functional independence—there is a difference when treating a patient with a cognitive disorder. Teaching is an essential element of physical therapy; therefore, memory loss will influence progress and the instructional approach. Awareness of the limitations imposed by cognitive dysfunction should result in modification of the treatment program. The baseline is the therapist's understanding of the cognitive aspect of aging, both normal and abnormal. Patients with cognitive disabilities can benefit from therapy and should have the opportunity to remain as functional as possible with the intervention of knowledgeable physical therapists.

REFERENCES

1. American Psychiatric Association: *Diagnostic and Statistical Manual of Mental Disorders,* ed 3, rev. Washington, DC, American Psychiatric Association, 1987.
2. Baltes PB, Lindenberger U: On the range of cognitive plasticity in old age as a function of experience: 15 years of intervention research. *Behav Ther* 1988; 19:283–300.
3. Bleeker ML, et al: Age-specific norms for the Mini Mental State Exam, *Neurology* 1988; 38:1565–1568.
4. Blessed G, Tominson BE, Roth M: The association between quantitative measures of dementia and of senile change in the cerebral grey matter of elderly patients. *Br J Psychiatry* 1968; 114:797–811.
5. Eisdorfer C, Cohen D: Dementing illness in middle and late life, in Ebaugh FG (ed): *Geriatric Medicine.* Menlo Park, Calif, Addison-Wesley, 1981.
6. Evans DA, et al: Prevalence of Alzheimer's disease in a community population of older persons: Higher than previously reported. *JAMA* 1989; 262:2551–2556.
7. Folstein MF, Folstein SE, McHugh PR: "Mini Mental State"—a practical method for grading the cognitive state of patients for the clinician. *J Psychiatr Res* 1975; 12:189–198.
8. Glickstein JK, Bottorf S: Alzheimer's disease: Providing a meaningful existence in the absence of definitive management, in Dwyer BJ (ed): *Focus on Geriatric Care and Rehabilitation.* Frederick, Md, Aspen Publishers, 1987.
9. Haggerty JR, et al: Differential diagnosis of pseudodementia in the elderly. *Geriatrics* 1988; 43:61–74.
10. Hartke RJ: The aging process: Cognition, personality and coping, in Hartke RJ (ed): *Psychological Aspects of Geriatric Rehabilitation.* Frederick, Md, Aspen Publishers, 1991.
11. Hertzog C, Schaie KW: Stability and change in adult intelligence: Simultaneous analysis of longitudinal means and covariance structures. *Psychol Aging* 1988; 3:122–130.
12. Keefe FJ, Williams DA: A comparison of coping strategies in chronic pain patients in different age groups. *J Gerontol* 1990; 45:161–165.
13. Mace NL, Hardy SR, Rabins PV: Alzheimer's disease and the confused patient, in Jackson O (ed): *Physical Therapy of the Geriatric Patient.* New York, Churchill Livingstone, 1989.
14. McKhann GD, et al: Clinical diagnosis of Alzheimer's disease: Report of the NINCDS-ADRDA work group under the auspices of the Department of Health and Human Services Task Force on Alzheimer's disease. *Neurology* 1984; 34:939–944.
15. Middaugh SJ, et al: Chronic pain: Its treatment in geriatric and younger patients. *Arch Phys Med Rehabil* 1988; 69:1021–1026.
16. Odenheimer GL: Acquired cognitive disorders of the elderly. *Med Clin North Am* 1989; 73:1383–1411.
17. Pearson JL, et al: Functional status and cognitive impairment in Alzheimer's patients with and without depression. *J Am Geriatr Soc* 1989; 37:1117–1121.
18. Peppard NR: Developing a special needs dementia unit, in Glickstein JK (ed): *Focus on Geriatric Care and Rehabilitation.* Frederick, Md, Aspen Publishers, 1990.
19. Pfeiffer E: A short portable mental status questionnaire for the assessment of organic brain deficit in elderly patients. *J Am Geriatr Soc* 1975; 23:433–441.
20. Pousada L, Leipzig RM: Rapid bedside assessment of postoperative confusion in older patients. *Geriatrics* 1990; 45:59–66.
21. Teri L, Hughes JP, Larson EB: Cognitive deterioration in Alzheimer's disease: Behavioral and health factors. *J Gerontol* 1990; 45:58–63.
22. Teri L, et al: Behavioral disturbance, cognitive dysfunction, and functional skill prevalence and relationship in Alzheimer's disease. *J Am Geriatr Soc* 1989; 37:109–116.
23. Teschendorf B: Cognitive impairment in the elderly: Delirium, depression or dementia?, in Dwyer BJ (ed): *Focus on Geriatric Care and Rehabilitation.* Frederick, Md, Aspen Publishers, 1987.
24. Tobias CR, Lippman S, Pary R: Dementia in the elderly. *Postgrad Med* 1989; 86:101–106.
25. Zarit S: *Aging and Mental Disorders: Psychological Approaches to Assessment and Treatment.* New York, Free Press, 1980.
26. Zillmer EA, et al: Comparison of two cognitive bedside screening instruments in nursing home residents: A factor analytic study. *J Gerontol* 1990; 45:69–74.

CHAPTER 10

Depression and Function in the Elderly

Ann K. Williams, Ph.D., P.T.

INTRODUCTION

Depression is the most common psychologic problem in the elderly.[14, 43, 51] While this is also true in other adult age-groups, depression remains a significant problem for professionals working with the elderly. Although depression is frequently neglected in the elderly, it is actually quite treatable.[14] There are many causes of depression; however, in the elderly one factor that is frequently associated with depression is loss of health. The stress of physical illness that may be associated with physical disability, pain, and life-style changes can result in the psychologic response of depression. Conversely, depression can dramatically affect the response of the elderly patient to rehabilitation. The hopelessness, apathy, and withdrawal of the depressed person make rehabilitation a challenge. While the assessment and treatment of depression are the responsibility of other health professionals, they constitute a problem that physical therapists must deal with frequently. This chapter will review the characteristics of depression, factors associated with it, common treatment approaches, and modifications of the physical therapist's treatment plan that are appropriate for the depressed elderly patient.

CHARACTERISTICS AND ASSESSMENT OF THE DEPRESSED OLDER PERSON

Characteristics of the Depressed Person

Most people think of the predominant characteristic of depression as depressed mood, that is, feelings of sadness, hopelessness, and loss of interest and pleasure in previously pleasurable activities. Although these emotions are a key feature of depression, experts agree that in order for depression to be a psychopathology or a "clinical depression," other characteristics must also be present. These include cognitive problems such as difficulty concentrating, memory complaints, slowed thinking, and indecisiveness. Feelings of low self-esteem, worthlessness, and excessive guilt also may be present. The depressed person has difficulties with interpersonal interactions, including withdrawal from family and friends and neglect of previously pleasurable activities. Finally, depression includes somatic symptoms such as problems with appetite, sleep, and psychomotor function. The disturbances of appetite usually involve loss of weight but may involve excessive eating. The sleep problems often involve insomnia and early morning wakening, but hypersomnia may also be demonstrated. Psychomotor functioning is usually retarded but may be agitated.

In order to help standardize the diagnosis of depression and the terminology associated with it, the *Diagnostic and Statistical Manual of Mental Disorders,* third edition, revised (*DSM* III-R) of the American Psychiatric Association describes specific criteria for various diagnoses of mood disorders that are generally accepted.[2] The two diagnoses that are important to this discussion of depression in the elderly are major depressive episode and adjustment disorder with depressed mood. According to the *DSM* III-R, as outlined in Table 10–1, the criteria for major depressive episode are either depressed mood or loss of pleasure in all activities and associated symptoms for a period of at least 2 weeks. These symptoms must be a change from previous functioning and relatively persistent. The associated symptoms include significant weight loss or gain when not dieting, insomnia or hypersomnia, psychomotor retardation or agitation, fatigue or loss of energy, feelings of worthlessness or excessive or inappropriate guilt, diminished ability to think or concentrate, and recurrent thoughts of death. The person must exhibit at least five of all these symptoms in order to be diagnosed as having a major depression.

Adjustment disorder with depressed mood is a subcategory of adjustment disorders in the *DSM* III-R.[2] Adjustment disorders are maladaptive reactions to an identifiable psychosocial stressor that occur within 3 months of the onset of the stressor and persist no longer than 6 months. The maladaptive nature of the reaction is signified by impairment of occupational functioning or usual social activities or relationships or by symptoms that are in excess of a normal and expected reaction. In an adjustment disorder with depressed mood the predominant symptoms are a depressed mood, tearfulness, and feelings of hopelessness. For example, a divorce may cause a person to have a depressed mood. This response would be classified as an adjustment disorder with depressed mood if the person's social relationship or job is affected. The depression response must be considered to be excessive.

When reading the numerous books and articles available on depression, the reader may become confused by the varied terminology that is sometimes different from that in the *DSM* III-R outlined above. For example, some authors will use the term *endogenous depression,* which is similar to a major depressive episode. Similarly, the term *reactive depression* is similar to an adjustment disorder with depressed mood. Finally, the term *dysphoria* is sometimes used to describe a milder depression characterized only by depressed mood.

Assessment of Depression

The various tools available for the assessment of depression are even more varied than the terms used to describe it. In the clinical setting, the diagnosis of various depressive disorders will usually be made by a health professional who is expert in this area, for example, a clinical

TABLE 10-1.

DSM III-R Criteria for Major Depressive Episode*

1. Depressed mood†
2. Markedly diminished interest or pleasure in all, or almost all, activities
3. Significant weight loss or weight gain when not dieting or decrease or increase in appetite
4. Insomnia or hypersomnia
5. Psychomotor agitation or retardation
6. Fatigue or loss of energy
7. Feelings of worthlessness or excessive or inappropriate guilt
8. Diminished ability to think or concentrate or indecisiveness
9. Recurrent thoughts of death, recurrent suicidal ideation, a suicide attempt, or a specific plan for committing suicide

*Adapted from American Psychiatric Association: *Diagnostic and Statistical Manual of Mental Disorders,* ed 3, rev. Washington, DC, American Psychiatric Association, 1987.
†Criteria: At least five of the following symptoms present during a 2-week period and represent a change from previous functioning. One of the symptoms must be either (1) depressed mood or (2) loss of interest or pleasure.

psychologist or a psychiatrist. The diagnosis is based on a careful interview with the client and close family and friends.

In research studies such as those referenced in this chapter where large numbers of persons in the community are involved, various self-report scales of depression are often used. The respondents will check off on a printed form whether or not they have experienced various of the symptoms of depression. While these self-report measures depend on the honesty of the respondent to truly report symptoms, they are frequently used in the interests of conserving time and money. These self-report scales are generally accepted as good screening devices to indicate individuals who are at risk for depression and may need further professional evaluation. It is beyond the scope of this chapter to give a detailed description of all the self-report scales used for depression. Some of the most commonly used scales are listed in the next paragraph with references to assist the reader who needs more information.

Four of the most commonly used depression scales are the Beck Depression Inventory, the Center for Epidemiological Studies Depression Scale (CES-D), the Geriatric Depression Scale (GDS), and the Zung Self-Rating Depression Scale (SDS).[30, 68, 72] Table 10-2 gives additional information about these depression scales, describing the number of items, total score, number of somatic items, and sample items. Generally, the scales make statements about feelings or situations, and the respondent indicates how frequently each item occurs.

An important issue in self-rating scales of depression is the degree of emphasis that they give to the somatic symptoms of depression.[4, 68] Many of these symptoms such as appetite or sleep disturbances may be a result of aging or the many physical illnesses that are more common in the elderly. Thus, a person may score high on the depression scale not because of depression but because of unrelated somatic symptoms. Scales that de-emphasize somatic signs of depression are generally considered more valid for the elderly.

Models of Depression

Numerous authors have speculated about the causes of depression, and various models have emerged. Four of the most frequently cited models are the cognitive model, the learned-helplessness model, the interpersonal model, and the neurobiologic model. Understanding these models is important because they help to explain various treatment approaches to depression.

The *cognitive model* of depression was proposed by Aaron Beck and is based on his empirical observation of depressed patients.[26] This model emphasizes the cognitive structure underlying depression including the negative views of the self, the environment, and the future. The depressed person employs a negative cognitive schema that influences the coding and organization of incoming stimuli. Errors of information processing occur, resulting in overestimation of negative input and underestimation of positive input. For example, a work supervisor's suggestions for improvement would be interpreted by the depressed person as an indication of unworthiness, inability to do the job, even dislike. Loss, grief, or dysphoric feelings then trigger depression in the person, with negative schemata. The perceptual bias then perpetuates the depression. In this model, the negative schemata are primary and the depressed effect is secondary.

In the *learned-helplessness model* of Seligman, uncontrollable negative events result in passive behaviors.[26] Although the research in this model was originally in animals, it has been applied to human depression. Emphasis is placed on the decreased motivation in depression and the perceptions of uncontrollability of events by the depressed person. This model may be particularly applicable to the medical patient. A series of negative health events

TABLE 10–2.

Common Self-Report Depression Scales

Scale	No. of items	Total Score	No. of Somatic Items	How Scored	Sample Item
Zung Self-rating Depression Scale (SDS)	20	80	8	Scored for frequency: e.g., some of the time, most of the time, etc.	"I feel downhearted and blue."
Beck Depression Inventory	21	63	6	Subject chooses one of four choices	"I do not feel sad." "I feel sad." I am sad all the time and can't snap out of it." "I am so sad or unhappy that I can't stand it."
Center for Epidemiological Studies Depression Scale (CES-D)	20	60	3	Scored for frequency	"I felt that I could not shake off the blues even with help from my friends and family."
Geriatric Depression Scale (GDS)	30	30	1	Scored yes/no	"Do you feel that your life is empty?"

may be perceived by the patient as uncontrollable. The sick role also promotes lack of control and passivity. The result may be excessively passive behavior, lack of motivation, and depression for the patient.

The *interpersonal model* for depression emphasizes overdependent personality traits that predispose the individual with a loss or negative life event to depression.[34] This vulnerability is often attributed to adverse childhood experiences or intrafamilial relations. This model focuses on personality rather than external causes for depression. For example, an overly protective parent might result in a child who is excessively dependent. This personality trait may then result in a depressive response to a negative life event later in life.

Finally, the *neurobiologic model* of depression suggests that the somatic symptoms of depression, such as the psychomotor retardation and temporal variation, indicate a biologic base for the illness.[41] Clinical observations that some drugs produced depressive symptoms, whereas other drugs relieved them, pointed to decreased neurotransmission or a disturbance of catecholamine transmission as the cause of depression. Deficient brain serotonergic transmission has been suggested because of the sleep disturbances that occur with depression.

Rates of Depression

Depression appears to be the most common psychopathology in all age groups.[14, 43] Two age-groups appear particularly vulnerable to depression: adolescents and very elderly males.[21] When the elderly are considered as one group including all persons over age 65, their rate of depression is no different than the rest of the adult population.[21, 49, 51] Thus, the commonly held stereotype of the elderly as lonely and depressed is not supported by research data. Selected subgroups of the elderly such as very

elderly males show higher rates of depression in some studies, although others have not confirmed this finding. The elderly as a whole, however, have about the same rates of depression as other adult groups.

Epidemiologic studies indicate a prevalence of depression in the elderly that ranges from 4% to 23%.[6, 15, 21, 49] This wide variation of results can be due to several factors. Some studies based their rates only on patients who had sought psychiatric treatment, a research method that could underestimate rates. A wide variety of scales and classification criteria have been used across studies, making comparison difficult. Inclusion of somatic symptoms as part of the criteria for the definition of depression is problematic in the elderly because these symptoms may occur in old age or disease.[4] Carefully designed studies indicate a rate of depression in the elderly of around 12%.[49, 61] Studies that use strict criteria for a major depression indicate lower rates around 5%. While these rates apply to all persons over age 65, certain special populations of the elderly would be expected to have higher rates of depression. These would include the institutionalized elderly[38] and, as will be discussed in detail later in this chapter, the physically ill elderly. Studies of the institutionalized elderly generally indicate higher rates of severe depression, around 12%.[38] This population is especially difficult to study because of their high rates of cognitive impairment and physical illness. Not surprisingly, newly admitted residents to a nursing home are more likely to be depressed.

Depression in the Elderly

An issue that is consistently debated is whether depression in the elderly is different from depression in other age-groups. A change of the characteristics of depression in the elderly is a common theme in the clinical literature.[48] Butler and Lewis suggested that feelings of guilt, self-derogation, and suicidal impulses are less common in the elderly.[8] More common in the elderly are symptoms of apathy, low motivation, low energy, sleep disturbances, and loss of appetite. Derogatis and Wise also noted increased apathy in the depressed elderly.[16] They point to an increased cognitive impairment in the depressed elderly as well as a reluctance to discuss feelings of dysphoria. Some authors believe that the elderly do not present as strongly with the somatic aspects of depression, whereas others indicate that somatization is the predominant symptom of depression in the elderly.

Unlike the clinical literature, epidemiologic studies of depression generally support a picture of depression in the elderly as basically similar to depression in other age-groups.[7, 20, 48] Somatic symptoms are especially problematic as they may be part of a coexisting physical illness.[4, 7] As will be discussed later in the chapter, this similarity of depression across the age span suggests that effective treatment strategies in younger age-groups may also be effective in the elderly.

Pseudodementia

Because the symptoms of depression may be confused with early dementia, depressed elderly persons are at risk to be diagnosed as having organic brain syndrome. This mistake is common enough to be given the name *pseudodementia* in clinical geriatric psychiatry. The apathy, decreased ability to concentrate, and memory complaints of the depressed elderly person may be misinterpreted as symptoms of dementia.[15, 31] Experts in geriatric psychiatry indicate that the differential diagnosis between depression and early dementia can be difficult. As guidelines for distinguishing between the two, they point out that the depressed person has poorer social skills than the person with early dementia. While the depressed older person usually has complaints of memory problems, when tested this individual shows few deficits.[31] Finally, symptoms of depression are usually worst in the morning and get better by the afternoon. In contrast, persons with dementia have more problems in the late afternoon.

As geriatric psychiatrists have noted, the distinction between depression and dementia is complicated by the fact that both can coexist in the same person. If there is a clear psychosocial stressor that could lead to depression, geriatric psychiatrists recommend that treatment should be first initiated for depression. Dementia should be a diagnosis of exclusion, that is, only given after other possible diagnoses have been eliminated.

Factors Associated With Depression

One factor consistently associated with depression in older persons is physical illness.[3, 12, 21, 32, 40, 54, 63, 69] This is clearly of import to health care professionals. While there are a few studies that indicate no association between physical illness and depression,[11, 62] numerous studies demonstrate an increased risk of depression in physically ill persons. Various studies of patients with heart disease, rheumatoid arthritis, diabetes, cancer, and multiple sclerosis show higher rates of depression than the average in the population.[42, 44–46, 54, 57, 67] In addition to studies of persons with specific diseases, studies that include persons with many different diagnoses also demonstrate an increased risk for depression.

While some psychologists theorize that all persons with a physical illness will experience a "stage" of depression,[35] clearly not all physically ill persons develop a *clinical* depression. At some point, dysphoric feelings may become excessive and maladaptive, which results in the cognitive, psychologic, and somatic symptoms of a major depression. The severity and number of symptoms as well as a previous history of depression are suggestive of a major depressive episode.[9, 60] Patients with an adjustment disorder with depressed mood will tend to have a decreased severity of psychologic symptoms, and increased severity of stressors, and recent functioning at a higher level.[60] Studies indicate the rate of severe depression in the physically ill elderly somewhere between 20% and 35%.[21, 32, 41, 54, 61]

Are older persons more or less likely to respond to the stress of physical illness with depression? The few studies that have investigated age as a factor in the relationship of physical illness to depression are about equally split on both sides of the issue. Some indicate that older physically ill persons are more likely to be depressed; others indicate no relationship to age or that older persons are less likely to be depressed.[10, 67] Given the high rates of physical illness in the elderly, the low overall rate of depression in this age-group suggests that older persons adapt at least as well as younger persons to the stress of physical illness.[68] Some experts have suggested that certain negative events may be more anticipated at certain times in life. Thus, older persons may expect health problems as a normal part of aging and therefore adjust better to them.[58] It remains critical to identify those whose response is maladaptive and to initiate treatment. The physical therapist may be instrumental in identifying those individuals who could benefit from referral to specialists in psychology.

Although depression in adults may be more common in women,[19, 52] studies of depression in the elderly have shown variable effects of gender.[7, 15, 40] Gurland et al. found the highest rate of depression in very elderly males.[24] Other studies of elderly persons with a medically related depression have not found gender to be a contributing factor.[6] Physical therapists might expect very elderly male patients to be at high risk for depression; however, generally, older male and female patients will be equally likely to be depressed.

Higher rates of depression are linked to lower income and socioeconomic status.[15, 28, 49] This remains the case for depressed physically ill older persons.[68] Not surprisingly, the stress of physical illness is confounded by the stress of limited resources, and physically ill older persons with low incomes are more likely to become depressed.

One would expect that a high degree of social support from family and friends would buffer the negative effects of an illness and result in a lower risk for depression. While research has generally supported this hypothesis, some studies have shown higher levels of anxiety and dependency in patients with more social support.[17] Social support, depression, and physical illness may form a complex web of interrelationships where persons who are ill and in pain become depressed and have difficulty mobilizing the social support that is available to them.[33, 71] Also, older persons with chronic physical illness may require support over long periods of time. This can stress any support system, so that expected support is not available, and this may contribute to or exacerbate a depression.

The increased risk of depression in physically ill older persons makes it critical to identify factors of an illness that increase the risk for depression. Several studies have indicated higher levels of functional incapacity and disability to be associated with higher levels of depression, and one would expect higher levels of physical dependency to result in more depression.[32, 45, 46] However, very elderly persons have high rates of physical dependency without correspondingly high rates of depression.[68] The very old may have different expectations regarding disability and are therefore more likely to accept it.

Chronic pain patients of all ages show high rates of depression, and level of pain would be expected to be related to depression.[16, 27, 55, 56, 69] Few studies have combined physical disability and pain when studying depression in the elderly. Williams and Schulz found that when control for other variables is added to the analysis, pain becomes a more important factor than physical disability in level of depression.[69]

Effect of Depression on Function in the Elderly

Because of the nature of depression, persons with depression will have a reduced functional capacity.[43, 47, 66] The apathy, loss of pleasure in activities, and psychomotor retardation will reduce the individual's capacity to participate in everyday activities and even perform activities of daily living. The depressed person perceives that even simple tasks require excessive amounts of energy, and these tasks become extremely difficult.[43] This decreased function is usually most evident in the morning.

For the physically ill elderly person with depression, this loss of functional capacity will become even more problematic. The deconditioning effects of age and illness will combine with depression to result in even more perceived effort required for minor everyday tasks. Long-term goals may appear unattainable. In a study of patients with hip fractures, Mossey et al. found increased depression to be associated with reduced functional recovery and reduced response to rehabilitation.[47] Depression and functional recovery are probably interactive, so that the depressed patient functions at a lower level, and this decreased function also reinforces the depression.

Motivation of the depressed older patient and the appropriate modifications of the rehabilitation plan will be a constant challenge to the therapist. The second part of this chapter on management of depression will discuss specific suggestions for this challenge. A case history will provide additional examples.

MANAGEMENT OF DEPRESSION IN THE OLDER PERSON

The management of depression in the older person has many aspects. Two of the most common treatment approaches are pharmacotherapy and psychotherapy, each of which is discussed in this section. While psychotherapy has demonstrated positive results with older persons, it is not as frequently used with the elderly as drug treatment.[26] Reasons for this bias may include resistance to and misunderstanding of psychotherapy on the part of the elderly, bias against the elderly on the part of psychotherapists, lower cost of drug treatment, and a bias toward drug treatment in the medical community. Some experts have suggested that psychotherapy may be more effective for adjustment disorder with depressed mood, whereas drug treatment may be more effective for a major depressive episode. Nevertheless, drug treatment remains the most common approach in managing elders with depression. The use of exercise in the treatment of depression has had limited research; however, as it is of particular interest to physical therapists, it will be discussed. Finally, practical suggestions for the physical therapist working with the depressed older patient will be described.

Pharmacotherapy

Pharmacologic treatment is the primary therapy for major depressive episodes in the elderly.[1, 65] Medications used to treat major depression can be divided into three major categories: tricyclics and tetracyclics, monoamine oxidase inhibitors, and psychostimulants.[29, 65] Table 10–3 indicates the common drug names in these categories of drugs that the therapist might find in the medical record.

The tricyclics and the newly developed tetracyclics are

TABLE 10–3.

Antidepressant Drug Names

Nonproprietary Name	Trade Name
Tricyclics and tetracyclics	
Amitriptyline	Amitril, Elavil
Amoxapine	Asendin
Desipramine	Norpramin, Pertofrane
Doxepin	Adapin, Sinequan
Imipramine	Janimine, Tofranil
Maprotiline	Ludiomil
Nortriptyline	Aventyl, Pamelor
Protriptyline	Vivactil
Trimipramine	Surmontil
Monamine oxidase inhibitors	
Isocarboxazid	Marplan
Phenelzine	Nardil
Tranylcypromine	Parnate
Psychostimulants	
Methylphenidate	Ritalin

the mainstay of the drug treatment of depression. Their mechanism of action is their ability to block the neuronal uptake of norepinephrine and serotonin and thereby affect the central nervous system amines implicated in depression.[22, 69] However, the tricyclics have numerous side effects, particularly in the elderly. These side effects are primarily anticholinergic and include dizziness, tachycardia, constipation, blurred vision, urinary retention, postural hypotension, and mild tremor.[22, 29, 65] Of particular concern to physical therapists are the side effects of dizziness and postural hypotension. Patients taking tricyclic antidepressants may have poorer balance, particularly after moving from supine to sitting or sitting to standing. These effects will be more pronounced in the period immediately after taking medication. While there are numerous drugs in the category of tricyclics, the differences between them are primarily in the degree of side effects produced.[1, 70] These side effects are more common in the elderly and could be especially troublesome in this age group.

The monoamine oxidase inhibitors also have major side effects similar to the tricyclics and are less frequently used in the elderly.[22, 29] Psychostimulants may be effective for adjustment disorders in the physically ill elderly.[29]

Psychotherapy

Older patients are seldom included in studies of the effectiveness of psychotherapy.[39] Older patients may be less likely to seek psychotherapy, but also, health professionals may be biased against older persons believing that elders will not benefit from psychotherapy. The few studies including older patients indicate that psychotherapy is an effective treatment for depression in the elderly.[18, 25, 39, 64] Psychotherapy treatments for the elderly include behav-

ioral, cognitive, and brief psychodynamic therapies. Behavioral treatments focus on modifying the behavioral components of depression, whereas cognitive approaches attempt to change the negative cognitive schemata that accompany depression. Psychodynamic therapies focus on the personality characteristics common in depression. Very few studies have compared medication and psychotherapy in the treatment of depression in the elderly, but some have indicated that psychotherapy may be at least as effective as medications in the elderly.[5, 18]

Exercise

Exercise has been occasionally used as an effective treatment for depression.[23, 37, 50, 53] However, the patients have usually been young or middle-aged persons, and the exercise was vigorous, aerobic exercise.[59] Such programs are therefore not suitable for most physically ill elderly.[59] Exercise programs for depressed elderly who are not seriously ill must also consider the high rates of cardiovascular disease in this age-group. While some studies indicate that heavy aerobic exercise reduces depression, others indicate that any activity including mild recreational activity will be associated with increases in feelings of well-being.[36, 70] This improvement may be caused by time-out from periods of psychologic stress, increased social interaction, or increased feelings of mastery. Some authors also hypothesize a psychologic effect of increased secretion of amines that would have an antidepressant effect.[53] While exercise is not a commonly accepted treatment for depression, its beneficial effects on well-being should be remembered by physical, occupational, and recreational therapists.

Working With the Depressed Older Patient

Suggestions for working with the depressed older patient are really little different than those for any adult who is depressed. Aerobic exercise may be a treatment modality that is less frequently used in the elderly. Also, elderly persons may be more likely to have experienced losses in their support networks, especially loss of a spouse. With a more limited support network, the stress of caring for a depressed ill person may be concentrated on a few individuals. Key support persons may also require extra assistance in dealing with the depressed patient.

Depression can affect many aspects of physical therapy treatment. The course of therapy would be expected to be longer, as the apathy and extra energy required will necessitate more time to accomplish goals. More time may need to be spent on activities of daily living, as these tasks will seem more difficult for the patient.

Physical therapists may need to modify their approach

when the patient is depressed. Some professionals may believe that being overly cheerful will "jolly" the patient out of feelings of sadness and low self-esteem. Generally, this is not the case, and the effect may be the opposite. The excessive cheerfulness of the therapist may only emphasize the separateness and depression of the patient and increase negative feelings. Anyone who remembers a time when he was quite depressed will recall that cheerfulness of others did not really decrease the depression but often only accentuated one's own sad feelings. Experts agree that a better approach to the depressed person is to be matter-of-fact and emphasize the patient's feelings of mastery rather than feelings of pleasure. It is important to acknowledge the great degree of effort required by the depressed person to accomplish even everyday tasks. Goals should be discussed in small, easily achievable steps. The depressed person will have difficulty visualizing goals far into the future. Achievement of short-term goals will enhance the person's sense of mastery and improve motivation.

Dealing with the depressed patient may be psychologically difficult for the therapist. These patients are not "fun" and may appear unmotivated. It is important to remember that these people are not lazy. For them, large amounts of energy are required to accomplish even simple tasks. Working with these patients also has its rewards. Depressed persons almost always get better and will achieve therapeutic goals. Most of us have experienced depression to some extent. Remembering our own sad times can help to develop empathy for the depressed patient.

Case Study

Mr. Clark is 84 years old. Prior to his present hospitalization, he lived alone in his suburban home; his wife of 45 years had died 6 months previously. He has two sons, one of whom lives in the same city. He was hospitalized because he fell in his home and fractured the subcapital area of his right femur. A hemiarthroplasty was performed, and Mr. Clark was referred to physical therapy. Laboratory tests also indicated a high blood sugar level, and he is being evaluated for possible diabetes. The therapist working with Mr. Clark notes that he appears quite sad, has cried several times during treatment, and has expressed hopelessness about his future. He also has difficulty remembering the precautions regarding his hip that have been repeatedly explained to him. He is apathetic, is hard to motivate, has a poor appetite, and has difficulty sleeping. The nursing and medical staff have noted similar problems. As his son indicated that these problems had been steadily getting worse since the death of Mrs. Clark, a psychiatric consult was requested. Although Mr. Clark's memory problems could have been due to early dementia, the consult indicated that the first treatment should be for depression with later reevaluation. Antidepressant medication and short-term therapy for depression were initiated. Mr. Clark was also started on insulin therapy and transferred to the rehabilitation unit.

Mr. Clark's progress in physical therapy was slower than expected, although he made steady improvement. His therapist established small short-term goals that could be accomplished in 2 to 3 days. Emphasis was placed on the mastery of these short-term goals rather than long-term goals. For example, Mr. Clark was given the goal of increasing his walking distance from 20 to 40 ft, rather than being given the long-term goal of independent ambulation. He was asked to be able to repeat one more precaution every other day, rather than learn all the precautions in 1 day. The extra effort required by Mr. Clark was acknowledged, but his negative expressions of low self-esteem and guilt were countered with more positive statements about his progress. Mr. Clark's depression gradually lifted, and he was discharged to his home. A home health agency continued his physical therapy and monitored the progress of his diabetes treatment. Antidepressant treatment was discontinued after 2 months.

SUMMARY

While depression is no more common in the elderly than in other adult age-groups, it remains the most common psychopathology of old age. The two categories of depression of greatest interest to physical therapists are major depressive episode and adjustment disorder with depressed mood. The characteristics of depression include problems with mood, cognition, self-esteem, interpersonal interactions, and somatic functions. Depression in the elderly is similar to depression in other adults, although some have suggested that the older depressed adult will show more apathy and lack of motivation. Difficulty in differentiating depression from early dementia is common enough to warrant a name, pseudodementia.

Factors that are commonly associated with depression in the elderly are the presence of physical illness, low income, and decreased social support. Among the physically ill elderly, high levels of pain and physical disability may be related to depression. Depression will reduce function in the physically ill elderly because of apathy, perceptions of low energy, and psychomotor retardation.

Pharmacotherapy is the primary treatment for a major depressive episode; however, psychotherapy has also been shown to be effective in the elderly. A few studies of exercise demonstrate some positive effect on depression, but the use of aerobic exercise is limited in the physically ill elderly.

Guidelines for working with the depressed older patient include establishing short-term goals, emphasizing achievement rather than pleasure, and avoiding excessive cheerfulness. Most depressed patients do get better with time and treatment. It is important to remember that many of us have experienced some degree of depression in our lives and can therefore be empathetic with these patients.

REFERENCES

1. Abrams WB, Berkow R: *Merck Manual of Geriatrics.* Rathway, NJ, Merck Sharp & Dome Laboratories, 1990.
2. American Psychiatric Association: *Diagnostic and Statistical Manual of Mental Disorders,* ed 3, rev. Washington, DC, American Psychiatric Association, 1987.
3. Ban T: Chronic disease and depression in the geriatric population. *J Clin Psychiatry* 1984, 45:18–24.
4. Berkman LF, et al: Depressive symptoms in relation to physical health and functioning in the elderly. *Am J Epidemiol* 1986; 24:372–388.
5. Beutler LE, et al: Group cognitive therapy and alprazolam in the treatment of depression in older adults. *J Consult Clin Psychol* 1987; 55:550–556.
6. Blazer D, Williams C: Epidemiology of dysphoria and depression in an elderly population. *Am J Psychiatry* 1980; 137:439–444.
7. Bolla-Wilson K, Bleecker ML: Absence of depression in elderly adults. *J Gerontol* 1989; 44:P53–55.
8. Butler RN, Lewis M: *Aging & Mental Health.* St Louis, CV Mosby, 1982.
9. Cameron OG: Guidelines for diagnosis and treatment of depression in patients with medical illness. *J Clin Psychiatry* 1990; 51(suppl):32–35.
10. Cappeliez P, Blanchet D: Strategies of the elderly in coping with depressive feelings. *Can J Aging* 1986; 5:125–134.
11. Cassileth B, et al: Psychosocial status in chronic illness, a comparative analysis of six diagnostic groups. *New Engl J Med* 1984; 311:506–511.
12. Cavanaugh S: Depression in the hospitalized inpatient with various medical illnesses. *Psychother Psychosom* 1986; 45:97–104.
13. Chaisson-Stewart GM: Depression incidence: Past, present, and future, in Chaisson-Stewart GM, (ed): *Depression in the Elderly: An Interdisciplinary Approach.* New York, J Wiley & Sons, 1985.
14. Chaisson-Stewart GM: The diagnostic dilemma, in Chaisson-Stewart GM (ed): *Depression in the Elderly: An Interdisciplinary Approach.* New York, J Wiley & Sons, 1985.
15. Comstock G, Helsing K: Symptoms of depression in two communities. *Psychol Med* 1976; 6:551–563.
16. Derogatis LR, Wise TN: Anxiety and depressive disorders in the medical patient. Washington, DC, American Psychiatric Press, 1989.
17. DiMatteo M, Hays R: Social support and serious illness, in Gottlieb BH (ed): *Social Networks and Social Support.* Beverly Hills, Sage, 1981.
18. Dobson KS: A meta-analysis of the efficacy of cognitive therapy for depression. *J Consult Clin Psychol* 1989; 57:414–419.
19. Dohrenwend B: Sociocultural and social psychological factors in the genesis of mental disorders. *J Health Soc Behav* 1975; 16:365–392.
20. Downes JJ, Davies AD, Copeland JR: Organization of depressive symptoms in the elderly population: Hierarchial patterns and Guttman scales. *Psychol Aging* 1988; 3:367–374.
21. Gatz M, Hurwicz M: Are old people more depressed? Cross-sectional data on Center for Epidemiological Studies—Depression Scale. *Psychol Aging* 1990; 5:284–290.
22. Goodman AG, et al: *Goodman & Gilman's the Pharmacological Basis of Therapeutics.* New York, Macmillan, 1985.
23. Griest JH, et al: Running as a treatment for non-psychotic depression. *Behav Med* 1978; 4:19–24.
24. Gurland B, et al: *The Mind and Mood of Aging.* New York, Haworth Press, 1983.
25. Gurland BJ, Toner JA: Depression in the elderly: A review of recently published studies, in Eisdorfer C (ed): *Annual Review of Gerontology and Geriatrics.* New York, Springer, 1982.
26. Haas GL, Fitzgibbon ML: Cognitive models, in Mann JJ (ed): *Models of Depressive Disorders.* New York, Plenum Press, 1989.
27. Hendler N: Depression caused by chronic pain. *J Clin Psychiatry* 1984; 45:30–38.
28. Hirschfeld R, Cross C: Epidemiology of affective disorders, psychosocial factors. *Arch Gen Psychiatry* 1982; 39:35–46.
29. Jenike MA: *Handbook of Geriatric Psychopharmacology.* Littleton, Mass, PSG, 1985.
30. Kane RA, Kane RL: *Assessing the Elderly: A Practical Guide to Measurement.* Lexington, Lexington Books, 1981.
31. Kasniak AW, Sadeh M, Stern LZ: Differentiating depression from organic brain syndromes in older age, in Chaisson-Stewart GM (ed): *Depression in the Elderly.* New York, J Wiley & Sons, 1985.
32. Kennedy GJ, Kelman HR, Thomas C: The emergence of depressive symptoms in late life. The importance of health and increasing disability. *J Community Health* 1990; 15:93–104.
33. Kessler R, Mcleod J: Social support in community samples, In Cohen, Syme (eds): *Social Support and Health.* Orlando, Academic Press, 1985.
34. Klerman G: The interpersonal model, in Mann JJ (ed): *Models of Depressive Disorders.* New York, Plenum Press, 1989.
35. Krueger DW: Psychological adjustment to physical trauma and disability, in Roessler, Decker (ed): *Emotional Disorders in Physically Ill Patients.* New York, Human Sciences Press, 1986.
36. Kugler J, et al: Hospital supervised versus home exercise in cardiac rehabilitation: Effects of aerobic fitness, anxiety, and depression. *Arch Phys Med Rehabil* 1990; 71:322–325.

37. Labbe EE: Effects of consistent aerobic exercise on the psychological functioning of women. *Percept Mot Skills* 1988; 67:919–925.

38. Lesher EL: Validation of the Geriatric Depression Scale among nursing home residents. *Clin Gerontol* 1986; 4:21–28.

39. Levy SM, et al: Intervention with older adults and the evaluation of outcome, in Poon LW (ed): *Aging in the Eighties*. Washington DC, American Psychological Association. 1980.

40. Magni G, de Leo D, Schifano F: Depression in geriatric and adult medical inpatients. *J Clin Psychol* 1985; 41:337–344.

41. Mann JJ: Neurobiologic models, in Mann JJ (ed): *Models of Depressive Disorders*. New York, Plenum Press, 1989.

42. Massei MJ, Holland JC: Depression and the cancer patient. *J Clin Psychiatry* 1990; 51(suppl):12–17.

43. Matteson M: Affective disorders, in Whanger AD, Myers AC (eds): *Mental Health Assessment and Therapeutic Intervention With Older Adults*. Rockville, Md, Aspen Systems Corporation, 1984.

44. Mayeux R: Depression in the patient with Parkinson's disease. *J Clin Psychiatry* 1990; 51(suppl):20–23.

45. McIvor G, Riklan M, Reznikoff M: Depression in multiple sclerosis as a function of length and severity of illness, age, remissions, and perceived social support. *J Clin Psychol* 1984; 40:1028–1033.

46. Moos R, Solomon G: Personality factors associated with rheumatoid arthritis. *J Chronic Dis* 1964; 17:41–55.

47. Mossey JM, Knott K, Craik R: The effects of persistent depressive symptoms on hip fracture recovery. *J Gerontol* 1990; 45:M163–168.

48. Newmann JP, Engel RJ, Jansen J: Depressive symptom patterns among older women. *Psychol Aging* 1990; 5:101–118.

49. Noll G, Dubinsky M: Prevalence and predictors of depression in a suburban county. *J Community Psychol* 1985; 13:13–19.

50. Palmer J, Vacc N, Epstein J: Adult inpatient alcoholics: Physical exercise as a treatment intervention. *J Stud Alcohol* 1988; 49:418–421.

51. Parmelee PA, Katz IR, Lawton MP: Depression among institutionalized aged: Assessment and prevalence estimation. *J Gerontol* 1989; 44:M22–29.

52. Radloff L, Rae D: Components of the sex difference in depression. *Res Community Ment Health* 1981; 2:111–137.

53. Ransford CP: A role for amines in the antidepressant effect of exercise: A review. *Med Sci Sports Exerc* 1982; 14:1–10.

54. Rodin G, Voshart K: Depression in the medically ill: An overview. *Am J Psychiatry* 1986; 143:696–703.

55. Romano J, Turner J: Chronic pain and depression: Does the evidence support a relationship? *Psychol Bull* 1985; 97:18–34.

56. Roy R: Chronic pain and depression: A review. *Compr Psychiatry* 1984; 25:96–105.

57. Rutter B: Some psychological concomitants of chronic bronchitis. *Psychol Med* 1977; 7:459–464.

58. Schulz R, Rau M: Social support through the life course, in Cohen S, Syme L (eds): *Social Support and Health*. New York, Academic Press, 1985.

59. Shisslah CM, Utic J: Exercise, in Chaisson-Stewart GM (ed): *Depression in the Elderly: An Interdisciplinary Approach*. New York, J Wiley & Sons, 1985.

60. Snyder S, et al: Differentiating major depression from adjustment disorder with depressed mood in the medical setting. *Gen Hosp Psychiatry* 1990; 12:159–165.

61. Stenbach A: Depression and suicidal behavior in old age, in Birren J, Sloan RS (eds): *Handbook of Mental Health and Aging*. Englewood Cliffs, NJ, Prentice-Hall, 1980.

62. Tennant C, Wilby J, Nicholson G: Psychological correlates of myasthenia gravis: A brief report. *J Psychosom Res* 1986; 30:575–580.

63. Teuting P, Koslow SH: Special report on depression research. *National Institutes of Mental Health Science Reports*. Rockville, Md, US Department of Health and Human Services, 1988.

64. Thompson LW, Gallagher E, Brechenridge JS: Comparative effectiveness of psychotherapies for depressed elders. *J Consult Clin Psychol* 1987; 55:383–390.

65. Veith RC: Depression in the elderly: Pharmacologic considerations in treatment. *J Am Geriatr Soc* 1982; 30:581–586.

66. Wade D, Legh-Smith J, Langton-Hewer R: Depressed mood after stroke: A community study of its frequency. *Br J Psychiatry* 1987; 151:200–205.

67. Westbrook M, Viney L: Psychological reactions to the onset of chronic illness. *Soc Sci Med* 1982; 16:899–905.

68. Williams A: *Physical Illness and Depression: Changes Over Time in Middle Aged and Elderly Persons* (thesis). Portland University, Portland, 1985.

69. Williams A, Schulz R: Association of pain and physical dependency with depression in physically ill middle-aged and elderly persons. *Phys Ther* 1988; 68:1226–1230.

70. Williams JM, Getty D: Effects of levels of exercise on psychological mood states, physical fitness, and plasma beta endorphin. *Percept Mot Skills* 1986; 63:1099–1105.

71. Wortman C, Conway T: The role of social support in adaption and recovery from physical illness, in Cohen S, Syme L (eds): *Social Support and Health*. New York, Academic Press, 1985.

72. Yesavage JA, et al: Development and validation of a Geriatric Depression Scale. *J Psychiatr Res* 1983; 17:31–49.

Laboratory Evaluation of the Geriatric Patient in the Planning of a Rehabilitation Program

Douglas P. Kiel, M.D., M.P.H.

INTRODUCTION

When planning rehabilitation for the geriatric patient, the physical therapist must carefully integrate the clinical history, physical examination, and laboratory evaluation. Whereas the physician member of the rehabilitation team may identify and evaluate abnormalities in laboratory tests, the actual impact of abnormal tests on the planning of rehabilitation may not be appreciated. It is thus important for the therapist to have some familiarity with commonly encountered laboratory tests to be able to appropriately design rehabilitation programs.

This chapter will discuss some of the more common laboratory tests encountered in aged patients who may be candidates for rehabilitation. A brief description of the physiologic implications of each selected laboratory test will be offered. The tests then will be discussed in the context of aging. Finally, the laboratory evaluation will be considered from the perspective of the physical therapist designing rehabilitation. The laboratory evaluation will include blood tests as well as tests of the urine, radiographic imaging tests, and electrocardiograms.

COMMONLY ENCOUNTERED LABORATORY TESTS

There has been a dramatic increase in laboratory testing in older patients for a number of reasons. First, older persons often have multiple pathologies that can be understood better by certain laboratory investigations. Second, the clinical history and examination may be more difficult to perform in older individuals, making the laboratory assessment even more important. Older persons tend to underreport symptoms and to underestimate the severity of symptoms when diseases are present. Finally, the geriatric patient is likely to be on multiple drugs that can act alone or together to affect laboratory parameters.

A great deal of information can be learned about an older person by measuring laboratory values for hematologic tests (complete blood cell count, or CBC count), biochemical tests (electrolytes such as sodium, enzymes, and other proteins such as alkaline phosphatase or albumin), urine tests, the chest radiograph, and the electrocardiogram.

LABORATORY TEST VALUES IN THE AGED

When assessing laboratory results in the aged, one must take into consideration that some "normal results" by the usual reference ranges are actually abnormal. On the other hand, some laboratory results that lie outside the traditional reference range may be "normal" in an older person. Since many test values show significant changes with age, the reference ranges used in test interpretation must be derived from subjects of the appropriate age. There are several reasons why reference ranges change with age. First, many physiologic functions (e.g., renal function) decline with aging. Hormonal changes such as those occurring at menopause may also influence laboratory values. Lifestyle patterns may account for additional changes in the reference ranges for older persons. For example, dietary preferences that change with age may influence laboratory assessment of parameters such as vitamin levels. There are some reference ranges that show an increase with age, making it difficult to separate true age change from the possibility of a rising prevalence of occult pathologies.

Usually, reference ranges are based on groups of appropriate age who are judged to be healthy.[6] A sample of normal reference ranges from a typical laboratory is found in Table 11–1. In older persons, this may be a problem because almost all elders have demonstrable pathologic abnormalities of some kind and usually cannot be judged as having no pathology. Furthermore, most older persons are taking some form of medication, which can also influence test results. These difficulties in determining reference ranges in the aged explain why age-adjusted reference ranges are usually not provided on the prototype computer printout of laboratory values. To properly assess the measured laboratory value in the aged patient, one must be aware of the changes in expected values with aging.

Complete Blood Count

The complete blood count (CBC) is a reflection of bone marrow function since the bone marrow is the source of red blood cells, white blood cells, and platelets. The CBC is done almost exclusively using an automated procedure that totals up the number of cells in a given volume of blood stained appropriately for the cellular elements. The red blood cell volume is commonly expressed as the *hemoglobin* (grams of hemoglobin/100 mL blood) or the *hematocrit* (percentage of the blood volume occupied by the red blood cells). These two measures are interchangeable, with the hematocrit being roughly three times the hemoglobin. The hemoglobin in the red cell is the primary site for oxygen transport, although a small amount of oxygen is dissolved in the blood. Any process that affects the production of red blood cells by the marrow (e.g., lack of iron) or that affects the survival of cells in the circulation (destruction of cells due to a drug reaction or blood loss from a gastrointestinal source) may result in anemia. On the other hand, certain stem cell disorders can lead to an excess production of red blood cells. If the hematocrit increases too much, there may be adverse consequences with

TABLE 11–1.

Reference Ranges for Laboratory Tests*

Laboratory Test	Reference Range
Complete blood count	
Hematocrit	Male 47 ± 5%
	Female 42 ± 5%
Hemoglobin	Male 16.2 ± 2 g/dL
	Female 14 ± 2 g/dL
White blood count	7.8 ± 3 × 10^9
Platelet count	140–400 × 10^9
Biochemical tests	
Potassium	3.6–5.1 mEq/dL
Calcium	9.0–10.5 mEq/dL
Magnesium	1.2–2.3 mg/dL
Glucose	67–109 mg/dL
Alkaline phosphatase	45–126 IU/L
Total protein	6.3–8.3 g/dL
Albumin	3.4–4.8 g/dL
T_4	5.0–12.5 mcg/dL
T_3 resin uptake	25%–35%
TSH	0.4–4.8 mcιu/mL

*Reference ranges may vary according to laboratory.
T_4 = thyroxine; T_3 = triiodothyronine; TSH = thyroid-stimulating hormone.

regard to blood circulation and coagulation. For example, polycythemia vera, a disorder of the stem cell for red blood cells, may result in elevated hematocrit and sludging of blood. In some instances, sludging of blood predisposes to the formation of a blood clot. If such a clot were to form in the cerebral circulation, a stroke may occur.

In studies of healthy aged populations there is a tendency for hemoglobin levels to be decreased compared with young adults.[2, 3, 16] This finding has been less consistent in older women than men.[2] Similar patterns have been noted for the hematocrit. With aging, there is a greater dispersion of values of hemoglobin and hematocrit about the mean, with a slight tail toward lower values for men. Despite these changes, the actual values of these tests in the elderly are well within the reference ranges for younger adults. In one study, when deficient hemoglobin was considered to be below 12.0 g/dL, no elderly persons had abnormally low values.[3]

The white blood cell, or leukocyte, is also counted in the automated analysis of blood. Leukocytes are divided into several varieties, including polymorphonuclear leukocytes (neutrophils), lymphocytes, and monocytes. Certain diseases such as infection or leukemia cause elevations in the leukocyte count, whereas declines in the count are also seen in certain leukemias, sepsis, tumors, or as a side effect of medication use. The total leukocyte count in aged individuals is not significantly different than in younger persons, although older men have slightly greater median leukocyte counts than do older women.

The third major cellular component of the CBC is the

platelet. The platelet primarily functions in the coagulation system to seal off disruptions in the blood vessel that would otherwise lead to blood loss. Platelet counts depend on the number produced in the marrow, and on the number lost, either through consumption or destruction. A decrease in the absolute numbers of circulating platelets or a defect in the qualitative function of existing platelets contributes to an increased risk of bleeding. Diseases such as essential thrombocytosis, resulting in an increase in the numbers of platelets, may lead to an increased tendency to form clots. Platelet counts in aged persons are not different than in younger groups.[2, 16]

Biochemical Tests

Biochemical tests commonly available from the clinical laboratory range from the very simple to the extremely complex. The more commonly encountered ones may be grouped into categories: electrolytes such as potassium, calcium, and magnesium; glucose; enzymes/proteins such as alkaline phosphatase, total protein, and albumin; and hormones such as thyroid hormone.

Potassium is the principal intracellular cation (positively charged ion). Extracellular potassium constitutes only a small part of total body potassium but greatly influences neuromuscular function. The ratio of the intracellular to extracellular potassium is influenced greatly when the concentration of the smaller extracellular concentration changes even slightly. The concentration of potassium is regulated by dietary intake, urinary and gastrointestinal losses mediated in part by hormones, the acid-base status of the blood, and other factors such as insulin and catecholamines (e.g., adrenaline).

Potassium depletion results in varying degrees of neuromuscular dysfunction. Many patients with hypokalemia complain of muscle weakness especially in the lower extremities that can be marked when the potassium deficiency is profound. Deep tendon reflexes can be diminished with potassium depletion. Very severe or rapid loss of potassium results in complete paralysis of muscles. In contrast, hyperkalemia has more dangerous effects on the electrical conduction system of the heart but occasionally may result in muscular weakness starting in the lower extremities and progressing upward.

Total body calcium is between 1 and 2 kg, with approximately 98% of the calcium found in the skeleton. The small fraction found in extracellular fluid plays a critical role in a variety of functions including neuromuscular irritability. As such, extracellular calcium is maintained in a very narrow range by several hormones including parathyroid hormone, calcitonin, and vitamin D. According to national nutrition surveys, the average American diet is deficient in calcium.[11] Since extracellular calcium is maintained at the expense of skeletal stores, dietary calcium deficiency may compromise skeletal integrity. The clinical implication for the elderly is the development of osteoporosis and related fractures.

Decreases in the concentration of free calcium ions in serum may lead to irritability of the neuromuscular system. The most dramatic illustration of this is tetany, characterized by paresthesias, spasm, anxiety, seizures, bronchospasm, and electrical problems affecting the heart. Increases in calcium usually do not lead to neuromuscular dysfunction but rather are associated with anorexia, nausea, vomiting, constipation, and delirium.

Serum calcium decreases in men with aging probably because of an age-related decline in serum albumin, the principal protein to which calcium is bound.[7] In women, there is a rise in serum calcium following the menopause that continues into old age.[7, 13] The higher serum calcium in older women may be related to the estrogen deficiency that occurs at menopause. Estrogen is thought to exert an antiresorptive effect on the skeleton, which at the menopause is absent, resulting in a diminished antagonism to the bone resorptive effects of either parathyroid hormone or local growth factors. This increase in calcium in women does not have any implications for interpreting calcium levels because it is usually insignificant on routine blood testing. However, total calcium values obtained by direct measurement should be interpreted in light of variations in the albumin level. Algorithms for correcting the total calcium values are available. When in question, the ionized calcium level may be measured and represents a more accurate assessment of calcium homeostasis than does total calcium.

Compared with calcium metabolism, less is known about magnesium. Magnesium levels are not maintained with the precision of calcium, and there are no hormone systems that regulate magnesium concentrations. Thus, the serum levels of magnesium depend on intake and on renal and gastrointestinal losses. These losses are small enough that over the short term, conditions associated with inadequate magnesium intake do not result in hypomagnesemia. Since magnesium is the predominant intracellular divalent cation, extracellular measurements do not correlate with total body stores. Nevertheless, the clinical manifestations of hypomagnesemia resemble those of hypocalcemia. Thus, depending on the degree of depletion, muscle weakness, tetany, tremors, cardiac arrhythmias, confusion, and even psychotic behavior can be symptoms of hypomagnesemia. Age-related changes in magnesium concentration have not been described, but diuretic use, which may be higher in older patients, is capable of lowering magnesium levels.

Glucose represents one of the major sources of energy for metabolic processes throughout the body. The liver functions to maintain normal levels of blood sugar by a combination of glycogenesis, glycogenolysis, glycolysis, and gluconeogenesis. Metabolic pathways of glucose metabolism are regulated by hormones such as insulin, glucagon, growth hormone, and certain catecholamines. Blood glucose levels are maintained within a relatively narrow range by these pathways. Deviations from normal often result in elevations of the blood glucose; however, abnormally low glucose levels may be caused by drug effects, alcoholism, neoplasms, sepsis, hypothermia, and malnutrition. The physical therapist is more likely to encounter elevated blood sugar secondary to diabetes than hypoglycemia from any cause. Elevated blood glucose levels may be asymptomatic or cause symptoms such as lethargy, thirst, polyuria, or blurry vision.

The age-related changes in glucose tolerance are best characterized by the response to a glucose challenge rather than the fasting blood level of glucose, which rises by only 1 to 2 mg/dL per decade.[8] A glucose challenge test is commonly performed by having an individual drink 75 g, of glucose dissolved in 300 mL of water consumed over 5 minutes. Postprandial blood glucose levels at 1 to 2 hours following a meal increase significantly with age in the range of 4 mg/dL per decade.[15] After an oral or intravenous glucose challenge test, serum glucose rises by 6 to 13 mg/dL per decade in measurements made 1 to 2 hours after the challenge.[8] Women tend to respond higher than men at all ages. With age the Hb A_{1c} level rises from about 7% at age 25 to over 9% after age 70.[8] The Hb A_{1c} measures the accumulation in red blood cells of hemoglobin that has been irreversibly transformed to a glycosylated form. The presence of high circulating levels of glucose over several weeks yields increased levels of this form of hemoglobin.

Given the above changes in glucose with aging, the interpretation of glucose levels in the aged remains problematic if one relies on the well-accepted recommendations of the National Diabetes Data Group (NDDG). In 1979, this group proposed that for the convenience of data comparison worldwide, glucose tolerance should be evaluated using an oral load of 75 g glucose dissolved in 300 mL of water consumed over 5 minutes. Normally, persons should not have a plasma glucose of 200 or greater during the subsequent 2 hours.[12] It has been suggested that the normal response to glucose loading (derived from studies in younger subjects) requires age adjustment because of the well-recognized age-related changes in glucose tolerance test curves. Without age adjustment, 50% to 60% of persons over age 60 would be considered to have diabetes.[8] Nevertheless, glucose tolerance tests are not routinely performed. Given the stability and reproducibility of fasting plasma glucose, some have suggested that a fasting value of 115 mg/dL should be used as the upper limit of normal in the elderly.[8]

One of the enzyme tests commonly encountered in clinical practice is the alkaline phosphatase level. Human serum contains several forms of alkaline phosphatase that arise from bone, intestine, liver, and placenta. Amounts of the enzyme are usually expressed in IU. If there is no underlying bone disease, elevated levels of alkaline phosphatase activity usually indicate impaired biliary tract function or other forms of hepatic parenchymal disease such as hepatitis. The physical therapist is likely to see elderly patients with underlying bone disorders, such as Paget's disease, osteomalacia, metastatic cancer, and hip fracture, who may have elevations of the alkaline phosphatase originating from bone.

Total serum alkaline phosphatase in the elderly may be a valuable indicator of disease of bone. Age-related changes, therefore, are particularly important in the interpretation of values outside the traditional reference range. The fact that total serum alkaline phosphatase increases with aging by as much as 40% in women and 10% in men means that reference ranges for young adults cannot be used to interpret serum alkaline phosphatase levels in the elderly.[14] This is especially true in elderly women.

Total serum protein and serum albumin are two of the commonly encountered serum protein measurements. Albumin is quantitatively the most important serum protein synthesized by the liver. Serum levels are influenced by a variety of factors including nutritional status, hormonal factors, and liver function. Most of the time, depressed serum albumin levels reflect synthetic liver problems. Nephrotic syndrome may deplete serum albumin by a combination of protein loss through the kidneys and inadequate compensatory hepatic synthesis. Albumin concentration falls in most chronic diseases. A patient confined to bed may also demonstrate lower albumin levels than when ambulatory. Low albumin levels clinically may lead to edema.

In the normal resting state the concentration of plasma proteins is maintained reasonably constant by the balance between synthesis and catabolism. These plasma proteins collectively form a circulating store of amino acids, maintain colloid osmotic pressure, act as transport for a variety of substances, and represent one of the body's buffering systems. The actual laboratory test measuring total protein historically has been divided into albumin and total globulin. Albumin is measured first, and globulin is estimated by subtracting from the total protein. The different proteins making up the globulin fraction may be individually quantitated with modern analytic techniques. In addition to albumin, other serum proteins include fibrinogen, other clotting proteins, transferrin (iron-carrying protein), and the immunoglobulins. Elevations of the latter may result in an increased serum total protein in chronic infections, autoimmune diseases, malignant conditions, and liver disease.

The changes in serum albumin and total protein with aging are also consistent across studies. Thus serum albumin concentrations decrease with age in both men and women.[2, 4, 9, 18] The difference between the established reference range and that in the elderly is usually between 7% and 10%.[18] In one study of 11,090 hospitalized medical patients ranging in age from less than 40 to more than 80 years, the mean serum albumin concentration fell significantly from 3.97 to 3.58 g/100 mL.[4] Despite the fall in serum albumin with aging, the total protein remains the same because there is a complementary rise in the globulin fraction of total protein measurements.

Amino acids, the basic components of the above proteins, also form polypeptide hormones. An example of a commonly encountered hormone is thyroid hormone, which consists of iodinated amino acids. The thyroid gland synthesizes and secretes two forms of the hormone referred to as thyroxine (T_4) and triiodothyronine (T_3). Thyroxine is the main form of the hormone produced by the thyroid, whereas only about one fifth of the daily requirement for T_3 is secreted by the thyroid. The remainder of the T_3 is derived from the peripheral conversion of T_4 to T_3. These hormones influence the growth and maturation of tissues, total energy expenditure, and the turnover of essentially all substrates, vitamins, and hormones, including the thyroid hormones themselves.

Disease processes that result in an underproduction of thyroid hormone lead to an insidious onset of lethargy, constipation, cold intolerance, stiffness and cramping of the muscles, carpal tunnel syndrome, slowing of intellectual and motor activity, appetite loss, and weight increase. Profound decreases in thyroid hormone production can be life threatening.

Disease processes that result in an overproduction of thyroid hormone produce symptoms of nervousness, emotional lability, insomnia, tremors, palpitations, tachycardia, frequent bowel movements, excessive sweating, and heat intolerance. Weight loss may occur, and loss of strength is often manifested by a weakness in proximal leg muscles resulting in difficulty climbing stairs or rising from chairs. In older subjects cardiovascular and myopathic symptoms predominate, although "apathetic" hyperthyroidism may also occur in the elderly. In such patients, there are a paucity of symptoms despite laboratory evidence of excessive thyroid production.

A detailed description of the laboratory evaluation of thyroid function is beyond the scope of this chapter. However, several basic laboratory tests may be encountered by the physical therapist. Four common tests are the T_4 level, the T_3 level, the T_3 resin uptake, and the thyroid-stimulating hormone (TSH) level. The T_4 and T_3 concentrations can be measured with a highly specific and sensitive radioimmunoassay. Alteration in the intensity of hormone binding by plasma proteins can influence the concentration of hormone in the blood. Thus, the measurement of free hormone levels is more reflective of the metabolic state than is measurement of total hormone concentrations, which also reflect carrier protein concentrations. However, when the free hormone levels are not measured directly, a test called the T_3 resin uptake may be performed to provide information about the most common carrier protein (thyroid-binding globulin). Multiplying the total T_4 level by the T_3 resin uptake yields the free thyroxine index. This index is high in hyperthyroidism and low in hypothyroidism.

In addition to the above tests of thyroid function, the TSH is commonly measured using a radioimmunoassay when thyroid disease is suspected. TSH is produced by the pituitary gland in response to the circulating levels of thyroid hormone. Low values of TSH generally indicate an overproduction of thyroid hormone, whereas high values of TSH reflect underproduction of hormone by the thyroid gland.

Thyroid function tests in the aged are required whenever the diagnosis of thyroid dysfunction is suspected since classical clinical symptoms may be absent. One of the most common tests of thyroid function is the T_4 level. Serum T_4 levels in the elderly have been reported as being unchanged, reduced, or increased.[1] One of the explanations for the disagreement between studies is the possibility that thyroxine-binding globulin (TBG), the main binding protein for T_4, may vary with clinically inapparent disease in old age. To account for this possibility, as mentioned above, the T_3 resin uptake test is performed to assess TBG indirectly. By multiplying the T_4 by the T_3 resin uptake, the free thyroxine index is produced. This index does not appear to change in any clinically significant way with normal aging.

Direct measurements of T_3 by radioimmunoassay reveal that this form of thyroid hormone decreases by between 10% and 50% with aging.[17] The reason for this decrease is probably a decrease in the peripheral conversion of T_4 to T_3. Thus, standard reference ranges for the direct measurement of T_3 cannot be used for assessment of this hormone in the elderly since mild hyperthyroidism caused by excess T_3 would remain undiagnosed.

The final thyroid function test commonly measured in the elderly is the TSH level. Although some studies of TSH levels with aging have found no age-related changes, the Baltimore longitudinal study on aging found serum TSH levels to be 38% higher in elderly men.[5] However, in another study the prevalence of elevated TSH in persons aged 60 to 89 was 5.9%, and was more common in women than men. When mean TSH levels in 20 to 59-year-olds were xcompared with those in persons over age 59, there were no differences, but a greater proportion of the older group had TSH levels greater than 10 $\mu U/mL$.[17] Approximately half of those with clearly elevated TSH levels were found to have low T_4 levels indicative of hypothyroidism.[19]

Urinalysis

Analysis of the urine historically has been included in the basic laboratory assessment of a patient. With the advent of the urine dipstick, the microscopic examination of the urinary sediment has become limited to those situations where dipstick abnormalities are detected or when renal disease is suspected. Current dipsticks are capable of measuring qualitative aspects of the urine. A complete review of this topic is available elsewhere.[10] For the physical therapist designing rehabilitation programs for the elderly, some familiarity with the basic testing is sufficient.

Dipsticks contain small pads impregnated with substances capable of detecting various components of the urine. The dipstick changes color in the presence of such components. Thus, the dipstick can detect the presence of glucose or protein (not normal findings), as well as blood. Two relatively new dipstick pads include leukocyte esterase and nitrite, used to predict the presence of urinary tract infection. The former measures an enzyme found in white blood cells that are commonly present in the urine during an infection. The latter detects the presence of nitrite, a substance produced from dietary nitrate in the presence of certain bacterial infections of the urine. If either of these two pads are "positive," a urine culture is commonly obtained to test for the presence of infection.

Several age-related changes in urine dipstick tests may be recognized. First, changes in the kidney with aging affect the older person's ability to maximally concentrate the urine. The specific gravity pad on the urine dipstick provides an approximation of urine concentration (higher specific gravity correlating with higher concentration). The inability to maximally concentrate the urine would not be clinically significant unless water loss was severe, or thirst was not intact. In fact, in most elderly, thirst is blunted. If dehydration occurs, the urine specific gravity increase may not be commensurate with the degree of dehydration, as it would be in a younger person.

With aging, the ability of the kidney to retain glucose is reduced because of the loss of nephrons, despite the fact that the renal glucose threshold (plasma glucose level at which urine glucose is present) is actually increased. In essence, the effect of nephron loss exceeds that of the increased threshold such that glucose in the urine occurs more commonly in nondiabetic older persons than it does in younger individuals.

Since asymptomatic bacteriuria is not uncommon in older women, the urinalysis may demonstrate a positive leukocyte test or nitrite test. However, if the incontinent patient has a positive test for leukocytes or nitrite, a urine culture is ordinarily performed to determine whether or not the urine is infected. Changes in the tissue lining the female urethra occur in elderly women who are not taking replacement estrogens and may cause mild degrees of positivity on the leukocyte test.

Radiographic Tests

The chest radiograph is the most commonly encountered X ray in clinical practice and may be available to the physical therapist designing rehabilitation programs in the elderly. Findings on the chest X ray may have implications for the therapist, requiring some fundamental understanding of common abnormalities.

The chest film contains information about the skeleton, soft tissues, heart, and lungs. The complete chest radiographic examination includes the anteroposterior (AP) film (indicating the direction of the X-ray beam) and the lateral film. When the patient is properly penetrated by the X-ray beam, and when the patient is correctly positioned, a chest radiograph may be of sufficient quality to provide information on all the above components.

The skeletal elements included in the chest X ray are the vertebrae, clavicles, scapulae, ribs, glenohumeral joint, and the proximal humeri. All skeletal elements on the chest X ray are ordinarily checked for signs of fracture. In addition, the vertebral column is examined for curvature. Osteopenia (loss of radio-opacity of the bone) often can be seen on lateral views of the spine. The spine and glenohumeral joint should be inspected for degenerative changes of arthritis (calcifications, loss of joint space). Calcified bursae or tendons may be evident in the region of the shoulder. Soft tissue findings are less common.

The heart and lungs are often the main focus of the chest X ray since they occupy the greatest portion of the film. The heart lies in the center of the chest cavity. The left side of the heart shadow from superior to inferior outlines the aortic knob, the left pulmonary artery, the left atrium, and the apex of the ventricle. The lung parenchyma appears as two radiolucent areas on either side of the heart. The lung parenchyma appears slightly radiodense due to vessels and connective tissue.

The chest radiograph may demonstrate several age-related changes. The vertebrae may appear osteopenic because of osteoporosis, osteomalacia, or both. Degenerative changes of the spine may appear as spurs at the corners of the vertebral bodies seen on the lateral chest X ray. Symptomatic or asymptomatic vertebral compression fractures are common in older women, sometimes resulting in an exaggeration of the normal thoracic kyphosis.

The heart shadow may look different in an older person. For example, the aortic knob that appears just to the left of the top portion of the cardiac silhouette may contain calcium that appears as a dense ring. The aorta itself may be tortuous, appearing as a separate shadow to the left of the heart shadow. Calcified coronary vessels and valve rings may sometimes be seen in the heart. As the prevalence of hypertension and other heart disease increases with aging, the size of the heart is more likely to be larger than it is in younger persons.

With aging, certain lung findings may be more common on the chest X ray. First, exposure to asbestos may eventually result in calcified diaphragmatic plaques that appear as dense lines at the inferior portion of the lungs. Over many years, smokers may develop large radiolucent lungs with flattened diaphragms. Calcified lesions in the lung indicate old infection with tuberculosis, healing of an old injury, or a malignancy. The increased prevalence of heart disease, pulmonary infections, and malignancies makes it more common to see patchy lung densities called infiltrates.

Electrocardiogram

A great deal of information is available from the electrocardiogram (ECG), and with newer computer technology, readings are often provided on the tracing for all health care providers. A complete guide to the interpretation of ECG findings is beyond the scope of this chapter, but some basic interpretive skills may be useful to the physical therapist designing a rehabilitation program for an elderly patient. Some of the basic elements of the ECG will be briefly reviewed, including rate rhythm and wave configuration.

The basic waveforms of the ECG are the P wave (indicative of atrial depolarization), the QRS complex (representing depolarization of the ventricles through the His-Purkinje conductive system), and the T wave (indicative of repolarization). The U wave, a small wave of low voltage, is sometimes seen following the T wave. A typical sequence is illustrated in Figure 11–1. Intrinsic diseases of the heart or other systems may alter the regular sequence of waveforms. This can lead to the absence of certain waves, prolongation of the intervals between waves, widening of waves, and changes in the polarity of the waves (above or below the isoelectric horizontal baseline).

The heart rate can be easily derived from the distance between QRS complexes (see Fig 11–1). Since the interval represented by one large box on the ECG paper is 0.2

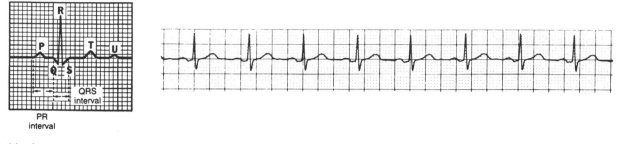

FIG 11–1.
Normal rhythm strip with P wave (atrial depolarization), QRS complex (ventricular depolarization), and the T wave (repolarization). (Adapted from Mammen BA: Basic electrocardiography, in Irwin S, Tecklin JS: *Cardiopulmonary Physical Therapy,* ed 2, St Louis, Mosby–Year Book, 1990.)

ms, heartbeats occurring on every large box line represent a rate of 300 beats/sec. Heartbeats occurring every other large box line signify a rate of 150 beats/sec; every third large box line, 100 beats/sec; and so on. Once the rate has been determined, the rhythm is next assessed. If every P wave is followed by a QRS complex, the rhythm is usually termed *normal sinus,* since the electrical activity is starting in an area of the atrium called the *sinus node* and is progressing down the conduction system to produce the QRS complex followed by the T wave. Many types of irregular rhythms can be identified. Occasional premature beats (Fig 11–2) must be distinguished from a consistently chaotic rhythm (Fig 11–3).

Related to the rate and rhythm are the intervals between the waves. The PR interval is the distance between the beginning of the P wave and the beginning of the QRS wave. The QRS duration is the distance from the beginning of the QRS complex to the end of the complex. The QT interval is the distance from the beginning of the QRS complex to the end of the T wave. These intervals vary in different diseases or metabolic disturbances, but each interval has a normal range. The PR interval is normally 0.21 seconds or less, the QRS duration is normally 0.08 seconds or less, and the QT interval varies with rate.

Having examined the above features of the ECG, attention is then focused on whether there are any signs of ischemia. Thus, a depression of the ST segment (the baseline between the end of the QRS complex and the begin-

ning of the T wave), an elevation of the ST segment, or the inversion of a T wave (position opposite the direction of the QRS complex) can indicate ischemia (Fig 11–4). Knowing these basic interpretive findings can be a useful screen for the presence of cardiovascular disease that may alter the therapist's treatment regimen.

Many physiologic changes that occur with aging may be reflected in the ECG. The conduction system of the aged heart undergoes histologic changes including an increase in fibrous and adipose tissue as well as degenerative calcification. The intrinsic sinus node rate decreases with age, but the heart rate can still increase with exercise. Nevertheless, the maximum heart rate that is achieved during exercise decreases with age. All these changes may lead to a slowing of the rate seen on ECG or a lengthening of the interval between atrial (P wave) and ventricular contraction (QRS complex). In addition to slowing of the rate, there is an increased incidence of ectopic activity (extra heartbeats) in the aging heart. The incidence of exercise-induced ventricular ectopy increases with age in otherwise healthy individuals.

Certain diseases of the cardiovascular system that are more common with aging can produce other ECG changes. For example, hypertensive heart disease may lead to an enlargement of the heart that is reflected in an increased height of the QRS complex (Fig 11–5) or a change in the appearance and polarity of the T wave (Fig 11–4). As mentioned above, ischemic changes appear as alterations of the ST segment (Fig 11–4).

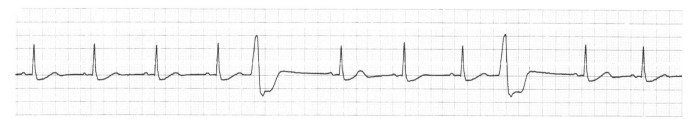

FIG 11–2.
Premature beats.

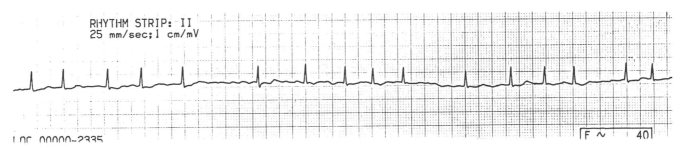

RHYTHM STRIP: II
25 mm/sec; 1 cm/mV

LnC 00000-2335   F ~ 40

FIG 11–3.
Chaotic irregular rhythm of atrial fibrillation.

CONSIDERATIONS FOR PHYSICAL THERAPISTS

From the above discussion, one can recognize that the laboratory assessment of the elderly is relevant to the design of rehabilitation programs. Relying on the history and examination may fail to identify abnormalities that might impede an effective program. This is because the elderly usually accept symptoms as being part of the aging process, rather than volunteering a complaint. There also may be cognitive deficits that prevent the communication of such symptoms to the therapist. The physician may not appreciate the effect of laboratory abnormalities on a therapist's program. In fact, the majority of physicians may have little understanding of physical therapy activities.

Reviewing the common laboratory values discussed above can provide insights into disease processes that may affect the rehabilitation program. To interpret these laboratory abnormalities, one must have an understanding of expected age-related changes that make traditional laboratory reference ranges derived from young health populations less useful. For example, since the alkaline phosphatase increases with age, the traditional reference range is not useful for interpreting results in older individuals, especially women. Similarly, by knowing that the age-related changes in albumin may affect the total calcium level, the therapist can interpret lower calcium levels in older persons. Low albumin and total protein levels, themselves, may indicate nutritional deficiencies that will influence successful participation in the rehabilitation program.

The tests reviewed in this chapter were chosen to be both representative and pertinent to the physical therapist's role. Thus, a review of the CBC may uncover important abnormalities that have the potential to impact on the rehabilitation program. Anemia may cause a decrease in stamina, limiting activity and requiring that the therapist modify tasks for the patient. Changes in mental status can be exacerbated by anemia in older patients who have marginal cognitive reserve. Changes in the normal white blood count are unlikely to affect the rehabilitation program, but low platelet counts may increase the tendency to bleed with minor trauma.

Muscular function can be affected by changes in the serum potassium, calcium, magnesium, or even thyroid hormone. Significant changes in the alkaline phosphatase may indicate bone pathology that has relevance to rehabilitation. For example, the alkaline phosphatase may be elevated in a patient with osteomalacia. This metabolic bone disease is characterized by deficiency in vitamin D and can predispose to fracture. The therapist who is aware of this possibility can recognize the need for adequate nutritional support during the rehabilitation process. On the other hand, alkaline phosphatase is commonly elevated following a fracture and hip repair as osteoblasts begin to make new bone matrix. The interpretation of these laboratory tests requires some familiarity with the normal reference

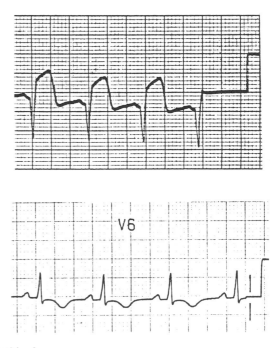

FIG 11–4.
Elevation of the ST segment and inversion of the T wave, suggesting ischemia.

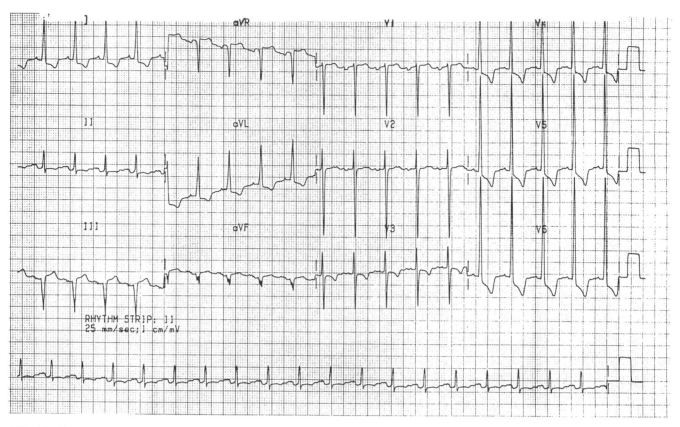

FIG 11–5.
Left ventricular hypertrophy with strain. This pattern is characterized by very tall R waves and deeply inverted T waves.

range for age, as well as some of the causes of abnormal values.

A basic familiarity with the ECG and chest X ray permits the therapist to approach the geriatric patient with a greater understanding of underlying disease processes that will influence rehabilitation. Thus, a patient with signs of ischemia (ST segment depression or elevation), with left ventricular hypertrophy, with atrial fibrillation, or with frequent disturbances in the normal rhythm may have less stamina or may develop chest pain or palpitations with exercise. The therapist can anticipate such events and alter the program appropriately. Similarly, a chest X ray with infiltrates or a large cardiac silhouette will indicate the potential for limitations in exercise capacity.

SUMMARY

The physical therapist planning rehabilitation programs for elderly patients must include the laboratory data in the initial assessment because the history and physical examination may not adequately reveal factors influencing an individual's capacity for such programs. Often the referring physician fails to appreciate the impact of these abnormal laboratory tests as they relate to physical therapy. Since the reference ranges for many laboratory tests change with age, and since the results of laboratory tests are often given with reference ranges obtained from young normals, the therapist must interpret laboratory test results against this background. This chapter has outlined expected age-related changes in several commonly encountered laboratory tests and has discussed the implications of the laboratory assessment in the planning and implementation of rehabilitation programs for the elderly.

REFERENCES

1. Denham MJ, Himsworth RL: Thyroid function tests, in Hodkinson MH (ed): *Clinical Biochemistry of the Elderly.* Edinburgh, Churchill Livingstone, 1984.
2. Dybkaer R, Lauritzen M, Krakauer R: Relative reference values for clinical chemical and haematological quantities in "healthy" elderly people. *Acta Med Scand* 1981; 209:1–9.
3. Garry PJ, Goodwin JS, Hunt WC: Iron status and anemia in the elderly: New findings and a review of previous studies. *J Am Geriatr Soc* 1983; 31:389–399.
4. Greenblatt DJ: Reduced serum albumin concentration in the elderly: A report from the Boston Collaborative Drug Surveillance Program. *J Am Geriatr Soc* 1979; 27:20–22.

5. Harman SM, Whemann RE, Blackman MR: Pituitary-thyroid hormone economy in health aging men: Basal indices of thyroid function and thyrotropin responses to constant infusions of thyrotropin releasing hormone. *J Clin Endocrinol Metab* 1984; 58:320–326.

6. Hodkinson MH: Basics of biochemical investigation of the elderly, in Hodkinson MH (ed): *Clinical Biochemistry of the Elderly*. Edinburgh, Churchill Livingstone, 1984.

7. Hodkinson MH: Calcium, phosphate and the investigation of metabolic bone disease, in Hodkinson MH (ed): *Clinical Biochemistry of the Elderly*. Edinburgh, Churchill Livingstone, 1984.

8. Jackson RA: Blood sugar and diabetes, in Hodkinson MH (ed): *Clinical Biochemistry of the Elderly*. Edinburgh, Churchill Livingstone, 1984.

9. Keating FR, Jones JD, Elveback LR, et al: The relation of age and sex to distribution of values in healthy adults of serum calcium, inorganic phosphorus, magnesium, alkaline phosphatase, total proteins, albumin, and blood urea. *J Lab Clin Med* 1969; 73:825–834.

10. Kiel DP: The urinalysis: A critical appraisal. *Med Clin North Am* 1987; 71:607–624.

11. Morgan KJ, Stampley GL, Zabik ME, et al: Magnesium and calcium dietary intakes of the US population. *J Am Coll Nutr* 1985; 4:195–206.

12. National Diabetes Data Group: Classification and diagnosis of diabetes mellitus and other categories of glucose intolerance. *Diabetes* 1979; 28:1039–1057.

13. Rochman H: Calcium and bone, in Rochman H (ed): *Clinical Pathology in the Elderly: A textbook of Laboratory Interpretations*. Basel, Karger, 1988.

14. Rochman H: Enzymes, in Rochman H (ed): *Clinical Pathology in the Elderly: A Textbook of Laboratory Interpretations*. Basel, Karger, 1988.

15. Rochman H: Glucose tolerance and diabetes mellitus, in Rochman H (ed): *Clinical Pathology in the Elderly: A Textbook of Laboratory Interpretations*. Basel, Karger, 1988.

16. Rochman H: Hematology, in Rochman H (ed): *Clinical Pathology in the Elderly: A Textbook of Laboratory Interpretations*. Basel, Karger, 1988.

17. Rochman H: Thyroid, in Rochman H (ed): *Clinical Pathology in the Elderly: A Textbook of Laboratory Interpretations*. Basel, Karger, 1988.

18. Rochman H: Total protein and albumin, in Rochman H (ed): *Clinical Pathology in the Elderly: A Textbook of Laboratory Interpretations*. Basel, Karger, 1988.

19. Sawin CT, Chopra D, Azizi F, et al: The aging thyroid increased prevalence of elevated serum thyrotropin levels in the elderly. *JAMA* 1979; 242:247–250.

Geriatric Pharmacology

Charles D. Ciccone, Ph.D., P.T.

INTRODUCTION

Physical therapists working with any patient population must be aware of the drug regimen used in each patient. Therapists must have a basic understanding of the beneficial and adverse effects of each medication and must be cognizant of how specific drugs can interact with various rehabilitation procedures. This seems especially true for geriatric patients receiving physical therapy. The elderly are generally more sensitive to the adverse effects of drug therapy, and many adverse drug reactions impede the patient's progress and ability to participate in rehabilitation procedures. An adequate understanding of the patient's drug regimen, however, can help physical therapists recognize and deal with these adverse effects as well as enable therapists to capitalize on the beneficial effects of drug therapy in their geriatric patients.

The purpose of this chapter is to discuss some of the pertinent aspects of geriatric pharmacology with specific emphasis on how drug therapy can affect older individuals receiving physical therapy. This chapter will begin by describing the pharmacologic profile of the geriatric patient, with emphasis on why adverse drug reactions tend to occur more frequently in the elderly. Specific adverse drug reactions that commonly occur in the elderly will then be discussed. Finally, the beneficial and adverse effects of specific medications will be examined along with how these medications can have an impact on the rehabilitation of the older adult.

PHARMACOLOGIC PROFILE OF THE GERIATRIC PATIENT

As a group, the elderly appear to be more susceptible to the toxic side effects of drug therapy. In general, the elderly are two to three times more likely to experience an adverse drug reaction.[47, 52, 78] The increased incidence of adverse drug effects in the elderly appears to be caused by two principal factors: the pattern of drug use that occurs in a geriatric population and the altered response to drug therapy in the elderly.[23, 117] A number of other contributing factors such as multiple disease states, lack of proper drug testing, and problems with drug education and compliance also increase the likelihood of adverse effects in older adults. The influence of each of these factors on drug response in the elderly is briefly discussed here.

Pattern of Drug Use in the Elderly: Problems of Polypharmacy

Although adults over age 65 currently compose 12% of the US population, they consume over 25% of all drugs.[119] By the year 2030, it is predicted that the elderly will account for 21% of the population and consume 40% of all drugs.[3] Hence, the elderly consume a disproportionately large amount of drugs relative to other age-groups.

A logical explanation for this disproportionate drug use is that the elderly take more drugs because they suffer more illnesses. Indeed, upward of 80% of individuals over age 65 suffer from one or more chronic conditions.[83, 104] Drug therapy is often the primary method used to treat many of the conditions typically seen in the elderly. Although it is difficult to determine precisely the extent of drug use in the elderly, it is clear that the use of prescription drugs is highest in individuals age 65 and older.[17, 53, 104] Use of nonprescription or over-the-counter products is also an important factor in geriatric pharmacology, especially in the community-dwelling elderly who have greater access to these products.

Hence, the elderly rely heavily on various prescription and nonprescription products, and medications are often essential in helping resolve or alleviate some of the illnesses and other medical complications that commonly occur in the elderly. A distinction must be made, however, between the reasonable and appropriate use of drugs and the phenomenon of *polypharmacy*. Polypharmacy is the excessive and unnecessary use of medications that can result in a geriatric patient[1] receiving large numbers of drugs that are unnecessary or even harmful.[104]

Polypharmacy can be distinguished from a more reasonable drug regimen by the criteria listed in Table 12–1. Of these criteria, the use of drugs to treat adverse drug reactions is especially important. The administration of drugs to treat adverse drug reactions often creates a vicious cycle where additional drugs are used to treat adverse drug reactions, thus creating more adverse effects, thereby initiating the use of more drugs, and so on (Fig 12–1). This

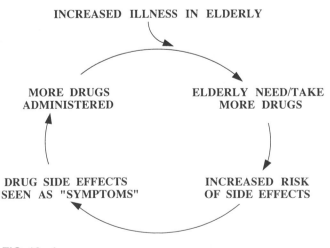

FIG 12–1.
Vicious cycle of drug administration that can lead to polypharmacy in the elderly.

TABLE 12–1.

Characteristics of Polypharmacy in the Elderly*

Characteristic	Example
1. Use of medications for no apparent reason	Digoxin use in patients who do not exhibit heart failure
2. Use of duplicate medications	Simultaneous use of two or three laxatives
3. Concurrent use of interacting medications	Simultaneous use of a laxative and an antidiarrheal agent
4. Use of contraindicated medications	Use of beta-blockers in congestive heart failure
5. Use of inappropriate dosage	Failure to use a lower dose of a benzodiazepine sedative-hypnotic in the older adult
6. Use of drug therapy to treat adverse drug reactions	Use of antacids to treat aspirin-induced gastric irritation
7. Patient improves when medications are discontinued	Withdrawal of a sedative-hypnotic results in clearer sensorium

*Adapted from Simonson W: *Medications and the Elderly: A Guide for Promoting Proper Use.* Rockville, Md, Aspen Publications, 1984.

cycle can rapidly accelerate until the patient is receiving a dozen or more medications.

In addition to the risk of creating the vicious cycle seen in Figure 12–1, there are several other obvious drawbacks to polypharmacy in the elderly. Since each drug will inevitably produce some side effects when used alone, the number of side effects will begin to accumulate when several agents are used concurrently. More important, the interaction of one drug with another (drug-drug interaction) increases the risk of an untoward reaction because of the ability of one agent to modify the effects and metabolism of another drug. If many drugs are administered simultaneously, the risk of adverse drug reactions increases exponentially.[13] Other negative aspects of polypharmacy are the risk of decreased patient compliance with the drug regimen and the increased financial burden of using large numbers of unnecessary drugs.

Polypharmacy can occur in the elderly for a number of reasons. In particular, physicians may rely on drug therapy to accomplish goals that could be achieved through nonpharmacologic methods. That is, it is often relatively easy to prescribe a medication to resolve a problem in the older adult even though other methods that do not require drugs could be used. For instance, the patient that has napped throughout the day will probably not be sleepy at bedtime. It is much easier to administer a sedative-hypnotic agent at bedtime rather than institute activities that keep the patient awake during the day and allow nocturnal sleep to occur naturally.

In some cases, the patient may also play a contributing role toward polypharmacy. Patients may obtain prescriptions from several different practitioners, thus accumulating a formidable list of prescription medications. Elderly individuals may receive medications from friends and family members who want to "share" the benefits of

their prescription drugs. Some older adults may also use over-the-counter and self-help remedies to such an extent that these agents interact with one another and with their prescription medications.

Polypharmacy can be prevented if the patient's drug regimen is reviewed periodically and any unnecessary or harmful drugs are discontinued. Also, new medications should only be administered if a thorough patient evaluation indicates that the drug is truly needed in that patient. When several physicians are dealing with the same patient, these practitioners should make sure that they communicate with one another regarding the patient's drug regimen. Physical therapists can play a role in preventing polypharmacy by recognizing any changes in the patient's response to drug therapy and helping to correctly identify these changes as drug reactions rather than disease "symptoms." In this way, therapists may help prevent the formation of the vicious cycle illustrated in Figure 12–1.

Altered Response to Drugs

There is little doubt that the response to many drugs is affected by age and that the therapeutic and toxic effects of any medication will be different in an older adult vs. a younger individual. Alterations in drug response in the elderly can be attributed to differences in the way the body handles the drug (pharmacokinetic changes) as well as differences in the way the drug affects the body (pharmacodynamic changes).[117] The effects of aging on drug pharmacokinetics and pharmacodynamics are discussed briefly here.

Pharmacokinetic Changes

Pharmacokinetics is the study of how the body handles a drug, including how the drug is absorbed, distributed, metabolized, and excreted. Several changes in physiologic function occur as a result of aging that alter pharmacokinetic parameters in the elderly. The principal pharmacokinetic changes associated with aging are summarized in Figure 12–2 and are briefly discussed here. The effects of aging on pharmacokinetics has been the subject of fairly extensive research, and the reader is referred to several excellent reviews for more information on this topic.[19, 22, 65, 116, 117]

Drug Absorption.—Several well-documented changes occur in gastrointestinal (GI) function in the older adult that could potentially affect the way drugs are absorbed from the GI tract. Such changes include decreased gastric acid production, decreased gastric emptying, decreased GI blood flow, diminished area of the absorptive surface, and decreased intestinal motility.[19, 27, 116] The effect of these changes on drug absorption, however, is often inconsistent. That is, aging does not appear to significantly alter the absorption of most orally administered drugs. This may be due in part to the fact that the changes listed above may offset one another. For instance, factors that tend to decrease absorption (decreased GI blood flow, decreased

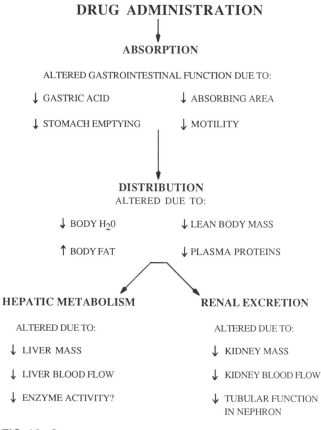

FIG 12–2.
Summary of the physiologic effects of aging that may alter pharmacokinetics in the elderly.

absorptive surface area) could be counterbalanced by factors that allow the drug to remain in the gut for longer periods (decreased GI motility), thus allowing more time for absorption. Hence, altered drug absorption does not appear to be a major factor in determining pharmacokinetic changes in the elderly.

Drug Distribution.—After a drug is absorbed into the body, it undergoes distribution to various tissues and body fluid compartments (vascular system, intracellular fluid, etc.). Drug distribution may be altered in the elderly due to several physiologic changes such as decreased total body water, decreased lean body mass, increased percent body fat, and decreased plasma protein concentrations.[116] Depending on the specific drug, these changes can affect how the drug is distributed in the body, thus potentially changing the response to the drug. For instance, drugs that bind to plasma proteins (aspirin, warfarin) may produce a greater response since there will be less drug bound to plasma proteins and more of the drug will be free to reach its target tissue. Drugs that are soluble in water (alcohol, morphine) will be relatively more concentrated in the body since there is less body water in which to dissolve the drug. Increased percentages of body fat can act as a reservoir for lipid-soluble drugs, and problems related to drug storage may occur with these agents. Hence, these potential problems in drug distribution must be anticipated, and dosages must be adjusted accordingly in elderly individuals.

Drug Metabolism.—The principal role of drug metabolism (biotransformation) is to inactivate drugs and create water-soluble by-products (metabolites) that can be excreted by the kidneys. Although some degree of drug metabolism can occur in tissues throughout the body, the liver is the primary site for metabolism of most medications. Several distinct changes in liver function occur with aging that affect hepatic drug metabolism. The total drug-metabolizing capacity of the liver decreases with age primarily because of reductions in liver mass and hepatic blood flow.[63, 68, 123, 124] Animal studies have also suggested that intrinsic activity of hepatic drug-metabolizing enzymes may decrease as a function of aging, but additional research is needed to document these findings in humans.[123] In any event, drugs that undergo inactivation in the liver will remain active for longer periods of time because of the general decrease in the hepatic metabolizing capacity seen in older adults.

Drug Excretion.—The kidneys are the primary route for drug excretion from the body. Drugs reach the kidney in either their active form or as a drug metabolite following biotransformation in the liver. In either case, it is the kidney's responsibility to filter the drug from the circulation and excrete it from the body via the urine. With aging, declines in renal blood flow, renal mass, and function of renal tubules result in a reduced ability of the kidneys to excrete drugs and their metabolites.[22, 64, 65, 116] These changes in renal function tend to be one of the most important factors affecting drug pharmacokinetics in the elderly, and reduced renal function should be taken into account whenever drugs are prescribed to these individuals.[56]

The cumulative effect of the pharmacokinetic changes associated with aging is that drugs are often allowed to remain active for longer periods of time, thus prolonging drug effects and increasing the risk for toxic side effects. This is evidenced by the fact that drug half-life (the time required to eliminate 50% of the drug remaining in the body) is often substantially longer in an older individual vs. younger adult.[13] For example, the half-life of certain medications such as the benzodiazepines (Valium, Librium) can be increased as much as fourfold in the elderly.[38] Obviously, this represents a dramatic change in the way the elderly body deals with certain pharmacologic agents. Altered pharmacokinetics in the elderly must be anticipated by evaluating changes in body composition (decreased body water, increased percentages of body fat) and monitoring changes in organ function (decreased hepatic and renal function) so that drug dosages can be adjusted and adverse drug reactions minimized in elderly individuals.[74, 122]

Finally, it should be noted that the age-related pharmacokinetic changes described here vary considerably from person to person within the geriatric population. These changes are, however, considered part of the "normal" aging process. Any disease or illness that affects drug distribution, metabolism, or excretion will cause an additional change in pharmacokinetic variables, thus further increasing the risk of adverse drug reactions in the elderly.

Pharmacodynamic Changes

Pharmacodynamics is the study of how drugs affect the body, including systemic drug effects as well as cellular and biochemical mechanisms of drug action. Changes in the control of different physiologic systems can influence the systemic response to various drugs in the elderly.[110, 116] For instance, deficits in the homeostatic control of circulation (decreased baroreceptor sensitivity, decreased vascular compliance) may change the response of the elderly patient to cardiovascular medications. Other age-related changes such as impaired postural control, decreased visceral muscle function, altered thermoregulatory responses, and declines in cognitive ability can alter the

pharmacotherapeutic response as well as the potential side effects that may occur when various agents are administered to the older adult.[110] The degree to which systemic drug response is altered will vary depending on the magnitude of these physiologic changes in each individual.

In addition to these systemic changes, the way a drug affects tissues on a cellular level may be different in the older adult. Most drugs exert their effects by first binding to a receptor that is located on or within the specific "target" cells that are influenced by each type of drug. This receptor is usually coupled in some way to the biochemical "machinery" of the target cell, so that when the drug binds to the receptor, a biochemical event occurs that changes cell function in a predictable way (Fig 12–3). For instance, binding of epinephrine (adrenaline) to beta-1-receptors on myocardial cells causes an increase in the activity of certain intracellular enzymes, which in turn causes an increase in heart rate and contractile force. Similar mechanisms can be described for other drugs and their respective cellular receptors. The altered response to certain drugs seen in the elderly may be caused by one or more of the cellular changes depicted in Figure 12–3. For instance, alterations in the drug-receptor attraction (affinity) could help explain an increase or decrease in the sensitivity of the older adult to various medications.[6, 54, 101, 110] Likewise, changes in the way the receptor is linked or coupled to the cell's internal biochemistry have been noted in certain tissues as a function of aging.[39, 81] Finally, the ac-

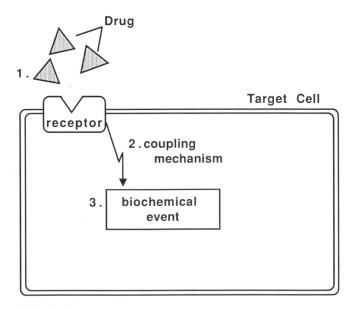

FIG 12–3.
Potential sites for altered cellular responses in the elderly. Changes may occur: (1) in drug-receptor affinity, (2) in the coupling of the receptor to an intracellular biochemical event, and (3) in the cell's ability to generate a specific biochemical response.

tual biochemical response within the cell may be blunted because of changes in cellular structure and function that occur with aging.[50, 110]

To date, many of the studies on cellular pharmacodynamic changes have been performed on animal models of aging. Hence, the significance of these changes in drug-receptor interactions is not fully understood for most medications used in elderly humans. Continued research in this area should begin to clarify how drug responses may be altered because of the age-related pharmacodynamic changes that occur on the cellular level in human tissues.

Consequently, pharmacodynamics may be altered in the elderly due to systemic physiologic changes acting in combination with changes in drug responsiveness that occur on a cellular or even subcellular level. These pharmacodynamic changes along with the pharmacokinetic changes discussed earlier help explain why the response of a geriatric individual to drug therapy will often differ from the analogous response in a younger individual.

Other Factors That Increase the Risk of Adverse Drug Reactions in the Elderly

In addition to the pattern of drug use and the altered response to drugs seen in the elderly, several other factors may also contribute to the increased incidence of adverse drug reactions seen in these individuals. Several of these additional factors are presented here.

Presence of Multiple Disease States
The fact that the elderly often suffer from several chronic conditions greatly increases the risk of adverse drug reactions. The presence of more than one disease often necessitates the use of several drugs, thus increasing the risk of drug-drug interactions. Even more important is the fact that various diseases and illnesses usually alter the pharmacokinetic and pharmacodynamic variables discussed earlier. For instance, the age-related changes in hepatic metabolism and renal excretion of drugs will be affected to an even greater extent if liver or kidney disease is present. Many elderly patients suffer from diseases that further decrease function in both of these organs as well as cause diminished function in other physiologic systems. The involvement of several organ systems, combined with the presence of several different drugs, makes the chance of an adverse drug reaction almost inevitable in the elderly patient with multiple disease states.

Lack of Proper Drug Testing
The Food and Drug Administration (FDA) is responsible for monitoring the safety and efficacy of all drugs marketed in the United States. The FDA requires all drugs to undergo extensive preclinical (animal) and clinical (human) trials before receiving approval. With regard to the elderly, some question has been raised about the evaluation of drugs specifically in geriatric individuals prior to FDA approval. It has been recognized that an adequate number of patients over age 65 should be included at various stages of the clinical testing, especially for drugs that are targeted for problems that occur in the elderly (e.g., Parkinson's disease and dementia).[3] It is unclear, however, if efforts to increase drug testing in geriatric subjects has been successful in providing improved information about drug safety in older adults.[1] Additional efforts on the part of the FDA and the drug-manufacturing companies may be necessary to help reduce the risk of adverse side effects through better drug testing.

Problems With Patient Education and Self-Adherence to Drug Therapy
Problems with patient education and self-adherence to drug therapy may result in an increased incidence of adverse side effects, especially if drugs are taken in excessive doses or for the wrong reason. Even the most appropriate and well-planned drug regimen will be useless if the drugs are not taken as directed. There can be, however, a number of factors that limit the ability of the older adult to understand and follow instructions regarding drug therapy. A decline in cognitive function in some older adults may impair their ability to understand instructions given by the physician, nurse practitioner, or pharmacist. This can hamper the ability of the geriatric patient to take drugs according to the proper dosing schedule, especially if several different medications are being administered, with a different dosing schedule for each medication. Other factors such as poor eyesight may limit the older person's ability to distinguish one pill from another, and arthritic changes may make it difficult to open certain "child-proof" containers.

The older adult may also stop taking a medication because of an annoying but unavoidable side effect. For instance, the elderly patient with hypertension may refuse to take a diuretic because this particular medication increases urinary output and may necessitate several trips to the bathroom in the middle of the night. To encourage patient self-adherence, it must be realized that these annoying side effects are not trivial and can represent a major source of concern to the patient. Hence, health care professionals should not dismiss these complaints but should make an extra effort to help the patient understand the importance of adhering to the drug regimen whenever such unavoidable side effects are present.

Additional Factors
Other factors including poor diet, excessive use of over-the-counter products, cigarette smoking, and consumption

of various other substances (caffeine, alcohol) may help contribute to the increased risk of adverse drug effects in the elderly.[5, 14, 98] These factors must be taken into consideration when implementing a prescription drug program for the elderly individual. For instance, it must be realized that the older adult with a protein-deficient diet may have extremely low plasma protein levels, thus further altering drug pharmacokinetics and increasing the risk of an adverse drug effect. Hence, it is important to consider all aspects of the life-style and environment of the older adult that may affect drug therapy in these individuals.

COMMON ADVERSE DRUG REACTIONS IN THE ELDERLY

An *adverse drug reaction* (ADR) is any unwanted and potentially harmful effect caused by a drug when the drug is given at the recommended dosage.[104] Listed here are some of the more common ADRs that may occur in older adults. Of course, this is not a complete list of all the potential ADRs, but these are some of the responses that physical therapists should be aware of when dealing with geriatric patients in a rehabilitation setting.

Sedation

The elderly seem especially susceptible to drowsiness and sleepiness as a side effect of many medications. In particular, drugs that produce sedation as a primary effect (sedative-hypnotics) as well as drugs with sedative side effects (narcotic analgesics, antipsychotics, others) will often produce excessive drowsiness in older adults.

Confusion

Various degrees of confusion ranging from mild disorientation to delirium may occur with a number of medications such as antidepressants, narcotic analgesics, and drugs with anticholinergic activity. Confusion can also indicate that certain drugs such as lithium and digoxin are accumulating and reaching toxic levels in the body. Elderly individuals who are already somewhat confused may be more susceptible to drugs that tend to further increase confusion.

Depression

Symptoms of depression (e.g. intense sadness and apathy, as described elsewhere in this text) may be induced in older adults by certain medications. Drugs such as barbiturates, antipsychotics, alcohol, and several antihypertensive agents (clonidine, reserpine, propranolol) have been implicated in producing depression as an ADR in the elderly.[10]

Orthostatic Hypotension

Orthostatic (postural) hypotension is described as a 20 mm Hg or greater decline in diastolic blood pressure that occurs when an individual assumes a more upright posture (e.g., moving from lying to sitting or sitting to standing). Owing to the fact that many older adults are relatively sedentary and have diminished cardiovascular function, these individuals tend to be more susceptible to episodes of orthostatic hypotension even without the influence of drug therapy.[51] A number of medications, however, augment the incidence and severity of this blood pressure decline. In particular, drugs that tend to lower blood pressure (antihypertensives, antianginal medications, others) tend to be a frequent cause of orthostatic hypotension in older adults. Orthostatic hypotension often leads to dizziness and syncope because blood pressure is too low to provide adequate cerebral perfusion and oxygen delivery to the brain. Hence, orthostatic hypotension may precipitate falls and subsequent injury (hip fractures, other trauma) in elderly individuals. Since elderly patients will be especially susceptible to episodes of orthostatic hypotension during certain rehabilitation procedures (gait training, functional activities), physical therapists should be especially alert for this ADR.

Fatigue and Weakness

Strength loss and muscular weakness may occur for a number of reasons in response to drug therapy. Some agents such as the skeletal muscle relaxants may directly decrease muscle contraction strength, whereas other drugs such as the diuretics may affect muscle strength by altering fluid and electrolyte balance. Elderly individuals who are already debilitated will be more susceptible to strength loss as an ADR.

Dizziness

Drug-induced dizziness can be especially detrimental in older adults because of the increased risk of loss of balance and falling. Problems with dizziness result from drugs that produce sedation or from agents that directly affect vestibular function. Examples of such agents include sedatives, antipsychotics, narcotic analgesics, and antihistamine drugs.[90, 115] Dizziness may also occur secondary to drugs that cause orthostatic hypotension (see above). Drug-induced dizziness may be especially prevalent in older adults who already exhibit balance problems, and physical therapists should be especially alert for this ADR in these individuals.

Anticholinergic Effects

Acetylcholine is an important neurotransmitter that controls function in the central nervous system and also affects peripheral organs such as the heart, lungs, and GI tract. A number of drugs exhibit anticholinergic side effects, meaning that these agents tend to diminish the response of various tissues to acetylcholine. In particular, antihistamines, antidepressants, and certain antipsychotics tend to exhibit anticholinergic side effects. Since acetylcholine affects several diverse physiologic systems throughout the body, drugs with anticholinergic effects are associated with a wide range of ADRs. Drugs with anticholinergic effects may produce central nervous system effects such as confusion, nervousness, drowsiness, and dizziness. Peripheral anticholinergic effects include dry mouth, constipation, urinary retention, tachycardia, and blurred vision. The elderly seem to be more sensitive to anticholinergic effects, possibly due to the fact that acetylcholine influence has already started to diminish as a result of the aging process. In any event, physical therapists should be aware that a rather diverse array of potentially serious ADRs may arise from drugs with anticholinergic properties.

Extrapyramidal Symptoms

Drugs that produce side effects that mimic extrapyramidal tract lesions are said to exhibit extrapyramidal symptoms. Such symptoms include tardive dyskinesia, pseudoparkinsonism, akathisia, and other dystonias. Antipsychotic medications are frequently associated with an increased risk of extrapyramidal symptoms. The problem of extrapyramidal symptoms as an antipsychotic ADR will be presented in more detail later in this chapter.

DRUG CLASSES COMMONLY USED IN THE ELDERLY: IMPACT ON PHYSICAL THERAPY

This section will provide a brief overview of drug therapy in the elderly. Included are some of the more common groups of drugs that are prescribed to older adults. For each group, the principal clinical indication or indications are listed along with a brief description of the mechanism of action of each type of drug. The primary adverse effects and any specific concerns for physical therapy in elderly patients receiving these drugs are also discussed. Examples of typical drugs found in each of the major groups are

indicated in several tables in this section. For additional information about specific agents listed here, the reader can refer to one of the sources listed at the end of this chapter.[18, 35, 88]

Psychotropic Medications

Psychotropic drugs include a variety of agents that affect mood, behavior, and other aspects of mental function. As a group, the elderly exhibit a high incidence of psychiatric disorders.[114] Hence, psychotropic drugs are frequently used in elderly individuals and are also associated with a high incidence of adverse effects that can have an impact on rehabilitation. The major groups of psychotropics are listed in Table 12–2, and pertinent aspects of each group are discussed here.

Sedative-Hypnotic and Antianxiety Agents

Sedative-hypnotic drugs are used to relax the patient and promote a relatively normal state of sleep. Antianxiety drugs are chemically similar to the sedative-hypnotics, but they are intended to decrease anxiety without producing excessive sedation. Insomnia and disordered sleep may occur in elderly individuals concomitant to normal aging or in response to medical problems and life-style changes that occur with advanced age.[37] Likewise, illness and other aspects of aging may result in increased feelings of fear and apprehension in older adults. Hence, use of sedative-hypnotic and antianxiety drugs will be encountered frequently in the elderly.

The primary group of agents used to promote sleep or decrease anxiety in the elderly is the benzodiazepines[48] (Table 12–2). Benzodiazepines are currently regarded as the principal sedative-hypnotic and anxiolytic drugs since they are somewhat safer and more effective than other agents such as the barbiturates and meprobamate (Miltown).[49] Benzodiazepines appear to exert their beneficial effects by increasing the central inhibitory effect of the neurotransmitter gamma-aminobutyric acid (GABA).[111] This increase in GABA-mediated inhibition seems to account for the decreased anxiety and increased sleepiness associated with these drugs.

Despite the relative safety of currently used agents, several problems still occur when benzodiazepines are used in the elderly. For instance, residual or "hangover" effects may occur, producing drowsiness and sluggishness the morning after a sedative-hypnotic is used. Addiction may also occur if these drugs are used indiscriminately for long periods. Also, a "rebound effect" may occur, where insomnia or anxiety increases when the drug is discontinued. Physical therapists should be especially aware of the residual effects of sedative-hypnotic drugs when scheduling elderly patients for rehabilitation first thing in the

TABLE 12–2.

Psychotropic Drug Groups

Group	Common Examples	
	Generic Name	Trade Name
Sedative-hypnotic agents		
Benzodiazepines	Flurazepam	Dalamane
	Temazepam	Restoril
	Triazolam	Halcion
Barbiturates	Pentobarbital	Nembutal
	Secobarbital	Seconal
Antianxiety agents		
Benzodiazepines	Chlordiazepoxide	Librium
	Diazepam	Valium
	Lorazepam	Ativan
Antidepressants		
Tricyclics	Amitryptyline	Elavil
	Imipramine	Tofranil
MAO* inhibitors	Isocarboxazid	Marplan
	Phenelzine	Nardil
Sympathomimetics	Dextroamphetamine	Dexedrine, others
Second-generation	Amoxapine	Asendin
agents	Maprotiline	Ludiomil
Antipsychotics		
Phenothiazines	Chlorpromazine	Thorazine
	Thioridazine	Mellaril
Thioxanthenes	Chlorprothixene	Taractan
	Thiothixene	Navane
Butyrophenones	Haloperidol	Haldol

*MAO = monoamine oxidase.

morning. Therapists should also realize that the use of antianxiety drugs in elderly patients is a two-edged sword. Decreased anxiety may enable the patient to be more relaxed and cooperative during rehabilitation, but any benefits will be negated if the patient experiences significant sedation and is unable to remain alert throughout the therapy session.

Antidepressants

In addition to being the most common form of mental illness in the general population, depression is the mental disorder most frequently observed in the elderly.[41] Feelings of intense sadness, hopelessness, and other symptoms may occur in the elderly following a specific event (loss of a spouse, acute illness) or in response to the gradual decline in health and functional status often associated with aging. Drug therapy may be instituted to help resolve these symptoms, along with other nonpharmacologic methods such as counseling and behavioral therapy.

There are several distinct groups of antidepressant medications known as the tricyclics, monoamine oxidase (MAO) inhibitors, sympathomimetics, and the newer "second-generation" drugs (see Table 12–2). Tricyclic antidepressants are often the drugs of choice in the elderly, although certain second-generation drugs such as mapro-

tiline (Ludiomil) may be more effective in some older patients.[40, 99] All antidepressant drugs share a common goal, which is to increase synaptic transmission in central neural pathways that use amine neurotransmitters such as norepinephrine. The rationale is that symptoms of depression are due to hypersensitivity of central amine receptors, and drugs that bring about overstimulation of these receptors will cause a compensatory decrease (down regulation) in the number of functioning receptors.[45] As receptor sensitivity stabilizes, the clinical symptoms of depression appear to be resolved.

Antidepressant use in the elderly may result in side effects such as sedation, lethargy, and muscle weakness. Certain antidepressants tend to have anticholinergic effects and may produce dry mouth, constipation, urinary retention, and confusion. Orthostatic hypotension may occur with the tricyclics, especially during the first few days after drug therapy is initiated. Physical therapists should be aware that antidepressants may help improve the patient's mood and increase the patient's interest in physical therapy. Certain side effects, however, such as sedation and confusion may impair the patient's cognitive ability and make it difficult for some elderly patients to participate actively in rehabilitation procedures.

Manic-Depression: Lithium Treatment

As the name implies, manic-depression is a form of mental illness characterized by mood swings from an excited, hyperactive state (mania) to periods of apathy and dysphoria (depression). Although the cause of manic-depression is unknown, this condition responds fairly well to the drug lithium. It is not exactly clear how lithium prevents episodes of manic-depression, but this drug may prevent the excitable or manic phase of this disorder, thus stabilizing disposition and preventing the mood swings characteristic of this disease.[103]

It is important to be aware of the use of lithium in treating elderly patients with manic-depression since this drug can rapidly accumulate to toxic levels in these individuals. Lithium is an element and cannot be degraded in the body to an inactive form. Hence, the body must rely solely on renal excretion to eliminate this drug. Since renal function is reduced in the elderly, the elimination of this drug is often impaired. Accumulation of lithium beyond a certain level results in lithium toxicity.[42] Symptoms of mild lithium toxicity include a metallic taste in the mouth, fine hand tremor, nausea, and muscular weakness and fatigue. These symptoms increase as toxicity reaches moderate levels, and other central nervous system (CNS) signs such as blurred vision and incoordination may appear. Severe lithium toxicity causes impaired consciousness that can lead to coma and even death.

Hence, physical therapists working with elderly patients who are taking lithium must continually be alert for any signs of lithium toxicity. This is especially important if there is any change in the patient's health or activity level that might cause an additional compromise in lithium excretion.

Antipsychotics

Antipsychotic medications are often used to help normalize behavior in older adults. *Psychosis* is the term used to describe the more severe forms of mental illness that are characterized by marked thought disturbances and altered perceptions of reality. Aggressive, disordered behavior may also accompany symptoms of psychosis. In the elderly, psychotic-like behavior may occur because of actual psychotic syndromes (schizophrenia, severe paranoid disorders) or may be associated with various forms of dementia.[120] In any event, antipsychotic drugs may be helpful in improving behavior and compliance in elderly patients.

There are several major chemical classifications of antipsychotic drugs (see Table 12–2). These drugs all share a common mechanism in that they impair synaptic transmission in central dopamine pathways.[30] It is theorized that psychosis may be due to increased central dopamine influence. Antipsychotic drugs are believed to reduce this dopaminergic influence, thus helping to decrease psychotic-like behavior.

Antipsychotic drugs are associated with several annoying but fairly minor side effects such as sedation and anticholinergic effects (dry mouth, constipation, etc.). Orthostatic hypotension may also occur, especially within the first few days after initiating drug treatment. A more serious concern with antipsychotic drugs is the possibility of extrapyramidal side effects. As discussed earlier in this chapter, motor symptoms that mimic lesions in the extrapyramidal tracts are a frequent ADR associated with these medications. For instance, patients may exhibit involuntary movements of the face, jaw, and extremities (tardive dyskinesia), symptoms that resemble Parkinson's disease (pseudoparkinsonism), extreme restlessness (akathisia), or other problems with involuntary muscle movements (dystonias). Early recognition of these extrapyramidal signs is important since they may persist long after the antipsychotic drug is discontinued, or these signs may even remain permanently. This seems especially true for drug-induced tardive dyskinesia, which may be irreversible if antipsychotic drug therapy is not altered when these symptoms first appear.

The use of antipsychotic drugs may have beneficial effects on rehabilitation outcomes since patients may become more cooperative and less combative during physical therapy. Therapists should be especially alert for the onset of any extrapyramidal symptoms because of the potential that these symptoms may result in long-term or permanent motor side effects.

Treatment of Dementia

Dementia is a term used to describe a fairly global decline in intellectual function, with marked impairments in cognition, speech, personality, and other skills.[94] Some forms of dementia may be due to specific factors such as a metabolic-hormonal imbalance (e.g., thyroid disease) or an adverse reaction to certain drugs that have psychoactive side effects.[120] These so-called reversible dementias are often resolved if the precipitating factor is identified and corrected. Irreversible dementia is typically associated with progressive degenerative changes in cortical structure and function such as those occurring in Alzheimer's disease. Drug treatment of irreversible dementia is discussed briefly here.

In the past, certain drugs have been reported to improve intellectual function or prevent further loss of cognitive abilities in patients with senile dementia. In particular, drugs known as ergoloid mesylates have been used extensively in patients with Alzheimer's disease due to their supposed ability to increase the uptake and utilization of oxygen in cerebral tissues.[46] The best known drug of this type, Hydergine, had previously been reported to slow the decline of cognitive function in such patients.[34, 46, 106] More recently, however, it was suggested that Hydergine lacked any effect (either beneficial or harmful) in patients with Alzheimer's disease.[113] Hence, the value of this medication in improving or maintaining intellectual function in these patients remains uncertain.

Agents that increase acetylcholine function in the brain have been suggested as possibly improving mental function in patients with Alzheimer's disease. In particular, physostigmine is a drug that inhibits the cholinesterase enzyme, thus decreasing acetylcholine breakdown and prolonging the activity of this neurotransmitter in the brain. Some reports have suggested that physostigmine is associated with some improvement in mental function in patients with primary degenerative brain disease.[7, 73, 121] Some evidence also exists that lecithin, a precursor to acetylcholine, may also help improve mental function when used alone or in combination with physostigmine.[112] However, the magnitude of the beneficial effects of these agents has been only modest at best. Also, physostigmine is associated with a number of side effects including diarrhea, bradycardia, bronchoconstriction, and visual disturbances. Hence, the actual value of drugs that attempt to increase acetylcholine function in patients with dementia remains unclear.

Consequently, there do not appear to be any drugs that will conclusively improve or maintain intellectual function in patients with irreversible dementia. However, some of the other drugs already discussed in this chapter may be used to help normalize and control behavior in patient's with Alzheimer's disease and other forms of dementia. In particular, antipsychotic drugs may improve certain aspects of behavior, such as decreased hallucinations and diminished feelings of hostility and suspiciousness.[92] However, response to these drugs is highly variable, and beneficial results from these medications may be inconsistent in patients with irreversible dementia.

Neurologic Agents

In addition to the drugs that affect mood and behavior, there are specific agents that are important in controlling certain neurologic conditions in the elderly. Drug treatment of two of these conditions, Parkinson's disease and seizure disorders, is discussed here.

Drugs Used for Parkinson's Disease

Parkinson's disease is one of the more prevalent disorders in the elderly, with over 1% of the population over 60 years of age being afflicted. This disease is caused by the degeneration of dopamine-secreting neurons located in the basal ganglia.[108] Loss of dopaminergic influence initiates an imbalance in other neurotransmitters, including an increase in acetylcholine influence. This disruption in transmitter activity ultimately results in the typical parkinsonian motor symptoms of rigidity, bradykinesia, resting tremor, and postural instability.[75]

Drug treatment of Parkinson's disease usually focuses on restoring the balance of neurotransmitters in the basal ganglia.[93] The most common way of achieving this is to administer dihydroxyphenylalanine (dopa), which is the immediate precursor to dopamine. Dopamine itself will not cross the blood-brain barrier, meaning that dopamine will not move from the bloodstream into the brain, where it is ultimately needed. However, levodopa (the L-isomer of dopa) will pass easily from the bloodstream into the brain, where it can then be transformed into dopamine and restore the influence of this neurotransmitter in the basal ganglia.

Levodopa is often administered orally with a drug known as carbidopa. Carbidopa inhibits the enzyme that transforms levodopa to dopamine in the peripheral circulation, thus allowing levodopa to cross into the brain before it is finally converted to dopamine. If levodopa is converted to dopamine before reaching the brain, the dopamine will not be of any use in Parkinson's disease since it is now trapped in the peripheral circulation. The simultaneous use of carbidopa and levodopa allows smaller doses of levodopa to be administered, since less of the levodopa will be wasted due to premature conversion to dopamine in the periphery.

Several other agents can be used in combination with or instead of levodopa to help alleviate the motor symptoms associated with Parkinson's disease (Table 12–3).

TABLE 12–3.

Drugs Used in Neurologic Disorders

	Generic Name	Trade Name
Drugs used in parkinson's disease		
Dopamine precursors	Levodopa	Sinemet*
Anticholinergic drugs	Biperiden	Akineton
	Ethopropazine	Parsidol
	Procyclidine	Kemadrin
Others	Amantadine	Symmetrel
	Bromocriptine	Parlodel
	Selegiline	Eldepryl
Drugs used in seizure disorders		
Barbiturates	Metharbital	Gemonil
	Phenobarbital	Luminal
Benzodiazepines	Clonazepam	Clonopin
	Clorazepate	Tranxene
Hydantoins	Ethotoin	Peganone
	Mephenytoin	Mesantoin
	Phenytoin	Dilantin
Succinimides	Ethosuximide	Zarontin
	Methsuximide	Celontin
Others	Carbamazepine	Tegretol
	Valproic acid	Depakene

*Indicates trade name for levodopa combined with carbidopa, a peripheral decarboxylase inhibitor.

Drugs such as bromocriptine (Parlodel) mimic the effects of dopamine and can be used to replace the deficient neurotransmitter. Anticholinergic drugs (biperiden, ethopropazine) act to decrease acetylcholine influence in the brain and can attenuate the increased effects of acetylcholine that tend to occur when dopamine influence is diminished. Amantadine (Symmetrel) is actually an antiviral drug that also exerts antiparkinsonian effects, presumably by facilitating the release of dopamine from storage sites in the basal ganglia. Selegiline (Eldepryl) inhibits the enzyme that degrades dopamine, thus prolonging the effects of any dopamine that exists in the basal ganglia.

Levodopa and the other drugs used in Parkinson's disease are often associated with some troublesome side effects. In particular, levodopa may cause symptoms such as GI distress (nausea, vomiting) and cardiovascular problems (arrhythmias, orthostatic hypotension), especially for the first few days after drug therapy is initiated. Behavioral and mood changes (confusion, depression, anxiety) and problems with involuntary movements (dyskinesias) have also been noted in patients on levodopa therapy. One of the most frustrating problems associated with levodopa therapy is the tendency for the effectiveness of this drug to diminish after 3 or 4 years of continuous use. The reasons for this diminished response are not fully understood and may relate to the patient's developing some sort of tolerance to this medication. Other fluctuations in the response to levodopa have been noted with long-term use. These fluctuations include a spontaneous decrease in levodopa effectiveness in the middle of a dose interval (on-off phenomenon) or loss of drug effects toward the end of a dose cycle (end-of-dose akinesia). The reasons for these fluctuations are poorly understood but may be related to problems in the absorption and metabolism of levodopa.

Physical therapists working with patients with Parkinson's disease should attempt to coordinate rehabilitation sessions with the peak effects of drug therapy whenever possible. For instance, scheduling physical therapy when levodopa and other antiparkinsonian drugs reach peak effects (usually 1 hour after oral administration) will often maximize the patient's ability to actively participate in exercise programs and functional training.

Therapists should also be cognizant of the potential side effects of levodopa, including the tendency for responses to fluctuate or diminish with prolonged use. Physical therapists may also play an important role in documenting any decline or alteration in drug effectiveness while working closely with patients with Parkinson's disease.

Drugs Used to Control Seizures

Seizure disorders such as epilepsy are characterized by the sudden, uncontrolled firing of a group of cerebral neurons.[102] This uncontrolled neuronal excitation is manifested in various ways, depending on the location and extent of the neuronal involvement, and seizures are classified according to the motor and sensory symptoms that occur during a seizure. In the general population, the exact cause of the seizure disorder is often unknown. In the elderly, however, seizure activity may be attributed to a fairly well defined cause such as a previous CNS injury (stroke, trauma), tumor, or degenerative brain disease. If the cause cannot be treated by surgical or other means, pharmacologic management remains the primary method of preventing recurrent seizures.

The primary goal of antiseizure drugs is to normalize the excitation threshold in the group of hyperexcitable neurons that initiate the seizure.[66] Ideally this can be accomplished without suppressing the general excitation level within the brain. Several groups of chemically distinct antiseizure drugs are currently in use, and each group uses a different biochemical mechanism to selectively decrease excitability in the seizure-prone neurons (see Table 12–3). The selection of a particular antiseizure drug depends primarily on the type of seizure present in each patient.

Sedation is the most common side effect that physical therapists should be aware of when working with elderly patients on seizure medications. Other annoying effects that may occur include GI distress, headache, dizziness, incoordination, and dermatologic reactions (rashes, etc.). Physical therapists working closely with elderly patients may also help assess the effectiveness of the antiseizure

medications by monitoring and documenting the incidence of any seizures that occur during the rehabilitation session.

Treatment of Pain and Inflammation

Pharmacologic treatment of pain and inflammation is used in the elderly to help resolve symptoms of chronic conditions (rheumatoid and osteoarthritis) as well as acute problems resulting from trauma and surgery. Drugs used for analgesic and anti-inflammatory purposes include the narcotic analgesics, non-narcotic analgesics, and glucocorticoids (Table 12–4). These are discussed briefly here.

Narcotic Analgesics

Narcotic or "opioid" analgesics compose the group of drugs used to treat relatively severe, constant pain. These agents are frequently used to reduce pain in elderly patients following surgery or trauma, or in more chronic situations such as cancer. These agents vary in terms of their relative analgesic strength, with drugs such as morphine and meperidine (Demerol) having strong analgesic properties, and drugs like codeine having a more moderate ability to decrease pain. These drugs are believed to exert their beneficial effects by binding to opioid receptors that are lo-

TABLE 12–4.

Drugs Used to Treat Pain and Inflammation

Category	Common Examples	
	Generic Name	Trade Name
Narcotic analgesics	Codeine	Many trade names
	Meperidine	Demerol
	Morphine	Duramorph
	Oxycodone	Percodan
	Propoxyphene	Darvon
Non-narcotic analgesics		
NSAIDs	Aspirin	Many trade names
	Ibuprofen	Advil, Motrin, others
	Piroxicam	Feldene
	Sulindac	Clinoril
Acetaminophen	—	Tylenol, Panadol
Corticosteroids	Betamethasone	Celestone
	Cortisone	Cortone
	Hydrocortisone	Hydrocortone
	Prednisone	Deltasone
Disease-modifying drugs*		
Gold compounds	Auranofin	Ridaura
	Aurothioglucose	Solganal
	Gold sodium thiomalate	Myochrysine
Antimalarials	Chloroquine	Aralen
	Hydroxychloroquine	Palquenil
Others	Penicillamine	Cuprimine, Depen
	Methotrexate	Mexate
	Azathioprine	Imuran

*Drugs used to slow the progression of rheumatoid arthritis.
NSAIDs = nonsteroidal anti-inflammatory drugs.

cated in the brain and spinal cord and impairing synaptic transmission in pain-mediating pathways.[25, 125] Narcotic analgesics are often characterized by their ability to alter pain perception rather than completely eliminating painful sensations. This allows the patient to focus on other things rather than being continually preoccupied by the painful stimuli.

Physical therapists should be aware that the analgesic effects of narcotic drugs tend to be accompanied by many side effects that can influence the patient's participation in rehabilitation. Adverse side effects such as sedation, mood changes (euphoria or dysphoria), and GI problems (nausea, vomiting, constipation) are quite common. Orthostatic hypotension and respiratory depression are also frequent side effects, especially for the first few days after beginning narcotic analgesic therapy. Confusion may be a problem, particularly in older adults. Finally, aspects of drug addiction including tolerance (the need for increased dosages to achieve a given effect) and physical dependence (the onset of withdrawal symptoms when the drug is stopped) are always a concern when narcotic analgesics are used for prolonged periods.

Non-narcotic Analgesics

Treatment of mild to moderate pain is often accomplished by using two types of non-narcotic agents: nonsteroidal anti-inflammatory drugs (NSAIDs) and acetaminophen. NSAIDs compose a group of drugs that are therapeutically similar to aspirin (see Table 12–4). These aspirin-like drugs produce four therapeutic effects: analgesia, decreased inflammation, decreased fever (antipyresis), and decreased platelet aggregation (anticoagulant effects). Acetaminophen appears to have analgesic and antipyretic properties similar to the NSAIDs, but acetaminophen lacks any significant anti-inflammatory or anticoagulation effects. NSAIDs and acetaminophen appear to exert most, if not all, of their beneficial effects by inhibiting the synthesis of a group of compounds known as the prostaglandins. Prostaglandins are produced locally by many cells and are believed to be involved in mediating some aspects of pain and inflammation.[20, 58] Aspirin and other NSAIDs inhibit the enzyme that synthesizes prostaglandins in the central nervous system as well as peripheral tissues, thus diminishing the painful and inflammatory effects of these compounds throughout the body.[95, 118] Acetaminophen also appears to inhibit prostaglandin biosynthesis, but this inhibition may only occur in the central nervous system, thus accounting for the differences in acetaminophen and NSAID effects.[28]

NSAID use in elderly patients tends to be fairly safe when these drugs are used in moderate doses for short periods.[79, 97] The most common side effect is gastric irritation, and this effect is seen more frequently with some NSAIDs such as aspirin than with others. More serious problems involving renal and hepatic toxicity may occur, especially if higher doses are used for prolonged periods or in patients with pre-existing kidney or liver disease. Acetaminophen does not produce any appreciable gastric irritation and may be taken preferentially by elderly patients for that reason. It should be noted, however, that acetaminophen may actually be more toxic to the liver than the NSAIDs in certain patients. Other problems with non-narcotic analgesics that may occur in elderly patients include allergic reactions (skin rashes) and possible CNS toxicity (confusion, hearing problems). In particular, tinnitus (a ringing or buzzing sound in the ears) may develop with prolonged aspirin use, and this side effect may be especially annoying and distressing to many elderly patients.

Glucocorticoids

Glucocorticoids are steroidal agents produced by the adrenal cortex that have a number of physiologic effects including a potent ability to decrease inflammation.[44] Synthetic derivatives of endogenously produced glucocorticoids can be administered pharmacologically to capitalize on the powerful anti-inflammatory effects of these compounds. These agents are used in rheumatoid arthritis and a variety of other disorders that have an inflammatory component. The anti-inflammatory effects of glucocorticoids appear to be a combination of several factors including the ability of these drugs to suppress leukocytic infiltration and inhibit the production of pro-inflammatory substances such as prostaglandins and leukotrienes at the site of inflammation.[44, 59, 95]

The powerful anti-inflammatory effects of glucocorticoids must be balanced against the risk of several serious adverse effects. In particular, physical therapists should be aware that these drugs produce a general catabolic effect on supporting tissues throughout the body. Breakdown of bones, ligaments, tendons, skin, and muscle occurs following prolonged systemic administration of glucocorticoids. This breakdown can be especially devastating in the elderly patient who already has some degree of osteoporosis or muscle wasting. Glucocorticoids also produce other serious adverse effects including hypertension, peptic ulcer, aggravation of diabetes mellitus, glaucoma, increased risk of infection, and suppression of normal corticosteroid production by the adrenal cortex. Adrenocortical suppression can have devastating or even fatal results if the exogenous (drug) form of the glucocorticoid is suddenly withdrawn, since the body is temporarily incapable of synthesizing adequate amounts of these important compounds. Finally, it should be realized that glucocorticoids often treat a disease manifestation (inflammation) without resolving the underlying cause of the disease. For instance, the elderly patient with rheumatoid arthritis may appear quite healthy due to this "masking" effect of glucocorticosteroids, whereas other sequelae of this disease (bone erosion, joint destruction) continue to worsen.

Other Drugs Used in Inflammatory Disease: Disease-Modifying Agents

Since glucocorticoids and other anti-inflammatory drugs do not appear to slow the disease process in rheumatoid arthritis, efforts have been made to develop drugs that do in fact try to curb the progression of this disease. These so-called disease-modifying drugs include an assortment of agents with different chemical and pharmacodynamic properties[82] (see Table 12–4). In general, these agents have immunosuppressive effects that blunt the autoimmune response, which is believed to underlie rheumatic joint disease.[61] The use and effectiveness of various drugs in this category remain under investigation, but it seems that certain agents such as the gold compounds and methotrexate have been successful in arresting or even reversing some of the arthritic changes in certain patients with this disease. Future studies should provide more information about the beneficial as well as potential adverse effects of these disease-modifying drugs.[71]

Cardiovascular Drugs

Cardiovascular disease is one of the leading causes of morbidity and mortality in elderly individuals. Hence, various drugs are used to prevent and treat cardiovascular problems in older adults, and many of these medications can directly affect rehabilitation of the elderly. Some of the more common cardiovascular drugs are listed in Table 12–5 and are discussed briefly here.

Beta-adrenergic Blockers

Beta-adrenergic antagonists, or "beta-blockers," are so named because they bind to beta-1-receptors on the heart and block the effects of catecholamines (epinephrine, norepinephrine) on myocardial tissues. Since catecholamines normally accelerate cardiac function, beta-blockers cause a decrease in heart rate (negative chronotropic effect) and a decrease in the force of myocardial contraction (negative inotropic effect). Owing to their ability to slow heart rate and contractile force, these drugs have become a mainstay in managing a number of cardiovascular problems such as hypertension, angina pectoris, and cardiac arrhythmias.[33]

TABLE 12–5.

Cardiovascular Drugs

Drug Group	Primary Indications	Common Examples	
		Generic Name	Trade Name
Alpha-blockers	Hypertension	Phenoxybenzamine	Dibenzyline
		Prazosin	Minipress
Angiotensin-converting enzyme inhibitors	Hypertension	Captopril	Capoten
	CHF	Enalapril	Vasotec
Anticoagulants	Overactive clotting	Heparin	Liquaemin
		Warfarin	Coumadin
Beta-blockers	Hypertension	Atenolol	Tenormin
	Angina	Metoprolol	Lopressor
	Arrhythmias	Nadolol	Corgard
		Propranolol	Inderal
Calcium channel blockers	Hypertension	Diltiazem	Cardizem
	Angina	Nifedipine	Procardia
	Arrhythmias	Verapamil	Calan, Isoptin
Centrally acting sympatholytics	Hypertension	Clonidine	Catapres
		Methyldopa	Aldomet
Digitalis glycosides	CHF	Digoxin	Lanoxin
Diuretics	Hypertension	Chlorothiazide	Diuril
	CHF	Furosemide	Lasix
		Spironolactone	Aldactone
Drugs that prolong repolarization	Arrhythmias	Amiodarone	Cordarone
		Bretylium	Bretylol
Organic nitrates	Angina	Nitroglycerin	Nitrostat, others
Presynaptic adrenergic depletors	Hypertension	Guanethidine	Ismelin
		Reserpine	Serpalan, others
Sodium channel blockers	Arrhythmias	Quinidine	Cardioquin, others
		Lidocaine	Xylocaine, others
Vasodilators	Hypertension	Hydralazine	Apresoline
		Minoxidil	Loniten

CHF = congestive heart failure.

Although beta-blockers are fairly well tolerated in younger adults, elderly individuals tend to be more susceptible to the side effects of these agents. In particular, CNS side effects including depression, lethargy, and sleep disorders are seen more often in older adults.[55] Other problems with beta-blockers occur because of the tendency of these drugs to attenuate cardiac pumping ability. For instance, heart rate will be lower at any given exercise workload in a patient taking beta-blockers. Orthostatic hypotension may occur due to the decreased ability of the heart to redistribute vascular fluid following a change in posture. Naturally, these cardiac effects will be exaggerated in the elderly patient with pre-existing cardiovascular problems or decreased cardiac function secondary to prolonged inactivity. Physical therapists working with the elderly should recall that beta-blockers will limit the cardiac response to exercise and postural changes, and some rehabilitation procedures (ambulation activities, various exercise regimens) may have to be changed accordingly.

Diuretics

Diuretic agents act on the kidneys to increase the excretion of water and sodium. This effectively decreases the amount of fluid in the vascular system, thus decreasing cardiac workload (i.e., the heart does not have to work as hard since there is less fluid to pump). Diuretics are classified according to their chemical structure (thiazides) or according to their mechanism of action (loop and potassium-sparing agents). Diuretic agents are used primarily in the treatment of hypertension and congestive heart failure.

The major problems with diuretics are associated with the tendency of these drugs to cause fluid volume depletion and electrolyte imbalances such as low blood sodium (hyponatremia) and low blood potassium (hypokalemia).[12, 29] This can be particularly harmful in the elderly patient with pre-existing volume depletion or hypokalemia due to poor diet.[76] Problems with fluid and electrolyte balance are often manifested through central symptoms (confusion, mood change) and peripheral problems involving skeletal muscle (weakness, fatigue). Orthostatic hypotension may also result due to inadequate intravascular fluid being available for redistribution on standing. Physical therapists working with the elderly can play an important role in recognizing these drug-related changes in function and alerting the medical staff of a potential problem in diuretic therapy.

Organic Nitrates

Organic nitrates such as nitroglycerin are used to prevent episodes of angina pectoris.[2] Angina typically occurs when myocardial oxygen demand exceeds myocardial oxygen supply. Nitroglycerin decreases myocardial oxygen demand by vasodilating the peripheral vasculature.[86] Peripheral vasodilation causes a decrease in the amount of blood returning to the heart (cardiac preload) as well as the amount of pressure in the vascular system that the heart must pump against (cardiac afterload).[2] Consequently, cardiac workload and oxygen demand are temporarily reduced, thus allowing the anginal attack to subside.

Nitrates are usually administered transdermally or by placing the drug under the tongue (sublingually). Oral administration of nitrates is not usually the preferred method of administration, since these drugs undergo extensive degradation in the liver when absorbed directly from the gastrointestinal tract. Patients who take nitrates sublingually at the onset of an anginal attack must be sure to bring their medications with them to physical therapy. This will allow the patient to self-administer the nitrate in case an attack of angina occurs during the rehabilitation session.

The primary adverse effects that may affect physical therapy are related to the peripheral vasodilatory effects of the nitrates. Blood pressure may fall in patients taking nitroglycerin, and dizziness due to hypotension is a common problem. Likewise, orthostatic hypotension may occur if the patient stands suddenly. Headache may also occur due to vasodilation of meningeal vessels. These side effects are most common immediately after the patient takes a rapid-acting sublingual dose. Hence, therapists should be especially concerned about hypotensive effects from the first minutes to an hour after a patient self-administers a sublingual dose of nitrates.

Antiarrhythmic Drugs

Disturbances in cardiac rhythm—that is, a heart rate that is too slow, too fast, or irregular—may occur in the elderly for various reasons. A variety of different drugs can be used to stabilize heart rate and normalize cardiac rhythm, and these agents are grouped into four categories.[8] Sodium channel blockers (lidocaine, quinidine) control myocardial excitability by stabilizing the opening and closing of membrane sodium channels. Beta-blockers (metoprolol, propranolol) normalize heart rate by blocking the effects of cardioacceleratory substances such as norepinephrine and epinephrine. Drugs that prolong cardiac repolarization (bretylium) stabilize heart rate by prolonging the refractory period of cardiac action potentials. Calcium channel blockers (diltiazem, verapamil) decrease myocardial excitability and conduction of action potentials by limiting the entry of calcium into cardiac muscle cells.

Although different antiarrhythmic drugs have various side effects, the most common adverse reaction is an increased risk of cardiac arrhythmias. That is, drugs used to treat one type of arrhythmia may inadvertently cause a different type of rhythm disturbance. Physical therapists should be alert for changes in cardiac rhythm by monitoring heart rate in elderly patients taking antiarrhythmic drugs.

Geriatric Hypertension

An increase in blood pressure is commonly observed in the elderly, and this increase is believed to be due to changes in cardiovascular function (decreased compliance of vascular tissues, decreased baroreceptor sensitivity) and diminished renal function (decreased ability to excrete water and sodium) that normally occur with aging.[4] A mild increase in blood pressure may not necessarily be harmful in the older adult and may in fact have a protective effect in maintaining adequate blood flow to the brain and other organs.[60, 105] However, blood pressure values above certain levels (e.g., systolic and diastolic values greater than 180 mm Hg and 100 mm Hg, respectively) are treated in elderly patients in order to reduce the risk of mortality and morbidity due to cardiovascular complications.[80, 84, 89, 107] The goal of antihypertensive therapy is not to reduce blood pressure in the older adult to levels equivalent to those seen in normotensive young adults who have systolic and diastolic values of 120 mm Hg and 80 mm Hg, respectively. Rather, target values of 160 mm Hg systolic and 90 mm Hg diastolic are recommended as much more realistic and safer goals in treating geriatric hypertension.[80, 89]

Fortunately, a large and diverse array of antihypertensive agents is available for treating geriatric patients with hypertension (see Table 12–5). Diuretic agents (discussed earlier) reduce blood pressure by diminishing the volume of fluid in the vascular system. Sympatholytic agents (beta-blockers, alpha-blockers, etc.) work in various ways to interrupt sympathetic stimulation of the heart and peripheral vasculature. Vasodilators reduce peripheral vascular resistance by directly relaxing vascular smooth muscle. Angiotensin-converting enzyme (ACE) inhibitors block the formation of angiotensin II, a potent vasoconstrictor. Finally, calcium channel blockers inhibit the entry of calcium into cardiac muscle cells and vascular smooth muscle cells, thus reducing contractility in these tissues.

Which antihypertensive agent or agents will be used in a given geriatric patient depends on several factors such as the magnitude of the hypertension and any other medical problems existing in that patient. Often, a "stepped-care" approach is used, where one drug is used initially, and other drugs are added sequentially until blood pressure is adequately reduced.[69] In the past, a diuretic was often the first drug used in the older adult, but more recent evidence has suggested that calcium channel blockers may be a more appropriate first choice, since they may be safer and more effective in managing geriatric hypertension.[11, 16, 26] In any event, a successful antihypertensive drug regimen is usually designed specifically for each patient and incorporates the "low-and-slow" philosophy of starting with low doses of each drug and slowly increasing dosages as needed.

The various drugs that could be used to manage hypertension are all associated with specific side effects. A common concern, however, is that blood pressure will be reduced pharmacologically to the point where symptoms of hypotension become a problem. Therapists should always be aware that dizziness and syncope may occur due to low blood pressure when the patient is stationary and especially when the patient stands (orthostatic hypotension). Also, any physical therapy intervention that causes an additional decrease in blood pressure should be used very cautiously in geriatric patients taking antihypertensive drugs. Treatments such as systemic heat (large whirlpool, Hubbard tank) and exercise using large muscle groups may cause peripheral vasodilation that acts synergistically with the antihypertensive drugs to produce a profound and potentially serious decrease in blood pressure.

Treatment of Congestive Heart Failure

Congestive heart failure is a common disorder in older adults characterized by a progressive decline in cardiac pumping ability.[70, 91] As the pumping ability of the heart diminishes, fluid often collects in the lungs and extremities (hence the term *congestive* heart failure). The most commonly used drugs in this disorder are the diuretics, ACE inhibitors, and digitalis glycosides.[70] Diuretics are used to relieve the strain on the failing heart by reducing vascular fluid volume. ACE inhibitors reduce peripheral vascular tone, thus decreasing the pressure the heart must pump against. The digitalis glycosides such as digoxin cause an increase in myocardial pumping ability by a complex biochemical mechanism that increases the calcium concentration in myocardial cells.[77]

The adverse effects of diuretics and ACE inhibitors were discussed earlier in this chapter. These agents are relatively safe when used in elderly patients compared with the third group, the digitalis glycosides. Digoxin and similar drugs often accumulate rapidly in the blood of an elderly patient, resulting in digitalis toxicity. Digitalis toxicity is characterized by gastrointestinal symptoms (nausea, vomiting, diarrhea), CNS disturbances (confusion, blurred vision, sedation), and cardiac arrhythmias. Arrhythmias can be quite severe and may result in cardiac fatalities if digitalis toxicity is not quickly rectified.[43] Physical therapists should be alert for signs of digitalis toxicity since early recognition is essential in preventing the more serious and potentially fatal side effects of these drugs.

Coagulation Disorders

Excessive hemostasis, or a tendency for the blood to clot too rapidly, is a common and serious problem in the older adult.[109] Formation of blood clots may result in thrombophlebitis and thromboembolism. These problems are especially important in the older patient following surgery and prolonged bed rest. The use of two anticoagulants, heparin and warfarin, is a mainstay in preventing excessive hemostasis. These agents work by different mechanisms to prolong and normalize the clotting time of the blood.[9, 85] Heparin must be administered parenterally, usually by intravenous injection, whereas warfarin can be taken orally. Typically, heparin is used initially to achieve a rapid decrease in blood clotting, followed by long-term management of excessive coagulation through oral warfarin administration.

The most common problem with anticoagulant drug therapy is an increased tendency for hemorrhage. Use of heparin and warfarin can result in too much of a delay in blood clotting, so that excessive bleeding occurs. Physical therapists should be cautious when dealing with open wounds or procedures that potentially induce tissue trauma (chest percussion, vigorous massage) because of the increased risk for hemorrhage.

Respiratory and Gastrointestinal Drugs

Drugs Used in Respiratory Disorders

Older adults may take drugs to treat fairly simple respiratory conditions associated with the common cold and seasonal allergies. Such drugs include cough medications (antitussives), decongestants, antihistamines, and drugs that help loosen and raise respiratory secretions (mucolytics and expectorants). Drugs may also be taken for more chronic, serious problems such as chronic obstructive pulmonary disease (COPD) and bronchial asthma. Drug therapy for asthma and COPD includes bronchodilators such as beta-adrenergic agonists (albuterol, epinephrine), xanthine derivatives (aminophylline theophylline), and anticholinergic drugs (atropine, ipratropium). Corticosteroids may also be given to treat inflammation in the respiratory tracts that is often present in these chronic respiratory problems.

These respiratory drugs are associated with various side effects that may affect physical therapy of the older adult. In particular, the elderly may be more susceptible to sedative side effects of drugs such as antihistamines and cough suppressants. For some of the prescription medications, side effects are often reduced if the medication can be applied directly to the respiratory tissues by inhalation.[24] For instance, even corticosteroids can be used fairly safely in the elderly if these drugs are inhaled rather than administered orally and distributed into the systemic circulation. If medications are administered systemically, however, lower doses of the prescription bronchodilators may be necessary in older adults. This is especially true in the elderly patient with reduced liver or kidney function, since metabolism and elimination of the active form of the drug will be impaired. Finally, some elderly patients may use excessive amounts of certain over-the-counter products. Physical therapists should question the extent to which their geriatric clients routinely take large doses of cough suppressants, antihistamines, and other over-the-counter respiratory drugs.

Drugs Used in Gastrointestinal Disorders

Gastrointestinal drugs such as antacids and laxatives are among the most frequently used medications in the elderly. Antacids typically consist of a base that neutralizes hydrochloric acid, thus helping to alleviate stomach discomfort caused by excess gastric acid secretion. These agents are often obtained as over-the-counter products. Prescription agents such as cimetidine (Tagamet) may also be used to decrease gastric acid secretion by blocking certain histamine receptors (H_2 receptors) that are located in the gastric mucosa. Laxatives stimulate bowel evacuation and defecation by a number of different methods, depending on the drug used. Drugs used to treat diarrhea are also used frequently in elderly patients. These drugs consist of agents such as opiate derivatives, which help decrease GI motility, and products such as the adsorbents, which help sequester toxins and irritants in the GI tract that may cause diarrhea.

The major concern for GI drug use in the elderly is the potential for inappropriate and excessive use of these agents. Many of these drugs are readily available as over-the-counter products. Elderly individuals may self-administer these agents to the extent that normal GI activity is compromised. For instance, the older person who relies on daily laxative use (or possibly even several laxatives per day) may experience a decline in the normal regulation of bowel evacuation. Drugs may also be used as a substitute for proper eating habits. Antacids may be taken routinely to disguise the irritant effects of certain foods that are not tolerated well by the older adult. Hence, physical therapists can often advise their geriatric patients that most GI drugs are meant to be used only for brief episodes of GI discomfort. Therapists can discourage the long-term use of such agents and advise their patients that proper nutrition and eating habits are a much safer and healthier alternative than prolonged use of GI drugs.

Hormonal Agents

General Strategy: Use of Hormones as Replacement Therapy

The endocrine glands synthesize and release hormones that travel through the blood to regulate the physiologic function of various tissues and organs. If hormonal production is interrupted, natural or synthetic versions of these hormones can be administered pharmacologically to restore and maintain normal endocrine function. This replacement therapy is commonly used in the elderly when endocrine function is diminished because of age-related factors (e.g., loss of ovarian hormones after menopause) or if endocrine function is lost following disease or surgery. Some of the more common hormonal agents used in the elderly are listed in Table 12–6 and are discussed here.

Estrogen Replacement

The primary female hormones, estrogen and progesterone, are normally produced by the ovaries from puberty until approximately the fifth or sixth decade when menopause occurs. Loss of these hormones is associated with a number of problems including vasomotor symptoms (hot flashes), atrophic vaginitis, and atrophic dystrophy of the vulva. Replacement of the ovarian hormones, especially estrogen, can help resolve all these symptoms. In addition, osteoporosis is quite common in older postmenopausal women, and estrogen used alone or with occasional cyclic doses of progesterone has been reported to reduce bone mineral loss in these individuals.[67] Also, there is considerable evidence that the risk of coronary heart disease is diminished in postmenopausal women receiving estrogen.[32]

The major problem associated with estrogen replacement is the increased risk of cancer reported by some studies.[32] However, the relationship between estrogen replacement and the risk of cancer remains uncertain, and estrogens continue to be used to reduce osteoporosis and other postmenopausal symptoms in elderly women.

Diabetes Mellitus

Insulin is normally synthesized by pancreatic beta cells, and this hormone regulates the metabolism of glucose and other energy substrates. Diabetes mellitus is a complex metabolic disorder caused by inadequate insulin production, decreased peripheral effects of insulin, or a combination of inadequate insulin production and decreased insulin effects. Diabetes mellitus consists of two principal types: type I (insulin-dependent diabetes mellitus) and type II (non–insulin-dependent diabetes mellitus). Type I diabetes mellitus is commonly associated with younger individuals, whereas type II diabetes mellitus occurs quite frequently in the elderly. As many as 10% to 20% of Americans over age 60 may be diagnosed with type II diabetes mellitus.[62] If diabetes mellitus is not managed appropriately, acute effects (impaired glucose metabolism, ketoacidosis) and chronic effects (neuropathy, renal disease, blindness) may occur.

In contrast to the younger type I diabetic, the older adult with type II diabetes mellitus may not require exogenous insulin to manage this disease. The principal methods of managing type II diabetes mellitus in the elderly are diet, exercise, and maintenance of proper body weight.[62] When drug therapy is required in the older type II diabetic, it is usually in the form of oral hypoglycemic drugs (see Table 12–6). These agents can be taken orally to lower blood glucose (hence the term *oral hypoglycemic*) and seem to work by enhancing the release of insulin from the pancreas as well as by increasing the sensitivity of peripheral tissues to insulin.

The principal problem associated with drug therapy in elderly diabetic patients is that blood glucose may be reduced too much, resulting in symptoms of hypoglycemia. Physical therapists should be alert for signs of low blood glucose such as headache, dizziness, confusion, fatigue, nausea, and sweating.

Thyroid Disorders

The thyroid gland normally produces two hormones, thyroxine and triiodothyronine. These hormones affect a wide

TABLE 12–6.

Drugs Used in Endocrine Disorders

Category	Indication	Common Examples	
		Generic Name	Trade Name
Estrogens	Osteoporosis	Conjugated estrogens	Premarin
	Severe postmenopausal symptoms	Estradiol	Estrace, others
	Some cancers		
Insulin	Diabetes mellitus	—	Iletin, Lente Iletin, Velosulin, others
Oral hypoglycemic agents	Diabetes mellitus	Chlorpropamide	Diabinese
		Glipizide	Glucotrol
		Tolbutamide	Orinase
Antithyroid agents	Hyperthyroidism	Methimazole	Tapazole
		Propylthiouracil	Propyl-Thyracil
Thyroid hormones	Hypothyroidism	Levothyroxine	Levothroid, Synthroid
		Liothyronine	Cytomel

variety of tissues and are primarily responsible for regulating basal metabolic rate and other aspects of systemic metabolism. Excess thyroid hormone production (hyperthyroidism, thyrotoxicosis) is quite prevalent in the elderly and produces symptoms such as nervousness, weight loss, muscle wasting, and tachycardia. Inadequate production of the thyroid hormones (hypothyroidism) is characterized by weight gain, lethargy, sleepiness, bradycardia, and other features consistent with a slow body metabolism.

Hyperthyroidism can be managed with drugs that inhibit thyroid hormone biosynthesis such as propylthiouracil, methimazole, or high doses of iodide. The primary problems associated with these drugs are transient allergic reactions (skin rashes, etc.) and blood dyscrasias such as aplastic anemia and agranulocytosis. A more permanent treatment of hyperthyroidism can be accomplished by administering radioactive iodine. The radioactive iodine is taken up by the thyroid gland, where it selectively destroys the overactive thyroid tissues.

Hypothyroidism is usually managed quite successfully by replacement therapy using natural and synthetic versions of one or both of the thyroid hormones. The most significant problem associated with thyroid hormone replacement in older patients is that the elderly require smaller doses of these hormones than younger individuals.[21, 100] Replacement doses that are too high will evoke symptoms of hyperthyroidism, such as nervousness, weight loss, and tachycardia. Physical therapists should be alert for these symptoms when working with elderly patients who are receiving thyroid hormone replacement therapy.

Treatment of Infections

Various microorganisms such as bacteria, viruses, fungi, and protozoa can invade and proliferate in the elderly individual. Often the immune system is able to combat these microorganisms successfully, thus preventing infection. Occasionally, however, various drugs must be used to supplement the body's normal immune response in combating infection caused by pathogenic microorganisms. The elderly are often susceptible to such infections, especially if their immune system has already been compromised by previous illness or a general state of debilitation. Two of the more common types of infections, bacterial and viral, are presented along with a brief description of the related drug therapy.

Antibacterial Drugs

Although some bacteria exist in the body in a helpful or symbiotic state, infiltration of pathogenic bacteria may result in infection. If the immune system is unable to contain or destroy these bacteria, antibacterial drugs must be ad-

ministered. Some of the principal groups of antibacterial drugs are shown in Table 12–7. These agents are often grouped according to how they inhibit or kill bacterial cells. For instance, certain drugs (penicillins, cephalosporins) act by inhibiting bacterial cell wall synthesis. Other drugs (aminoglycosides, tetracyclines) specifically inhibit the synthesis of bacterial proteins. A group of drugs that includes norfloxacin and rifampin works by selectively inhibiting the function and replication of bacterial DNA and RNA. Finally, drugs such as the sulfonamides inhibit the synthesis of folic acid, a substance needed to manufacture nucleic acids and other essential metabolites in the bacterial cell. The selection of a specific agent from one of these groups is based primarily on the type of bacterial infection present in each patient.

The side effects that tend to occur with these agents vary from drug to drug, and it is not possible in this limited space to discuss all the potential antibacterial ADRs. With regard to their use in elderly patients, many of the precautions discussed earlier tend to apply. For instance, adverse drug reactions tend to occur more frequently because of the decreased renal clearance of antibacterial drugs in older adults.[36, 72] Hence, physical therapists should be alert for any suspicious reactions in elderly patients taking antibacterial drugs, especially if renal function is already somewhat compromised.

TABLE 12–7.
Treatment of Infection

Antibacterial Drugs		
	Common Examples	
Major Groups	Generic Name	Trade Name
Aminoglycosides	Gentamicin	Garamycin
	Streptomycin	—
Cephalosporins	Cefaclor	Ceclor
	Cephalexin	Keflex
Erythromycins	Erythromycin	E-Mycin, many others
Penicillins	Penicillin G	Bicillin, others
	Penicillin V	V-Cillin K, others
	Amoxicillin	Amoxcil, others
	Ampicillin	Amcill, others
Sulfonamides	Sulfadiazine	Silvadene
	Sulfisoxazole	Gantrisin
Tetracyclines	Doxycycline	Vibramycin, others
	Tetracycline	Sumycin, others

Antiviral Drugs		
Generic Name	Trade Name	Principal Indication
Acyclovir	Zovirax	Herpes simplex infections
Amantadine	Symmetrel	Influenza A
Vidarabine	Vira-A	Herpes virus infections
Zidovudine	Retrovir	Human immunodeficiency virus (HIV) infections

Antiviral Drugs

Viruses are small microorganisms that can invade human (host) cells and use the biochemical machinery of the host cell to produce more viruses. As a result, the virus often disrupts or destroys the function of the host cell, causing specific symptoms that are indicative of viral infection. Viral infections can cause disease syndromes ranging from the common cold to serious conditions such as acquired immunodeficiency syndrome (AIDS). Since the viral invader usually functions and coexists within the host cell, it is often difficult to administer a drug that will kill the virus without simultaneously destroying the host cell. Hence, the number of antiviral agents is limited (see Table 12-7), and these drugs often attenuate viral replication rather than actually destroy a virus that already exists in the body.

Due to the relatively limited number of effective antiviral agents, pharmacologic management of viral disease often focuses on preventing viral infection through the use of vaccines. Vaccines are usually a modified, inactive form of the virus that stimulates the patient's immune system to produce specific antiviral antibodies. When exposed to an active form of the virus, these antibodies help destroy the viral invader before an infection is established.

The antiviral agents shown in Table 12-7 are often poorly tolerated and produce a number of adverse side effects, especially in elderly or debilitated patients. Hence, prevention of viral infection through the use of vaccines is especially important in the elderly. For instance, influenza vaccines are often advocated for elderly individuals prior to seasonal outbreaks of the "flu."[31, 96] Of course, some vaccines are not always completely effective in preventing viral infections, and an appropriate vaccine has yet to be developed for certain viral diseases such as AIDS. Still, vaccines represent the most effective method of dealing with viral infections in elderly individuals.

Cancer Chemotherapy

Cancer is the term used to describe diseases that are characterized by a rapid, uncontrolled cell proliferation and conversion of these cells to a more primitive and less functional state. Cancer is often treated aggressively using a combination of several different techniques such as surgery, radiation, and one or more cancer chemotherapeutic agents.

The elderly represent the majority of patients who will ultimately require some form of anticancer medication.[87] In general, the cancer chemotherapy regimens in older adults are similar to those used in younger individuals, with the exception that dosages are adjusted according to changes in liver and kidney function or other changes that affect drug pharmacokinetics. The results of cancer chemotherapy in the older patient also parallel those seen in the younger individual with the possible exception that some hematologic malignancies (certain leukemias) do not appear to respond as well to drug therapy in the elderly.[87] The principal chemotherapeutic strategies and types of anticancer agents are presented here.

Basic Strategy of Cancer Chemotherapy

Most anticancer drugs work by inhibiting the synthesis and function of DNA and RNA. This impairs the proliferation of cancer cells since they must rely on the rapid replication of genetic material in order to synthesize new cancer cells. Of course, DNA and RNA function is also impaired to some extent in healthy noncancerous cells, and this accounts for the many severe side effects and high level of toxicity associated with cancer chemotherapeutic agents. However, cancer cells should suffer to a relatively greater degree, since cancer cells typically have a greater need to replicate their genetic material in order to sustain a high rate of cell reproduction. Still, most of the common adverse effects discussed here occur because of the nonselective effect of many anticancer drugs on normal cell function.

Types of Anticancer Drugs

The two principal types of anticancer medications are the alkylating agents and the antimetabolites (Table 12-8). Alkylating agents work by cross-linking nucleic acids in the DNA double helix so that the DNA is essentially tied

TABLE 12-8.

Cancer Chemotherapeutic Agents

Alkylating Agents
  Busulfan (Myleran)
  Carmustine (BCNU, BiCNU)
  Chlorambucil (Leukeran)
  Cyclophosphamide (Cytoxan, Neosar)
  Dacarbazine (DTIC-Dome)
  Lomustine (CeeNU)
  Mechlorethamine (Mustargen)
  Melphalan (Alkeran)
  Streptozocin (Zanosar)
  Thiotepa
  Uracil mustard
Antimetabolites
  Cytarabine (Cytosar-U)
  Floxuridine (FUDR)
  Fluorouracil (Adrucil)
  Mercaptopurine (Purinethol)
  Methotrexate (Mexate)
  Thioguanine (Lanvis)
Others
  Antineoplastic antibiotics
  Hormones
  Interferons
  Plant alkaloids
  Miscellaneous cytotoxic agents

up in knots. The DNA strands within the helix are unable to unwind and allow replication of the cell's genetic code. Hence, the cell cannot reproduce or continue to function properly since replication of DNA and synthesis of RNA are no longer possible. Antimetabolites are drugs that impair the normal biosynthesis of nucleic acids and other important cellular metabolic components. Basically, antimetabolites resemble the normal cellular biochemical components (metabolites). However, these drugs either directly inhibit the steps involved in nucleic acid synthesis or substitute themselves for the normal metabolite, resulting in an incomplete or nonfunctional version of the finished product (nucleic acid). In either case, replication and function of the cancer cell are attenuated because the cell is unable to synthesize the nucleic acid building blocks needed for synthesizing more DNA and RNA.

In addition to the alkylating agents and antimetabolites, various other drugs have been used to treat cancer (see Table 12–8). Certain antibiotics, hormones, antiviral agents, and a variety of other drugs have all been used to treat specific forms of cancer. In general, these agents also attempt to impair cell division and replication, but the exact drug mechanism varies from agent to agent. For more information on these agents or the other anticancer drugs discussed here, the reader is referred to several references at the end of this chapter.[15, 18, 57]

Adverse Effects and Concerns for Rehabilitation

As mentioned, patients receiving cancer chemotherapy typically experience a number of severe adverse drug effects. Side effects such as GI distress (anorexia, vomiting), blood disorders (anemia, thrombocytopenia), skin reactions (hair loss, rashes), and toxicity of various other organs are extremely common. Unfortunately, these adverse effects must be tolerated because of the serious nature of cancer and the fact that death will ensue if these drugs are not used. In terms of rehabilitation of elderly patients, the physical therapist must recognize that these adverse effects will inevitably interfere with rehabilitation procedures. There will be some days that the patient is simply unable to participate in any aspect of physical therapy. Still, the therapist can provide valuable and timely support for the elderly patient on cancer chemotherapy and reassure the patient that these drug-related effects are often unavoidable because of the cytotoxic nature of these drugs.

GENERAL STRATEGIES FOR COORDINATING PHYSICAL THERAPY WITH DRUG TREATMENT IN THE ELDERLY

Based on the preceding discussion, it is clear that various medications can produce beneficial and adverse effects that may affect physical therapy of the elderly in many different ways. There are, however, some basic strategies that therapists can use to help maximize the beneficial aspects of drug therapy and minimize the detrimental drug effects when working with geriatric individuals. These general strategies are summarized here.

Distinguishing Drug Effects From Symptoms

When evaluating a geriatric patient, therapists must try to account for the subjective and objective findings that may be due to ADRs rather than true disease sequelae and the effects of aging. For instance, the patient who appears confused and disoriented during the initial physical therapy evaluation may actually be experiencing an adverse reaction to a psychotropic drug, cardiovascular medication, or some other agent. The correct distinction of true symptoms from ADRs allows better treatment planning and clinical decision making.

As discussed earlier, therapists can also take steps to prevent inappropriate drug use and polypharmacy by helping distinguish ADRs from true disease symptoms. Distinguishing drug-related signs from true patient symptoms may require careful observation and consultation with family members or other health professionals to see if these signs tend to increase following each dosage. Periodic reevaluation should also take into account any changes in drug therapy, especially if new medications are added to the patient's regimen. Finally, the medical staff should be alerted to any change in the patient's response that may indicate an ADR.

Scheduling Physical Therapy Sessions Around Dosage Schedule

Physical therapy should be coordinated with peak drug effects if the patient's active participation will be enhanced by drug treatment. For instance, drugs that improve motor performance (antiparkinsonian agents), improve mood and behavior (antidepressants, antipsychotics), and decrease pain (analgesics) may increase the older patient's ability to take part in various rehabilitation procedures. Conversely, physical therapy should be scheduled when drug effects are at a minimum for elderly patients receiving drugs that produce excessive sedation, dizziness, or other adverse effects that may impair the patient's cognitive or motor abilities. Unfortunately, there is often a trade-off between desirable effects and adverse effects with the same drug, such as the narcotic analgesic that also produces sedation. In these cases, it may take some trial and error in each patient to find a treatment time that capitalizes on the drug's benefits with minimum interference from the adverse effects.

Promoting Synergistic Effects of Physical Therapy Procedures With Drug Therapy

One must not lose sight of the fact that many of the rehabilitation procedures employed with geriatric clients may augment drug therapy. For instance, the patient with Parkinson's disease may experience an optimal improvement in motor function through a combination of physical therapy and antiparkinsonian drugs. In some cases, drug therapy may be reduced through the contribution of physical therapy procedures (e.g., reduction of pain medications through the simultaneous use of TENS, physical agents, etc.). This synergistic relationship between drug therapy and physical therapy can help achieve better results than if either intervention is used alone.

Avoiding Potentially Harmful Interactions Between Physical Therapy Procedures and Drug Effects

Some physical therapy interventions used in the elderly could potentially have a negative interaction with some medications. For instance, the use of rehabilitation procedures that cause extensive peripheral vasodilation (e.g., large whirlpool, some exercises) may produce severe hypotension in the patient receiving certain antihypertensive medications. These negative interactions must be anticipated and avoided when working with geriatric patients.

Improving Education and Compliance With Drug Therapy in the Elderly

Proper adherence to drug therapy is one area in which physical therapists can have a direct impact. Therapists can reinforce the need for adhering to the prescribed regimen, and therapists can help monitor whether or not drugs have been taken as directed. Therapists can also help educate their geriatric patients and their families as to why specific drugs are indicated and what side effects should be expected and tolerated as opposed to side effects that may indicate drug toxicity.

CASES

Case 1: Parkinson's Disease

Brief History

A 71-year-old male patient was diagnosed with Parkinson's disease 15 years ago. Drug therapy was initiated in the form of the anticholinergic drug trihexyphenidyl (Artane). Levodopa therapy was added to the anticholinergic drug approximately 5 years ago when symptoms became incapacitating. Levodopa dosage was progressively increased over the next few years as the patient's condition gradually worsened. Recently, symptoms of bradykinesia

and rigidity increased to the point that the patient's spouse was no longer able to care for him, and he was admitted to a nursing home. At the time of admission, the patient was receiving 1,500 mg of levodopa given in combination with 150 mg of carbidopa three times per day. Dosages were administered at mealtimes to decrease stomach irritation caused by these drugs. Upon admission, the patient began receiving daily physical therapy to help maintain mobility and joint range of motion.

Problem/Influence of Medication

The therapist began seeing the patient each morning in the physical therapy clinic at the nursing home. Although symptoms of rigidity and bradykinesia were fairly marked, the therapist found that the patient was able to actively participate to some extent in range-of-motion exercises and some ambulation activities. During the second session, however, the patient suddenly became extremely rigid and exhibited a complete loss of all voluntary movement. The therapist found this surprising since the patient had started the physical therapy session with a reasonable amount of voluntary motor activity. The patient had also completed the entire session on the preceding day without any such akinetic episodes. Upon further consideration, the therapist realized that the patient was seen later in the morning on the second day and that the akinetic episode occurred about 1 hour before the patient's next dose of levodopa.

Decision/Solution

The therapist realized that the patient was exhibiting end-of-dose akinesia. Patients who have been on levodopa therapy for several years often exhibit this phenomenon where the effectiveness of levodopa appears to wear off prior to the next dose. To prevent a recurrence of this problem, the therapist made a point of scheduling this patient about 1 hour after his initial (breakfast) dose of antiparkinsonian medications. This at least allowed the patient to participate as much as possible in his daily exercise regimen. The therapist also notified the patient's physician of the end-of-dose akinesia. This problem was ultimately resolved by increasing the levodopa dosage so that a sufficient amount of drug was available to maintain motor function throughout each dosing cycle.

Case 2: Lithium Toxicity

Brief History

A 76-year-old woman living at home fell and fractured her right hip. She was admitted to the hospital, where she underwent total hip arthroplasty. The patient had been in relatively good health prior to her fall but had been receiving treatment for bipolar syndrome (manic-depression) for several years. At the time of admission, she was maintained on a dosage of 300 mg of lithium taken three times daily. The patient began receiving physical therapy in the hospital on the day following her hip surgery and was ambulating independently with a walker within 1 week after admission to the hospital. She was discharged to her home, but physical therapy was recommended at home to ensure continued progress and full recovery.

Problem/Influence of Medication

The physical therapist visiting this patient at home initially found her to be alert and enthusiastic about resuming her rehabilitation. By the second visit, however, the therapist noticed some confusion and slurred speech in this patient. Upon closer inspection, the therapist also observed symptoms such as hand tremors and muscle weakness. When ambulating, the patient exhibited some incoordination and became fatigued very easily.

Decision/Solution

The therapist became concerned of the potential for lithium toxicity in this patient. Apparently the hip surgery and subsequent change in activity level in this patient had altered renal excretion of lithium to the extent that this drug was slowly accumulating in the patient's body. The therapist immediately notified the patient's physician. Laboratory tests revealed a serum concentration of 2.1 mEq/L, indicating moderate levels of lithium toxicity. The patient's dosage of lithium was decreased until serum levels returned to values that were within the therapeutic range. The patient continued to receive physical therapy at home and completed her recovery from hip surgery without any further incidents.

SUMMARY

Drug intervention in geriatric individuals can be regarded as a two-edged sword: the beneficial and therapeutic effects of any given medication must be balanced against the risk that the older adult will experience an adverse reaction to that drug. There is no doubt that many illnesses and afflictions that typically occur in a geriatric population can be alleviated through appropriate pharmacologic measures. However, the risk of adverse drug reactions is increased in the elderly due to factors such as disproportionate drug use and an altered response to many medications. Hence, the potential for beneficial drug effects coexists with an increased chance for serious adverse effects in the older adult.

Physical therapists must be aware of the drug regimen used in their geriatric patients and how the beneficial and adverse effects of each medication can affect rehabilitation of these individuals. Physical therapists can also play an important role in recognizing adverse drug reactions in the elderly. Finally, therapists can help encourage proper compliance with drug therapy and discourage the excessive and inappropriate use of unnecessary medications in their geriatric clients.

Acknowledgment

I would like to thank Jan Coy and Tom DiMatteo for their time and expert assistance in reviewing this chapter.

REFERENCES

1. Abernethy DR, Azarnoff DL: Pharmacokinetic investigations in elderly patients: Clinical and ethical considerations. *Clin Pharmacokinet* 1990; 19:82–93.
2. Abrams J: Nitroglycerin and long-acting nitrates in clinical practice. *Am J Med* 1983; 74(suppl 6b):85–94.
3. Abrams WB: Introduction: The concept of geriatric clinical pharmacology. *Clin Pharmacol Ther* 1987; 42:659–662.
4. Abrams WB: Pathophysiology of hypertension in older patients. *Am J Med* 1988; 85(suppl 3b):7–13.
5. Anderson KE: Influence of diet and nutrition on clinical pharmacokinetics. *Clin Pharmacokinet* 1988; 14:325–346.
6. Baker SP, Marchand S, O'Neil E, et al: Age-related changes in cardiac muscarinic receptors: Decreased ability of the receptor to form a high affinity agonist binding state. *J Gerontol* 1985; 40:141–146.
7. Beller SA, Overall JE, Swann AC: Efficacy of oral physostigmine in primary degenerative dementia: A double-blind study of response to different dose levels. *Psychopharmacology* 1985; 87:147–151.
8. Bigger JT, Hoffman BF: Antiarrhythmic drugs, in Gilman AG, Goodman LS, Rall TW, et al. (eds): *The Pharmacological Basis of Therapeutics,* ed 7. New York, Macmillan, 1985.
9. Bjork I, Lindahl U: Mechanism of the anticoagulant action of heparin. *Mol Cell Biochem* 1982; 48:161–182.
10. Blumenthal MD: Depressive illness in old age: Getting behind the mask. *Geriatrics* 1980; 35:34–43.
11. Busse JC, Materson BJ: Geriatric hypertension: The growing use of calcium-channel blockers. *Geriatrics* 1988; 43:51–58.
12. Byatt CM, Millard PH, Levin GE: Diuretics and electrolyte disturbances in 1000 consecutive geriatric admissions. *J R Soc Med* 1990; 83:704–708.
13. Cadieux RJ: Drug interactions in the elderly: How multiple drug use increases risk exponentially. *Postgrad Med* 1989; 86:179–186.
14. Cartwright A: Medicine taking by people aged 65 or more. *Br Med Bull* 1990; 46:63–76.
15. Chabner BA, Meyers CE: Clinical pharmacology of cancer chemotherapy, in DeVita VT, Hellman S, Rosenberg SA (eds): *Cancer: Principles and Practice of Oncology, vol 1.* New York, Lippincott, 1985.

16. Chalmers JP, Smith SA, Wing LM: Hypertension in the elderly: The role of calcium antagonists. *J Cardiovasc Pharmacol* 1988; 12(suppl 8):147–155.

17. Chien CP, Townsend EJ, Ross-Townsend A: Substance use and abuse among the community elderly: The medical aspect. *Addict Dis* 1978; 3:357–372.

18. Ciccone CD: *Pharmacology in Rehabilitation*. Philadelphia, FA Davis, 1990.

19. Cohen JL: Pharmacokinetic changes in aging. *Am J Med* 1986; 80(suppl 5a):31–38.

20. Davies P, Bailey PJ, Goldenberg MM: The role of arachadonic acid oxygenation products in pain and inflammation. *Annu Rev Immunol* 1984; 2:335–357.

21. Davis FB, LaMantia RS, Spaulding SW, et al: Estimation of a physiologic replacement dose of levothyroxine in elderly patients with hypothyroidism. *Arch Intern Med* 1984; 144:1752–1754.

22. Dawling S, Crome P: Clinical pharmacokinetic considerations in the elderly. An update. *Clin Pharmacokinet* 1989; 17:236–263.

23. Denham MJ: Adverse drug reactions. *Br Med Bull* 1990; 46:53–62.

24. Dow L, Holgate ST: Assessment and treatment of obstructive airway disease in the elderly. *Br Med Bull* 1990; 46:230–245.

25. Duggan AW, North RA: Electrophysiology of the opioids. *Pharmacol Rev* 1983; 35:219–281.

26. Elliott HL: Calcium antagonists in the treatment of hypertension and angina pectoris in the elderly. *J Cardiovasc Pharmacol* 1989; 13(suppl 4):12–16.

27. Evans MA, Triggs EJ, Cheung M, et al: Gastric emptying rate in the elderly: Implications for drug therapy. *J Am Geriat Soc* 1981; 29:201–205.

28. Flower RJ, Vane JR: Inhibition of prostaglandin synthetase in brain explains the anti-pyretic action of paracetamol (4-acetamidophenol). *Nature* 1972; 240:410–411.

29. Freis ED: The cardiovascular risks of thiazide diuretics. *Clin Pharmacol Ther* 1986; 39:239–244.

30. Friedhoff AJ: A strategy for developing novel drugs for the treatment of schizophrenia. *Schizophr Bull* 1983; 9:504–527.

31. Galbraith AW: Influenza: Recent developments in prophylaxis and treatment. *Br Med Bull* 1985; 41:381–385.

32. Gambrell RD: Estrogen-progesterone replacement and cancer risk. *Hosp Pract* 1990; 25:81–91.

33. Gerber JG, Nies AS: Beta-adrenergic blocking drugs. *Annu Rev Med* 1985; 36:145–164.

34. Geriatrics Panel Discussion: Practical considerations in managing Alzheimer's disease. *Geriatrics* 1987; 42:55–65.

35. Gilman AG, Goodman LS, Rall TW, et al (eds): *The Pharmacological Basis of Therapeutics*, ed 7, New York, Macmillan, 1985.

36. Gleckman RA, Czachor JS: Reviewing the safe use of antibiotics in the elderly. *Geriatrics* 1989; 44:33–39.

37. Gottlieb GL: Sleep disorders and their management: Special considerations in the elderly. *Am J Med* 1990; 88(suppl 3a):29–33.

38. Greenblatt DJ, Shader RI, Harmatz JS: Implications of altered drug disposition in the elderly: Studies of benzodiazepines. *J Clin Pharmacol* 1989; 29:866–872.

39. Guarnieri T, Filburn CR, Zitnik G, et al: Contractile and biochemical correlates of beta-adrenergic stimulation of the aged heart. *Am J Physiol* 1980; 239:H501–H508.

40. Gwirtsman HE, Ahles S, Halaris A, et al: Therapeutic superiority of maprotiline versus doxepin in geriatric depression. *J Clin Psychiatry* 1983; 44:449–453.

41. Hall RCW, Beresford TP: Tricyclic antidepressants in the treatment of the elderly. *Geriatrics* 1984; 39:81–93.

42. Harris E: Lithium. *Am J Nurs* 1981; 81:1311–1315.

43. Haustein K-O: Cardiotoxicity of digitalis. *Arch Toxicol* 1986; 59(suppl 9):197–204.

44. Haynes RC, Murad F: Adrenocorticotropic hormone; adrenocortical steroids and their synthetic analogs; inhibitors of adrenocortical steroid biosynthesis, in Gilman AG, Goodman LS, Rall TW, et al (eds): *The Pharmacological Basis of Therapeutics*, ed 7. New York, Macmillan, 1985.

45. Hollister LE: Current antidepressants. *Annu Rev Pharmacol Toxicol* 1986; 26:23–37.

46. Hollister LE, Yesavage J: Ergoloid mesylates for senile dementias: Unanswered questions. *Ann Intern Med* 1984; 100:894–898.

47. Hurvitz N: Predisposing factors in adverse reactions to drugs. *Br Med J* 1969; 1:536–539.

48. Jenike MA: Treating anxiety in elderly patients. *Geriatrics* 1983; 38:115–119.

49. Jenike MA: Psychoactive drugs in the elderly: Antipsychotics and anxiolytics. *Geriatrics* 1988; 43:53–65.

50. Johnson JE: *Aging and Cell Structure*, 2 vols. New York, Plenum Press, 1984.

51. Jonsson PV, Lipsitz LA: Cardiovascular factors contributing to falls in the older adult. *Top Geriatr Rehabil* 1990; 5:21–33.

52. June SG: Adverse drug reactions in the elderly, in Vestal RE (ed): *Drug Treatment in the Elderly*. Sydney, ADIS Health Science Press, 1984.

53. Kalchthaler DO, Coccaro E, Lichtiger S: Incidences of polypharmacy in a long-term care facility. *J Am Geriatr Soc* 1977; 25:308–313.

54. Kelliher GJ, Conahan ST: Changes in vagal activity and response to muscarinic receptor agonists with age. *J Gerontol* 1980; 35:842–849.

55. Koella WP: CNS-related (side) effects of beta-blockers with special reference to mechanism of action. *Eur J Clin Pharmacol* 1985; 28(suppl 1):55–63.

56. Lamy PP: Special features of geriatric prescribing. *Geriatrics* 1981; 36:42–52.

57. Lane M: Chemotherapy of cancer, in del Regato JA, Spjut HJ, Cox JD (eds): *Cancer: Diagnosis, Treatment, and Prognosis*, ed 6. St Louis, CV Mosby, 1985.

58. Larsen GL, Henson PM: Mediators of inflammation. *Annu Rev Immunol* 1983; 1:335–359.

59. Lewis GD, Campbell WB, Johnson AR: Inhibition of prostaglandin synthesis of glucocorticoids in human endothelial cells. *Endocrinology* 1986; 119:62–69.

60. Libow LS, Butler RN: Treating mild diastolic hypertension in the elderly: Uncertain benefits and possible dangers. *Geriatrics* 1981; 36:55–62.

61. Lipsky PE: Remission-inducing therapy in rheumatoid arthritis. *Am J Med* 1983; 75(suppl 4b):40–49.

62. Lipson LG: Diabetes in the elderly: Diagnosis, pathogenesis, and therapy. *Am J Med* 1986; 80(suppl 5a):10–21.

63. Loi C-M, Vestal RE: Drug metabolism in the elderly. *Pharmacol Ther* 1988; 36:131–149.

64. Lonergan ET: Aging and the kidney: Adjusting treatment to physiologic change. *Geriatrics* 1988; 43:27–33.

65. Lowenthal DT: Drug therapy in the elderly: Special considerations. *Geriatrics* 1987; 42:77–82.

66. Macdonald RL, McLean MJ: Anticonvulsant drugs: Mechanisms of action, in Delgado-Escueta AV, Ward AA, Woodbury DM, et al (eds): *Basic Mechanisms of the Epilepsies*. New York, Raven Press, 1986.

67. MacLennan WJ: Osteoporosis. *Br Med Bull* 1990; 46:94–112.

68. Marchesini G, Bua V, Brunori A, et al: Galactose elimination capacity and liver volume in aging man. *Hepatology* 1988; 8:1079–1083.

69. McDonald RH: The evolution of current hypertension therapy. *Am J Med* 1988; 85(suppl 3b):14–18.

70. McMurray L, McDevitt DG: Treatment of heart failure in the elderly. *Br Med Bull* 1990; 46:202–229.

71. Melnyk V: Geriatric rheumatology: Safe use of potentially toxic antirheumatics. *Geriatrics* 1988; 43:83–90.

72. Meyers BR, Wilkinson P: Clinical pharmacokinetics of antibacterial drugs in the elderly: Implications for selection and dosage. *Clin Pharmacokinet* 1989; 17:385–395.

73. Mohs RC, Davis BM, Johns CA, et al: Oral physostigmine treatment of patients with Alzheimer's disease. *Am J Psychiatry* 1985; 142:28–33.

74. Montamat SC, Cusack BJ, Vestal RE: Management of drug therapy in the elderly. *N Engl J Med* 1989; 321:303–309.

75. Newman RP, Calne DB: Parkinsonism: Physiology and pharmacology, in Shah NS, Donald AG, (eds): *Movement Disorders*. New York, Plenum Press, 1986.

76. Nicholls MG: Age-related effects of diuretics in hypertensive subjects. *J Cardiovasc Pharmacol* 1988; 12(suppl 8):51–59.

77. Noble D: Mechanism of action of therapeutic levels of cardiac glycosides. *Cardiovasc Res* 1980; 14:495–514.

78. Nolan L, O'Malley K: Prescribing for the elderly. Part I: Sensitivity of the elderly to adverse drug reactions. *J Am Geriatr Soc* 1988; 36:142–149.

79. Nuki G: Pain control and the use of non-steroidal analgesic antiinflammatory drugs. *Br Med Bull* 1990; 46:262–278.

80. O'Brien DK, Pattee JJ: Hypertension in older patients—what drugs to use and when. *Geriatrics* 1981; 36:111–120.

81. O'Connor SW, Scarpace PJ, Abrass IB: Age-associated decrease of adenylate cyclase activity in rat myocardium. *Mech Ageing Dev* 1981; 16:91–95.

82. O'Duffy JD, Luthra HS: Current status of disease-modifying drugs in progressive rheumatoid arthritis. *Drugs* 1984; 27:373–377.

83. O'Hara NM, White D: Drugs and the elderly, in Lewis CB (ed): *Aging: The Health Care Challenge*. Philadelphia, FA Davis, 1985.

84. Oparil S: Introduction: Treating the older hypertensive patient—an overview. *Am J Med* 1988; 85(suppl 3b):1.

85. O'Reilly RA: Vitamin K and the oral anticoagulant drugs. *Annu Rev Med* 1976; 27:245–261.

86. Paratt JR: Nitroglycerin—the first one hundred years: New facts about an old friend. *J Pharm Pharmacol* 1979; 31:801–809.

87. Phister JE, Jue SG, Cusack BJ: Problems in the use of anticancer drugs in the elderly. *Drugs* 1989; 37:551–565.

88. *Physician's Desk Reference,* ed 45. Oradell, NJ, Medical Economics Co, 1991.

89. Potter JF, Haigh RA: Benefits of antihypertensive therapy in the elderly. *Br Med Bull* 1990; 46:77–93.

90. Ray WA, Griffin MR: Prescribed medications and the risk of falling. *Top Geriatr Rehabil* 1990; 5:12–20.

91. Remme WJ: Congestive heart failure—pathophysiology and medical treatment. *J Cardiovasc Pharmacol* 1986; 8(suppl 1):36–52.

92. Risse SC, Barnes R: Pharmacologic treatment of agitation associated with dementia. *J Am Geriatr Soc* 1986; 34:368–376.

93. Robertson DRC, George CF: Drug therapy for Parkinson's disease in the elderly. *Br Med Bull* 1990; 46:124–146.

94. Robinson BE: Dementia: A 3-pronged strategy for primary care. *Geriatrics* 1986; 41:75–86.

95. Robinson DR: Prostaglandins and the mechanism of action of antiinflammatory drugs. *Am J Med* 1983; 75(suppl 4b):26–31.

96. Ruben FL: Prevention and control of influenza: Role of vaccine. *Am J Med* 1987; 82(suppl 6a):31–33.

97. Sack KE: Update on NSAID's in the elderly. *Geriatrics* 1989; 44:71–90.

98. Salerno E: Psychopharmacology and the elderly. *Top Geriatr Rehabil* 1986; 1:35–45.

99. Salzman C: Clinical guidelines for the use of antidepressant drugs in geriatric patients. *J Clin Psychiatry* 1985; 46:38–44.

100. Sawin CT, Herman T, Molitch ME, et al: Aging and the thyroid: Decreased requirement for thyroid hormone in older hypothyroid patients. *Am J Med* 1983; 75:206–209.

101. Scarpace PJ, Abrass IB: Decreased beta-adrenergic agonist affinity and adenylate cyclase activity in senescent rat lung. *J Gerontol* 1983; 38:143–147.

102. Scheuer ML, Pedley TA: Current concepts: The evaluation and treatment of seizures. *N Engl J Med* 1990; 323:1468–1471.

103. Sheard MH: The biological effects of lithium. *Trends Neurosci* 1986; 3:85–86.

104. Simonson W: *Medications and the Elderly: A Guide for Promoting Proper Use*. Rockville, Md. Aspen Publications, 1984.

105. Smith WF: Epidemiology of hypertension in older patients. *Am J Med* 1988; 85(suppl 3b):2–6.

106. Spiegel R, Huber F, Koberle S: A controlled long-term study with ergoloid mesylates (Hydergine) in healthy, elderly volunteers: Results after 3 years. *J Am Geriatr Soc* 1983; 31:549–555.

107. Staessen J, Fagard R, VanHoof R, et al: Antihypertensive drug treatment in elderly hypertensive subjects: Evidence of protection. *J Cardiovasc Pharmacol* 1988; 12(suppl 18):33–38.

108. Stahl SM: Neuropharmacology of movement disorders: Comparison of spontaneous and drug-induced movement disorders, in Shah NS, Donald AG (eds): *Movement Disorders.* New York, Plenum Press, 1986.

109. Stults BM, Dere WH, Caine TH: Long-term anticoagulation: Indications and management. *West J Med* 1989; 151:414–429.

110. Swift CG: Pharmacodynamics: Changes in homeostatic mechanisms, receptor and target organ sensitivity in the elderly. *Br Med Bull* 1990; 46:36–52.

111. Tallman JF, Gallager DW: The GABA-ergic system: A locus of benzodiazepine action. *Annu Rev Neurosci* 1985; 8:21–44.

112. Thai LJ, Fuld PA, Masur DM, et al: Oral physostigmine and lecithin improve memory in Alzheimer's disease. *Ann Neurol* 1983; 13:491–496.

113. Thompson TL, Filley CM, Mitchell WD, et al: Lack of efficacy of Hydergine in patients with Alzheimer's disease. *N Engl J Med* 1990; 323:445–450.

114. Thompson TL, Moran MG, Nies AS: Psychotropic drug use in the elderly. *N Engl J Med* 1983; 308:134–138, 194–199.

115. Tinetti ME, Speechley M, Ginter SF: Risk factors for falls among elderly persons living in the community. *N Engl J Med* 1988; 319:1701–1707.

116. Tregaskis BF, Stevenson LH: Pharmacokinetics in old age. *Br Med Bull* 1990; 46:9–21.

117. Tsujimoto G, Hashimoto K, Hoffman BB: Pharmacokinetic and pharmacodynamic principles of drug therapy in old age: Part 1. *Int J Clin Pharmacol Ther Toxicol* 1989; 27:13–26.

118. Vane JR: Inhibition of prostaglandin synthesis as a mechanism of action for aspirin-like drugs. *Nature* 1971; 231:232–235.

119. Vestal RE, Dawson GW: Pharmacology and aging, in Finch CE, Schneider EL (eds): *Handbook of the Biology of Aging,* ed 2. New York, Van Nostrand Reinhold, 1985.

120. Whalley LJ, Bradnock J: Treatment of the classical manifestations of dementia and confusion. *Br Med Bull* 1990; 46:169–180.

121. Whitehouse PJ: Reviewing the "breakthroughs" in Alzheimer's research. *Geriatrics* 1987; 42:107–111.

122. Wieman HM: Avoiding common pitfalls of geriatric prescribing. *Geriatrics* 1986; 41:81–89.

123. Woodhouse KW, James OF: Hepatic drug metabolism and aging. *Br Med Bull* 1990; 46:22–35.

124. Wynne HA, Cope LH, Mutch E, et al: The effect of age upon liver volume and apparent liver blood flow in healthy men. *Hepatology* 1989; 9:297–301.

125. Yaksh TL, Noueihed R: The physiology and pharmacology of spinal opiates. *Annu Rev Pharmacol Toxicol* 1985; 25:433–462.

PART III

Problems and Procedures

CHAPTER 13

Endurance Training of the Older Adult

Marybeth Brown, Ph.D., P.T.
Wendy M. Kohrt, Ph.D.

INTRODUCTION

Changes in cardiovascular functional capacity occur with aging, regardless of life-style. Unfortunately, the sedentary life-style that is typical of older adults in the United States accelerates the decline in functional capacity and increases the risk for losing independence at a relatively young age. Some older adults, particularly women, are so debilitated that they use nearly 100% of their cardiovascular functional capacity just to perform the basic activities of daily living. This magnitude of deterioration in functional capacity need not occur with successful aging and would not occur if our society engaged in routine physical activity.

Even though cardiovascular fitness declines with aging, it appears that most older adults have the potential to improve fitness markedly through endurance exercise training. Although the primary benefit of training is an improvement in maximal cardiovascular functional capacity, there are secondary benefits that are of significant practical importance. For example, an activity that demands 100% of functional capacity prior to training may require only 80% of post-training capacity, thereby reducing the fatigue and discomfort associated with the activity. The improvement of endurance also is likely to provide a margin of safety; activities requiring 90% to 100% of functional capacity may be too taxing for the cardiovascular system. Furthermore, the potential health benefits associated with habitual exercise translate into an improved quality of life, by reducing the risk of developing such age-related diseases as atherosclerosis, hypertension, non–insulin-dependent diabetes, and osteoporosis.

Studies conducted to determine the potential of older adults to adapt to endurance exercise training have yielded conflicting results. However, recent studies strongly support the hypothesis that older men and women are as trainable as young people; that is, relative improvement in cardiovascular fitness does not appear to be limited by age, at least through the eighth decade.

Before discussing some of the normal age-related changes that occur in the cardiovascular system with aging, it is necessary to review a few concepts of physiology. The best index of cardiovascular functional capacity is maximal oxygen uptake, or $\dot{V}O_2$max. Briefly, $\dot{V}O_2$max is the maximal rate at which the body can utilize oxygen (O_2) or, in other words, the maximal rate at which energy can be produced aerobically. Usually, $\dot{V}O_2$max is expressed as the volume of O_2 consumed (mL) relative to body weight (per kg) and time (per minute)—or mL/min/kg. To provide some degree of perspective, a world-class endurance athlete may have a $\dot{V}O_2$max of 75 mL/min/kg whereas a debilitated 75-year-old may have a $\dot{V}O_2$max of 15 mL/min/kg. For additional perspective, the energy cost of walking 3 mph is approximately 12 mL/min/kg. Thus, walking 3 mph would require only 16% of the elite endurance athlete's $\dot{V}O_2$max, whereas the same activity would require 80% of the 75-year-old's $\dot{V}O_2$max. The fatigue and discomfort associated with an activity depends on the intensity of the exercise relative to an individual's $\dot{V}O_2$max. Walking would be perceived as easy by the elite athlete but as difficult by the debilitated 75-year-old. Thus, the higher a person's $\dot{V}O_2$max, the greater the opportunity to enjoy a large variety of physical activities without undue fatigue.

There are three physiologic determinants of $\dot{V}O_2$max: maximal heart rate (HR); stroke volume (SV); and arteriovenous oxygen difference (a-$\bar{v}O_2$ diff), or the ability of tissues to extract oxygen from the blood. In terms of aging, the most important of these contributors to $\dot{V}O_2$max is maximal HR, which declines steadily with age. Each of these determinants of $\dot{V}O_2$max will now be examined.

CHANGES IN CARDIOVASCULAR FUNCTION WITH AGING

Maximal Oxygen Consumption

Oxygen consumption rate ($\dot{V}O_2$) increases linearly as exercise or work intensity increases and is a function of the rate at which oxygen is delivered to (cardiac output, or $\dot{Q}$) and extracted by the tissues (arteriovenous oxygen difference, or a-$\bar{v}O_2$ diff). The maximal $\dot{V}O_2$ ($\dot{V}O_2$max) an individual may reach is determined by such factors as heredity, sex, age, body composition, and endurance exercise training.[7] In most individuals, $\dot{V}O_2$max is limited by $\dot{Q}$, which is the product of HR and SV. For this reason, $\dot{V}O_2$max is considered the best available index of cardiovascular fitness. It is usually measured during a treadmill or cycle ergometer protocol, during which exercise intensity is progressively increased. The objective determination of $\dot{V}O_2$max is a person's failure to increase $\dot{V}O_2$ even though the workload is getting more difficult (i.e., there is a plateau in $\dot{V}O_2$). Because this criterion is difficult to attain, other indices of a near-maximal effort include a respiratory exchange ratio greater than 1.10, an HR within ten beats per minute of the age-predicted maximal HR, or a blood lactate level greater than 8 mmol/L.[7, 53, 72, 115] Using these criteria, it has been shown that healthy older men and women up to 80 years of age reach $\dot{V}O_2$max values during treadmill exercise that are reproducible.[53] When $\dot{V}O_2$ is measured during cycle ergometer exercise, however, individuals are often limited by muscular fatigue and attain peak $\dot{V}O_2$ values that are approximately 10% below the treadmill value.[58] This deficit may be exaggerated in the elderly due to declining quadriceps muscle mass and/or strength.

Average $\dot{V}O_2$max values in healthy, sedentary 25-year-old men and women are 46 to 48 mL O_2/min/kg and

34 to 36 mL O_2/min/kg, respectively.[46, 63, 72] The rate at which $\dot{V}O_2$max declines with age is difficult to determine due to the increasing level of adiposity[42, 73] and declining level of physical activity[117] that usually occur with aging; both will accelerate the decline in $\dot{V}O_2$max. It is also questionable whether $\dot{V}O_2$max declines in a linear or curvilinear fashion.[22] Cross-sectional and longitudinal studies indicate that $\dot{V}O_2$max decreases approximately 4 to 5.5 mL/min/kg/decade in men and 2.0 to 3.5 mL/min/kg/decade in women, or approximately 12% to 13% per decade.* This rate probably represents the average loss due to the combined effects of age, increasing body fat level, and a sedentary life-style. In men and women who remain relatively lean, the estimated rate of decline in $\dot{V}O_2$max is about 9% per decade,[57, 72] and in master athletes, who remain lean and maintain a vigorous level of physical activity, the estimated rate of decline is approximately 5% per decade.[45, 57, 101]

It has been suggested that the age-related decline in $\dot{V}O_2$max in sedentary people is due in large part to the loss of muscle mass that occurs with aging.[45] However, the decline of $\dot{V}O_2$max in well-trained athletes does not appear to be linked to changes in body composition but rather to a decline in maximal HR.[45, 52, 57, 101] Other factors that may contribute to the loss of aerobic power with advancing age include a decline in mitochondrial volume,[89] a reduced ability to shunt blood to exercising muscle,[127] or an increased proportion of connective tissue in muscle.[131]

DETERMINANTS OF $\dot{V}O_2$max

Heart Rate

Maximal HR (HR_{max}) is determined primarily by age, as evidenced by the equation recommended for its estimation ($HR_{max} = 220 - $ age).[7] However, a number of studies of exercise capacity of the elderly have found that HR at maximal exercise is actually greater than predicted.[52, 72, 115] For example, among groups of healthy people whose age averaged 58 years,[52] 65 years,[72] and 72 years,[53] maximal HR averaged 176, 165, and 157 beats per minute (bpm), respectively, or approximately 10 bpm higher than the age-predicted values. HR_{max} is not different between older men and women[59, 72] and is not markedly altered by endurance exercise training.[8, 40, 53, 55, 72, 115]

To determine the effect of age per se on cardiovascular responses to exercise, researchers have studied master athletes, who remain lean and maintain a high level of physical activity. These studies[52, 56, 101] indicate that HR_{max} plays a major role in the age-related decline of $\dot{V}O_2$max.

Rivera and colleagues found that HR_{max}, SV, and $\bar{v}O_2$ diff were all lower in older compared with young distance runners.[101] However, others[52, 56] have found that O_2 pulse (defined as $\dot{V}O_2$max divided by HR_{max}), SV, and a-$\bar{v}O_2$ diff were similar in young and older athletes, indicating that a slower HR was responsible for the lower $\dot{V}O_2$max in older athletes. In comparisons of master athletes and age-matched sedentary controls,[52, 56] HR_{max} was similar in master athletes and age-matched sedentary controls, yet $\dot{V}O_2$max values were 40% to 50% lower in the untrained men due to reductions in both SV and a-$\bar{v}O_2$max diff. These differences are probably related to differences in both physical activity level and genetic potential. There is a strong likelihood that the master athletes had a higher $\dot{V}O_2$max and larger values for SV and a-$\bar{v}O_2$ diff than their sedentary controls at much younger ages.

The cause of the age-related decline in maximal HR is not fully understood. Sympathetic drive appears adequate, since higher catecholamine levels are typically observed in older people than in young in response to stress.* With aging, however, there does appear to be a decreased sensitivity[65, 109, 134] and responsiveness[45, 92, 124, 127, 128, 133] to the effects of catecholamines. Thus, the chronotropic response to a given plasma catecholamine concentration is reduced with aging.

Stroke Volume

SV is the difference between end-diastolic and end-systolic volumes. Maximal SV may be maintained or actually increased with aging to help offset the decline in maximal $\dot{Q}$ (cardiac output) due to the reduction in HR_{max}. From studies of men and women aged 20 to 75 years,[59, 63] it has been determined that there is no relationship between age and stroke index (SV per m^2 body surface area). These studies reported significant declines in $\dot{V}O_2$max with aging due to the decline in maximal $\dot{Q}$ that occurred as a result of a slower HR_{max}. It is possible, however, that this apparent decline in cardiac function was complicated by the high prevalence of occult coronary artery disease.[82, 104] Indeed, when people were rigorously screened to eliminate those with cardiovascular disease,[119] older subjects had a greater increase in SV during vigorous exercise than did younger subjects. This was accomplished by an increase in end-diastolic volume rather than a reduction in end-systolic volume. This increased reliance on the Frank-Starling mechanism in older people has also been observed by others.[49, 132]

Although end-diastolic volume may increase with age in healthy people, end-systolic volume apparently also increases and ejection fraction is reduced.[119] The decline

*References 4–6, 15, 26, 27, 29, 35, 40, 57, 60, 62–66, 71–73, 78–82, 97, 98, 102, 103, 105, 116, 126.

* References 45, 65, 92, 109, 124, 127, 133, 134.

with aging in ejection fraction at peak exercise has been attributed to an increase in aortic stiffness[47, 64] and/or peripheral vascular resistance,[33, 55] both of which may be related to altered autonomic modulation.

Arteriovenous Oxygen Difference

The extraction of O_2 across a working muscle is expressed as the difference in the arterial and venous O_2 content measured in mL of O_2 per 100 mL of blood. At rest, O_2 content in arterial and venous blood is approximately 20 and 15 mL/100 mL, and the a-$\bar{v}O_2$ diff is 5 mL/100 mL. During maximal exercise, the a-$\bar{v}O_2$ diff increases to 16 to 17 mL/100 mL in both young and master athletes.[104] Therefore, age per se does not seem to alter the ability of skeletal muscle to extract O_2. However, in sedentary populations, there is a decline with advancing age in a-$\bar{v}O_2$ diff,[33, 55] which is most likely associated with disuse rather than aging.

The decrease in O_2 extraction that has been reported to occur with aging does not appear to be due to a reduction in O_2-carrying capacity of arterial blood[33, 62] or to a decline in the metabolic potential of skeletal muscle.[3, 28, 50] There is, however, a decreased capillary/fiber ratio in aged muscle[28, 93] as well as a reduction in maximal peripheral blood flow[83] that could contribute to the decrease in a-$\bar{v}O_2$ diff.

PULMONARY FUNCTION

Lung Volumes and Capacities

Although total lung capacity does not change with aging, there is a decrease in vital capacity that is countered by an increase in residual volume (dead air space).[111] Between ages 20 and 60 years there is approximately a 1-L loss of vital capacity,[78] due primarily to decreased compliance of the chest wall. A prolongation of muscle contraction and relaxation times also occurs, leading to a deterioration in timed ventilatory functions.[66] The forced expiratory volume in 1 second (FEV_1), for example, declines in a linear fashion with advancing age. Both static[14] and dynamic[88] measures of pulmonary function appear to be unaltered by endurance exercise training.

Ventilatory Responses to Exercise

In healthy young adults, exercise performance is rarely limited by ventilation. Indeed, during low to moderate intensity exercise, the ventilatory equivalent for oxygen, which is the ratio of minute ventilation ($\dot{V}E$, L/min) to $\dot{V}O_2$ (L/min), is approximately 25:1, but during moderate to high-intensity exercise the ventilatory rate increases to a greater degree than does $\dot{V}O_2$, leading to a rise in the ventilatory equivalent ($\dot{V}E/\dot{V}O_2$) to 30:1 or higher. Further evidence that ventilation does not limit exercise performance comes from the observation that 15-second and 4-minute maximal voluntary ventilation (MVV) rates are substantially higher than the ventilation rate during maximal exercise ($\dot{V}E_{max}$).[66] Thus, there is a ventilatory "reserve" that is not usually called on during maximal aerobic exercise, although there are exceptions. For example, in people with obstructive airway disease, $\dot{V}E$ at peak exercise may be 95% of the 12-second MVV, indicating that exercise capacity in these patients may be limited by pulmonary function.[80]

There is a decline with aging in $\dot{V}E_{max}$ that parallels the decline in $\dot{V}O_2$max. The question, therefore, is whether the decline in pulmonary function contributes to the decline in $\dot{V}O_2$max, or whether $\dot{V}E_{max}$ is merely lower because of the reduced maximal cardiovascular function. Support for the latter comes from the observation that the ventilatory equivalent at maximal exercise is similar in old and young people[55, 86, 130] as well as in trained and untrained older people,[55, 86, 88, 127] indicating adequate ventilation. $\dot{V}E$ at maximal exercise in older sedentary people has also been found to be only 55% of the 15-second MVV rate,[88] indicating a ventilatory reserve in older people similar to that seen in young people. Furthermore, the increase in $\dot{V}E_{max}$ that occurs with exercise training in older people is proportional to the increase in $\dot{V}O_2$max (i.e., the ventilatory equivalent is unchanged).[72, 81, 130] Thus, it does not appear that healthy older people are limited in exercise capacity by pulmonary function.

It has been suggested that ventilatory rate at submaximal exercise intensities is higher in older compared with young people, as evidenced by a higher ventilatory equivalent.[81, 94, 130] It must be noted, however, that although ventilatory rate increases linearly with increasing $\dot{V}O_2$ at low to moderate intensities, a relative hyperventilation occurs as lactate (a by-product of anaerobic metabolism) begins to accumulate in the blood. This event is sometimes referred to as the *ventilatory threshold*. Because the ventilatory threshold occurs at a higher relative intensity in people who are aerobically trained compared with those who are not trained, differences between young and old in $\dot{V}E$ at submaximal intensities may reflect differences in training status rather than ventilatory function per se. When young and older trained and sedentary men exercised at the same relative intensity (approximately 70% of $\dot{V}O_2$max), ventilatory equivalent was similar in all groups except the young trained men, in whom it was reduced,[86] indicating that age does not markedly alter the ventilatory response to exercise.

EXERCISE TRAINING

Cardiorespiratory Fitness

Early studies of the effect of endurance exercise training on aerobic power in the elderly led to equivocal results. On one hand was a report[12] that older men and women increased $\dot{V}O_2$max by 38% with training, a large increase in comparison with the 15% to 25% improvement that typically occurs in young people.[5, 7] On the other hand, however, were studies[1, 13, 38, 39, 51] showing little or no increase in $\dot{V}O_2$max in older people in response to training. Because more recent studies indicate that the relative increase in aerobic power with training is not age dependent, at least through the eighth decade, the lack of a marked training response in the aforementioned studies may have been the result of an insufficient training stimulus (i.e., training duration and/or intensity). Conversely, the 38% improvement in $\dot{V}O_2$max reported by Barry and colleagues[12] was probably an overestimation of the adaptability of older people, since maximal heart rate, respiratory exchange ratio, and blood lactate concentration were all markedly higher after training than before, indicating that a true $\dot{V}O_2$max had not been attained in the pretraining assessments.

Recent studies indicate that older people can increase $\dot{V}O_2$max with endurance exercise training to the same relative degree as young people, that is, 15% to 25%.[53, 72, 114, 123, 125] While no significant gender difference in the adaptability to training has been reported, a tendency toward less improvement in women was noted by Blumenthal and colleagues[17] (9% in women vs. 14% in men) and by Seals and coworkers[114] (19% in women vs. 27% in men). It is not known whether the exercise training prescriptions were similar for men and women in these studies. However, a recent report by Kohrt and colleagues[72] indicated that the increases in $\dot{V}O_2$max in older men (26%) and women (23%) were not different when the exercise stimulus was of similar frequency (4 days per week), duration (45 minutes per day), and relative intensity (80% HR_{max}). In this study, the individual improvements in $\dot{V}O_2$max for the 53 men and 57 women who completed the exercise program varied markedly, ranging from 0% to 54%. Earlier studies suggested that the degree to which $\dot{V}O_2$max could be improved was dependent on the intensity of the exercise—higher intensity, larger improvement[54, 114, 125]—and on the initial level of fitness—lower fitness, larger improvement.[30, 110, 125] However, the study by Kohrt and coworkers[72] found that the magnitude of improvement in $\dot{V}O_2$max with training was not related to any specific component of the exercise prescription (i.e., frequency, duration, or intensity), nor was it related to the initial fitness level of the participant. Thus, it seems likely that most older men and women, whether they lead very sedentary or fairly active lives, could improve cardiovascular fitness through regular endurance exercise training. The level of cardiovascular function that the average 65-year-old man or woman can attain through vigorous exercise is equivalent to that of someone 15 to 20 years younger.[72]

Besides improvements in cardiovascular function, there are a number of other health benefits of exercise for older men and women. It has been estimated that people who are sedentary are twice as likely to develop coronary artery disease (CAD) as people who exercise regularly.[77, 87, 90, 91] At least part of this protective nature of exercise is probably due to its effects on the coronary risk factor profile. Risk factors for CAD that can be improved through exercise include hypercholesterolemia,[115, 129] hypertension,[54] hyperinsulinemia,[56, 61] glucose intolerance,[61, 107, 108] and obesity.[74, 112] Exercise is also one of the few interventions that can successfully increase plasma high-density lipoprotein (HDL) cholesterol, which is negatively correlated with CAD.[107, 129]

Aging is often associated with a decline in glucose tolerance that may progress to non–insulin-dependent diabetes mellitus (NIDDM). This deterioration is not due to insulin deficiency, as in insulin-dependent diabetes mellitus, but rather to the resistance of peripheral tissues (primarily skeletal muscle) to the actions of insulin.[34, 100] Thus, as insulin resistance develops, there is typically an excess of insulin secreted to try to maintain glucose homeostasis. Insulin resistance and hyperinsulinemia are very common in older people, particularly in those who have an abdominal fat pattern (i.e., apple-shaped) as opposed to a gluteal-femoral fat pattern (i.e., pear-shaped), and there is accumulating evidence that hyperinsulinemia is associated with the development not only of NIDDM but also of hypertension[44, 99–101] and CAD.[10, 95] Exercise is very important in this regard, since some of the short-term effects of exercise are a blunted insulin response to a glucose challenge[67, 70, 106] and an increase in the sensitivity of muscle to the action of insulin.[68, 69, 84] Thus, exercise may play a major role in both the treatment and prevention of NIDDM, CAD, and hypertension.

Many of the effects of exercise are only short term. For example, the increased sensitivity of muscle to the action of insulin persists for approximately 48 hours after a bout of exercise.[24, 84] The long-term benefits of exercise are believed to be mediated through the reduction in fat mass, particularly in the abdominal region, that may occur with training. Although obesity in general is known to be associated with an increased risk for a number of diseases and/or metabolic disorders, the emphasis in research over the past decade has been on the associations of these disorders with regional obesity, specifically accumulation of fat in the visceral region. Fat stored in the visceral region is unique in that it is highly sensitive to lipolytic stimuli, and it is also drained by the portal circulation.[16, 37] Thus, it is hypothesized that as fat accumulates in the visceral region, there is an increased flux of free fatty acids and glycerol through the liver, and that this condition leads to a cascade of metabolic consequences that may be associated with the development of NIDDM, CAD, and hypertension.[16, 37] The accumulation of intra-abdominal fat appears to begin in young- to middle-aged men and progress with advancing age, whereas women appear to be somewhat resistant to this until the menopause, at which time they, too, accumulate visceral fat.[19, 36, 43, 118] Furthermore, although premenopausal women are at far lower risk for developing CAD than age-matched men, the risk profile of postmenopausal women that are not on replacement hormone therapy becomes more like that of their male counterparts.[11, 21, 23] It is not known to what degree the accumulation of intra-abdominal fat mediates this change in risk profile, but abdominal obesity appears to be a common factor in a cluster of metabolic disorders associated with the development of NIDDM, CAD, and hypertension.[16, 37]

There is preliminary evidence that exercise training results in a preferential loss of fat from the central,[74] and possibly the visceral,[37, 112] regions of the body. There is also some evidence that a reduction in intra-abdominal fat is predictive of improvements in plasma insulin and cholesterol concentrations.[37] However, it is unknown to what extent regular exercise training can prevent the accumulation of fat that typically occurs with advancing age. Although master athletes are generally not as lean as young athletes,[73] they are typically much leaner than age-matched nonathletes and seem to be largely protected against the usual age-related changes in coronary risk factors.[55, 113] Clearly, the potential role of exercise in the prevention of abdominal obesity and the associated metabolic disorders is encouraging and must be studied in more depth.

Another benefit of exercise training, of particular importance for older women, is an increase in bone mineral density (BMD).[75, 122] It is well known that reductions in physical activity, such as bed rest[76] or space flight,[85] result in a rapid loss of bone mineral. The finding that exercise performed in space does not fully prevent the loss of calcium during space flight has been taken as evidence that exercise must be weight bearing in nature in order to have a beneficial effect on the skeleton. However, it is unlikely that relatively short duration exercise sessions in space could fully compensate for the marked reduction in gravitational and load-bearing forces that occur in space flight. The effects of non–weight-bearing exercise on bone min-

eral status remain to be elucidated. There is encouraging evidence from a study by Dalsky and colleagues[31] that weight-bearing exercise can increase BMD of the spine by 5% to 10%, which is substantial considering that the age-related loss of mineral is typically approximately 1% per year. It should be noted, however, that some studies that have employed weight-bearing exercise[25, 48, 103] have not yielded positive results. Although the discrepant results may be due to a number of factors, the study by Dalsky et al. was unique in that a variety of exercise modes were employed and the intensity of the exercise was vigorous. To date, there have been no prospective studies of the effectiveness of exercise on increasing BMD of the proximal femur in older women. Moreover, there is relatively little information regarding the type of exercise regimen that would optimize the osteogenic effects. From the information available, it seems prudent to recommend fairly vigorous weight-bearing exercise using a variety of exercise modes (e.g., walking, jogging, stair climbing, weight lifting) as a means of preventing osteoporosis.

SPECIAL CONSIDERATIONS FOR EXERCISING THE ELDERLY

Exercise prescription for older adults is challenging, as often there are factors that may limit activity or narrow the range of possibilities for exercise. Factors to consider may include, but are not limited to, heart disease, medications that alter heart rate or blood pressure responses, severe osteoarthritis, lung disease, osteoporosis, and diabetes. Additionally, obesity, painful feet, postural deformity, insensitive feet, claudication, and incontinence are other factors that may limit the scope of participation. Taking all these factors into consideration and designing a program that is adequately challenging, enjoyable, easy to perform, and reasonably inexpensive will tax the most creative of minds.

By definition, endurance exercise will challenge the cardiovascular system, resulting in an increased HR and blood pressure (BP). Selecting the activities appropriate for each individual is based in large measure on initial fitness or $\dot{V}O_2max$. Thus, for those who are unfit, with low $\dot{V}O_2max$ values, simple range-of-motion exercises, slow walking, or gentle calisthenics may be appropriate for the desired increase in fitness. Men and women with higher $\dot{V}O_2max$ values, without orthopedic or other limitations, may be able to walk briskly, bicycle, or even jog. Above all, the exercises should be safe.

The American College of Sports Medicine recommends the following for developing cardiovascular fitness in older *healthy* adults: an exercise frequency of 3 to 5 days a week, a training intensity of 60% to 85% of $\dot{V}O_2max$ or

50% to 85% of maximum heart rate reserve, and 20 to 60 minutes of continuous aerobic activity (Table 13–1).[2] In general, lower-intensity activity should be performed for a longer duration. The mode of exercise can be any activity that uses a large proportion of available muscle mass, can be maintained continuously, and is aerobic. Aerobic exercise may include walking, brisk walking, treadmill walking, bicycling, hiking, dancing, running, rowing, stair climbing, indoor ski machine, cross-country skiing, swimming, calisthenics, and skating.

Our experience suggests that for older adults an activity program with multiple forms of endurance exercise is less likely to cause muscle and joint overuse and fatigue than a program that features only one activity (e.g., bicycling), particularly when exercise is being performed four to six times per week. Also, warm-up and cool-down periods seem to be important to keep muscle strain to a minimum and to maintain flexibility. One exercise session of 60 minutes' duration may include a warm-up, brisk walking, riding a stationary bicycle, and rowing, while maintaining a comparable HR for all three activities, and a cool-down.

If the same endurance activity, such as running, is performed routinely, alternating days of reduced or less intense activity with days of rigorous activity appears to reduce the risk of injury and allow an adequate recovery.[96] For example, a 6-mile run may be performed Monday, Wednesday, Friday, whereas swimming or walking may be the mode of exercise on Tuesday and Thursday. All exercisers, regardless of age, need adequate rest cycles, which should be incorporated into a fitness program. In general, the older the individual, the longer the period of recovery from an intense exercise bout needs to be.

Thomas Jefferson once said, "Of all exercises, walking is the best." Walking, brisk walking, treadmill walking, hill walking, and mall walking have become popular forms of endurance exercise for men and women of all ages, particularly older adults. If this form of activity is to be prescribed, attention to proper footwear is important. Name-brand walking shoes may provide adequate comfort for most people, but if feet are unusually wide, foot deformities are present, or if the plantar fat pad is diminished in thickness, a running shoe may be more comfortable. There is more impact absorption built into a running shoe than into a walking shoe. Thus, even though your client may never run, a running shoe might be a better investment. For the runner, a proper running shoe is imperative. A quick physical therapy evaluation of the foot is helpful to determine if a brand of shoe that has, for example, a curved last, rigid hindfoot control, or other features should be recommended.

Physical therapy evaluation is also highly recommended to identify clients with postural abnormalities or orthopedic conditions that might predispose a client toward injury or pain. If a long history of knee arthritis is present, for example, and the client has obvious joint involvement, a program of swimming or other form of activity that does not load the knees should be suggested. Components of a physical therapy evaluation are covered elsewhere in this text. Many of these evaluation tools should be utilized for determining an endurance exercise program that is appropriate for the client. The stimulus for exercise training needs to be based on level of cardiovascular fitness and musculoskeletal capability.

Before World War II, women did not receive postpartum care designed to return abdominals and pelvic musculature to former strength levels. Consequently, the pelvic floor and lower abdominals, in particular, are weak in many older women, resulting in stress incontinence during some forms of exercise. Most women are embarrassed to admit having difficulty with urine retention but will confess to problems if asked. If stress incontinence is present, appropriate strengthening exercises may help. Prescribing endurance exercise that does not exacerbate the problem will likely enhance adherence to the exercise program. Generally, nonimpact exercise such as bicycling, rowing,

TABLE 13–1.

American College of Sports Medicine Position Stand: Recommended Quantity and Quality of Exercise for Developing and Maintaining Cardiorespiratory and Muscular Fitness in Healthy Adults*

1. *Frequency of training*—3 to 5 days per week.
2. *Intensity of training*—60% to 90% of maximum heart rate (HR_{max}) or 50% to 85% of maximum oxygen uptake ($V_{O_2}max$) or HR_{max} reserve.
3. *Duration of training*—20 to 60 minutes of continuous aerobic activity. Duration is dependent on the intensity of the activity; lower-intensity activity should be conducted over a longer period of time.
4. *Mode of activity*—any activity that uses large muscle groups, can be maintained continuously, and is rhythmic and aerobic in nature.
5. *Resistance training*—strength training of a moderate intensity should be an integral part of an adult fitness program.

*From American College of Sports Medicine: *Med Sci Sport Exerc* 1990; 22:265–275. Used by permission.

and swimming will be more successful than loading activities (e.g., jogging, aerobics), which may cause fear of an accident.

Women also may have low bone mass, another factor that will influence the choice of endurance activity. If osteoporosis is known to be present, or a family history or other risk factors suggest a strong possibility of osteoporosis, exercise without pounding is strongly recommended, as spontaneous fractures have occurred. Jogging would be inappropriate; stair climbing, stationary bicycling, or walking might be more acceptable forms of training. We have been experimenting with having women with low bone mass wear a weighted vest (10 to 15 lb) while walking to see if bone mass can be enhanced. Results are still too preliminary to know if this form of loading the long bones is successful. Wearing the vest may increase lower extremity strength, particularly the more proximal musculature.

Heart disease is not a contraindication to exercise in most instances. Stress testing will reveal the presence of heart disease and provide guidelines on the degree to which the cardiovascular system can be stressed. Physician input is imperative, providing information on target HR or BP responses that are safe but adequately challenging. All clients with heart disease should be well aware of the danger signs—shortness of breath, profuse sweating, lightheadedness, and so forth—and be able to monitor their own HRs. If the exercise program is of high intensity, perhaps a physician should be present or nearby and on call. Unless a physician feels endurance training is unsafe, clients with heart disease generally can exercise rigorously, often increasing $\dot{V}O_2max$ significantly.

Age, per se, is not a contraindication to endurance exercise. Advancing age will limit the choices for endurance training, given the decline in $\dot{V}O_2max$ that occurs with each successive decade. A wide range of possibilities (jogging, dancing, bicycling, cross-country skiing, and hiking, to name a few) exist for the healthy "young old" adult. For a man or woman in their latter 70s or 80s, or even 90s, jogging and hiking become less likely as options. Musculoskeletal complaints become more commonplace with advancing age, and fewer individuals are capable of activities as rigorous as jogging. Age, however, is but one factor that determines the choice of endurance exercise.

To summarize, selection of an exercise program to enhance aerobic capacity is based primarily on level of fitness as determined by a treadmill or other test to determine $\dot{V}O_2max$. Other factors such as strength, flexibility, postural deviations, painful joints, osteoporosis, and stress incontinence, as revealed by evaluation, also must be considered in the design of exercise. Finally, the client's desire for a particular form of activity needs to be considered carefully and seriously. It should be borne in mind that 90-year-old men and women have scaled some of the major mountains in the world and completed marathons and that desire can result in remarkable achievements at any age. Above all, the program chosen should be prudent, reasonable, and safe.

SCREENING TOOLS

Stress testing the older adult before exercise is imperative for identifying those with cardiac disease. Incorrect or thoughtless exercise programming can result in a tragic outcome. Stress testing also provides the required information to distinguish between those who are "young" old vs. "old" old and at what level to start training. The risks of physical activity, if present, need to be balanced with the risks of physical inactivity, and stress testing will provide insight as to what the risks may be.

Maximum oxygen intake, or aerobic power, provides the most definitive information available about the performance capability of the cardiorespiratory system. Many older adults, however, cannot or should not be maximally tested, and a submaximal test must serve as a proxy. Although perhaps not as accurate as a maximal examination, a submaximal test at least provides some insight as to what a subject can or cannot do. Multiple tests of aerobic capacity exist, but what tool is chosen will depend on the client's ability to walk or run, how deconditioned they are, existing medical conditions, how much muscle mass is available to work with, the age of the person being tested, and safety.

Treadmill Testing

By far, the most popular and best-evaluated form of testing is conducted on a treadmill. Most clinics utilize the Bruce or modified Bruce protocol for treadmill testing, which is a progressive, multistage examination designed to elicit maximal oxygen intake.[20] The modified protocol is presented in Table 13–2.

Most healthy men and women in their 60s and 70s are able to accomplish at least the first stage or two. For men and women who are advanced in age or quite deconditioned, an alternative treadmill test exists called the *modified Balke protocol*.[9] This examination requires subjects to walk at a constant speed while increasing the grade every 2 minutes. In our facility, treadmill speed varies from 1.0 mph for particularly deconditioned people up to 2.5 mph. Whether the chosen walking speed is 1.0 mph, 2.0 mph, or 2.5 mph, treadmill incline is increased to the point where 80% of predicted HR_{max} (220 − age) is reached. This protocol is interminable for the well-conditioned person, so care should be taken in choosing an ap-

TABLE 13–2.

Modified Bruce Protocol

Stage	Treadmill Speed (mph)	Treadmill Grade (%)
½	1.7	5
1	1.7	10
2	2.5	12
3	3.4	14
4	4.2	16
5	5.0	18

propriately difficult test. A third alternative was developed by Sidney and Shepard [20] and consists of walking at between 2.5 and 3.5 mph and adjusting the slope of the treadmill (incline) every 3 minutes. This test was devised so that 75% to 85% of HR_{max} would be reached during the ninth minute of exercise. This method of testing permits enough time for most subjects to stabilize at each work level.

During treadmill testing, expired air usually is collected and subsequently analyzed to provide information on the amount of oxygen being utilized at each level of difficulty. Not many exercise facilities have oxygen analysis capability and use instead HR response at each treadmill level achieved. The formula (220 − age) is used to estimate $\dot{V}O_2max$ (Fig 13–1). Assuming a linear relationship between an increase in HR in response to exercise and an increase in $\dot{V}O_2$, 80% of HR_{max} is equivalent to approximately 80% of $\dot{V}O_2max$.

BP and HR must be monitored continuously during

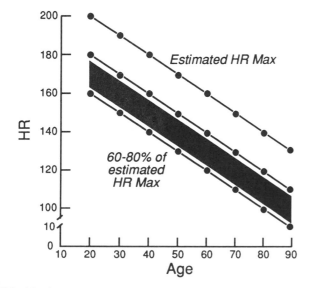

FIG 13–1.
Top line, estimated HR_{max} reflecting the decline in maximum HR aging. *Bottom Line*, estimated exercise HR range for each decade give a program intensity of 60% to 80% of HR_{max}.

the test. Ideally, the client is hooked up to an electrocardiogram (ECG) machine, permitting analysis of heart rate response while the examination is in process. A physician must interpret ECG changes and take responsibility for terminating the test if indicated. Systolic BP is expected to rise during the entire examination and if pressure fails to rise or decreases, the test must be stopped. Other reasons for stopping a stress test include excessive tachycardia or bradycardia, ischemic deviation of ST segments and other ECG abnormalities, anginal pain, breathlessness, dizziness or lightheadedness, leg pain, and clinical signs (pallor, mottling of skin, cyanosis, cold sweat, ataxis, excessive fatigue, glassy stare, gallop heart sounds).

Many older adults are limited by musculoskeletal disorders, balance problems, fear, lack of coordination, lightheadedness, or pain and cannot perform a treadmill test well enough for results to be meaningful. Consequently, an alternative form of testing must be used.

Cycle Ergometer Testing

If an older adult is fearful of a continuously moving treadmill belt, has a history of dizziness, has joint pain while walking, walks poorly, or is not well balanced, cycle ergometer testing may be indicated. The cycle has the advantages of being weight supporting while allowing the subject to hold on to the handlebars. There is also a greater sense of security knowing that the test can be terminated by the participant, rather than the examiner. Also, a cycle ergometer is much less expensive than a treadmill. Cycle ergometer testing is not indicated if a subject has quadriceps weakness, suffers from leg pain, particularly with exertion, or is poorly coordinated.

A typical cycle ergometer test is continuous, has multiple stages, and should be completed within 6 to 9 minutes.[121] The subject should work up to 75% to 85% of predicted HR_{max}. BP and ECG responses are monitored continuously. A typical bicycle test progression is presented in Table 13–3. Work intensity is presented both in "W" and "Kgm/min" as cycles typically have one or the other. The increment in intensity should approximate a metabolic cost of 3 to 4 mL/min kg. The oxygen cost (mL/min kg) of cycling exercise can be estimated using the following equations, where body weight is expressed in kg:

$$\dot{V}O_2 = W \times 12.24 + 250/ \text{ body weight}$$

$$\dot{V}O_2 = Kgm/min \times 2 + 250/ \text{ body weight}$$

Because there is more localized muscular fatigue, particularly quadriceps, associated with cycling than with walking or jogging, it may be preferable to use smaller, more frequent increments in intensity to avoid fatigue. For

TABLE 13-3.

Cycle Ergometer Stress Test

Estimated $\dot{V}_{O_2}$ (L/min)	Work Intensity (W)	Work Intensity (Kgm/min)	Duration (min)
0.5	25	150	3
0.9	50	300	3
1.2	75	450	3
1.5	100	600	3
1.8	125	750	3

example, rather than increasing power output by 30 W every 3 minutes, a 10-W increase each minute can be selected instead.

Additional levels or stages may be added as indicated. If a subject is obviously well conditioned, the test may start at 100 W and go up 25 W every 3 minutes. The average deconditioned older adult will probably need to start at 25 or 50 W. Starting at a lower level is recommended if there is a question of safety.

One-Mile Walk Test

Although the One-Mile Walk Test was developed fairly recently, its reliability and validity have been established.[71] As the name implies, the subject walks continuously at a self-chosen "brisk" pace that is perceived as appropriate for the distance required. For the final quarter of a mile, the time required to cover this distance and the heart rate during the final quarter mile are recorded. $\dot{V}_{O_2}$max is estimated from the following formula:

$$\dot{V}_{O_2}max = 6.9652 + (0.0091 \times wt) - (0.0257 \times age) + (0.5955 \times sex) - (0.2240 \times T_1) - (0.0115 \times HR_{1/4})$$

Where

wt = body weight in pounds
age = age in years
sex = 0 for females; 1 for males
T_1 = time in minutes to complete the final ¼ mile
$HR_{1/4}$ = HR at the end of the final ¼ mile

Obvious advantages of this form of testing include cost, performing an activity most people can do, and ease of administration. Disadvantages are that not many old-old adults can walk that far, people with dizziness or balance deficits may be at risk for falling, and fatigue may overcome the subject before the end of the test.

Step Tests

Bench stepping or step testing is a fairly popular form of field testing, as large numbers of subjects can be tested at

a time and it is easy to administer. Disadvantages outweigh the advantages for most older adults, as quadriceps strength or quadriceps fatigue limits performance. In addition, the correlation between HRs elicited with step testing and $\dot{V}_{O_2}$max are barely acceptable ($r = 0.76$ for Harvard step test and $r = 0.75$ for McArdle's test). Correlations were obtained for young subjects; the possibility of lower correlations for older adults exists. The utility of this form of testing for the older adult simply has not been established.

The test requires stepping up and down a step of standard height, usually 6 or 8 in., to the beat of a metronome, for 3 minutes. The next stage requires stepping up and down a stair that is 10 to 12 in. tall. Holding on to a handrail is not permitted, as heart rates become artificially high. For many older adults, the energy demand of the test exceeds their potential, even at the first stage of testing (i.e., a step 6 or 8 in. high). Consequently, it is not possible to increment intensity very precisely. Although not validated as yet, some clinics are using steps of smaller heights, 2 to 3 in., and increasing step height by 2 in. to increase demand in a more reasonable fashion for older adults.

Chair Step Test

In an attempt to accommodate for the older adult who has limited muscle strength, is very deconditioned $\dot{V}_{O_2}$max of 12 mL O_2/kg/min or less), and may be unsafe on a bicycle or treadmill, Smith and Gilligan[121] developed the chair step test. This examination is primarily for the nursing home population or the old-old adult. A chair, metronome, stopwatch, and adjustable bar are all that are required for the test. Subjects are positioned comfortably in a chair and, to the beat of a metronome, are asked to place a foot on the bar, which is positioned 6 in. above the ground. Feet are alternated for 3 minutes, at which time the bar is raised to 12 in. off the ground, and the test is repeated for another 3 minutes. The third stage requires alternate "stepping" up to a bar that is 18 in. above the ground. The fourth stage is a repeat of the third stage except the arms are raised overhead each time a foot is raised to the bar. HR_{max} is used to determine approximate $\dot{V}_{O_2}$max.

Perceived Exertion

If time, resources, and subject capability are limited, a walking test can be used. There is a close relationship between perceived exertion and $\dot{V}_{O_2}$ uptake.[41] Thus, perceived exertion during a walking trial of at least 3 to 5 minutes[1] duration will provide insight as to the approximate percentage of $\dot{V}_{O_2}$max being utilized. The perceived exertion scale as designed by Borg[18] is presented in Table

TABLE 13-5.

Classification of Intensity of Exercise Based on Perceived Exertion*

Rating of Perceived Exertion	Classification of Intensity	Relative Intensity (%)	
		HR_{max}	$\dot{V}O_2max$ or HR_{max} Reserve
<10	Very light	<35	<30
10–11	Light	35–59	30–49
12–13	Moderate (somewhat hard)	60–79	50–75
14–16	Heavy	80–89	75–84
>16	Very heavy	≥90	≥85

*From Pollock ML, Wilmore JH: *Exercise in Health and Disease: Evaluation and Prescription for Prevention and Rehabilitation,* ed 2. Philadelphia, WB Saunders, 1990. Used by permission.

13–4. Perceived exertion also may be used to estimate the relative intensity of an exercise (Table 13–5).

A walk test can simply be a slow, moderate, and briskly paced walk, self-selected by the client, and performed for 3 to 5 minutes at each velocity. The client walks until HR plateaus at each velocity—thus, the 3- to 5-minute window of time. HR is taken after 3 to 5 minutes of slow walking, after 3 to 5 minutes of moderately paced walking, and after 3 to 5 minutes of brisk walking. The estimated HR_{max} is drawn from the three data points provided by each walk.

EXERCISE PRESCRIPTION

Choice of an endurance training program for older adults is based on four factors: fitness level ($\dot{V}O_2max$), presence or absence of cardiovascular disease, musculoskeletal limitations, and the individual's goals and determination. Information from the history sheet, physical examination, stress test, and interview are integrated to design a program that is optimal for the individual. Initially, a great

TABLE 13-4.

Borg Scale of Perceived Exertion*

6	
7	Very, very light
8	
9	Very light
10	
11	Fairly light
12	
13	Somewhat hard
14	
15	Hard
16	
17	Very hard
18	
19	Very, very hard
20	

*From Borg G: *Scand J Rehabil Med* 1970; 2:92. Used by permission.

deal of exercise prescription is trial and error until experience is gained, as is often the case with some forms of physical therapy intervention. Practice is imperative to gain skill in this complex and challenging arena. It is not uncommon to have two clients of relatively the same age who present with vastly differing capabilities. For example, in our clinic we have prescribed exercise training programs for two 80-year-old individuals, one with no physical or cardiac limitations who desired to participate in the Senior Olympics (fast-walking event) and the other with strength, balance, heart disease, fitness, and pain limitations. Both are exercising successfully, but the expectations and mode of activity are considerably different—moderate, fast, and "sprint" walking for distances of up to ½ mile for the Senior Olympiad, chair exercises and wall walking 25 ft at a moderately brisk pace for the other. More in-depth examples of exercise prescription follow.

CASE STUDIES

Lottie D.

This 67-year-old retired teacher had never exercised but was interested in becoming active to prevent the deterioration that she had observed in her aged mother. Initially, she was screened by her physician and declared free of cardiac disease. Physical therapy evaluation did not reveal any musculoskeletal abnormalities or other physical problems that would be a source of concern. Lottie was not overweight, standing 5 ft 2 in. and weighing 118 lb. She had an interest in a walking program that could be conducted in her neighborhood or some form of exercise that could be performed at home. In addition to her mother, Lottie also had an unwell husband at home—thus, the need for activity that could be performed close to or in the home.

A maximal graded treadmill exercise test was performed that revealed that Lottie had a $\dot{V}O_2max$ of 20.0 mL/kg/min and HR_{max} of 158 bpm. Thus, Lottie was judged to be moderately unfit. Her training HR range was determined to be between 95 and 126 bpm, and a walking/ bicycling program was begun that elicited a HR that was close to this range. Before Lottie began her exercise program, she was taught stretches to maintain adequate hip and ankle range of motion. She was also taught how to monitor her own HR, and she was checked periodically to ensure the veracity of her determinations. During week 1, Lottie began her exercise by stretching, doing a 5-minute warm-up walk, and then walking at a moderate pace for 30 minutes, riding a stationary bicycle at 150 Kgm/min for 5 minutes, riding the bike for 5 minutes at 300 Kgm/min, and then cooling down. This program took approximately an hour to complete and included 40 minutes of aerobic activity. BP was checked both before and after her workouts, and once a week, BP was checked 20 minutes after exercise cool-down.

Initially, Lottie found she was very fatigued by the end of the week and unable to maintain the training pace. Consequently, her program was modified so that she was performing the activities described above on Monday, Wednesday, Friday and eliminating the 10 minutes of bicycle on Tuesday and Thursday.

Lottie realized that she looked forward to exercise on the days that did not include the bicycle. She did not like the bicycle, and thus this mode of activity was dropped.

Lottie quickly progressed as she became quite exercise oriented. She observed that some of the exercises around her were jogging, and she wanted to try jogging in lieu of bicycling, which was done. Thus, by week 5 Lottie's activity program was as follows: stretching, 5-minute warm-up walk, 1½ miles of fast walking, and 1½ miles of two jogs/two walks (each revolution around the track was ½₀ mile. Lottie jogged two laps, walked two laps, jogged two laps, walked two laps, etc.), followed by a cooldown.

At the end of 3 months, Lottie's program consisted of stretching, 5 minutes of warm-up walking, 40 minutes of one jog/one walk (approximately 3 miles covered), 5 minutes of moderate walking, and a cool-down. At this point, she had a repeat maximal treadmill exercise test that revealed that a significant increase in $\dot{V}o_2$max had occurred with 3 months of training.

Lottie continued to progress and experienced only one painful episode during her training. She had begun to neglect her stretches and developed adductor tightness that resulted in a groin pull. Once this problem was alleviated, Lottie went on to perform the following program: stretching, 5-minute warm-up, 2 miles of slow jogging, walk five laps, 1 mile of slow jogging, walk five laps, cool down. Exercise HR was 124 bpm.

As Lottie gained confidence in herself and her abilities, she exercised at home more and more, coming into our facility perhaps 1 day per week. Now, as she approaches her 70th birthday, Lottie is still performing the same program on an average of three to four times per week.

Mary P.

Mary was 97 years of age when she came in for exercise testing and a program of activity. She had been sedentary for 7 years because of an osteoarthritic knee but had decided she wished to become sufficiently active to take a trip to Ireland, her native country, for her 100th birthday. Mary was cleared for exercise by her physician, and baseline testing was initiated. Mary performed a very modified treadmill walking test, beginning at 0.75 mph and progressing to a symptom-limited (fatigue) 1.25 mph. On the basis of Mary's treadmill heart rate response of 110 bpm, her $\dot{V}o_2$max was estimated to be approximately 8 mL O_2/kg/ min, which is extremely low. By comparison, a $\dot{V}o_2$max of 4 to 5 mL O_2/kg/min is required for quiet sitting. Physical therapy evaluation revealed a woman in remarkable physical condition for her stated age, with no postural abnormalities or range-of-motion deficits. Lower extremity strength was good with the exception of knee extension on the right, which was limited by her painful arthritis. Mary walked with a cane, as she did not trust her knee, which exhibited 30 degrees of valgus deformity during stance. Mary was able to accomplish all personal activities of daily living (ADL) but could not get out of a bathtub, get off the floor, reach into low cupboards, ascend or descend stairs without a railing, or walk more than 100 ft. Mary's 67-year-old daughter lived with her and did all the housekeeping, food shopping and preparation, and chores. Apparently, Mary had become depressed when her knee began interfering with her ability to walk and get out, and she had not been out of the house, prior to her exercise appointment, for 7 years. Her daughter figured prominently in the decision to seek assistance.

Mary's very low $\dot{V}o_2$max and unstable knee precluded participation in any kind of conventional aerobic training, and thus a simple low-intensity activity program was chosen. Exercises consisted of general conditioning while sitting in a chair or standing while holding on to the back of the chair or wall. Examples of activity are (1) partial sit to stand and hold the position midway, slowly lower down; and (2) reaching toward the floor, first side to side and then frontwards. Exercises were done at a reasonably brisk pace, sometimes to music, and HR was kept at approximately 100 bpm. Exercises were done in blocks, starting with easy warm-ups and progressing to activities eliciting an HR in the desired range of 95 to 105 bpm. Typically, a rest would be given after 10 minutes of "aerobic" activity.

As an adjunct, Mary was fitted with a knee brace that did not correct her deformity but did give her more confidence in using her knee. The brace or the exercises (or possibly both) reduced the knee pain substantially, and Mary was able to walk further. As part of her program, Mary was encouraged to walk in from the car instead of being pushed in a wheelchair by her daughter.

Mary could have progressed to performing a home program but chose instead to continue coming in for activity. She enjoys the social nature of the program and looks forward to getting out of the house. Now she must decide between spending her 100th birthday in exercise class or going to Ireland.

Repeat treadmill testing reveals that Mary has increased her $\dot{V}o_2$max by an estimated 25%.

Ethel L.

Ethel L. had no real interest in exercise but wanted to accompany her husband on walks that had been prescribed for him as part of a cardiac rehabilitation program. She came in for testing as she wanted to be sure she was safe to exercise, and she did not know how to begin. Ethel was found to have limited exercise endurance, in part because of a low $\dot{V}o_2$max (18 mL O_2) and in part because of obesity. Ethel was 63 in. tall and weighed 246 lb. Physical therapy evaluation did not reveal any musculoskeletal abnormalities or other physical problems. She did have flat feet, for which appropriate shoes and orthotics were prescribed, and hip range of motion limited to -25 degrees of extension, which was reduced with selected stretches. Lower extremity strength was probably adequate, but given the heaviness of Ethel's legs, she could not get up and down from the ground nor climb stairs readily.

Ethel was taught how to take her own pulse and was given a program designed to elicit an HR response of between 93 and 116 bpm. A simple walking program on flat ground (no hills) at her normal or self-selected pace was adequate for the first 4 weeks to elicit the desired target HR response. Walking time was increased from 20 to 40 minutes over that 4-week period. The next phase of activity included walking for 40 minutes, walking up and down three flights of stairs, and 5 minutes of moderate-paced walking. Over the next month Ethel progressed to walking 35 minutes at a self-selected pace, walking 15 minutes at a moderate pace (brisk) and six flights of stairs. By the fourth month Ethel was able to progress to walking 40 minutes at a moderate pace, or 3 mph. Currently, Ethel is walking at a brisk pace for 20 minutes, walking at a "fast" pace for 30 minutes, and walking up and down six flights of stairs. Her heart rate response for this program is 125 bpm. She is enjoying her activity, typically walks 4 or 5 days a week at a local track, and finds she has the energy to do much more than she did previously. Ethel did have two bouts of knee pain during the first year of activity that were treated successfully by conservative means: ice, rest,

compression bandage, and ibuprofen. She must replace her shoes every 6 months as the foam bottoms out, causing foot fatigue and discomfort.

Liz F.

This 83-year-old client had a long history of osteoarthritis of the knees and hips, hypertension, asthma, and falling. She lived alone in a large apartment complex in which the majority of tenants were pensioners. Liz wanted an exercise program to improve her walking; she could not cross the street quickly enough to beat the stoplight, and she was exhausted by the time she reached the church where she did volunteer work. Additionally, Liz had fallen on numerous occasions while walking to the church and had sustained fractures of the wrist and coccyx.

Treadmill testing (symptom-limited) revealed an estimated $\dot{V}o_2$max of 12 mL O_2/min/kg. Dizziness and fatigue were problems during the stress test, where HR reached 108 bpm and BP rose to 165/95. The client also felt quite breathless for perhaps 5 minutes after the test was terminated.

Physical therapy evaluation revealed lower extremity strength of F+ to good, with deficiencies primarily in the muscles of weight bearing: plantar flexors, quadriceps, and hip abductors and extensors. Standing balance was diminished, with Liz accomplishing only two of the six stages of the sharpened Romberg. A cane was used during all walking activities inside the home and out. Range of motion was within normal limits with the exception of knee flexion, which was 110 degrees, and ankle dorsiflexion, which was 0. The client was able to dress herself and take care of the easier day-to-day chores. She had help with procuring groceries, cleaning, and laundry. She could not get out of the tub, get up from the floor, step up more than a 6-in. step, or ascend/descend stairs without a railing.

For the first 3 weeks, training consisted of relatively easy chair exercises to enhance strength and challenge balance while sitting or holding on to the chair while standing. Target HR range was 95 to 100 bpm. A walking program was initiated that started with a distance of 25 ft. Liz stood from a chair, walked 25 ft, rested a few seconds, and then returned to the chair while walking at a faster-than-normal pace. Walking was done next to the wall so that Liz could hold on to her cane with one hand and use the wall for balance as necessary. For the first few weeks, chair exercises for 20 minutes and three to four repetitions of the 50-ft walk were all that the client could tolerate. After a month, she could walk 50 ft without resting and at a slightly faster pace four times. After 2 months Liz walked 75 ft without resting, first at her self-selected pace, then 75 ft "briskly," then normally, and again "briskly." Ultimately the client progressed to walking briskly around the entire apartment complex, a distance of 220 ft, without resting and at a faster-than-normal pace. Walking on carpeted surfaces and up and down stairs will be added to the program in time. Liz is able to walk further without undue fatigue a little more quickly, *safely,* but still cannot get across the street before the light turns green, the ultimate goal of the program.

These case histories exemplify typical real-life situations in which clients are interested in exercise but do not know how to begin a safe and effective program, have some physical difficulties to accommodate, and have varying levels of ability. Exercise prescription was successful for each of these individuals because programs were tailored to their needs, physical capabilities, and desires. Significant gains in fitness have been made by all that have made a difference in functional capacity. Exercise works for nearly everyone.

EXERCISE AND INJURY

For the past 6 years, data related to the incidence of injury with exercise, in our in-house program, have been collected. Of the approximately 230 men and women over age 60 who have completed 3 months of stretching, strengthening, and flexibility exercise (low-intensity activity), only 3 have left the program because of painful conditions that developed secondary to exercise. Twenty percent of the participants developed some form of orthopedic discomfort, usually at the knee. Discomfort was transient, related, in all probability, to the novelty of the activity. With conservative measures—cessation of an activity for a day or two, modifying the activity, or icing—pain soon went away. Rarely was an exercise class missed because of a painful episode. Thus, low-intensity activities produced no discomfort in the vast majority of exercisers, most of whom were rather deconditioned.

High-intensity training, on the other hand, resulted in some form of painful episode in 72% of all participants. To date, 128 men and women between the ages of 60 and 72 years have completed at least 6 months of training (jogging, brisk walking, rowing, stationary bicycle). Most painful episodes were classified as nonspecific joint pain, probably of osteoarthritic origin, usually at the knee or foot-ankle complex. Again, conservative measures were successful for managing almost all complaints: icing, rest, elastic wrapping, modification of the exercise program, and nonsteroidal anti-inflammatory drugs. Seven people dropped out of the program because of a painful condition. The remainder either continued exercising even though a painful condition was present (we modified the exercise program to accommodate for the problem) or rested until the pain went away and then resumed training.

Results suggest that some form of orthopedic discomfort should be expected when endurance training older adults. If clients are told up front to expect an orthopedic problem, they will not become afraid of exercise when a problem arises. Additionally, if physical therapy care is provided immediately, fears are allayed and small painful episodes do not blossom into significant concerns. Thus, older adults in training need to understand that endurance training will probably result in some form of orthopedic discomfort and, when pain arises, that someone is there to provide needed care.

Do we feel the high incidence of orthopedic discomfort is a contraindication to exercise training? Absolutely not. The overwhelmingly positive effects of exercise far surpass the incidental and (usually) transient problems associated with increased activity. Proper exercise planning, which takes into account the physical capabilities of the client, previous history, fitness level, and interests, will likely promote change that has the potential to impact on physical and functional performance, fatigue, and numerous risk factors associated with cardiac disease. Exercise should be part of the daily routine for all adults, regardless of age.

SUMMARY

One of the factors that is most responsible for changes in cardiovascular functional capacity is a sedentary life-style. Older adults do have the ability to improve their cardiovascular condition by undertaking a systematic program of exercise, which can have a substantial impact on their functional status. Data from appropriate cardiac testing and measurements from a physical therapy evaluation can be used by physical therapists to design and implement a safe and effective training program for an older person.

REFERENCES

1. Adams GM, deVries HA: Physiological effects of an exercise training regimen upon women aged 52 to 79. *J Gerontol* 1973; 28:50–55.
2. American College of Sports Medicine: The recommended quantity and quality of exercise for developing and maintaining cardiorespiratory muscular fitness in healthy adults. *Med Sci Sports Exerc* 1990; 22:265–275.
3. Aniansson A, Hedberg M, Henning GB, et al: Muscle morphology, enzymatic activity, and muscle strength in elderly men: A follow-up study. *Muscle Nerve* 1986; 9:585–591.
4. Astrand I: The physical work capacity of workers 50–64 years old. *Acta Physiol Scand* 1958; 42:73–86.
5. Astrand I: Aerobic work capacity in men and women with

special reference to age. *Acta Physiol Scand* 1960; 49(suppl 169):92.

6. Astrand I, Astrand P-O, Hallback I, et al: Reduction in maximal oxygen intake with age. *J Appl Physiol* 1973; 35:649–654.

7. Astrand P-O, Rodahl K: *Textbook of Work Physiology.* New York, McGraw-Hill, 1986.

8. Badenhop DT, Cleary PA, Schaal SF, et al: Physiological adjustments to higher- or lower-intensity exercise in elders. *Med Sci Sports Exerc* 1983; 15:496–502.

9. Balke B: An experimental study of physical fitness of Air Force personnel. *US Armed Forces Med J* 1965; 20:745–750.

10. Barnard RJ, Ugianskis EJ, Martin DA, et al: Role of diet and exercise in the management of hyperinsulinemia and associated atherosclerotic risk factors. *Am J Cardiol* 1992; 69:440–444.

11. Barrett-Connor E, Wingard DL, Criqui MH: Postmenopausal estrogen use and heart disease risk factors in the 1980s. *JAMA* 1989; 261:2095–2100.

12. Barry AJ, Daly JW, Pruett EDR, et al: The effects of physical conditioning on older individuals. I. Work capacity, circulatory-respiratory function, and work electrocardiogram. *J Gerontol* 1966; 21:182–191.

13. Benestad AM: Trainability of old men. *Acta Med Scand* 1965; 178:321–327.

14. Berglund E, Birath G, Burke J, et al: Spirometric studies in normal subjects. I. Forced expirograms in subjects between 7 and 70 years of age. *Acta Med Scand* 1963; 173:185–206.

15. Binkhorst RA, Pool J, VanLeeuwen P, et al: Maximum oxygen uptake in healthy nonathletic men. *Int A Angew Physiol Einschl Arbeitsphysiol* 1965; 22:10–18.

16. Björntorp P: "Portal" adipose tissue as a generator of risk factors for cardiovascular disease and diabetes. *Arteriosclerosis* 1990; 10:493–496.

17. Blumenthal JA, Emery CF, Madden DJ, et al: Cardiovascular and behavioral effects of aerobic exercise training in healthy older men and women. *J Gerontol* 1989; 44:M147–157.

18. Borg G: Perceived exertion as an indicator of somatic stress. *Scand J Rehabil Med* 1970; 2:92–97.

19. Borkan GA, Hults DE, Gerzof SG, et al: Age changes in body composition revealed by computed tomography. *J Gerontol* 1983; 38:673–677.

20. Bruce RA: Maximal oxygen uptake and nonographic assessment of functional aortic impairment in cardiovascular disease. *Am Heart J* 1973; 85:545–557.

21. Bush TL, Barrett-Connor E, Cowan LD, et al: Cardiovascular mortality and noncontraceptive use of estrogen in women: Results from the Lipid Research Clinics Program Follow-up Study. *Circulation* 1987; 75:1102–1109.

22. Buskirk ER, Hodgson JL: Age and aerobic power: The rate of change in men and women. *Fed Proc* 1987; 46:1824–1829.

23. Campos H, Wilson PWF, Jiménez D, et al: Differences in apolipoproteins and low-density lipoprotein subfractions in postmenopausal women on and off estrogen therapy: Results from the Framingham Offspring Study. *Metabolism* 1990; 39:1033–1038.

24. Cartee GD, Young DA, Sleeper MD, et al: Prolonged increase in insulin-stimulated glucose transport in muscle after exercise. *Am J Physiol* 1989; 256:E494–E499.

25. Cavanaugh DJ, Cann CE: Brisk walking does not stop bone loss in postmenopausal women. *Bone* 1988; 9:201–204.

26. Cempla J, Szopa J: Decrease of maximum oxygen consumption in men and women during the fourth to sixth decades of life, in the light of cross-sectional studies of Cracow population. *Biol Sport* 1985; 2:45–59.

27. Chiang BN, Montoye HJ, Cunningham DA: Treadmill exercise study of healthy males in a total community—Tecumseh, Michigan: Clinical and electrocardiographic characteristics. *Am J Epidemiol* 1970; 91:368–377.

28. Coggan AR, Spina RJ, King DS, et al: Skeletal muscle adaptations to endurance training in 60–69 year old men and women. *J Appl Physiol,* 1992; 72:1780–1786.

29. Convertino VA, Goldwater DJ, Sandler H: Bedrest-induced peak Vo_2 reduction association with age, gender and aerobic capacity. *Aviat Space Environ Med* 1986; 57:17–22.

30. Cunningham DA, Rechnitzer PA, Howard JH, et al: Exercise training of men at retirement: A clinical trial. *J Gerontol* 1987; 42:17–23.

31. Dalsky GP, Stocke KS, Ehsani AA, et al: Weight-bearing exercise training and lumbar bone mineral content in postmenopausal women. *Ann Intern Med* 1988; 108:824–828.

32. Davidson MB: The effect of aging on carbohydrate metabolism: A review of the English literature and a practical approach to the diagnosis of diabetes mellitus in the elderly. *Metabolism* 1979; 28:688–705.

33. Davies CTM: The oxygen transporting system in relation to age. *Clin Sci* 1972; 42:1–13.

34. DeFronzo RA: Glucose intolerance and aging: Evidence for tissue insensitivity to insulin. *Diabetes* 1979; 28:1095–1101.

35. Dehn MM, Bruce RA: Longitudinal variations in maximal oxygen intake with age and activity. *J Appl Physiol* 1972; 33:805–807.

36. Després J-P, Moorjani S, Lupien PJ, et al: Regional distribution of body fat, plasma lipoproteins, and cardiovascular disease. *Arteriosclerosis* 1990; 10:497–511.

37. Després J-P, Pouliot MC, Moorjani S, et al: Loss of abdominal fat and metabolic response to exercise training in obese women. *Am J Physiol* 1991; 24:E159–E167.

38. deVries HA: Physiological effects of an exercise training regimen upon men aged 52 to 88. *J Gerontol* 1970; 25:325–336.

39. deVries HA, Adams GM: Comparison of exercise responses in old and young men: II. Ventilatory mechanics. *J Gerontol* 1972; 27:349–352.

40. Drinkwater BL, Horvath SM, Wells CL: Aerobic power in females, ages 10 to 68. *J Gerontol* 1975; 30:385–394.

41. Dunbar CC, Robertson RJ, Baun R, et al: The validity of regulating exercise intensity by ratings of perceived exertion. *Med Sci Sports Exerc* 1992; 24:94–99.

42. Durnin JV, Wormesly J: Body fat assessed from total body density and its estimation from skinfold thickness: Measurements on 481 men and women aged from 16 to 72 years. *Br J Nutr* 1974; 32:77–97.

43. Enzi G, Gasparo M, Biondetti PR, et al: Subcutaneous and visceral fat distribution according to sex, age, and overweight, evaluated by computed tomography. *Am J Clin Nutr* 1986; 44:739–746.

44. Flack JM, and Sowers JR: Epidemiologic and clinical aspects of insulin resistance and hyperinsulinemia. *Am J Med* 1991; 91(suppl 1A): 11S–21S.

45. Fleg JL, Lakatta EG: Role of muscle loss in the age-associated reduction in Vo_2max. *J Appl Physiol* 1988; 65:1147–1151.

46. Fleg JL, Tzankoff SP, Lakatta EG: Age-related augmentation of plasma catecholamines during dynamic exercise in healthy males. *J Appl Physiol* 1985; 59:1033–1039.

47. Gerstenblith G, Lakatta EG, Weisfeldt ML: Age changes in myocardial function and exercise response. *Progr Cardiovasc Dis* 1976; 19:1–21.

48. Gleeson PB, Protas EJ, LeBlanc AD, et al: Effects of weight lifting on bone mineral density in premenopausal women. *J Bone Miner Res* 1990; 5:153–158.

49. Gonza ER, Marble AE, Shaw A, et al: Age-related changes in the mechanics of the aorta and pulmonary artery of man. *J Appl Physiol* 1974; 36:407–411.

50. Grimby G, Danneskiold-Samsoe B, Hvid K, et al: Morphology and enzymatic capacity in arm and leg muscles in 78–81 year old men and women. *Acta Physiol Scand* 1982; 115:125–134.

51. Grimby G, Saltin B: Physiologic analysis of physically well-trained middle-aged and old athletes. *Acta Med Scand* 1968; 179:513–523.

52. Hagberg JM, Allen WK, Seals DR, et al: A hemodynamic comparison of young and older endurance athletes during exercise. *J Appl Physiol* 1985; 58:2041–2046.

53. Hagberg JM, Graves JE, Limacher M, et al: Cardiovascular responses to 70- to 79-year-old men and women to exercise training. *J Appl Physiol* 1989; 66:2589–2594.

54. Hagberg JM, Montain SJ, Martin WHI, et al: Effect of exercise training in 60- to 69-year-old persons with essential hypertension. *Am J Cardiol* 1991; 64:348–353.

55. Hagberg JM, Seals DR, Yerg JE, et al: Metabolic responses to exercise in young and older athletes and sedentary men. *J Appl Physiol* 1988; 65:900–908.

56. Heath GW, Gavin JR III, Hinderliter JM, et al: Effects of exercise and lack of exercise on glucose tolerance and insulin sensitivity. *J Appl Physiol* 1983; 55:512–517.

57. Heath GW, Hagberg JM, Ehsani AA, et al: A physiological comparison of young and older endurance athletes. *J Appl Physiol* 1981; 51:634–640.

58. Hermansen L, Saltin B: Oxygen uptake during maximal treadmill and bicycle exercise. *J Appl Physiol* 1969; 26:31–37.

59. Higginbotham MB, Morris KG, Williams RS, et al: Physiologic basis for the age-related decline in aerobic work capacity. *Am J Cardiol* 1986; 57:1374–1379.

60. Hodgson JL, Buskirk ER: Physical fitness and age, with emphasis on cardiovascular function in the elderly. *J Am Geriatr Soc* 1977; 25:385–392.

61. Holloszy JO, Schultz J, Kusnierkiewicz J, et al: Effects of exercise on glucose tolerance and insulin resistance. *Acta Med Scand Suppl* 1986; 711:55–65.

62. Horvath SM, Borgia JF: Cardiopulmonary gas transport and aging. *Am Rev Respir Dis* 1984; 129(suppl):568–571.

63. Hossack KF, Bruce RA: Maximal cardiac function in sedentary normal men and women: comparison of age-related changes. *J Appl Physiol* 1982; 53:799–804.

64. Julius S, Antoon A, Whitlock LS, et al: Influence of age on the hemodynamic response to exercise. *Circulation* 1967; 36:222–230.

65. Kaijser L, Sachs C: Autonomic cardiovascular responses in old age. *Clin Physiol* 1985; 5:347–357.

66. Kenney RA: *Physiology of Aging: A Synopsis*. Chicago, Year Book Medical Publishers, 1982, p 42.

67. King DS, Dalsky GP, Clutter WE, et al: Effects of exercise and lack of exercise on insulin secretion. *Am J Physiol* 1988; 254:E537–E542.

68. King DS, Dalsky GP, Clutter WE, et al: Effects of exercise and lack of exercise on insulin sensitivity and responsiveness. *J Appl Physiol* 1988; 64:1942–1946.

69. King DS, Dalsky GP, Staten MA, et al: Insulin action and secretion in endurance trained and untrained people. *J Appl Physiol* 1987; 63:2247–2252.

70. King DS, Staten MA, Kohrt WM, et al: Insulin secretory capacity in endurance-trained and untrained young men. *Am J Physiol* 1990; 259:E155–E181.

71. Kline G, Parcari JP, Hintermeister R, et al: Estimated Vo_2max from a one-mile track walk, gender, age, and body weight. *Med Sci Sports Exerc* 1987; 19:253–259.

72. Kohrt WM, Malley MT, Coggan AR, et al: Effects of gender, age, and fitness level on response of Vo_2max to training in 60- to 71-year-olds. *J Appl Physiol* 1991; 71:2004–2011.

73. Kohrt WM, Malley MT, Dalsky GP, et al: Body composition of healthy sedentary and trained, young and older men and women. *Med Sci Sports Exerc*, 1992; 24:832–837.

74. Kohrt WM, Obert KA, Holloszy JO: Exercise training improves fat distribution patterns in 60- to 70-yr-old men and women. *J Gerontol* 1992; 47:M99–105.

75. Kohrt WM, Snead DB: Effect of exercise on bone mass in the elderly, in Perry HM III, Morley JE, Coe RM (eds): *Aging, Musculoskeletal Disorders and Care of the Frail Elderly*. New York, Springer, in press.

76. LeBlanc AD, Schneider VS, Evans HJ, et al: Bone mineral loss and recovery after 17 weeks of bed rest. *J Bone Miner Res* 1990; 5:843–850.

77. Leon AS, Connett J, Jacobs DRJ, et al: Leisure-time physical activity levels and risk of coronary heart disease and death. *JAMA* 1987; 258:2388–2395.

78. Lynne-Davies P: Influence of age on the respiratory system. *Geriatrics* 1977; 32:57–62.

79. MacKeen PC, Rosenberger JL, Slater JS, et al: A 13-year follow-up of a coronary heart disease risk factor screening and exercise program for 40- to 59-year-old men: Exercise

habit maintenance and physiologic status. *J Cardiac Rehabil* 1985; 5:510–523.

80. Mahler DA, Harver A: Prediction of peak oxygen consumption in obstructive airway disease. *Med Sci Sports Exerc* 1988; 20:574–578.

81. Makrides L, Heigenhauser GJF, Jones NL: High-intensity endurance training in 20- to 30- and 60- to 70-yr-old healthy men. *J Appl Physiol* 1990; 69:1792–1798.

82. Mann DL, Deneberg BS, Gash AK, et al: Effects of age on ventricular performance during graded supine exercise. *Am Heart J* 1986; 111:108–115.

83. Martin WH III, Kohrt WM, Malley MT, et al: Exercise training enhances leg vasodilatory capacity of 65-year-old men and women. *J Appl Physiol* 1990; 69:1804–1809.

84. Mikines KJ, Sonne B, Farrell PA, et al: Effect of physical exercise on sensitivity and responsiveness to insulin in humans. *Am J Physiol* 1988; 254:E248–E259.

85. Morey ER, Baylink DJ: Inhibition of bone formation during space flight. *Science* 1978; 201:1138–1141.

86. Morgan DW, Kohrt WM, Bates BJ, et al: Effects of respiratory muscle endurance training on ventilatory and endurance performance of moderately trained cyclists. *Int J Sports Med* 1987; 8:88–93.

87. Morris JN, Everitt MG, Pollard R, et al: Vigorous exercise in leisure-time: Protection against coronary heart disease. *Lancet* 1980; 2:1207–1210.

88. Niinimaa V, Shephard RJ: Training and oxygen conductance in the elderly. I. The respiratory system. *J Gerontol* 1978; 33:354–361.

89. Orlander J, Kiessling K-H, Larson L, et al: Skeletal muscle metabolism and ultrastructure in relation to age in sedentary men. *Acta Physiol Scand* 1978; 104:249–261.

90. Paffenbarger RS, Hyde RT, Wing AL, et al: A natural history of athleticism and cardiovascular health. *JAMA* 1984; 252:491–495.

91. Paffenbarger RS, Hyde RT, Wing AL, et al: Physical activity, all cause mortality and longevity of college alumni. *N Engl J Med* 1986; 314:605–613.

92. Palmer GH, Ziegler MG, Lake CR: Response of norepinephrine and blood pressure to stress increases with age. *J Gerontol* 1978; 33:482–487.

93. Pariskova J, Eiselt E, Sprynarova S, et al: Body composition, aerobic capacity and density of muscle capillaries in young and old men. *J Appl Physiol* 1971; 31:323–325.

94. Patrick JM, Bassey EJ, Fentem PH: The rising ventilatory cost of bicycle exercise in the seventh decade: A longitudinal study of nine healthy men. *Clin Sci* 1983; 65:521–526.

95. Peiris AN, Sothmann MS, Hoffmann RG, et al: Adiposity, fat distribution, and cardiovascular risk. *Ann Intern Med* 1989; 110:867–872.

96. Pollock ML, Carroll JF, Craves JE, et al: Injuries and adherence to walk/jog and resistance training programs in the elderly. *Med Sci Sports Exerc* 1991; 23:1194–1200.

97. Pollock ML, Foster C, Knapp D, et al: Effect of age and training on aerobic capacity and body composition of master athletes. *J Appl Physiol* 1987; 62:725–731.

98. Profant GR, Early RG, Nilson KL, et al: Responses to maximal exercise in healthy middle-aged women. *J Appl Physiol* 1972; 33:595–599.

99. Reaven GM: Insulin resistance and compensatory hyperinsulinemia: Role in hypertension, dyslipidemia, and coronary heart disease. *Am Heart J* 1991; 121:1283–1288.

100. Reaven GM: Insulin resistance, hyperinsulinemia, and hypertriglyceridemia in the etiology and clinical course of hypertension. *Am J Med* 1991, 90(suppl 2A):7S–12S.

101. Rivera AM, Pels AE III, Sady SP, et al: Physiological factors associated with the lower maximal oxygen consumption of master runners. *J Appl Physiol* 1989; 66:949–954.

102. Robinson S, Dill DB, Tzankoff SP, et al: Longitudinal studies of aging in 37 men. *J Appl Physiol* 1975; 38:263–267.

103. Rockwell JC, Sorensen AM, Baker S, et al: Weight training decreases vertebral bone density in premenopausal women: A prospective study. *J Clin Endocrinol Metab* 1990; 71:988–993.

104. Rodeheffer RJ, Gerstenblith G, Becker LC, et al: Exercise cardiac output is maintained with advancing age in healthy human subjects: Cardiac dilatation and increased stroke volume compensate for diminished heart rate. *Circulation* 1984; 69:203–213.

105. Rogers MA, Hagberg JM, Martin WH III, et al: Decline in Vo_2max with aging in master athletes and sedentary men. *J Appl Physiol* 1990; 68:2195–2199.

106. Rogers MA, King DS, Hagberg JM, et al: Effect of 10 days of inactivity on glucose tolerance in master athletes. *J Appl Physiol* 1990; 68:1833–1837.

107. Rogers MA, Yamamoto C, Hagberg JM, et al: The effect of 7 years of intense exercise training on patients with coronary artery disease. *J Am Coll Cardiol* 1987; 10:321–326.

108. Rogers MA, Yamamoto C, King DS, et al: Improvement in glucose tolerance after one week of exercise in patients with mild NIDDM. *Diabetes Care* 1988; 11:613–618.

109. Rubin CP, Scott PJ, McLean K, et al: Noradrenaline release and clearance in relation to age and blood pressure in man. *Eur J Clin Invest* 1982; 12:121–125.

110. Saltin B, Hartley L, Kilbom A, et al: Physical training in sedentary middle-aged and older men. *Scand J Clin Lab Invest* 1969; 24:323–334.

111. Schmidt CD, Dickman ML, Gardner RM, et al: Spirometric standards for healthy elderly men and women. *Am Rev Respir Dis* 1973; 108:933–939.

112. Schwartz RS, Shuman WP, Larson V, et al: The effect of intensive endurance exercise training on body fat distribution in young and older men. *Metabolism* 1991; 40:545–551.

113. Seals DR, Hagberg JM, Allen WK, et al: Glucose tolerance in young and older athletes and sedentary men. *J Appl Physiol* 1984; 56:1521–1525.

114. Seals DR, Hagberg JM, Hurley BF, et al: Effects of endurance training on glucose tolerance and plasma lipids in older men and women. *JAMA* 1984; 252:645–649.

115. Seals DR, Hagberg JM, Hurley BF, et al: Endurance training in older men and women. I. Cardiovascular re-

sponses to exercise. *J Appl Physiol* 1984; 57:1024–1029.

116. Shephard RJ: World standards of cardiorespiratory performance. *Arch Environ Health* 1966; 13:664–672.

117. Shephard RJ: Assessment of physical activity and energy needs. *Am J Clin Nutr* 1989; 50(suppl):1195–1200.

118. Shimokata H, Tobin JD, Muller DC, et al: Studies in the distribution of body fat: I. Effects of age, sex, and obesity. *J Gerontol* 1989; 44:M66–M73.

119. Shocken DD, Blumenthal JA, Port S, et al: Physical conditioning and left ventricular performance in the elderly; assessment by radionuclide angiocardiography. *Am J Cardiol* 1983; 52:359–364.

120. Sidney KH, Shephard RJ: Maximum and submaximum exercise tests in men and women in the seventh, eighth and ninth decades of life. *J Appl Physiol* 1977; 43:280–287.

121. Smith EL, Gilligan C: Physical activity prescription for the elderly. *Phys Sports Med* 1983; 11:91–101.

122. Snow-Harter C, Marcus R: Exercise, bone mineral density, and osteoporosis, in Holloszy JO (ed): *Exercise and Sport Sciences Reviews,* Baltimore, Williams & Wilkins, 1991, pp 351–388.

123. Suominen H, Hiekkinen E, Liesen H, et al: Effects of 8 weeks' endurance training on skeletal muscle metabolism in 56–70-year-old sedentary men. *Eur J Appl Physiol* 1977; 37:173–180.

124. Tejada C, Strong JP, Montenegro MR, et al: Distribution of coronary and aortic atherosclerosis by geographic location, race, and sex. *Lab Invest* 1968; 18:509–526.

125. Thomas SG, Cunningham DA, Rechnitzer PA, et al: De-terminants of the training response in elderly men. *Med Sci Sports Exerc* 1985; 17:667–672.

126. Vogel JA, Patton JF, Mello RP, et al: An analysis of aerobic capacity in a large United States population. *J Appl Physiol* 1986; 60:494–500.

127. Wahren J, Saltin B, Jorfeldt L, et al: Influences of age on the local circulatory adaptation to leg exercise. *Scand J Clin Lab Invest* 1974; 33:79–86.

128. Weisfeldt ML: Aging of the cardiovascular system. *N Engl J Med* 1980; 303:1172–1173.

129. Wood PD, Stefanick ML, Williams PT, et al: The effects on plasma lipoproteins of a prudent weight-reducing diet, with or without exercise, in overweight men and women. *N Engl J Med* 1991; 325:461–466.

130. Yerg JE II, Seals DR, Hagberg JM, et al: Effect of endurance exercise training on ventilatory function in older individuals. *J Appl Physiol* 1985; 58:791–794.

131. Yiengst MJ, Barrows CH Jr, Shock NW: Age changes in the chemical composition of muscle and liver in the rat. *J Gerontol* 1959; 14:400–404.

132. Yin FCP, Spurgeon HA, Kallman CH: Age associated decrease in viscoelastic properties of canine aortic strips. *Circ Res* 1983; 53:464–472.

133. Young JB, Rowe JW, Pallotta JA, et al: Enhanced plasma norepinephrine response to upright posture and oral glucose administration in elderly human subjects. *Metabolism* 1980; 29:532–539.

134. Ziegler MG, Lake CR, Kopin IJ: Plasma noradrenaline increases with age. *Nature* 1976; 261:333–335.

Posture in the Older Adult

Carolee Moncur, Ph.D., P.T.

INTRODUCTION

When one is asked to imagine a picture of the posture of an elderly person, too often the image visualized is that of a bent or stooped individual who, more often than not, is of the female gender and of fragile constitution (Fig 14–1). Often, previous experience as a student or clinician has created a picture of the posture of only those elderly persons who are confined to nursing homes or similar circumstances.

Posture can be a statement about an individual. It may be an outward demonstration of wellness, illness, self-esteem (or the lack thereof), the vicissitudes of life, or simply the processes of development or aging. As physical therapists, it is important to decipher between the circumstances to be expected as a result of aging and those conditions extraneous to growing old, thereby altering upright posture.

The purpose of this chapter is to review these parameters and to demonstrate the process of designing and implementing a physical therapy plan of care for common postural problems seen in the elderly person. It is imperative that posture be evaluated on an individual basis as, in the case of other human characteristics, the upright position has great variability among this population of people.

POSTURE THROUGH THE LIFE SPAN

Development of Upright Posture

During fetal life, childhood, and adolescence, increase in the number of cells is of prime importance to growth of the body systems responsible for the development of posture. The central nervous system matures concurrent with the continuous changes occurring in the musculoskeletal system. Martin suggests that children develop postural control in various stages corresponding with their ability to integrate sensory information.[65] In the early years, vision is the primary source used to reinforce upright orientation, with the proprioceptive systems being of secondary importance. In order to effectively develop proprioception as a mode of input, the child must continue to practice motor skills to perfect the system.

Aging of the child, as well as increased use of the somatosensory and vestibular systems, enhances the adaptation of the individual to the upright position. The somatosensory systems continue to be the primary sources used by both children and adults to achieve postural stability.[36] It is important to appreciate that, notwithstanding the importance of the nervous system, other factors must develop parallel with the development of movement such as strength and endurance against gravity. This of course requires the appropriate integration of healthy cardiopulmo-

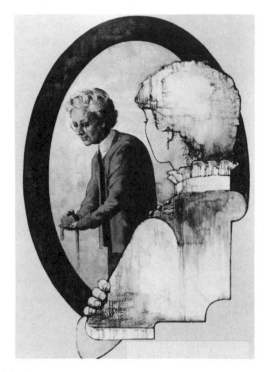

FIG 14–1.
Traditional perception of elderly posture. (Adapted from *Osteoporosis: Is It in Your Future?* Kansas, Mo, Marion Laboratories, Pharmaceutical Division, 1986. Used by permission.)

nary, musculoskeletal, and neuromuscular systems. In essence, posture is derived from the relationship of body parts to one another as well as the maturation and interaction of a number of body systems.[56, 104, 105] Once postural control has been established, the child can begin coordinated, sequential movements about the environment.[65]

A brief description of the development of posture would not be complete if some comment were not made regarding the influence of psychosocial factors on the upright position. In the pre–school-age youngster, parental and sibling influences affect the mobility of the child and can give rise to the intensity, duration, and selection of activity in which the child participates. When boys and girls enter school, obvious differences begin to appear with respect to motor behavior, as demonstrated by Hayes and coworkers.[45] Physical growth during adolescence, as well as other changes associated with that time period, can have an important effect on the individual's belief in oneself. Fears of being different from peers may interfere with self-image and be reflected in the youth's posture.[45]

Since it is outside the scope of this chapter to elaborate on the theories of aging, we will assume for our purposes that growth, development, and differentiation of the human continues throughout life and does not stop at young adulthood.[98] Furthermore, it will be assumed that the elderly are those who have had long lives with varied experiences that demonstrate great differentiation. How the elder person maintains the capacity to adapt to the growth and changes of life will decide how the individual will master the tasks of later maturity and old age, including optimizing upright posture.[16]

Factors Influencing Postural Changes During Senescence

It is clear that one person who is elderly is not the same as another person who is elderly. *Variability* is the important word to keep in mind as we discuss postural changes characteristic of aging. The description here will be of what one might find to be typical or reflective of the aging process; however, it should be recognized that the posture of the individual may be altered or changed by disease, medication, trauma, state of mind, or the setting and time of day when you are evaluating the person.

Musculoskeletal Changes

Some authors draw a fine line between decreases occurring in the density of long bones and the vertebral column due to aging changes in bone mineral balance and decreases that result in osteopenic or more severe osteoporotic bone. Results of scientific studies have demonstrated that a decrease of height or stature can generally be expected due to senescence.[25, 96]

Age-related changes in bone density differ from site to site. Bone mineral at peripheral sites (such as the radius) remains relatively stable until menopause, but bone loss of the spine and neck of the femur occurs 5 to 10 years earlier, respectively. Simply stated, bone changes during aging occur earlier in the spine than in the limbs.[69] Bone loss in men occurs at a rate of about 0.4% per year, beginning at age 50, and does not characteristically become problematic until the male is in his 80s.[68,69] In both men and women between the ages of 60 and 80 years, the average rate of decrease in height is about 2 cm per decade and may be as much as a total of 12 cm in extreme cases of bone loss.[24]

These changes commence around age 40 and are more noticeable in women than in men, likely due to the increased vulnerability for women to lose bone mass. In aging women, bone loss begins at 0.75% to 1% per year beginning at age 30 to 35 years. A higher rate (2% to 3%) of bone mineral loss occurs after menopause. A greater loss occurs in the spine the first 5 years after menopause than during the subsequent 15 years of the woman's life.[41] At this rate, women may lose 30% of bone mineral mass of the spine by 70 years of age. Interestingly, bone mineral loss does not occur as readily in overweight women.[86] Longcope et al. suggested that this is a consequence of peripheral estrogen production by adipose tissue.[62]

Since the upright posture of an individual is reflected dramatically in the spine and related structures, discussion will concentrate on the life span changes in the musculoskeletal properties of these structures. The focus will be limited to the intervertebral disks, spine ligaments, vertebrae, ribs, articular cartilage, entheses, muscles, and related biomechanics.

Age-related change in the *intervertebral disk* is a well-known phenomenon occurring throughout the life span, beginning about 30 years of age.[77, 113] Briefly, the intervertebral disks are composed of fibroblasts, collagen, elastin, and a polysaccharide ground substance consisting of hyaluronic acid and proteoglycans. While serving various functions, the individual disk is subjected to considerable forces and moments throughout the life span. In concert with the facet joints, it is responsible for responding to the compressive loads placed on the trunk.[46, 85] Nachemson et al.[74, 76, 113] have described these forces, stating that the forces on a disk are greater during the standing anatomic position than the weight of the portion of the body above it. Sitting position is another matter. When it comes to the forces on the lumbar disks, the summation of forces on the lumbar spine during sitting is greater than three times the weight of the trunk.[74, 76] Dynamic loads such as jumping or running will obviously increase the forces to perhaps twice as high as those in standing or sitting.[10] Not only are intervertebral disks subjected to compressive stresses[17, 30, 46, 47, 64, 87, 109]; they must also endure tensile stress[17, 39, 113] and axial rotation of the trunk, which results in shear stresses.[17, 30, 31, 47, 52, 64]

Anatomically, the intervertebral disk constitutes 20% to 30% of the cumulative height of the spinal column.[113] The disk is composed of a nucleus pulposus, an annulus fibrosus, and the cartilaginous end plates. Centrally located, the nucleus pulposus is composed of a loose, translucent network of fibers that lie in a mucoprotein gel containing a variety of mucopolysaccharides. The water content of the nucleus ranges from 70% to 90%, being highest at birth and diminishing in amount with age. The relative size of the nucleus to the total disk area depends on where it is located in the bony column, with the nuclei of the lumbar spine being 30% to 50% of the disk area.

The annulus fibrosus is composed of fibroelastic tissue arranged in concentrically laminated bands that are arranged in a helicoid fashion. Any two adjacent bands demonstrate fibers that run in opposite directions from each other (Fig 14–2) such that the fibers of two bands are oriented at 120 degrees to each other. The annulus fibers are attached to the cartilaginous end plates on the inner zone of the vertebral body, while peripherally they are attached by Sharpey's fibers to the edges of the body. The cartilaginous end plate is composed of hyaline cartilage and separates the nucleus and annulus from the vertebral body.[113]

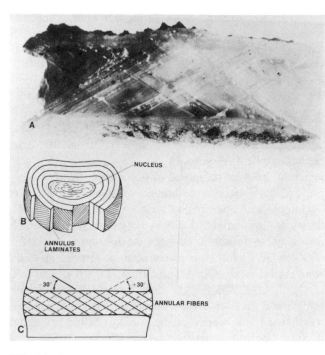

FIG 14–2.
Components of the intervertebral disc. **A,** photograph of a disk showing the annular fibers and their orientation. **B,** drawing of the lamellar configuration of the annular fibers. **C,** orientation of fibers at about 30 degrees with respect to placement of the disk. (From White AA, Panjabi MM: *Clinical Biomechanics of the Spine.* Philadelphia, JB Lippincott, 1978. Used by permission.)

In general, aging alters both the properties and the relative proportion of the connective tissue elements of the disk. Specifically, there is an increase in the stability and density of collagen with the exception of some tissues such as the skin.[67] With aging, elastin becomes less distensible and can undergo fragmentation. Collagen molecules forming elastin may change either by degradation or by incorrect synthesis, resulting in an intermediate form of elastin called pseudoelastin.[96] This departure from normal collagen fibers is predominantly found in the exposed dermis of the neck of the elderly person.

The nucleus pulposus contains considerable water and mucopolysaccharides that coalesce as a gelatinous mass up to about age 25 to 30. This anatomic feature is significant in protecting the spinal elements when the vertebrae are subjected to stress and loads. Alterations of these constituents found in the disk may cause it to collapse, thus diminishing the height of the individual as well as decreasing the soft yellow core of pulpy elastic material that forms the nucleus pulposus.[76]

The *ligaments of the spine* are depicted in Fig 14–3. Ligaments surrounding any anatomic structure act much like guy wires and/or rubber bands with respect to their function. In the spine, one might conceptualize that the ligaments respond to tensile forces by becoming taut. The reverse is true when the spine is subjected to compressive loads; namely, the collagen fibers in ligaments buckle and become slack. Ligaments allow mobility in the spine while maintaining fixed postural relationships between vertebrae. Additionally, they need to do this with the least amount of effort. This suggests that as long as the spinal column is healthy, properly aligned, and supported by strong musculature and ligaments, upright posture will be sustained. However, should the ligaments be maintained in a slackened position, changes will occur in postural patterns. The tensile ability of the ligaments of the spine degenerates with age. In an extensive study on 484 samples, Tkaczuk determined that the tensile characteristics of both the anterior and posterior ligaments of the lumbar spine decreased with age.[106] This was particularly true of the ligaments' ability to respond to shock absorption. Likewise, Nachemson and Evans determined that the ligamentum flavum declines in its ability to perform "resting" tension upon the spine. This duty is important in lending to the stability of the spine.[75] Without the tensile strength in ligaments and resultant laxity, it seems apparent that these changes might contribute to the flexed forward posture of the elderly person.

Studies of the strength characteristics of the *human vertebra* began over 100 years ago and have received considerable attention since that time.[1, 8, 72, 84, 110] It has been observed that the vertebra decreases in strength with age, particularly beyond age 40. Figure 14–4 depicts the results of an investigation by Bell and associates that demonstrates that there is a definite relationship between the strength (stress of failure) and relative ash content (osseous tissue) of the vertebra.[8] These data indicate that vertebral strength is lost with age and is directly related to the decrease in the amount of bone. Furthermore, a small loss of osseous tissue produces considerable decrease in vertebral bone strength. As seen in Fig 14–4, a 25% loss in osseous tissue results in a greater than 50% decrease of strength of a vertebra.[8]

The separate components of the vertebra—including the body,[8, 83, 110] cortical shell,[7, 8, 88, 110] cancellous core,[61, 88] endplates,[84,89] neural arch,[57, 90, 111] and facets[30, 32, 54, 74, 81, 112, 114]—have been investigated to determine the response of each to compressive loads on the spine. To summarize this literature, it has been determined that cancellous bone contributes 25% to 55% of the strength to the lumbar vertebrae. Under 40 years of age, 55% of the load is carried by the cancellous core, and after 40 years, this share decreases to about 35%.[66] Failure patterns in the end plates of vertebrae can be central or peripheral or involve the entire end plate.[84, 89] Strength in the neural arch decreases with age, and when loaded with compressive forces, the arch is most likely to fail through

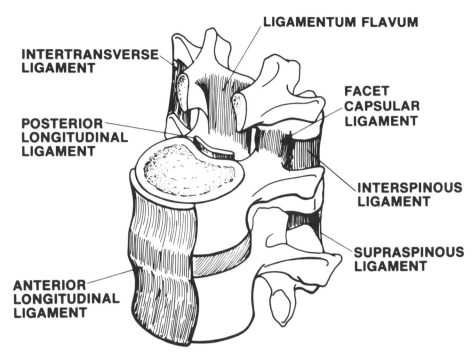

FIG 14–3.
Ligaments of the spine. (From White AA, Panjabi MM: *Clinical Biomechanics of the Spine.* Philadelphia, JB Lippincott, 1978. Used by permission.)

the pedicles.[57] The facet joints appear to carry about 18% of the total compressive load borne by a motion segment.[74] However, King and colleagues determined that the share of the load carried by the facets could be from 33% to 0%, depending on the spinal postures.[54]

Atkinson et al.[6, 26] evaluated the vertebral trabecular bone to determine the age-related patterns. The earliest changes seen were related to the orientation of the trabeculae from horizontal to vertical structures. The horizontal trabeculae were decreased first; however, there was a concomitant thickening of some of the vertical trabeculae. Therefore, there was no appreciable loss of osseous tissue on the whole until age 50 but rather a decrease in the mechanical strength of the vertebral body due to the loss of the horizontal trabeculae.

Not only was there a loss in the horizontal trabeculae; the loss was in the central region of the vertebral body, whereas the peripheral trabeculae were largely unaltered. The implication is that the loss of strength with age is preferential to the center of the vertebrae. Microcollapse of the vertebral body, not sufficient to be diagnosed as osteoporosis, may contribute to the reduction in height that an elderly person experiences. Extensive collapse correlates well with the clinical findings of central collapse of the body in individuals who have developed osteoporosis.[68,69]

It is difficult to determine the contribution of the *rib cage* or its components to the inherent stability of the

spine. The individual components of the rib cage may be quite flexible. However, using mathematical modeling on a computer, Andriacchi and colleagues studied a variety of simulations to determine the effects of the rib cage on the stiffness properties of the normal spine, on the stability of the normal spine under axial compression, and on the scoliotic spine subjected to traction.[3] Essentially, the results demonstrated that the stiffness properties of the spine were found to be greatly increased by the presence of the rib cage during various spinal motions. The rib cage was also found to increase the mechanical stability of the spine by four times when a compression load was placed on it. Finally, while traction increased axial stiffness in the normal spine 40% due to the presence of a rib cage, this was not the case in a scoliotic spine. Flexibility in the scoliotic spine with a rib cage was found to be 2½ times greater, which might be attributed to the abnormal geometric curvature found in scoliosis.[3] One might conjecture that changes occurring in the geometric relationship of the ribs and the spinal column due to aging could reduce its stiffness and ability to maintain an upright position.

Articular cartilage, with similar components found in other connective tissues, likewise undergoes change. Healthy cartilage in fresh cadavers is translucent, glistening, and pearl-like, whereas the cartilage of older cadavers is opaque and yellow and may have undergone some decrease in thickness. So a reduction in the thickness of the articular cartilage of the lower extremities in particular will

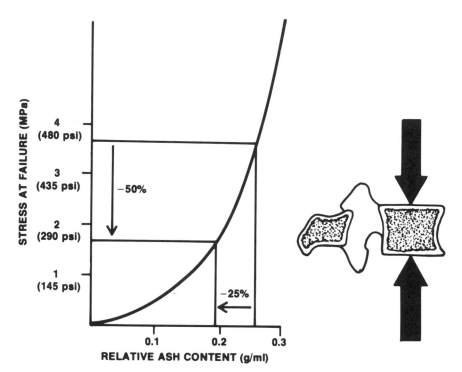

FIG 14–4.
Relationship between osseous tissue and vertebral strength. (From Bell GH, et al: *Calcif Tissue Res* 1967; 1:75–86. Adapted from White AA, Panjabi MM: *Clinical Biomechanics of the Spine.* Philadelphia, JB Lippincott, 1978. Used by permission.)

contribute to the decrease of upright height. Degenerative joint disease may be present in some specimens but should not be equated with age-related changes in the cartilage. Rather, while there are age-related changes in the structure of the collagen—including a loss of resilience, decreases in the content and aggregation of the hydrophilic proteoglycans (chondroitin and keratin sulfate side chains), and a decrease in the length of the chondroitin chains in articular cartilage[11]—this does not mean that joint disease will occur. It does mean that there is an increased possibility that the articular cartilage could sustain microfractures or damage[19] from forces such as overuse, obesity, trauma, metabolic disease, or hereditary factors.

For practicing physical therapists, it is not uncommon to see older individuals who have participated in a physical activity that has caused a sprain, strain, or rupture of a muscle or tendon. Age-related changes modify not only the tendon but also the *entheses.* These changes unfortunately make the older person more vulnerable to injury of tendons by reducing the distensibility of the collagen and elastic fiber when pressed to complete vigorous activity. Indirectly, the tendinous age-related changes may contribute to the alterations in upright posture.

Last and extremely important are the aging changes that occur in *muscular tissue.* It has been demonstrated for quite some time by various authors[2, 4, 5, 35, 42, 58, 60, 107] that muscle strength peaks at about 30 years of age and re-

mains constant to about 50 years, whereupon it begins to show an accelerating loss somewhat parallel to the decline of lean body tissue (Fig 14–5). It has been demonstrated that there is a reduction of myosin adenosine triphosphatase (ATPase) activity as well as a selective decrease in the number of fast twitch, type II muscle fibers as one ages. This tends to explain why there is a lengthening of the time to peak tension, a decrease in peak tension of muscle, and a lengthening of the half-relaxation time. The functional consequences of the prevertebral and postvertebral muscle becoming atrophied could result in some of the postural and biomechanical changes seen in some older persons.

Neurologic Changes

Distinguishing between uncomplicated aging of the nervous system and comorbid factors such as cerebrovascular disease is sometimes difficult to accomplish. Aging of the nervous system does not affect all neural structures in the same fashion.* Of particular importance is the contribution that degeneration of the nigrostriatal pathways makes to decreasing motor performance and posture in the elderly. Extensive degeneration of these same monoaminergic neuronal systems occurs in Parkinson's disease,[59, 78, 108] lead-

*References 3, 16, 18, 44, 63, 71, 79, 105.

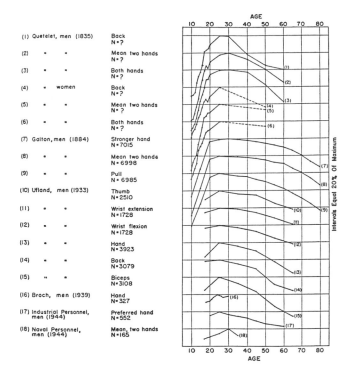

(1) Quetelet, men (1835)	Back N=?	
(2) " "	Mean two hands N=?	
(3) " "	Both hands N=?	
(4) " women	Back N=?	
(5) " "	Mean two hands N=?	
(6) " "	Both hands N=?	
(7) Galton, men (1884)	Stronger hand N=7015	
(8) " "	Mean two hands N=6998	
(9) " "	Pull N=6985	
(10) Ufland, men (1933)	Thumb N=2510	
(11) " "	Wrist extension N=1728	
(12) " "	Wrist flexion N=1728	
(13) " "	Hand N=3923	
(14) " "	Back N=3079	
(15) " "	Biceps N=3108	
(16) Broch, men (1939)	Hand N=327	
(17) Industrial Personnel, men (1944)	Preferred hand N=552	
(18) Naval Personnel, men (1944)	Mean, two hands N=165	

FIG 14–5.
Relationship of strength to age. (From Fisher MB, Birren JE: *J Appl Psychol* 1947; 31:628–630. Used by permission.)

ing to flexed posture, muscular rigidity, tremor, and slow movement.

While the clinical appearance of some elderly individuals bears a remarkable similarity to Parkinson's disease, one should not presume that all elderly persons have the disease.[103] Minor extrapyramidal signs may be present in the elderly and are often overlooked as due to the aging process. Pyramidal tract and cerebellar signs are less common in the younger elderly. The significance of the age-related imbalances between the motor systems that may occur in aging are not clearly understood. It is possible that when one observes the older person who is flexed forward, has a slight tremor, weak voice, and shuffling gait, it could be related to the aging process occurring in the basal ganglia and associated nuclei.[103] Postural tremor occurring in the elderly[29, 94] and impairment of balance may be due to cerebellar degeneration[23] or to any of its connections.[103] Therefore, neurologic causes of postural change should also be examined.

Decreases in voluntary movement control and reaction time occur in the elderly.[22, 50, 91, 101, 102, 115] It has been reported that the effects of age are more marked when the individual is asked to accomplish complex reaction time tasks,[35, 80, 97, 116] complicated motor responses,[90] or sudden postural adjustments.[50, 115] Muscular atrophy of the postural muscles in the elderly has been discussed previously in this chapter and elsewhere.[14, 90]

Although the foregoing events occur with aging, it appears that some of the decline in motor performance, including postural control, may be more related to a decrease in physical activity on the part of the elder. Various authors have demonstrated that individuals who are physically active and continue to maintain maximal oxygen uptake during senescence enjoy the benefits derived from an improved heart rate, cardiac output, blood pressure,[4, 9, 21, 27, 37, 43, 95] joint mobility,[20] and increased flexibility.

Psychosocial Factors

The impact of psychosocial factors on the posture of elderly individuals has not been well documented; therefore, this discussion will be mostly anecdotal from observations made by the author of elderly individuals with arthritis and associated psychosocial concerns. It is beyond the scope of this chapter to address the multiple psychosocial problems that could affect posture. Three of the more common phenomena seen in a physical therapy practice are depression,[13, 15] delirium (acute confusional state),[92] and dementia[40, 48, 49, 55, 73] and are covered in detail in other chapters.

Depression is the single-most common problem of mental health occurring in the elderly and is the most treatable.[12] The following case study demonstrates how depression altered both the posture and the general affect of one of the author's recent patients.

Mrs. VJ is a 73-year-old woman who lives with her husband, a recently retired obstetrician, in an affluent high-rise condominium. She has a 25-year history of osteoarthritis of the lumbar spine including both the disks and the facet joints of L1 to L5. On X ray the L4–5 segment has collapsed and fused, and there are large osteophytes protruding into the intervertebral foramina. The facet joints of these segments are fused.

Mrs. VJ is overweight by 50 lbs. About 8 months ago (about the same time her husband completely retired from his practice), she developed intolerable low back pain. She responded initially to a nonsteroidal anti-inflammatory drug and a carefully planned therapeutic exercise and walking program. She was seen weekly for 1 month, then once a month thereafter. Each time she returned for her monthly appointment, it was noted that her complaints of fatigue and lack of sleep increased. She also seemed apathetic about her appearance and about 4 months ago began to wear the same workout clothes for treatment along with her fur coat. Her complaints about her low back pain increased as did the complaints of fatigue and low endurance, and she began to sleep for 2 to 4 hours during the day. She walked lethargically and with a more stooped, bent-forward posture. She claimed to be compliant at home with her home program of exercises.

When confronted with the question as to whether she was depressed, she openly admitted she was and burst into tears. Multiple problems were bothering her, including unresolved feelings and beliefs about a daughter who had died 20 years ago, resentment that her husband was home "under my feet all day," and feeling that she had no freedom. She was referred to a psychiatrist who prescribed an antidepressant and counseling for her. Although she was seeing a psychiatrist, the author continued to follow her monthly to monitor her exercise program as well as to provide support during her initial counseling sessions. In 1 month her entire demeanor, depression, countenance, and posture improved. She continued with counseling and her exercise program and has been discharged from physical therapy to be followed ad libitum.

Pharmaceutical Factors

Many drug groups may change posture. Pepper and Robbins have suggested that the major mechanisms by which drugs impair mobility and alter posture are sedation (decreased motivation), postural instability (imbalance that contributes to falls and fear of falling that causes elders to limit activity), sensory or psychomotor impairment (alter visual, proprioceptive, or vestibular compensatory mechanisms necessary for balance), and postural hypotension (syncope, dizziness, weakness).[83] Learning what drugs the patient is taking can be valuable information prior to making any final evaluative decisions regarding the posture of the elder.

Comorbidity Factors

Comorbidity factors that may alter the posture and postural control of the elder person might be tinnitus, visual impairment, deafness, headaches, hypertension, or hypoten-

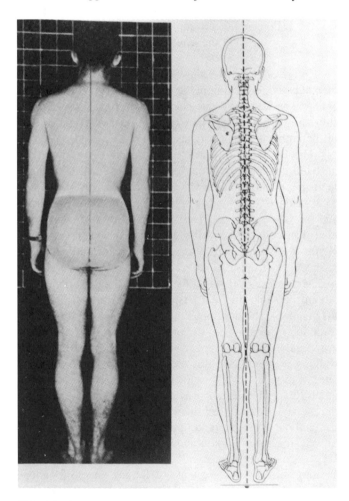

FIG 14–6.
Posture in the standing position viewed from the posterior. (From Kendall EP, McCreary EK: *Muscles: Testing and Function.* Baltimore, Williams & Wilkins, 1983, p 290. Used by permission.

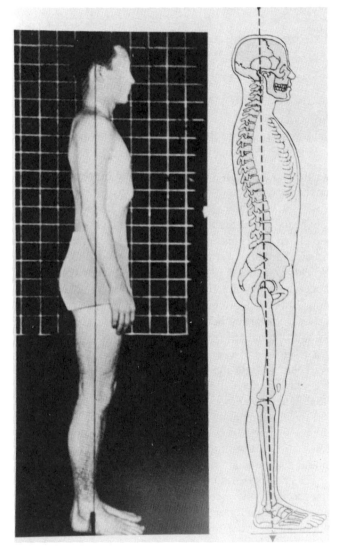

FIG 14–7.
Posture in the standing position viewed from the side. (From Kendall EP, McCreary EK: *Muscles: Testing and Function.* Baltimore, Williams & Wilkins, 1983, p 280. Used by permission.)

sion. Control of the posture is governed by the vestibular system in the inner ear, by the visual system, and by proprioceptive information from the peripheral nervous system. Degenerative changes or other insult to these mechanisms could impair postural control. Alterations in the cerebral regulatory function probably contribute an important part in postural disturbances in old people.[99] The list of comorbid factors could be lengthy, and to explain each is outside the scope of this chapter. The physical therapist must be cognizant of any comorbid factors that may be present in the elder, no matter how subtle or unimportant they appear when taking an initial history.

EVALUATION OF POSTURE AND POSTURAL CHANGES

Before beginning a discussion on the evaluation process, a precautionary note should be emphasized again. The model for correct postural alignment is a young, healthy individual who has a well-integrated neuromusculoskeletal system and postural control, as reflected in Figures 14–6

and 14–7.[53] While this information is important in general, it may not be specific to the elder person. Figures 14–8 and 14–9 are more reflective of the postural changes particular to the elderly.[51] As can be seen, with advancing age the head moves forward, the thoracic spine is more kyphotic, and there is a loss of the normal lumbar lordosis. One should remember, however, that postural alignment in elderly persons can be highly individualized in appearance.

Alignment

To assess the total body alignment, visual inspection should occur in the sagittal, coronal, and horizontal planes as well as from anterior, posterior, and lateral views. Typically, one uses a plumb line or a posture grid to determine a reference point for inspection from each view. Although the proximal fixation points for the plumb line are (1) mental protuberance of the mandible for the anterior view, (2) anterior margin of the mastoid process of the temporal bone for the lateral view, and (3) the external occipital protuberance on the occipital bone for the posterior view

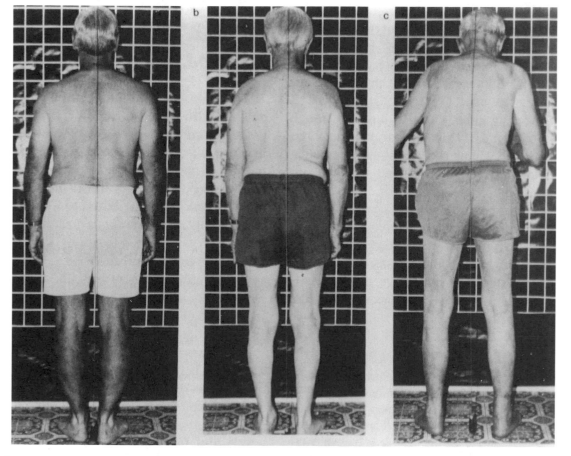

FIG 14–8.
Posterior posture of **(A)** a 60-year-old man, **(B)** a 78-year-old man, and **(C)** a 93-year-old man. (From Kauffman T: *Top Geriatr Rehabil* 1987; 2(4):13–28. Used by permission.)

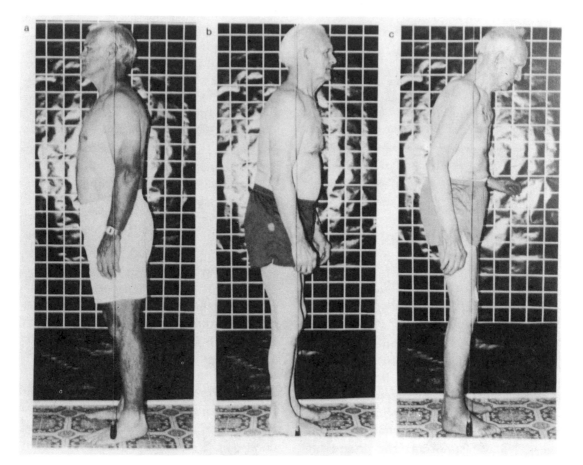

FIG 14–9.
Lateral posture of **(A)** a 60-year-old man, **(B)** a 78-year-old man, and **(C)** a 93-year-old man. (From Kauffman T: *Top Geriatr Rehabil* 1987; 2(4):13–28. Used by permission.)

as in the young adult, deviations from what is expected in younger persons should be anticipated.

For example, Friedenburg and Miller identified that 70% of their subjects had appreciable degenerative changes in the cervical spine by the seventh decade of life.[38] Likewise, Brain reported that spondylosis of the cervical spine was present in 80% of subjects in his study older than age 55.[11] These cervical changes can restrict motion in the cervical spine and contribute to the forward head posture seen in older persons. Furthermore, it might be observed that the pelvis tends to tilt posteriorly more often than is seen in younger patients. This might be due to prolonged sitting postures and hypokinesis of the postural muscles. Deviations of the posture in the posterior and lateral views can be seen in Figures 14–10 and 14–11.[70]

While assessing the alignment of the body, it is also important to determine the extent to which the person is able to maintain the posture (posture holding) or position of the body without extraneous movements (equilibrium or postural sway). Maintaining postural control in a static po-

sition decreases with age and is potentially problematic for the elder, as the loss of postural control increases the risk of falling.[10, 34] Sample tests for determining disturbances in posture are depicted in Table 14–1. Suggested tests for assessing equilibrium coordination are outlined in Table 14–2.[93] Assessment of postural sway may be as simple as observation by the therapist or as complex as objective data that may be generated from a computer-assisted force plate as the subject stands on it.

TABLE 14–1.

Tests for Disturbances of Posture*

1. Fixation or position holding (upper and lower extremities).
2. Displace balance unexpectedly in sitting or standing positions.
3. Standing, alter base of support.
4. Standing, one foot directly in front of the other.
5. Standing on one foot.

*From Schmitz TJ: Coordination assessment, in Sullivan SB, Schmitz TJ (eds): *Physical Rehabilitation: Assessment and Treatment*, ed 2. Philadelphia, FA Davis, 1988. Used by permission.

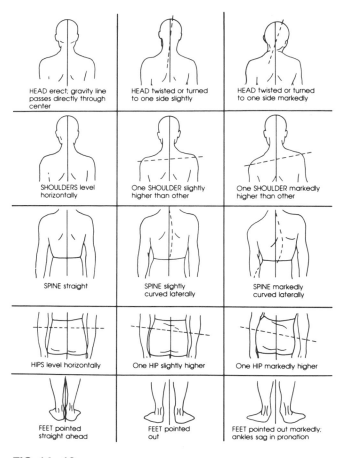

FIG 14–10.
Postural deviation from the posterior view. (Redrawn from McGee DJ: Assessment of posture, in McGee DJ (ed): *Orthopedic Physical Assessment.* Philadelphia, WB Saunders, 1987.

It should be noted that elders with significant sensory losses of vision and proprioception may have difficulty maintaining a stable posture.[10, 28] It is an important component of assessment to view posture as a total integration of multiple systems. Hence, while static positions are important to assess, it is equally important to assess posture in terms of dynamic balance and coordination by asking the subject to execute a sit-to-stand movement, establish immediate standing balance, react to a nudge by the examiner when standing, turn in a circle, perform a one-legged stance, and sit down.

The "get up and go" test was described by Mathias et al.[66] The purpose is to have the person complete a series of postural adjustments in sequence, including sitting in a chair, standing up, maintaining static bipedal stance, walking a distance, turning around without touching any object for support, walking back to the chair, and turning around and sitting down in the chair. The subject's performance is scored using a five-point Likert scale, with 1 being normal and 5 being a severely abnormal performance.

Joint alignment, joint stability, and range-of-motion examinations are generic tests used in physical therapy but applied with consideration given for age-related changes previously mentioned. Soft tissue changes, stiffness, and stretch weakness of muscles are not uncommon in the elder person.

Respiratory Function

While the primary goal of a postural assessment is not necessarily to determine how the respiratory apparatus is functioning, it is an opportunity to determine whether or not the posture of the individual has the potential of compromising how one breathes. Speads and Leong[100] suggest that while some disturbances in breathing are quite obvious, others will require close observation to determine whether posture is impairing the air flow of the patient. For example, these authors suggest that the observer should watch the patient in the supine position and observe whether the patient experiences difficulty breathing or is able to lie comfortably. Sitting postures will also reveal whether the thorax is able to move air appropriately. If the person bends forward while sitting, this may compress the

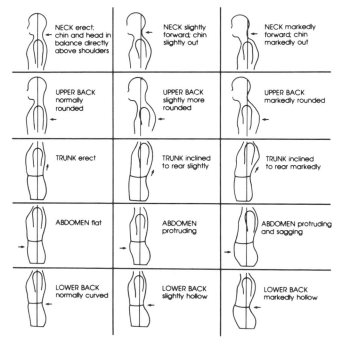

FIG 14–11.
Postural deviations from the lateral view. (Redrawn from McGee DJ: Assessment of posture, in *Orthopedic Physical Assessment.* Philadelphia, WB Saunders, 1987.

TABLE 14–2.

Equilibrium Coordination Tests*

1. Standing in a normal, comfortable posture.
2. Standing, feet together (narrow base of support).
3. Standing, with one foot directly in front of the other (toe of one foot touching heel of opposite foot).
4. Standing on one foot.
5. Arm position may be altered in each of the above postures (i.e., arms at side, over head, hands on waist, etc.).
6. Displace balance unexpectedly (while carefully guarding patient).
7. Standing, alternate between forward trunk flexion and return to neutral.
8. Standing, laterally flex trunk to each side.
9. Walking, placing the heel of one foot directly in front of the toe of the opposite foot.
10. Walk along a straight line drawn or taped to the floor; or place feet on floor markers while walking.
11. Walk sideways and backward.
12. March in place.
13. Alter speed of ambulatory activities (increased speed will exaggerate coordination deficits).
14. Stop and start abruptly while walking.
15. Walk in a circle, alternate directions.
16. Walk on heels or toes.
17. Normal standing posture. Observe patient both with patient's eyes open and with patient's eyes closed (or vision occluded). If patient is able to maintain balance with eyes open but not with vision occluded, it is indicative of a proprioceptive loss. This inability to maintain an upright posture without visual input is referred to as a positive *Romberg's sign.*

*From Schmitz TJ: Coordination assessment, in Sullivan SB, Schmitz TJ (eds): *Physical Rehabilitation: Assessment and Treatment,* ed 2. Philadelphia, FA Davis, 1988. Used by permission.

contents of the abdomen against the diaphragm, causing breathing to be restricted. Observations should be made of the rhythm of breathing as well as the movement of the whole thorax. Is the rhythm regular? Is the movement of the thorax too fast or too slow? Does the patient sigh more often than is necessary? Does the person execute Valsalva's maneuver when changing positions or when doing a task? It is important that the air is moving freely, without strain and without interference.[100]

It is useful also to watch for signs of fatigue or lack of endurance as the patient changes positions or completes the posture examination. Casual and routine questions such as "Do you sleep well at night?" and "How long could you walk outdoors before you would have to sit down because you were tired?" may be interspersed into a conversation with the patient during the examination. Answers to these questions can provide direction for further endurance and fatigue testing.

Muscle Strength

Given the variability in changes of the muscular tissue in the elder person, traditional manual muscle testing may be both spurious and disinclined to provide a true picture of what the person is able to accomplish. Performance-based assessment is much more useful as a global indicator of what the person can accomplish, whereas isolated manual muscle testing or isokinetic testing may be used when there are questions about specific muscle groups.

Coping With Postural Change

Having assessed the person's posture and having determined that there are some noticeable variations from what would be considered normal posture for an elderly person, several questions need to be answered before a plan of care for the patient can be formulated. Some questions are:

1. Does the patient agree that there is a problem with his posture?
2. Are the postural deformities flexible or fixed in nature?
3. Is the patient suffering from a comorbidity? What effect would correcting the posture problem have on the comorbidity? Which is more important to the person: the comorbidity or the posture problem?
4. What is the extent of the person's ability to care for himself at home?
5. What are the home conditions of the patient?
6. What occupational or recreational activities does the person enjoy? Would a correction in posture result in the individual's ability to enjoy them more?

Once you have determined that the answers to these questions reflect that the person is motivated, willing to commit to taking charge of the plan of care (with supervision as necessary from a physical therapist), and believes that he can succeed for the most part, it is appropriate to develop the plan of care.

THE PLAN OF CARE

Four different postural disorders of primarily musculoskeletal origin (commonly seen by this author in elderly persons) will be used to illustrate how to develop and implement a physical therapy plan of care. The postural disorders to be discussed are those occurring in hypokinetics, osteoporosis, cervical spine dysfunction, and degenerative joint disease. As these patients are typically seen in an outpatient setting in a tertiary care hospital, they rarely present with a simple clinical problem but rather have several comorbid conditions.

Hypokinesis

Hypokinesis is a decrease in activity that results in an accentuation of the age-related changes that may be seen in the elder person such as increased flexed posture, decreased flexibility, decreased muscle strength, decreased endurance, and decreased functional ability. Hypokinesis may occur separately or with comorbidity.

Mr. HS is an 85-year-old Caucasian male who was first seen in physical therapy for lower extremity strengthening and aerobic and balance exercises in July 1986. His past medical history was remarkable for hypertension, tinnitus, and occasional bouts with syncope. He was able to execute the "get up and go" test, with mild difficulty getting up and down out of a chair. He exhibited decreased one-legged stance balance on each leg but did not exhibit rigidity, cerebellar signs, or tremor. His home exercise routine consisted of walking with his wife through his neighborhood and caring for a very large flower garden. His chief complaint in 1986 was the difficulty he was experiencing with getting up from a chair or the toilet and up and down stairs. He was retired and financially secure and lived with his wife who was 4 years his senior in age.

In November 1990, he reported to his physician that he was falling more often, had "the shakes" when he ate his food, and was easily fatigued with just walking from his home to the garage to get into his car. His wife had died suddenly in 1988, and in 1989, he remarried. Over the past year he has not been able to do any kind of air travel, which he previously could do, nor can he play golf. He complained of being house bound because he had become so weak and shaky. He was not able to complete the "get up and go" test and demonstrated a positive Romberg's sign. He walked with a shuffling flat-footed gait, taking short steps. Although he was now using a cane for balance, he tended to walk in a flexed position reminiscent of an individual with Parkinson's. His physician referred him to a neurologist for a complete workup, which was only remarkable for symptoms compatible with 85 years of age.

In this particular case, he was described as having hypokinesis and referred to physical therapy for a "tune-up" on his exercise program. Since it was thought that he might also be depressed, he was referred to a physical therapist who worked in a sports physical therapy setting. The therapist was also trained with a gerontologic background and worked with elder exercisers. Mr. HS joined with the group of elders and young athletes doing exercise in the clinic. While his improvement physically is slow, his increase in morale has given him some zest to be more active.

What is important to note here is that the aging process, along with inactivity and depression, can accentuate the elder person's decreased functional ability and loss of freedom to move around. In this case, Mr. HS was carefully matched in an environment for physical therapy where he might experience success in his physical functioning, however modest. Since he loved athletics as a young person, he greatly enjoyed interacting with the young and elder athletes.

Osteoporosis

Mrs. TB is a 68-year-old Caucasian female who is widowed and has a 35-year history of rheumatoid arthritis. Considering her numerous upper extremity joint deformities, particularly the instability of the right shoulder and the left elbow, she does very well functionally. Over the past 10 years she has developed severe scoliosis of the spine with a right thoracic and left lumbar curvature. Associated with these changes, she has degenerative joint disease of the lumbosacral spine involving both the facet joints and the intervertebral disks. Her current medical problems are degenerative joint disease, osteoporosis, rheumatoid arthritis, scleritis, and hypertension. Her medications list includes: azathioprine (Imuran), prednisone (Decadron), estrogens (Premarin), medroxyprogesterone (Provera), acetaminophen (Tylenol 3), enalapril (Vasotec), and ranitidine (Zantac). She has been using some form of corticosteroid in various dosages for over 30 years. Her current dosage is 5 mg orally per day, which is considered a maintenance dose.

Her risk factors for osteoporosis are postmenopausal female, Caucasian, light skeletal mass, and steroid dependence for over 30 years. She presented herself to the physical therapy clinic because of our long-standing client-therapist association. Her chief complaint was of localized back pain that seemed to start at her spine and follow around her rib cage. She also felt that she was twisting more and was having great difficulty getting up and down from the bed, chairs, and toilet. Asked when the symptoms began, she reported that they had been ongoing for about 2 weeks. The only activity she could attribute it to was straining to close the door on her car, which had become caught on a grassy curb.

Anterolateral assessment of her back revealed the dramatic scoliotic curvature of her spine. Upon visual inspection it could not be determined if the scoliotic curves were increasing; however, she did complain of greater difficulty breathing, sometimes having sharp, stabbing pain on forced inhalation and upon coughing. Palpation of her spine revealed point tenderness at the level of the 12th thoracic vertebra toward the right side of the spine within the mass of the sacrospinalis muscles. The pain followed the dermatome out to approximately the midaxillary line on the right side. Mrs. TB was unable to bend the trunk to the right or rotate the trunk to either side because of pain. She demonstrated a positive straight leg test (Lasègue's sign) on the right.

Given the results of Mrs. TB's evaluation and her history of steroid dependency, she was referred to her rheumatologist for a medical workup, which revealed that she had sustained a compression fracture of the 11th thoracic vertebra on the 12th. She was placed on bed rest for 3 weeks, with subsequent home visits from the physical therapist to instruct her in deep-breathing and bed mobility exercises and to help her put on a soft spinal corset. Owing to the instability and deformities of her upper extremities, she was unable to care for herself and hence stayed with a daughter. She was gradually progressed to weight-bearing exercises and returned to independence.

The significance of this case is that Mrs. TB had more than one diagnosis that could have caused her back pain. Because of her osteoporosis, risk factors, the type of event that could have elicited her pain, as well as the distribution of the pain, a vertebral compression fracture is a strong alternative diagnosis that requires confirmation before an appropriate physical therapy plan of care can be devised or implemented.

Cervical Spine Dysfunction

Mr. MJ is a 63-year-old custodian who was referred to physical therapy with a diagnosis of cervical spondylosis and radiculopathy to the right upper extremity. Cervical spine X rays demonstrated moderate degenerative changes in C5 and C6, with anterior osteophytes from the margins of the vertebral bodies. There was narrowing of the cartilage space of the facet joints, with sclerosis and osteophytes encroaching the right neuroforamina of C5 and C6.

Upon physical examination of the cervical spine, it was noted that rotation to the right was limited to 45 degrees. Forward flexion was within the normal limits; however, hyperextension was limited to 20 degrees, with the presence of pain and crepitus. Rotation to the left was 50 degrees, with crepitus. Palpation revealed point tenderness over the coracoid process and tendon of the supraspinatus on the right. Postural examination of the cervical spine revealed a forward head posture. Mr. MJ reported that he had a history of migraine headaches and has become addicted to triazolam (Halcion) and propoxyphene napsylate (Darvocet). His addiction is currently being medically managed to get him off these drugs.

When asked about his job and work style, Mr. MJ described himself as a workaholic and a perfectionist. He claimed to exercise his neck every day to strengthen the muscles. When asked to demonstrate the exercises, he executed rapid rotatory motions of the neck as well as rapid flexion and extension exercises. His upper extremity exercises were demonstrated at the same velocity.

Given his diagnosis, forward head, work style, drug addiction, and methods of exercise, our treatment plan centered around his taking the responsibility to modify the way he was working, standing, and exercising. He was instructed to do long, slow stretching motions of the neck, to perform shoulder shrug exercises at a slow pace, to assess his workplace, and to pace himself so he did not mechanically aggravate his neck. At night he was to use a cervical pillow, and during the day he was to use a cervical traction unit at home at least once a day. The traction was attached to his bed, which allowed him to lie down to do his treatment. Furthermore, he agreed to begin a swimming program of aerobic work to help his arthritis and to reduce stress.

In this particular case, the forward head posture could not be substantially reversed. Mr. MJ was, however, able to realize the value of gentle exercise on sore joints, relaxation techniques, life-style modifications, and aerobic conditioning. Too often cervical exercises are performed incorrectly by the elder person, resulting in greater pain and immobility. Careful attention to avoid "overkill" in performing the exercise program can reap significant pain relief.

Degenerative Joint Disease of the Lumbosacral Spine

Mrs. HJ is a 78-year-old widow who was referred to the clinic with a diagnosis of degenerative joint and disk disease of the lumbosacral spine. She also has degenerative disease of the distal interphalangeal joints of both hands (Heberden's nodes), the carpometacarpal joint of the right thumb, the right hip, and both knees. Her X-ray findings of the lumbosacral spine revealed that she also had diffuse osteoporosis, discogenic sclerosis between T11 and T12 and L1 through S1 disk spaces, abundant osteophyte formation, spondylolisthesis of L4 on L5, and sacralization of L5, all of which are consistent with degenerative joint disease of the spine. Her right knee X ray demonstrated degenerative changes in the patellofemoral compartment with cartilage loss in both the lateral and medial compartments of the knee. The left knee X rays revealed mild osteophyte formation and subchondral sclerosis of the medial compartment of the knee.

Examination of the back revealed a kyphosis of the lumbar spine, decreased mobility in all active ranges of motion, bilateral positive straight leg raise signs, pain on palpation of the central low back region, and pain when asked to hyperextend the back. Assessment of her functional status revealed Mrs. HJ to be a very active 78-year-old person, particularly when one observed her X rays. She noted that sitting or standing too long exacerbated her symptoms; however, if she intermingled rest with activity, she was able to get many things accomplished during the day. Mrs. HJ is highly active in managing her arthritis on a personal level. She is a positive individual with many hobbies, including having sung for 20 years with an internationally acclaimed religious choir.

Evaluation of her posture demonstrated that she had a slight forward head without any concurrent thoracic kyphosis, no scoliosis, and a lumbar kyphosis. She had a leg length difference of one half in., which was easily corrected by an insole she wore in her right shoe. She commented that when she did not wear her orthosis, she noticed that her back would become more painful. She has been advised to have surgery in the past but has chosen to use exercise and other means of conservative treatment rather than take the risk of a surgical failure.

Her treatment in the clinic included heat, gentle flexion exercises (since hyperextension aggravates her symptoms), riding a stationary bike, and instruction in the use of a home transcutaneous electrical nerve stimulation (TENS) unit for pain control. Because of the arthritis in her knees and back, the stationary bicycle had to be adjusted so that she did not bend forward over the handlebars. The seat also had to be raised so that her knees were extended as much as possible when she peddled the bike. She was instructed to avoid flexion of the knee to 90 degrees.

Mrs. HJ's case is instructive because a hasty conclusion, based only on her X rays, would project a life of severe disability. This serves to point out that all patients have a different level of self-efficacy and handle low back pain quite differently. Because of her mental and emotional outlook and careful incorporation of energy-conserving techniques in her daily life-style, Mrs. HJ was able to increase her quality of life, which could have been quite different if she had had a lesser sense of mastery over the impact of arthritis on her life or if she had avoided consulting physical therapy at the appropriate time.

SUMMARY

This chapter has reviewed the posture and postural changes found in elderly persons. Evaluation and treatment of posture are accomplished by using the generic skills of physical therapy and adapting them to the elderly patient. What is most important for the physical therapist to consider and remember is that not all elderly persons are alike—not all are stooped forward; not all are unmotivated to change their posture. With professional guidance, they can make changes in their posture that will enhance the positive process of getting older.

REFERENCES

1. Amstutz HC, Sisson HA: The structure of the vertebral spongiosa. *J Bone Joint Surg* 1969; 51B:540–550.
2. Amussen E, Freunsgaard K, Norgaard S: A follow-up longitudinal study of selected physiologic functions in former physical education students: After forty years. *J Am Geriatr Soc* 1975; 23:442–450.
3. Andriacchi TP, et al: A model for studies of mechanical interactions between the human spine & rib cage. *J Biomech* 1974; 7:497–507.
4. Anianson A, et al: Muscle function in 75-year-old men and women: A longitudinal study. *Scand J Rehabil Med Suppl* 1983; 90:92–102.
5. Anianson A, Grimby G: Muscle strength and endurance in elderly people with special reference to muscle morphology, in Amussen E, Jorgensen R (eds): *Biomechanics VI-A*. Baltimore, University Park Press, 1977.
6. Atkinson PJ: Variation in trabecular structure of vertebrae with age. *Calcif Tissue Res* 1967; 1:24–32.
7. Bartley MH, et al: The relationship of bone strength and bone quantity in health, disease and aging. *J Gerontol* 1966; 21:517–521.
8. Bell GH, et al: Variation in strength of vertebrae with age and their relation to osteoporosis. *Calcif Tissue Res* 1967; 1:75–86.
9. Benestad AM: Trainability of older men. *Acta Med Scand* 1965; 178:321–327.
10. Bohannon RW, Larkin P, Cook A, et al: Decrease in timed balance test scores with aging. *Phys Ther* 1984; 64:1067–1070.
11. Brain L: Some unsolved problems of cervical spondylosis. *Br Med J* 1963; 1:771–777.
12. Brandt K, Palmoski M: Organization of ground substance proteoglycans in normal and osteoarthritic knee cartilage. *Arthritis Rheum* 1976; 19:209–215.
13. Bressler R: Treating geriatric depression: current options. *Drug Ther* 1984; 9:129–144.
14. Briggs RC, et al: Balance performance among noninstitutionalized elderly women. *Phys Ther* 1989; 69:748–756.
15. Brody EM: Aging and family personality: A developmental view. *Fam Process* 1974; 13:23–39.
16. Brody H: An examination of cerebral cortex and brainstem aging, in Terry RD, Gershon S (eds): *Neurobiology of Aging*. New York, Raven Press, 1976.
17. Brown T, Hanson RJ, Yorra AJ: Some mechanical tests on the lumbosacral spine with particular reference to the intervertebral discs: A preliminary report. *J Bone Joint Surg* 1957; 39A:1135–1164.
18. Bugiani O, et al: Nerve cell loss with aging in the putamen. *Eur Neurol* 1978; 17:286–291.
19. Calkins E, Challa HR: Disorders of the joints and connective tissue, in Andres R, Bierman EL, Hazzard WR (eds): *Principles of Geriatric Medicine*. New York, McGraw-Hill, 1985.
20. Chapman EA, DeVries HA, Swezey R: Joint stiffness: Effects of exercise on young and old men. *J Gerontol* 1972; 27:218–221.
21. Choquette G, Ferguson RJ: Blood pressure reduction in "borderline" hypertensives following physical training. *Can Med Assoc J* 1973; 108:699–703.
22. Clarkson PM: The effect of age and activity level on simple and choice fractionated response time. *Eur J Appl Physiol* 1978; 40:17–25.

23. Corsellis JAN: Some observations on the Purkinje cell population and on brain volume in human aging, in Terry RD, Gershon S (eds): *Neurobiology of Aging*. New York, Raven Press, 1976.

24. Courpron P, Meunier PJ: Osteopénie et pathologie osscusc, in Bourliere F (ed): *Gerontologie. Biologie et clinique*. Paris, Flammarion, 1982.

25. Damon A, et al: Age and physique in healthy white veterans at Boston. *J Gerontol* 1972; 27:202–208.

26. Dunhill MS, Anderson JA, Whitehead R: Quantitative histological studies on age changes in bone. *J Pathol Bacteriol* 1967; 94:275.

27. Ekblom B: Effects of physical training on oxygen transport in man. *Acta Physiol Scand Suppl* 1969; 328:9.

28. Era T, Heikkinen E: Postural sway during standing and unexpected disturbance of balance in random sample of men of different ages. *J Gerontol* 1985; 40:287–295.

29. Fahn S: Differential diagnosis of tremors. *Med Clin North Am* 1972; 56:1363–1375.

30. Farfan HF: *Mechanical Disorders of the Low Back*. Philadelphia, Lea & Febiger, 1973.

31. Farfan HF, et al: The effects of torsion on the lumbar intervertebral joints, the role of torsion in the production of disc degeneration. *J Bone Joint Surg* 1970; 52A:468–497.

32. Farfan HF, Sullivan JD: The relationship of facet orientation to intervertebral disc failure. *Can J Surg* 1967; 10:179–185.

33. Fernie G, et al: The relationship of postural sway in standing to the incidence of falls in geriatric subjects. *Age Ageing* 1982; 11:11–16.

34. Ferris S, et al: Reaction time as a diagnostic measure in senility. *J Am Geriatr Soc* 1976; 24:529–533.

35. Fisher MB, Birren JE: Age and strength. *J Appl Psychol* 1947; 31:628–630.

36. Forssberg H, Nashner LM: Ontogenic development of postural control in man: Adaptation to altered support and visual conditions during stance. *J Neurosci* 1982; 2:545–552.

37. Frick MH, Konttinen A, Sarajas HSS: Effects of physical training at rest and during exercise. *Am J Cardiol* 1963; 12:142–147.

38. Friedenburg ZB, Miller WT: Degenerative disc disease of the cervical spine. *J Bone Joint Surg* 1963; 43A:1171–1178.

39. Galante JO: Tensile properties of the human lumbar annulus fibrosus. *Acta Orthop Scand* 1967; (Suppl 100): 1–91.

40. Galasko D, et al: Neurological findings in Alzheimer's disease and normal aging. *Arch Neurol* 1990; 47:625–627.

41. Gallagher JC, Goldgar D, Moy A: Total bone calcium in normal women: Effect of age and menopausal status. *J Bone Miner Res* 1987; 2:491–496.

42. Grimby G, et al: Morphology and enzymatic capacity in arm and leg muscles in 78–81 year old men and women. *Acta Physiol Scand* 1982; 115:125.

43. Hartley LH, et al: Physical training in sedentary middle-aged and older men. III. Cardiac output and gas exchange at submaximal and maximal exercise. *Scand J Clin Lab Invest* 1969; 24:335–344.

44. Hassler R: Extrapyramidal control of the speed of behavior and its change by primary age processes, in Welford AT, Birren JE (eds): *Behaviour, Aging and the Nervous System*. Springfield, Charles C Thomas, 1965.

45. Hayes SC, et al: The development of the display and knowledge of sex-related motor behavior in children. *Child Behav Ther* 1981; 3:1.

46. Hirsch C: The reaction of intervertebral discs to compressive forces. *J Bone Joint Surg* 1955; 37A:1188–1196.

47. Hirsch C, Nachemson A: New observations on the mechanical behavior of lumbar discs. *Act Orthop Scand* 1954; 23:254–283.

48. Huff FJ, et al: The neurologic examination in patients with probable Alzheimer's disease. *Arch Neurol* 1987; 44:929–932.

49. Huff FJ, Growdon JH: Neurological abnormalities associated with severity of dementia in Alzheimer's disease. *Can J Neurol Sci* 1986; 21:403–405.

50. Inglin B, Woollacott M: Age-related changes in anticipatory postural adjustments associated with arm movements. *J Gerontol* 1988; 43:105–113.

51. Kauffman T: Posture and age. *Top Geriatr Rehabil* 1987; 2(4):13–28.

52. Kazarian LE: Creep characteristics of the human spinal column. *Orthop Clin North Am* 1975; 6:3–18.

53. Kendall EP, McCreary EK: *Muscles: Testing and Function*. Baltimore, Williams & Wilkins, 1983, pp 280,290.

54. King AI, Prasad P, Ewing CL: Mechanism of spinal injury due to caudocephalad acceleration. *Orthop Clin North Am* 1975; 6:19–31.

55. Koller WC, et al: Motor signs are infrequent in dementia of the Alzheimer's type. *Ann Neurol* 1984; 16:514–515.

56. Kugler PN, Turvey MT: *Information, Natural Law and the Self Assembly of Rhythmic Movement*. Hillsdale, NJ, Erlbaum, 1987.

57. Lamy C, et al: The strength of the neural arch and the etiology of spondylolysis. *Orthop Clin North Am* 1975; 6:215–231.

58. Larsson L, Grimby G, Karlsson J: Muscle strength and speed of movement in relation to age and muscle morphology. *J Appl Physiol* 1979; 46:451–456.

59. Lewis PD: Parkinsonism-neuropathology. *Br Med J* 1971; 3:690–692.

60. Lexell JK, Henriksson-Larsson E, and Sjostrom M: Distribution of different fiber types in human skeletal muscles. A study of cross-sections of whole muscle vastus lateralis. *Acta Physiol Scand* 1983; 117:115–122.

61. Lindahl O: Mechanical properties of dried defatted spongy bone. *Acta Orthop Scand* 1976; 47:11–19.

62. Longcope C, et al: Aromatization of androgens by muscle and adipose tissue in vivo. *J Clin Endocrinol Metab* 1978; 46:146–152.

63. Mann DMA, Yates PO: The effects of aging on the pigmented nerve cells of the human locus caeruleus and substantia nigra. *Acta Neuropathol (Berl)* 1979; 47:93–97.

64. Markolf KL, Morris JM: The structural components of the intervertebral disc. *J Bone Joint Surg* 1974; 56A:675–687.

65. Martin T: Normal development of movement and function: Neonate, infant and toddler, in Scully RM, Barnes MR (eds): *Physical Therapy*. Philadelphia, JB Lippincott, 1989.

66. Mathias S, Nayak U, Isaacs B: Balance and elderly patients: The "get up and go" test. *Arch Phys Med Rehabil* 1986; 67:387–389.

67. Maurel E, et al: Age dependent biochemical changes in dermal connective tissue. Relationship to histological and ultrastructural observations. *Connect Tissue Res* 1980; 8:33–39.

68. Mazess RB: Measurement of skeletal status by noninvasive methods. *Calcif Tissue Int* 1979; 28:89–92.

69. Mazess RB: Bone densiometry in osteoporosis. *Intern Med Specialist* 1987; 8:133.

70. McGee DJ: Assessment of posture, in McGee DJ (ed): *Orthopedic Physical Assessment*. Philadelphia, WB Saunders,.1987.

71. McGeer PL, McGeer EG, Suzuki JS: Aging and extrapyramidal function. *Arch Neurol* 1977; 34:33–35.

72. Messerer O: *Über Elasticitat und Festigkeit Meuschlichen Knochen*. Stuttgart, JG Cottaschen Buchhandling, 1880.

73. Molsa PK, Marttila RJ, Rinne UK: Extrapyramidal signs in Alzheimer's disease. *Neurology* 1985; 34:1114–1116.

74. Nachemson A: The influence of spinal movements on the lumbar intradiscal pressure and on the tensile strength in the annulus fibrosus. *Acta Orthop Scand* 1963; 33:183–207.

75. Nachemson AL, Evans JH: Biomechanical study of human lumbar ligamentum flavum. *J Anat* 1969; 105:188–189.

76. Nachemson A, Morris JM: In vivo measurements of intradiscal pressure. Discometry, a method for determination of pressure in the lower lumbar discs. *J Bone Joint Surg* 1964; 46A:1077–1092.

77. Naylor A, Happy F, MacRae T: Changes in the human intervertebral disc with age: A biophysical study. *J Am Geriatr Soc* 1955; 3:964–973.

78. Ohama E, Ikuta F: Parkinson's disease: Distribution of Lewy bodies and monoaminergic neuron system. *Acta Neuropathol (Berl)* 1976; 34:311–319.

79. Pakkenberg H, Brody H: The number of nerve cells in the substantia nigra in paralysis agitans. *Acta Neuropathol (Berl)* 1965; 5:320–324.

80. Panek PE: Age differences in perceptual style, selective attention and perceptual-motor reaction time. *Exp Aging Res* 1978; 4:377–387.

81. Panjabi MM, White AA, Johnson RM: Cervical spine mechanics as a function of transection components. *J Biomech* 1975; 8:327–336.

82. Peng MT, Lee LR: Regional differences of neuron loss of rat brain in old age. *Gerontology* 1979; 25:205–211.

83. Pepper GA, Robbins LJ: Improving geriatric drug therapy. *Generations* 1987; 12:57–61.

84. Perry O: Fracture of the vertebral end-plate in the lumbar spine. *Acta Orthop Scand* 1957; 25(suppl):1.

85. Prasud P, King AI, Ewing CL: The role of the articular facets and +Gz acceleration. *J Appl Mech* 1974; 41:321.

86. Ribot C, et al: Obesity and postmenopausal bone loss: The influence on vertebral density and bone turnover in postmenopausal women. *Bone* 1988; 8:327–331.

87. Roaf R: A study of the mechanics of spinal injuries. *J Bone Joint Surg* 1960; 42B:810–823.

88. Rockoff SD, Sweet E, Bleustein J: The relative contribution of trabecular and cortical bone to the strength of human lumbar vertebrae. *Calcif Tissue Res* 1969; 3:163–175.

89. Rolander SD, Blair WE: Deformation and fracture of the lumbar vertebrae end-plate. *Orthop Clin North Am* 1975; 6:75–81.

90. Rothschild BM: Age-related changes in skeletal muscle. *Geriatr Med Today* 1986; 5:87–95.

91. Salthouse TA: Speed and age: Multiple rates of age decline. *Exp Aging Res* 1976; 2:349–359.

92. Saylor C: Stigma, in Lubkin IM (ed): *Chronic Illness: Impact and Intervention*. Boston, Jones and Bartlett, 1990.

93. Schmitz TJ: Coordination assessment, in Sullivan SB, Schmitz TJ (eds): *Physical Rehabilitation: Assessment and Treatment*, ed 2. Philadelphia, FA Davis, 1988.

94. Scott TR, Netsky MG: The pathology of Parkinson's syndrome: A critical review. *Int J Neurol* 1961; 2:51–60.

95. Shepherd RJ: *Fitness of a Nation—The Canada Fitness Survey*. Basel, Karger, 1986.

96. Shephard RJ: Gross changes of form and function, in Shephard RJ (ed): *Physical Activity and Aging*, ed 2. Rockville, Md, Aspen Publishers, 1987.

97. Simon JR, Pouraghabagher AR: The effect of aging on the stages of processing in a choice reaction time task. *J Gerontol* 1978; 33:553–561.

98. Sinclair D: *Human Growth After Birth*. London, Oxford University Press, 1973.

99. Sixt E, Landahl S: Postural disturbances in a 75-year-old population: I. Prevalence and functional consequences. *Age Ageing* 1987; 16:393–398.

100. Speads CH, Leong MJ: Breathing: An approach for facilitating movement, in Jackson OL (ed): *Therapeutic Considerations for the Elderly*. New York, Churchill Livingstone, 1987.

101. Stelmach GE, Diewert GL: Aging information processing and fitness, in Borg G (ed): *Physical Work and Effort*. Oxford, Pergamon Press, 1977.

102. Surwillo WW, Titus TG: Reaction time and the psychological refractory period in children and adults. *Dev Psychobiol* 1976; 9:517–527.

103. Teravainen H, Calne DB: Motor system and normal aging, in Katzman R, Terry RD (eds): *The Neurology of Aging*. Philadelphia, FA Davis, 1983.

104. Thelen E, Kelso JAS, Fogel A: Self organizing systems and infant motor development. *Dev Rev* 1987; 7:39–65.

105. Thelen E, Ulrich B, Jenson J: The developmental origins of locomotion, in Woollacott MH, Shumway-Cook A (eds): *The Development of Posture and Gait Across the Lifespan*. Columbia, University of South Carolina Press, 1989.

106. Tkaczuk H: Tensile properties of human lumbar longitudinal ligaments. *Acta Orthop Scand Suppl* 1968; 115:1.

107. Viitsala JJ, et al: Muscular strength profiles and anthro-

pometry in random samples of men aged 31–35, 51–55 and 71–75 years. *Ergonomics* 1985; 28:1563–1574.

108. Vijayashankar N, Brody H: A quantitative study of the pigmented neurons in the nuclei locus coeruleus and sub-coeruleus in man as related to aging. *J Neuropathol Exp Neurol* 1979; 38:490.

109. Virgin W: Experimental investigations into physical properties of the intervertebral disc. *J Bone Joint Surg* 1951; 33B:607–611.

110. Weaver JK, Chalmers K: Cancellous bone: Its strength and changes with aging and an evaluation of some methods for measuring mineral content. *J Bone Joint Surg* 1966; 48A:289–298.

111. Weiss EB: Stress at the lumbosacral junction. *Orthop Clin North Am* 1975; 6:83–103.

112. White AA, Hirsch C: The significance of the vertebral posterior elements in the mechanics of the thoracic spine. *Clin Orthop* 1971; 81:2–14.

113. White AA, Panjabi MM: *Clinical Biomechanics of the Spine*. Philadelphia, JB Lippincott, 1978.

114. White AA, et al: Biomechanical analysis of clinical stability in the cervical spine. *Clin Orthop* 1975; 109:85–96.

115. Woollacott M, Inglin B, Manchester D: Response and posture control: Neuromuscular changes in the older adult. *Ann N Y Acad Sci* 1988; 515:42–53.

116. Wright GR, Shephard RJ: Brake reaction time-effects of age, sex, and carbon monoxide. *Arch Environ Health* 1978; 33:141–150.

CHAPTER 15

Balance and Falls in the Elderly: Issues in Evaluation and Treatment

Julie M. Chandler, M.S., P.T.
Pamela W. Duncan, Ph.D., P.T.

INTRODUCTION

Everybody falls. Regardless of age, falling is a ubiquitous event experienced by all throughout life. Most falls, especially in children and young adults, are of minor consequence, are readily forgotten, and have no impact on subsequent function. Falls in the elderly, by contrast, are a major cause of morbidity and mortality, the consequences often extending far beyond minor injury to significant loss of functional independence and even death. The reason that falling becomes a major health hazard in persons over age 65 is a result of the complex and poorly understood interaction of biomedical, physiologic, psychosocial, and environmental factors.

The overall objective of this chapter is to provide the reader with an understanding of the complex issues in the evaluation and treatment of the older person with instability. To meet this objective, we will follow a five-step process. First, we will define the problem of falls in the elderly from an epidemiologic perspective. Then we will delineate the multiple interacting factors in falls. Because the contribution of physiologic impairment to falls is particularly important for the therapist to assess, we will review the role of postural control in instability. Based on the above information, we will present a strategy for the comprehensive assessment of the older faller, and finally, we will discuss the principles of intervention.

DEFINING THE PROBLEM OF FALLS

Falls are a major cause of morbidity and mortality in persons over age 65. They are the leading cause of death from injury, a rate that increases with advancing age. In persons over age 85, approximately two thirds of injury-related deaths are due to falls.[1] It is estimated that 30% of community-dwelling elders over age 65, 40% of those over 80 years, and 66% of institutionalized elders fall each year. There is a greater-than-linear increase in the rate of falls between the ages of 60 to 65 and 80 to 85.[36] Because most falls do not result in injury requiring medical attention, it is likely that many falls go unreported and that fall rates are grossly underestimated.[34]

Major morbidity from falls includes hip and other fractures and serious soft tissue injuries that require immobilization or hospitalization. The majority of falls in the elderly, however, result in minor or no injury.[55] Regardless of injury severity, sequelae from even a benign fall can be devastating. A single fall often results in a fear of falling, which leads to a loss of confidence in one's ability to perform routine tasks, restriction in activities, social isolation, and increased dependence on others. The ensuing deconditioning, joint stiffness, and muscle weakness that result

from immobility can lead to more falls and further mobility restriction.[27, 34]

Risk Factors

Seriousness of the consequences of falls coupled with the recognition of falling as an escalating problem in an aging population has prompted many investigators in the field of geriatrics to examine risk factors associated with falls. The US Public Health Service estimates that two thirds of falls by the elderly are potentially preventable. Identification of significant risk factors is an important step toward fall prevention.

Risk factors associated with falls can be classified as either intrinsic (host) or extrinsic (environmental).[39] Host factors include symptoms such as dizziness, weakness, difficulty walking, or confusion, whereas environmental factors include conditions such as a slippery surface, loose rug, poor lighting, and obstacles. Tinetti et al. found that intrinsic factors such as sedative use, cognitive impairment, lower extremity disability, palmomental reflex, and foot problems increase the likelihood of falling in community-dwelling elders over age 75.[54] Not surprisingly, the likelihood of falling increases as risk factors accumulate. Overwhelming medical or environmental events such as stroke, syncope, or slipping on the ice account for a very small percentage of falls in the elderly and are usually eliminated from falls rate and risk factor analysis. Lach et al. found that intrinsic factors such as dizziness, weakness, difficulty walking, and confusion accounted for 45% of falls in community-dwelling elders, whereas slippery surfaces, loose rugs, loose objects, or poor lighting accounted for 39% of falls.[23] For most falls in the elderly, however, it is difficult to distinguish between those that are intrinsically and extrinsically precipitated. It is likely that most falls are a result of the complex interaction of host and environmental factors.[24, 51, 52] Multisystem failure can lower one's threshold for environmentally precipitated falls. In the 80-year-old diabetic with severe osteoarthritis of the hip, peripheral neuropathy, and failing vision, the likelihood of tripping over a carpet edge or raised threshold increases dramatically.

Aging Theory: Concepts Pertinent to Falls in the Elderly

While it is useful to identify potential markers of physical frailty that may contribute to falls risk, one must be careful not to simply treat a "laundry list" of host and environmental conditions with the hope that falls risk will diminish. The reason for this is that the process of aging itself is a complex event; several important axioms in gerontology should be considered in the comprehensive evaluation and treatment of the frail elder.[50]

The first of these axioms is the notion of functional reserve. *Functional reserve* refers to the excess or redundant function that is present in virtually all physiologic systems such that a significant degree of physiologic function can be lost long before clinical symptoms appear. In the older adult, functional reserve is markedly diminished, and the threshold for clinically observable loss of function is lowered. For the older faller, it may be that redundant functions within the postural control system are lost gradually. As losses accumulate, a critical threshold is reached, and clinical signs and symptoms such as falling and instability are observed.

The second important axiom is that aging is heterogeneous. Variability between individuals increases with age, and the discrepancy between biologic age and chronologic age widens. It is therefore difficult to examine the effect of age on any one physiologic system because individuals have different combinations of subtle and interacting pathologies.

Third, an elderly person's function may represent more or less than the sum of losses in his physiologic systems. Results of a recent study suggest that function is likely to be maintained when only one sensory component is compromised.[9] When additional subtle losses occur across other domains (e.g., central processing or effector), compensatory capacity may become compromised and function lost. In other words, function is the outcome produced by the integration of the system's physiologic components. When a single component is lost, function can be maintained by compensatory mechanisms through other components. When multiple subtle losses accumulate across other components, compensatory capacity may become compromised. It is therefore critical when interpreting diagnostic and physiologic information to examine integrated measures of functional performance in order to understand the functional consequences of physiologic losses.

Finally, the consequences of impaired mobility and poor balance in the older person may vary depending on his social, emotional, and behavioral resources. A strong social support network and sound judgment in risk-taking behavior may mitigate the effect of poor balance control and reduce falls risk.

MULTIFACETED APPROACH TO THE FALLS PROBLEM

Falls themselves are a heterogeneous phenomenon. Falls represent a failure of the body to remain upright but do not necessarily signal a disruption in the integrity of the postural control system. For some, a fall or series of falls may be a marker of an acute illness or other overwhelming medical event. For others, a fall or falls can occur in the presence of extreme environmental conditions or unusual activity. In most cases, however, falls represent the failure of the person with impaired functional capacity to meet the intrinsic and extrinsic demands of mobility within specific environments.[34] In general, as one ages, falls risk shifts from being spread out over many diverse activities, situations, and environments to being focused on basic movements required for routine daily activities.[36, 38]

Because of the complexity of falls themselves and of interpreting falls risk, a multifaceted approach to examining the falls phenomenon in the geriatric patient is useful. Studenski suggests four approaches to assessing the falling syndrome in the geriatric patient: ecologic, biomedical, physiologic, and functional (Fig 15–1).[47] The ecologic approach focuses on the extrinsic components of a fall event, that is, the interaction between the organism and the environment. A fall can occur in the presence of an unusual environment (e.g., icy surface) in a person with minimal impairment. A fall can also occur in a mildly impaired person attempting to negotiate a gravel pathway in unfamiliar territory. Or a severely impaired person may fall while walking in his home. Such an approach allows the examiner to assess the contribution and potential modification of environmental factors in fall events.

The biomedical component of the assessment focuses on medical events that are potentially contributory to falls. It is important for the practitioner to identify acute and chronic diseases that result in instability. For example, acute illnesses and conditions such as electrolyte abnormalities, infections, drug side effects, dehydration, orthostatic hypotension, blood loss, and hypoxemia can all

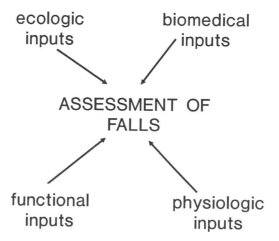

FIG 15–1.
Four approaches to the assessment of falls. (Adapted from Studenski S: Falls, in Calkins E (ed): *The Practice of Geriatrics,* ed 2. Philadelphia, WB Saunders, 1992.)

cause weakness, lightheadedness, and falls. The possibility of an acute process in the chronic faller can be signaled by a sudden, unexplained change in fall frequency.

Diseases that cause falls can be classified by organ system. For example, cardiovascular conditions include arrhythmias, aortic stenosis, and carotid sinus sensitivity. Neuromuscular diseases such as cerebrovascular accidents (CVAs), seizures, Parkinson's disease, myelopathies, cerebellar disease, normal pressure hydrocephalus, brain tumors, myopathies, peripheral neuropathies, and vestibular disease can also cause instability and falling. While it is relatively rare for a single diagnosis to account wholly for falls in the geriatric patient (with the exception of Parkinson's disease), this approach is useful for identifying treatable disease components of the falls syndrome.

The pathophysiologic component of geriatric falls assessment allows for identification of deficits in postural control that contribute to instability. Components of the postural control system that are assessed include sensory, effector (strength, range of motion, biomechanical alignment, flexibility), and central processing. Current postural control theory as outlined in the next section of this chapter forms the conceptual basis for the physical therapist's assessment and treatment of the geriatric faller.

Finally, the functional components of the assessment allow the examiner to identify important routine movements with which the patient has difficulty. These movements represent the integrated function of the postural control system and signal how the "output" of the system is affected by deficits in its components.

POSTURAL CONTROL THEORY

Physiology of Balance

Adequate postural control requires keeping the center of gravity over the base of support during both static and dynamic situations. The body must be able to respond to translations of the center of gravity voluntarily imposed (e.g., intentional movement) and involuntarily or unexpectedly imposed (e.g., slip, trip).

Physiologically speaking, how does the body maintain balance? First, a person must continually acquire information about the body's position and trajectory in space. This is done through the sensory system. Second, the body must determine, in advance, an effective and timely response (central processing). And third, the body must carry out that response via the effector system (strength, range of motion, flexibility, endurance).

Sensory data critical to balance are provided primarily from visual, vestibular, and somatosensory systems. Vision helps to orient the body in space by referencing vertical and horizontal axes of objects around them. In stand-

ing, vision helps to detect slight postural shifts by providing information to the central nervous system (CNS) about the position and movements of the body parts in relation to each other and the external environment. Components of vision that are clinically important to consider include (1) acuity, (2) contrast sensitivity, (3) peripheral vision, and (4) depth perception. *Acuity* refers to the ability to detect subtle differences in shapes and letters, whereas contrast sensitivity is the ability to detect subtle differences in shading and patterns (e.g., the ability to discriminate steps covered with a heavily patterned carpet). *Peripheral vision* is the ability to see from the side while looking straight ahead, and *depth perception* is the ability to distinguish distances.

The vestibular system also provides key sensory data for balance control. This system provides the CNS with information (via the otoliths and semicircular canals) regarding head movement and position. Vestibular input is used to generate compensatory eye movements and postural responses during head movements and helps to resolve conflicting information from visual images and actual movement. Information from sensory receptors in the vestibular apparatus interacts with visual and somatosensory information to produce proper body alignment and postural control.

Somatosensation is the third important input to the sensory system for balance control. Proprioceptive input provided to the CNS by joint, tendon, and muscle receptors gives information regarding the motion of the body with respect to the support surface and motion of the body segments with respect to each other.

Sensory information provided from visual, vestibular, and somatosensory systems is somewhat redundant in balance control. Blind people can stand and walk without losing balance. Nevertheless, it is well documented that in the absence of diagnosable disease, visual (especially contrast sensitivity),[13] vibratory, and proprioceptive input are frequently diminished in the older adult.[25, 28] Specifically, Lord et al. found that clinical loss of contrast sensitivity was associated with a higher incidence of falls in older adults.[26] Thus, redundancy in sensory input may be compromised either as a result of aging alone or as a result of subclinical disease processes to which elders are particularly prone.[18, 58]

Central processing is the second major physiologic component of balance control. It can be regarded as the process of "setting up" the postural response. Horak and Nashner's systems approach to balance control proposes that the central nervous system maps the location of the center of gravity and adaptively organizes its response to disequilibrium by preprogramming postural sensorimotor strategies. The preprogrammed strategies are based on the body's biomechanical constraints, available sensory infor-

information, the environmental context, and prior experience.[17]

In simpler terms, the CNS receives sensory information provided by the visual, vestibular, and somatosensory systems, processes it in the context of previously learned responses, and executes a corrective automatic postural response that is guided by or expressed through the mechanical structure in which it sits. Such responses are elicited in both feedback and feedforward situations. *Feedback* refers to situations where the body is perturbed by an external event, such as slipping on a rug, tripping, or being pushed. The center of gravity is displaced, and the CNS, based on the sensory information it has received, sets up a postural response to bring the center of gravity back over the base of support. Responses can be either protective or corrective. *Feedforward* describes a situation where the CNS sets up a postural response in anticipation of a disturbance of the center of gravity, such as catching a ball or simply raising the arms. The movement of reaching to catch a ball is a voluntary displacement of the center of gravity, but the automatic postural responses must precede the voluntary movement in order to stabilize the center of gravity and allow the movement to take place.

Recent research in automatic postural responses has focused on neurophysiologic responses to postural perturbations in feedback paradigms. Movable platforms have been used to create perturbations (forward, backward, or rotatory) as the patient stands in his normal stance. In this paradigm, the base of support is displaced, and a postural response to restore normal upright alignment is elicited. Using electromyography (EMG), muscle responses to such perturbations have been identified. The primary variables examined are latency (time to muscle response) and sequence (the order in which muscles respond). Based on his original work in this area, Nashner has proposed a model to interpret postural responses using this paradigm.[30–33] Though recent research in this area suggests that postural response mechanisms are more complex than originally proposed by this model, it does provide a framework from which to understand postural responses better. Nashner describes three basic strategies as "normal" responses to unexpected postural perturbations:

1. An *ankle strategy* is used with relatively small disturbances of the base of support. The center of gravity is perturbed backward or forward, and the body moves as a relatively rigid mass about the ankle joints, like an inverted pendulum, to bring the center of gravity back over the base of support. The latency is approximately 100 to 120 ms for healthy young adults, and the typical muscle sequence follows a distal to proximal pattern of lower extremity activation. For example, a forward movement of the platform induces a posterior displacement of the center

of gravity, similar to a slip on a rug. Because this perturbation is relatively mild on a wide stable base of support, the response is subtle and corrective movement occurs primarily around the ankle joint. In a typical healthy young adult, the tibialis anterior would be activated first (about 100 ms), followed by a quadriceps response as the center of gravity is pulled back over the base of support. A perturbation in the opposite direction (induced forward sway) would stimulate a gastrocnemius-hamstring response.

2. For more forceful perturbations, or for perturbations that occur while standing on a narrow or unstable base of support, a *hip strategy* is typically seen. In this response, primary movement occurs at the hip (flexion or extension) as the center of gravity moves rapidly back and forth over a relatively short distance. Instead of distal to proximal sequencing, the reverse is typically seen, that is, a proximal to distal pattern.

3. The third major classification is the *stepping strategy,* which occurs in situations where the center of gravity is displaced beyond the limits of the base of support. A stepping or stumbling strategy is necessary to regain equilibrium because neither the ankle nor hip strategy is sufficient to move the center of gravity back over the base of support.

Investigation in this area has expanded immensely during the past decade. Continued attempts to elucidate postural control mechanisms have included examination of EMG responses along the axial skeleton to the neck[22] as well as assessment of kinematic responses during postural perturbation.[40] Normal postural control mechanisms as evaluated electromyographically are more complex and variable than originally postulated in the Nashner model. Keshner found that response patterns do not always ascend in a distal to proximal sequence, even to subtle perturbations.[21] She postulates that sequences vary because muscles are activated either by a combination of inputs from different sensory components (vestibular, visual, neck proprioceptors) activated by the perturbation or by proprioceptive inputs at each joint. It appears that people have distinct muscle response patterns but that response patterns are variable among individuals. Her work suggests that the CNS should provide multiple alternatives for attaining the goal of postural stability. The key to success in developing balance is to develop adaptable and flexible strategies that will meet the demands of a complex and constantly changing environment.

Influence of Age on Postural Control

Many investigators have examined the effects of age on postural responses.[19, 28, 44, 59–61] While distal to proximal sequencing in response to platform perturbation appears to

Response Sequency

be the predominant pattern, a higher incidence of proximal to distal sequencing in the older adult has been observed. Such altered sequencing may be an indicator of altered postural control in the older adult.[60] Other studies, however, have shown similar variability in response patterns in healthy elders and older fallers.[48] It is thus not clear exactly what significance EMG sequence has in the postural response of the aging adult.

Response Latency & Age

Findings from studies of response latencies have been more consistent. Investigators have consistently found that responses are delayed in the healthy older adult by approximately 20 to 30 ms.[45, 48, 59, 60] It has been postulated that specific timing, if delayed sufficiently, may significantly affect one's ability to produce an effective response. Thus, inability to fire fast enough, regardless of activation sequence, may be a significant factor in the patient who presents with instability. Studenski and colleagues reported evidence of delayed latency in older fallers when compared with age-matched nonfallers. Latencies are not only delayed in the healthy older adult but are even further delayed in the older person with a history of unexplained falls.[48]

In summary, the variables of sequence and latency are currently used to describe central-processing mechanisms in both feedback and feedforward paradigms. The information available in this area has not clarified which exact EMG sequence is the most effective for a given perturbation. Furthermore, the relationship between responses to artificially imposed perturbations and responses to balance disturbances in everyday life is not known. Nevertheless, it would appear that a patient with significantly delayed latencies or a patient who demonstrates cocontraction instead of an organized distal to proximal or proximal to distal response to a platform perturbation is likely to also respond ineffectively to mild or moderate center of gravity displacements during functional activities. The CNS should be able to provide multiple alternatives for attaining the single goal of postural stability.[21] The key to successful balance control is to develop adaptable strategies that will meet the demands presented in a complex environment.

Effector Δ's

The third major physiologic component of balance is the effector component, which constitutes the biomechanical apparatus through which the centrally programmed response must be expressed. Factors such as range of motion, muscle torque and power, postural alignment, and endurance can all affect the capacity for a person to effectively respond to a disturbance of balance. Studenski and her coworkers determined that elderly fallers produce significantly weaker distal lower extremity torque than healthy elders.[48] Similarly, Whipple et al. found that nursing home residents with a history of recurrent falls

demonstrated diminished torque production of both the ankle and knee.[56] Sufficient muscle power of the lower extremity muscles is a key element in effective balance control.

Less is known about the influence of joint limitations on righting reactions and falls. Back extension and neck range of motion may be reduced and arthritis more common in elderly fallers.[54] Intuitively, sufficient flexibility in the mechanical structure is needed for effective execution of the balance response. Loss of flexibility may lead to a less efficient or ineffective response strategy.[41]

Relationship Between Postural Control and Falls: A Model

It is clear from the previous discussion that the issue of balance impairment and falls is a complex and multifaceted problem in the aging adult. With the exception of overwhelming medical or environmental events, falls in the elderly usually occur in those with physical impairment.[20, 43] Yet the relationship between physical impairment and falls is not linear. Factors outside of physical function—psychosocial, cognitive, environmental—can modify the risk of falling in persons with severely impaired mobility. Thus, physical impairment may be a necessary but not sufficient condition for falling.[50]

At the highest levels of physical mobility and balance control, falls risk is very low. At very low levels of physical mobility and balance control, falls risk is also low because the person is unable to displace his center of gravity. The relationship between falls risk and physical impairment between those two extremes is not clear. In a person with moderately impaired mobility, the risk of falling may be modified if he has social support to help with risky tasks. A person's risk-taking behavior can also affect his falls risk. If a person recognizes that he is at risk for falling in a particular situation and modifies his behavior, falls risk will be minimized. If, on the other hand, he recognizes the risk of falling but prefers to take the risk by performing the task, the risk of falling is heightened. Another important consideration is that improved physical function may not necessarily reduce falls risk but may simply alter the types of activities during which falls occur. Finally, cognitive impairment can include a loss of judgment in risk-taking behavior and has been strongly associated with falls risk.[54]

Comprehensive assessment of the older faller must include not only evaluation of physiologic impairments and physical performance deficits but also an assessment of cognitive, behavioral environmental, and social factors.

ASSESSMENT

Comprehensive assessment of the older faller requires a multidisciplinary team effort, of which the physical therapist is an integral part. Other members include a physician, a social worker, a nurse, and possibly a psychologist or counselor. Medical screening crucial to the evaluation process includes (1) examination of the patient's current and past medications for potential interactions and side effects (hypnotics, sedatives, tricyclic antidepressants, tranquilizers, and antihypertensive drugs have all been associated with falls and instability)[3, 4, 39, 54] and (2) identification of medical conditions that may contribute to unsteadiness (focal neurologic lesion, cardiovascular conditions, orthostasis), diseases manifesting with balance disorders, and metabolic causes of instability.

The social worker or psychologist can gather information from the patient and family about social and financial resources, depression, cognitive function, and family dynamics. The physical therapist gathers information about impairments in the postural control system and about functional performance deficits that contribute to the person's disability. Successful management of the geriatric faller, then, is based on input from all sources of the evaluation.

How should you approach the older patient referred for instability and falls? Because of the complex nature of the problem, a systematic approach to the evaluation procedure is useful (Table 15–1).

History

It is useful to have a clear idea of the patient's perception of his unsteadiness problem before gathering other relevant historical information. Knowing how the unsteadiness is primarily affecting the patient or family member provides a useful framework from which to proceed with the evaluation. It is important to gather specific information regarding the patient's falls, such as onset of falls, environmental conditions, activities at the time of falls, direction of falls, and medications. For example, it is useful to know whether the onset of falls is sudden (acute medical condition) or gradual (slowly deteriorating compensatory mechanisms). In addition, it is important to know what environmental conditions are associated with falls. Was the fall inside the home (consider factors such as lighting, chair height, steps) or outside the home (review factors such as unfamiliar territory, uneven surfaces, more vigorous activities)? Finding out about the activity at the time of the fall can give insight into how much the postural control system was being stressed. The presence of vertigo or dizziness at the time of the fall can signal a circulatory or vestibular function problem. Information regarding the direction of

TABLE 15–1.
Elements in the Assessment of Instability in the Older Faller

I. Falls history
  A. Onset—sudden vs. gradual, frequency
  B. Environmental factors
  C. Activities at time of fall
  D. Presence of dizziness, vertigo, lightheadedness
  E. Current medications, past medications
  F. Direction of falls
II. Etiologic assessment
  A. Sensory
    1. Vision
    2. Proprioception, vibration
    3. Vestibular
  B. Effector
    1. Strength
    2. Range of motion, flexibility
    3. Endurance
  C. Central processing
    1. Feedback
    2. Feedforward
    3. Response to changing conditions
III. Functional assessment
  A. Standing reach
  B. Mobility skills
  C. Varied conditions of performance
IV. Environmental assessment
  A. Functional home assessment—interaction of patient and home

falls (forward, backward, to the side) is useful because reproducible circumstances of falls may signal specific postural control deficits. Finally, the patient's current and past medications should be noted for their possible contribution to unsteadiness (e.g., antidepressants, sedatives, tranquilizers, and antihypertensives).

Etiologic Assessment

The etiologic assessment allows identification of deficits in the sensory, effector, and central-processing systems that may contribute to the falls problem.

Sensory

Sensory examination should include vision, vestibular, and somatosensory systems. Important aspects of vision to consider include acuity, contrast sensitivity (ability to discriminate fine details in a cluttered environment), peripheral fields, and depth perception. Acuity, peripheral fields, and depth perception can be easily screened in the clinic. For acuity, having the patient read a pocket-size Snellen chart (Fig 15–2) can give a quick gross estimate of his ability to discriminate fine detail. A score of 20/200 may signal that vision is contributing to the patient's instability. For peripheral fields, the examiner brings his fingers from

SNELLEN CHART (hold card in good light
14 in. from eye)

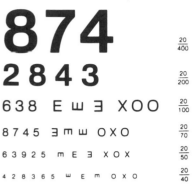

874	20/400
2843	20/200
638 E ॥ Ǝ XOO	20/100
8745 Ǝ ᴍ ॥ OXO	20/70
63925 ᴍ E Ǝ XOX	20/50
428365 ॥ E ᴍ OXO	20/40

FIG 15-2.
Pocket-sized Snellen chart for gross visual acuity screening.

behind the patient's head at eye level while the patient stares straight ahead. The patient identifies when he first notices the examiner's finger in his side view. A significant field cut unilaterally or bilaterally would be noteworthy. For depth perception, the examiner holds his index fingers parallel and pointing upward in front of the patient at eye level. As the examiner moves his fingers apart (one forward, one back), the patient identifies when the fingers are back together (parallel). If the patient is off by 3 in. or more, then depth perception may be a problem. Examination of existing lenses may also be useful. Bifocals magnify objects and can be very disorienting during activities such as stair climbing and descent.

Vestibular function should also be assessed. Vestibulo-ocular and vestibulospinal reflexes are critical in balance control. Vestibulospinal input is particularly important for maintaining upright body position during movement. Because of the complexity of the pathway, few good clinical tests of vestibulospinal function exist. Vestibulo-ocular tests are therefore used more frequently to assess vestibular function. Vestibulo-ocular function can be tested by having the patient maintain gaze on a fixed object (e.g., examiner's finger) while he turns his head rapidly to the right or left. Normally, a person should be able to maintain gaze without difficulty. In the presence of vestibular dysfunction the patient's eyes will move off target and will make a corrective saccade to regain fixation. Other clinical tests of dynamic stability that grossly assess integrated vestibular function include (1) reading a book while walking or (2) marching in place with eyes closed. In the first test, the patient should be able to read while walking without losing balance. The patient with vestibular dysfunction will be unable to maintain visual fixation on the reading material and move at the same time. Marching in place with eyes closed is also difficult for the patient with a vestibular lesion. When asked to perform

this test, he will deviate markedly from his initial position.[16]

Somatosensory examination includes proprioception and vibration. Both should be assessed in a distal to proximal sequence. A patient with normal proprioception should be able to detect very subtle motion of the great toe (less than 5 mm). Vibratory sense can be assessed by placing a tuning fork at the first metatarsal head. If vibratory sense and proprioception are present distally, there is no need to proceed proximally.

The Sensory Integration Test (SIT) developed by Shumway-Cook and Horak can also be used clinically to assess the influence of vision, somatosensation, and vestibular function on standing balance.[42] The SIT includes a series of six tests under varying sensory conditions during which the patient is timed and standing balance is assessed. Visual, proprioceptive, and vestibular inputs are manipulated in various combinations to provide six different sensory conditions. It is important to note that as sensory conditions change, the expected response also changes. That is, under conditions of diminished sensory input, increased sway is anticipated. The patient with severe joint motion loss or weakness may be unable to maintain his balance under the conditions of increased sway. This patient may not have a problem with sensory integration but rather with a faulty effector system that is unable to execute a sufficient motor response to maintain stability under those conditions. While the SIT cannot identify specific causes of balance dysfunction, it can be useful in identifying conditions under which the patient may have difficulty.

Effector
Effector components that should be evaluated are strength, range of motion, and endurance.

Strength.—Traditional methods of manual muscle testing may not provide the most useful information with regard to balance control. This is especially true in muscle groups for which large displacements and fast, forceful movements are required (i.e., quadriceps, hamstrings). Isokinetic testing of the quadriceps, hamstring, dorsiflexors, and plantarflexors at both slow and moderate speeds gives a more accurate picture of the patient's torque-generating capacity under different conditions. In the more proximal hip and trunk muscles, whose primary function is stabilization, an isometric muscle test may be more appropriate.

Range of Motion.—Measurement of range of motion and flexibility using standard goniometric methods is an important component of the etiologic evaluation. Important musculoskeletal regions to be assessed include ankle, knee, hip, trunk, and cervical spine. While it is not known to what extent limited flexibility contributes to instability in the frail elderly, it is clear that a patient with severe limitation of trunk, neck, or lower extremity motion will be constrained by the biomechanical apparatus through which his postural response must be expressed. The variety of postural response strategies that are required to function in a complex environment may be restricted as a result of a stiff body segment.

Endurance.— Another effector component to consider in overall stability and function is endurance. A patient may be able to generate adequate force during a few repeated contractions but may have difficulty during tasks that require continued efforts. One useful quantitative test for assessing endurance in frail elders is the 6-minute walk. In this test, the patient walks up and down a premeasured walkway (e.g., a hospital corridor) at his normal pace for 6 minutes, resting as needed. The distance covered after 6 minutes is recorded.[7, 14]

Central Processing

Central processing can be grossly assessed in both feedforward and feedback situations. The examiner looks for (1) the effectiveness of the patient's response to induced, unexpected perturbations (feedback) and (2) the ability of the patient to maintain stability during movements that intentionally displace the center of gravity (feedforward). It is important to note, however, that responses to such tests represent integrated function of the postural control system and not just central processing. Because responses are ultimately expressed through the effector system, an ineffective response to a perturbation may be the result of weakness or stiffness rather than faulty central processing.

A simple semiquantitative method of testing responses to induced posterior perturbation is the Postural Stress Test (PST).[57] In this test, motor responses to postural perturbations of varying degrees are measured during normal standing using a simple pulley-weight system that displaces the center of gravity behind the base of support. The PST measures an individual's ability to withstand a series of destabilizing forces applied at the level of the subject's waist. Scoring of the postural responses is based on a nine-point ordinal scale where a score of 9 represents the most efficient postural response, and a score of 0 represents complete failure to remain upright. Mild perturbations should require minimal response (corresponding to a score of 8 or 9), whereas larger perturbations may require a stepping strategy (corresponding to a score of 4, 5, or 6). Studies have shown that healthy elders demonstrate effective balance responses during this test but that elderly fallers are likely to show ineffective responses (corresponding to scores of 0, 1, or 2).[6] The test is useful in grossly as-

sessing the patient's capacity to withstand mild unexpected perturbations.

An alternative to the PST is a simple manual test that can be performed in any clinic setting. In this test, the therapist stands behind the patient and pulls him backward at waist level several times with varying degrees of force (mild to moderate). The therapist looks for the appropriateness of the patient's responses to a given level of perturbation. For example, the patient should be able to maintain upright stance using minimal postural response (ankle dorsiflexion only) when the pull backward is very mild. With a more forceful pull backward, the patient should be able to recover his balance using a hip or stepping strategy. The patient who cannot execute an effective response will require intervention by the therapist to keep from falling. Similarly, the patient who requires multiple steps to recover balance when given a very mild perturbation will likely lose his balance with more forceful balance disturbances.

Feedforward postural responses can be assessed by having the patient perform voluntary movements that require mild to moderate displacements of his center of gravity. For example, in his normal standing position, asking the patient to raise his arms in front of him requires subtle postural stabilization by the lower extremity and trunk muscles in preparation for mild displacement of the center of gravity caused by arm raising. Varying the speed of the task can give further information regarding the patient's ability to organize his preparatory postural responses in a timely fashion. Catching a ball thrown slightly off center, slowly, then faster, is an example of a higher-level feedforward task that further stresses the postural control system.

Reaction time is another element of central processing that may be useful to assess. Tests involving simple lower or upper extremity movements in response to a light cue are examples of reaction time tests and may be abnormally slowed in the older faller.[35, 46] Patla et al. developed a lower extremity reaction time test in which the subject takes a step forward, backward, or to the side in response to the appropriate light cue.[37] This task may be particularly relevant in the older faller because it requires movements that are initiated to avoid collision and potential falls and requires weight transfer to the other limb before the initiation of movement. Total reaction time in this test reflects the process of stimulus detection, response selection, and planning and movement execution.

Functional Assessment

While identification of defective components of the postural control system can help to guide specific treatment planning, more critical is the assessment of the patient's functional performance. It is during this part of the evaluation that the therapist must determine how specific deficits in the system affect the patient's overall function. Given a significant level of hip abductor and hip extensor weakness, for example, one would expect the patient to demonstrate instability during activities such as walking, stair climbing, or rising from a chair. If the patient's balance problems are not manifested during those activities but rather during simple reaching tasks or when turning to change direction, then hip weakness may not be a key component of the patient's instability and may not need to be addressed in treatment.

A series of progressively challenging mobility tasks can be used to screen for functional balance deficits. The progressive mobility skills protocol takes the patient through a series of increasingly complex tasks from sitting unsupported to stair climbing (Table 15–2).[49] Failure to perform a task at any point during the test theoretically precludes further testing. Overall performance can be scored and used as baseline information against which to measure change. Performance on individual tasks in the protocol can be used to identify specific functional deficits that can be addressed in treatment. Other quantitative performance-oriented scales have also been developed and tested.[2, 29, 53]

Another quantitative and informative measure of functional performance is the functional reach measure.[11] During this test the patient is asked to reach forward as far as possible from a comfortable standing posture. The excursion of the arm from start to finish is measured via a yardstick affixed to the wall (Fig 15–3). This measure tests the ability and willingness of the patient to move to the margins of his base of support voluntarily. Duncan and her colleagues have shown that frail persons with reaches under 6 in. have four times the likelihood of falling than persons with a reach greater than 18 in.[10]

While quantitative tests are useful for measurement and documentation purposes, qualitative description and observation are also important. During the functional assessment process, the therapist should vary the conditions under which the patient performs the tasks. For example, it is useful to see how the patient responds to changes in gait speed and direction, negotiates obstacles, and handles changing surfaces and other environmental distractions and conditions.

Environmental Assessment

Another aspect of functional performance that is important to consider is how the patient functions at home. Often, decisions are made to modify a person's environment based on performance deficits that may have been observed during evaluation in a hospital room or clinic. Not surprisingly, the unstable patient is often able to maneuver around his own home much more steadily and safely than he can in an unfamiliar hospital or clinic environment. Chandler and coworkers have developed an instrument that allows the therapist to assess performance-based environmental risk (Table 15–3).[5] Ideally, home modifications or other interventions should be designed based on the patient's performance during routine activities within his home. The therapist can perform the assessment by asking the patient to show him how he maneuvers around his home on a typical day. Getting in and out of a favorite chair; turning on the television; opening high and low cabinets and the refrigerator; getting on and off the commode,

TABLE 15–2.

Progressive Mobility Skills Assessment Task*

Task	Performance (scoring)
Sitting balance	Subjects sit in firm-surfaced chair with arms crossed, unsupported
Sitting reach	Subjects grasp ruler held at shoulder level 12 in. from outstretched arm
Chair rise	Subjects rise from standard straight chair with arms folded
Standing balance	Subjects stand steadily, without support, for 60 seconds
Pick up object	Subjects pick up ruler placed on the floor 2 ft in front of them without holding on for support
Walking	Subjects walk 10 ft with a safe, stable gait without assistive device
Abrupt stop	Subjects walk as fast as they can for several steps and then, on command, stop abruptly without stumbling or grabbing for support
Turning	Subjects walk at normal pace, then turn around with smooth, continuous steps
Obstacle	Subjects step over shoebox in walking path without hesitating or stumbling over box
Standing reach	Subjects grasp ruler held at shoulder level 12 in. beyond outstretched arm without taking a step
Stairs	Subjects ascend and descend stairs, step over step, without support

*Adapted from Studenski S, Duncan P, Hogue C, et al: Progressive mobility skills. Presented at the American Geriatrics Society Annual Meeting, Boston, Massachusetts, May 12, 1989, p 41.

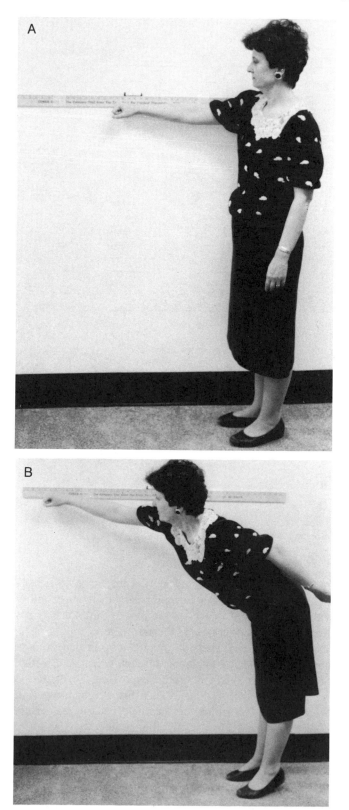

FIG 15–3.
A, functional reach—starting position. **B,** functional reach—ending position.

in and out of the shower or bath, and in and out of bed are examples of typical activities that should be assessed. Access to lighting and illumination is important to assess. It is unnecessary to suggest bathroom modification if the patient has no difficulty with such transfers. Obstacles, cords, and clutter become particularly relevant in the patient with serious visual deficits or gait abnormality but need to be addressed only to the extent that they pose a threat to the patient's safe function. Using this instrument, environmental risk can be quantified by evaluating both the *degree* of environmental hazard and the *frequency* with which it is encountered.

Psychosocial Assessment

Factors outside of physical performance that should be covered in the comprehensive evaluation of the geriatric faller include social support and behavioral/cognitive function. While other members of the interdisciplinary team are better equipped to identify specific problems in these areas, the therapist should be aware of how these factors may influence falls risk. The presence of a strong social support network may minimize falls risk because other people may be available to perform the "risky" activities for the patient. The patient that is no longer able to climb ladders or do yardwork safely must first recognize that these activities are no longer safe. Then one must decide the willingness to restrict activities or whether to take the risk of falling. Patients with severe cognitive loss are generally unable to recognize risk and consequently do not make sound judgments regarding safe activity.

INTERVENTION

Comprehensive multidisciplinary evaluation should guide the management of the geriatric patient with instability. The universal goal of intervention is to maximize independence in mobility and function. Within the limits of safety, it is always preferable to improve mobility and function than to restrict activity. Indeed, the consequences of immobilization and restricted activity can be more devastating that the instability itself. The typical sequelae of restricted activity include decreased life space, fear of movement, deconditioning, depression, and often a high financial and emotional cost to family and society.

The goal of maximum functional independence can be achieved by using the following principles to guide treatment planning:

1. Identify and treat modifiable deficits.
2. Identify and compensate for fixed deficits.

TABLE 15–3.

Functional Home Assessment Profile*

Pathways	Potential Risk Items	Frequency		Hazard		Sum
1. Entrance into home	Access (railing)	_____	X	_____	=	_____
	Door	_____	X	_____	=	_____
	Threshold	_____	X	_____	=	_____
	Other	_____	X	_____	=	_____
				Total	=	_____
2. Living room	Lighting	_____	X	_____	=	_____
3. Kitchen	Floor	_____	X	_____	=	_____
4. Bedroom	Storage	_____	X	_____	=	_____
5. Bathroom	Furniture	_____	X	_____	=	_____
	Other	_____	X	_____	=	_____
				Total†	=	_____
6. Other (hallway)	Floor	_____	X	_____	=	_____
	Lighting	_____	X	_____	=	_____
	Other	_____	X	_____	=	_____
				Total	=	_____

Variables (for each potential risk item)

Hazard
  0 = No risk
  1 = Low to moderate risk (patient would likely have difficulty 10% to 40% of time hazard is encountered)
  2 = Moderate to high risk (patient would likely have difficulty 50% to 100% of time hazard is encountered)
Frequency (frequency of encounter)
  0 = Never
  1 = < 1× / month
  2 = < 1× / week
  3 = 2–3×/week
  4 = 1–2× / day
  5 = > 2× / day
Total = Sum (frequency × hazard)

*Adapted in part from Chandler JM, Duncan PW, Prescott BL, et al: The functional home profile (F/HAP): Reliability of a new instrument. (in review).
†The sum (frequency × hazard) should be totaled for each of the rooms: living room, kitchen, bedroom, and bathroom.

Based on the evaluation, the therapist should first be able to identify possible etiologic components of the patient's instability. For example, major visual dysfunction is a fixed deficit but can be potentially treated by altering eyewear. Glasses with prisms can compensate for peripheral field deficits, tinted glasses can increase contrast sensitivity, and different glasses for near and far vision can reduce problems caused by bifocals. A referral to a geriatric optometrist can be extremely useful.

Loss of proprioception is also a fixed deficit and may be a potential contributor to the patient's instability. Because the probability of reversing proprioceptive loss is low, training the patient to compensate with increased visual input may be the most effective strategy. Patients with vestibular lesions can be potentially treated with specific exercises to improve vestibular function or can be taught compensatory techniques using vision.[15, 16]

When irreversible neurologic disease is the basis for instability, it is necessary to address the treatable aspects of the condition in order to improve or maintain mobility within the limits of safety. In the patient with Parkinson's disease, emphasis on flexibility and range of motion, particularly of the axial skeleton, may help to provide a more supple biomechanical apparatus through which an effective balance strategy might be better expressed. Teaching the Parkinson's disease patient to keep his weight forward in both standing and sitting can facilitate walking and rising from a chair, respectively. A rolling walker may be a useful tool to facilitate this movement strategy and provide additional safety.

To the extent that strength, range of motion, and endurance are contributing to the patient's instability they need to be addressed in treatment. Research has indicated that lower extremity weakness, especially at the ankle and knee, is significantly associated with recurrent falls in the elderly.[48, 56] It has also been well established that strength gains can be made in all age-groups, even in nonagenarians, by applying the physiologic exercise principles of overload and specificity.[12]

No treatment will be effective without specifically addressing the patient's functional deficits. Just as in treating the young orthopedic patient, vigorous strength training will not improve function unless specific functional training is incorporated into the exercise program. The functional assessment allows the therapist to identify specific functional limitations, so treatment should focus on similar activities. If, for example, reaching is limited, the therapist might incorporate functional activities that stress the patient's margin of stability, such as reaching for a glass, leaning forward, reaching behind self (as if to put arm in coat sleeve), and catching a ball off center. Weakness of the hip musculature can be effectively addressed by incorporating chair rising and stair climbing into the exercise program. Similarly, teaching the most biomechanically efficient chair-rise strategy can lead to immediate functional improvement.

For the patient who demonstrates poor balance responses to either feedforward or feedback displacements of the center of mass, it may be useful to practice effective balance responses, such as weight-shifting techniques. However, there is little evidence that balance training carries over to improved functional performance.[8] Evidence does suggest that balance is highly task specific and that muscles respond differently to different center-of-mass displacements. Interventions for balance deficits should therefore be functionally driven and task specific.

Compensatory treatment strategies must be applied when balance deficits cannot be changed. Such strategies must include environmental modification (e.g., grab bars, railings, improved lighting, altered chair heights), assistive devices, and increased external support (e.g., home health aide).

SUMMARY

Falls in the elderly are a multifaceted and heterogeneous problem. The most effective management strategy requires a multidisciplinary approach where pathophysiologic, functional, and environmental issues can be thoroughly evaluated and treated. The goal of intervention should always be to maximize functional independence within the margins of safety.

REFERENCES

1. Baker SP, Harvey AH: Fall injuries in the elderly. *Clinics in Geriatric Medicine*. Philadelphia, WB Saunders, 1985.

2. Berg K, Wood-Dauphinee S, Williams J, et al: Measuring balance in the elderly: Preliminary development of an instrument. *Physiother Can* 1989; 41:304–311.

3. Blake AJ, Morgan K, Bendall MJ, et al: Falls by elderly people at home: Prevalence and associated factors. *Age Ageing* 1988; 17:365–372.

4. Campbell JA, Borrie MJ, Spears GF: Risk factors for falls in a community-based prospective study of people 70 years and older. *J Gerontol* 1989; 44:M112–M117.

5. Chandler JM, Duncan PW, Prescott BL, et al: The functional home assessment profile (F-HAP): Reliability of a new instrument. (in review).

6. Chandler JM, Duncan PW, Studenski SA: Comparison of postural responses in young adults, healthy elderly and fallers using postural stress test. *Phys Ther* 1990; 70:410–415.

7. Cooper KH: A means of assessing maximal oxygen intake: Correlation between field and treadmill testing. *JAMA* 1968; 203:201–204.

8. Daleiden S: Weight shifting as a treatment for balance deficits: A literature review. *Physiother Can* 1990; 42:81–87.

9. Duncan PW, Chandler JM, Prescott BL, et al: How do physiologic components of balance affect function in elders?, in review.

10. Duncan PW, Studenski SA, Chandler JM: Functional reach: Predictive validity. *J Gerontol* 1992; 47 (3):M93–98.

11. Duncan PW, Weiner D, Chandler JM, et al: Functional reach: A new measure of balance. *J Gerontol* 1990; 45:M192–197.

12. Fiatarone MA, Marks EC, Ryon ND, et al: High intensity strength training on nonagenarians. *JAMA* 1990; 263:3029–3034.

13. Greene HH, Madden DJ: Adult age difference in visual acuity, stereopsis and contrast sensitivity. *Am J Optom Physiol Opt* 1986; 63:724–732.

14. Guyatt G, Thompson PJ: How should we measure function in patients with chronic heart and lung diseases? *J Chronic Dis* 1985; 38:517–524.

15. Herdman SJ: Exercise strategies in vestibular disorders. *Ear Nose Throat J* 1989; 68:961–964.

16. Herdman SJ: Assessment and treatment of balance disorders in the vestibular deficient patient, in Duncan P (ed): *Balance*. Proceedings of the American Physical Therapy Association Forum. Alexandria, Va, APTA Publications, 1990, pp 87–94.

17. Horak FB, Nashner LM: Central programming of postural movements: Adaptations to altered support-surface configurations. *J Neurophysiol* 1986; 55:1369–1381.

18. Horak FB, Shupert CL, Mirka A: Components of postural dyscontrol in the elderly: A review. *Neurobiol Aging* 1989; 10:727–738.

19. Inglin B, Woollacott M: Age-related changes in anticipatory postural adjustments associated with arm movements. *J Gerontol* 1988; 43:M105–M113.

20. Kauffman T: Impact of aging-related musculoskeletal and postural changes on falls. *Top Geriatr Rehabil* 1990; 5(2):34–43.

21. Keshner EA: Reflex, voluntary, and mechanical process in postural stabilization, in Duncan PW (ed): *Balance*. Proceedings of the American Physical Therapy Association Forum. Alexandria, Va, APTA Publications, 1990, pp 13–21.

22. Keshner EA, Allum JHJ, Pfaltz CR: Postural coactivation and adaptation in the sway stabilizing responses of normals and patients with bilateral peripheral vestibular deficit. *Exp Brain Res* 1987; 69:66–72.

23. Lach HW, Reed AT, Arfken CL, et al: Falls in the elderly: Reliability of a classification system. *J Am Geriatr Soc* 1991; 39:197–202.

24. Lipsitz LA, Jonsson PV, Kelley MM, et al: Causes and correlates of recurrent falls in ambulatory frail elderly. *J Gerontol* 1991; 46:M114–M122.

25. Lord SR, Clark RD, Webster IW: Postural stability and associated physiological factors in a population of aged persons. *J Gerontol* 1991; 46:M69–M76.

26. Lord SR, Clark RD, Webster IW: Visual acuity and contrast sensitivity in relation to falls in an elderly population. *Age Ageing* 1991; 20:175–181.

27. Maki BE, Holliday PJ, Topper AK: Fear of falling and postural performance in the elderly. *J Gerontol* 1991; 46:M123–M131.

28. Manchester D, Woollacott M, Zederbauer-Hylton N, et al: Visual, vestibular and somatosensory contributions to balance control in the older adult. *J Gerontol* 1989; 44:M118–M127.

29. Mathias S, Nayak USL, Isaacs B: Balance in elderly patients: The "get-up and go" test. *Arch Phys Med Rehabil* 1986; 67:387–389.

30. Nashner LM: Fixed patterns of rapid postural responses among leg muscles during stance. *Exp Brain Res* 1977; 30:13–24.

31. Nashner LM, McCollum G: The organization of human postural movement: A formal basis and experimental synthesis. *Behav Brain Sci* 1985; 8:135–172.

32. Nashner LM, Woollacott MH: The organization of rapid postural adjustments of standing humans: An experimental-conceptual model, in Talbott RE, Humphrey DR (eds): *Posture and Movement*. New York, Raven Press, 1979.

33. Nashner LM, Woollacott M, Tuma G: Organization of rapid response to postural and locomotor-like perturbation of standing man. *Exp Brain Res* 1979; 36:463–476.

34. Nevitt MC: Falls in older persons; Risk factors and prevention, in Berg RL, Cassells JF (eds): *The Second Fifty Years: Promoting Health and Preventing Disability*. Washington DC, Institute of Medicine National Academy Press, 1990, pp 263–290.

35. Nevitt MC, Cummings SR, Kidd S, et al: Risk factors for recurrent nonsyncopal falls: A prospective study. *JAMA* 1989; 261:2663–2668.

36. Nickens H: Intrinsic factors in falling among the elderly. *Arch Intern Med* 1985; 145:1089–1093.

37. Patla A, Winter D, Frank J, et al: Identification of age-related changes in the balance control system, in Duncan PW (ed): *Balance*. Proceedings of the American Physical Therapy Association Forum. Alexandria, Va, APTA Publications, 1990, pp 43–53.

38. Prudham D, Evans J: Factors associated with falls in the elderly: A community study. *Age Ageing* 1981; 10:141–146.

39. Robbins AS, Rubenstein LZ, Josephson DR, et al: Predictors of falls among elderly people: Results of two population-based studies. *Arch Intern Med* 1989; 149:1628–1633.

40. Romick-Allen R, Schultz AB: Biomechanics of reactions to impending falls. *J Biomech* 1988; 21:591–600.

41. Schenkman M: Interrelationship of neurological and mechanical factors in balance control, in Duncan PW (ed): *Balance*. Proceedings of the American Physical Therapy Association Forum. Alexandria, Va, APTA Publications, 1990 pp 29–41.

42. Shumway-Cook A, Horak F: Assessing the influence of sensory interaction on balance. *Phys Ther* 1986; 66:1548–1550.

43. Speechley M, Tinetti M: Assessment of risk and prevention of falls among elderly persons: Role of the physiotherapist. *Physiother Can* 1990; 42:75–79.

44. Stelmach GE, Phillips J, Difabio RP, et al: Age, functional postural reflexes and voluntary sway. *J Gerontol* 1989; 44:B100–106.

45. Stelmach GE, Teasdale N, Difabio RP, et al: Age related decline in postural control mechanisms. *Int J Aging Hum Dev* 1989; 23:205–223.

46. Stelmach GE, Worringham CJ: Sensorimotor deficits related to postural stability: Implication for falling in elderly. *Clinics in Geriatric Medicine*. Philadelphia, WB Saunders, 1985.

47. Studenski S: Falls, in Calkins E (ed): *The Practice of Geriatrics,* ed 2. Philadelphia, WB Saunders, 1992.

48. Studenski SA, Duncan PW, Chandler JM: Postural responses and effector factors in persons with unexplained falls: Results and methodologic issues. *J Am Geriatr Soc* 1991; 39:229–234.

49. Studenski S, Duncan P, Hogue C, et al: Progressive mobility skills. Presented at the American Geriatric Society Annual Meeting, May 12, 1989, p 41.

50. Studenski S, Duncan P, Weiner D, et al: The role of instability in falls among older persons, in Duncan PW (ed): *Balance*. Proceedings of the American Physical Therapy Association Forum. Alexandria, Va, APTA Publications, 1990, pp 57–60.

51. Tideiksaar R: Geriatric falls in the home. *Home Health Nurse* 1986; 4:14–23.

52. Tideiksaar R: Geriatric falls: Assessing the cause, preventing recurrence. *Geriatrics* 1989; 44:57–64.

53. Tinetti ME: Performance oriented assessment of mobility problems on elderly patients. *J Am Geriatr Soc* 1986; 34:119–126.

54. Tinetti ME, Speechley M, Ginter SF: Risk factors for falls among elderly persons living in the community. *N Engl J Med* 1988; 319:1701–1707.

55. Waller JA: Falls among the elderly—human and environmental factors. *Accid Anal Prev* 1978; 10:21–33.

56. Whipple RH, Wolfson LI, Amerman P: The relationship of knee and ankle weakness to falls in nursing home residents: An isokinetic study. *J Am Geriatr Soc* 1987; 35:13–20.

57. Wolfson LI, Whipple R: Stressing the postural response. *J Am Geriatr Soc* 1986; 34:845–850.

58. Wolfson LI, Whipple R, Amerman P, et al: Gait and balance in the elderly. *Clinics in Geriatric Medicine*. Philadelphia, WB Saunders, 1985, pp 649–659.

59. Woollacott MH: Changes in posture and voluntary control in the elderly: Research findings and rehabilitation. *Top Geriatr Rehabil* 1990; 5(2):1–11.

60. Woollacott H, Shumay-Cook A, Nashner L: Aging and posture control: Changes in sensory organs and muscular coordination. *Int J Aging Hum Dev* 1986; 23:97–114.

61. Woollacott MH, Shumway-Cook A, Nashner L: Postural reflexes and aging, in Mortimer J, Rorozzolo F, Maletta G (eds): *The Aging Nervous System*. New York, Praeger Publishers, 1989.

CHAPTER 16

Ambulation: An Integrated Framework to Achieve a Functional Outcome

Patricia E. Sullivan, Ph.D, P.T.

INTRODUCTION

One of the primary purposes of physical therapy is to enhance the physical ability of individuals to interact within the environment by improving, restoring, or maintaining ambulatory status. Thus, the mission of the profession can be seen to be tied intimately to the physical independence of elders.

Independent ambulation and walking at a functional speed are two of the most important factors in maintaining an independent life-style for older individuals. There are several reasons for the importance of these functional activities.[50] The ability to walk at an adequate speed for a reasonable time without undue fatigue certainly contributes to a comfortable and independent life.[6] Furthermore, the loss of independent ambulation and reduced safety while walking are common reasons for admission to nursing homes or other residential facilities.[17] Ambulation, however, is hazardous for some elders. Although falls occur during many activities, a large percentage of falls occur while walking,[50] and some falls result in injury.[38] Of those who enter a hospital because of a hip fracture, estimates suggest that as many as 25% will die within 1 year.[25] The evaluation of ambulation and intervention to preserve or restore skill in walking are critical if the physical therapist's goals are to decrease the number of falls, to reduce the need for nursing home placement, and to improve or maintain functional independence in the elderly.

In the older population, physical capability is influenced both by changes in the aging systems, compounded by acute or chronic conditions and medications, and by changes resulting from a less active life-style with altered nutrition and dehydration.[14, 38] A sedentary life-style for elders is not uncommon.[41] It has been estimated that only 45%[14] to 66% of older persons participate in regular exercise.[12] An active life-style seems to be critical to maintaining mental and physical function.[41, 43]

Interpreting the literature related to physical ability in the elderly is difficult because many factors, which have not been or cannot be statistically controlled, influence physical functioning. In addition to the physical and medical factors, psychologic,[5] social, and environmental factors can greatly affect independence.[38] It is not clear which changes occurring in an elder are due to the aging process and which should be attributed to a sedentary life-style. Despite their importance to physical therapy, many of the changes found in older persons have not been studied in relation to functional ability and, particularly, ambulation.

The focus of this chapter will be to explore the physical impairments that seem to influence ambulation in the general aging population and to use this information as a basis for evaluation and intervention. Therefore, common changes in the ambulatory pattern that occur in elders will be reviewed and an outline of their environmental and social significance presented. A specific framework for the analysis of clinical practice will be used to focus the evaluation of the physical systems and to classify the impairments into an intervention strategy that integrates factors related to the control of movement and the capacity to sustain activity (Fig 16–1). Finally, suggestions on how to adapt this general model to the individual patient will be made.

CHANGES IN AMBULATION WITH AGING

Gait Characteristics

Gait analysis of elderly individuals is similar to gait analysis of younger persons. The therapist should observe the elderly person's movement, in both the sagittal and frontal planes, systematically reviewing the stability and excursion of each body part as the individual walks at a self-chosen speed. General kinematic changes in ambulation that are associated with aging are slower velocity, decreased stride length, and increased cadence.[6, 10, 32] With respect to the stance phase of gait, elders generally employ a wider base of support and exhibit a shorter step length and thus spend a longer time in double support. During the early swing phase, greater hip and knee flexion is associated with greater toe clearance; however, there is less dorsiflexion. At late swing, when the compensatory increase in knee flexion seen in early swing becomes impossible, there is less toe clearance. With respect to the trunk and the proximal joints, there are less pelvic rotation and trunk counter-rotation, increased shoulder extension and elbow

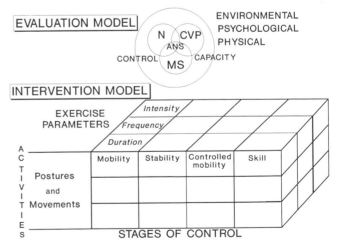

FRAMEWORK OF CLINICAL PRACTICE

FIG 16–1.
Framework of clinical practice with the evaluation and intervention models.

flexion, increased hip abduction, greater toeing out, and less vertical projection of the trunk and pelvis at toe-off.[7, 16, 22, 32, 54]

Changes in the capacity to sustain movement for a given speed of ambulation, as measured by oxygen consumption, are known to become more pronounced with advancing age.[4] The energy expenditure in ambulation over level ground and in stair climbing is similar for many elders and younger persons because elders regulate their energy consumption by walking more slowly.[7, 16, 22] Even when performed more slowly, the energy cost of stair climbing can easily exceed the maximum voluntary ability of some elders.[14] The association between the changes noted during walking and various physical impairments, including decreased range in the trunk and limbs and decreased muscular strength, has not been documented clearly. In addition, decrements in aerobic capacity that accompany aging require consideration. Changes in motor control during ambulation, as shown in kinematic and kinetic analyses, and reduced control of postural sway contribute to the decreased efficiency of ambulation in the elderly. For example, decreased trunk counter-rotation, decreased pelvic forward rotation, shorter step length, wider base of support, and decreased vertical projection at heel-off have all been attributed to the attempt by the older individual to improve stabilization during ambulation.[16, 32] However, these findings can have additional interpretations, not merely as causes of gait changes in the elderly but as the secondary effects of other common impairments associated with aging. These impairments, which are often noted in gait evaluation, may themselves be due to decreased range in the trunk, hips, and ankles and decreased force production in the postural extensors and plantarflexors.[53] Similarly, the altered speed of walking, especially during stair climbing, may be due to a decrease in the number of type II muscle fibers,[51] a decreased ability to perform unilateral stance, or a decreased aerobic capacity. The increased shoulder extension noted during gait[32, 54] may be a mechanism to counterbalance the increased kyphosis and forward head that move the center of mass anteriorly.

During the evaluation, the impairments that lead to functional limitation with ambulation are identified so that an effective treatment plan can be developed. For example, while decreased toe-off is an important clinical finding in a gait analysis, the therapist must determine whether this finding is a result of loss of range of motion (ROM) at the ankle, weak plantarflexors, or poor motor control, or any combination of these factors, before an effective intervention can be designed. When gait changes are considered functional limitations that can be associated with specific physical impairments, such as decreased ROM, strength, stability, and exercise capacity, treatment should address these specific impairments, in addition to encouraging an increased speed of ambulation.

Sex Differences

Variations in ambulation related to sex differences in elders have also been found. Women take shorter steps than men. To increase their speed, women take more steps, whereas men increase step length.[6, 22] It is not clear whether these sex differences are related to variations in leg length, flexibility, strength, general physical condition, or some combination of these factors.

EVALUATION

The purpose of the evaluation is to determine the patient's capability to perform functional activities. Although the therapist needs to focus the physical therapy assessment on the parameters within the physical and physiologic systems, the environmental, social, psychologic, and medical factors require consideration as well.[49]

Categorization of Age-Related Physical Impairments by System

The kinetic and kinematic characteristics of ambulation in elders may be associated with changes that occur in any of the physical systems. Of most concern to physical therapists are changes in the nervous, musculoskeletal, and cardio-vascular-pulmonary (CVP) systems. In addition to the anatomic changes that occur with aging in each of these systems, the interrelationships among these systems are important to the evaluation and intervention of limitations in ambulation. The control of movement is based on the physiologic relationship between the nervous and musculoskeletal systems. The overall capacity for movement is determined by the link between the CVP and musculoskeletal systems. Fear of falling and a general increase in anxiety are psychologic states that may also influence ambulation patterns. These states influence physical ability through the functions of the autonomic nervous system (Fig 16–2).

Nervous System

Many changes in the nervous system may contribute to alterations in ambulation. Sensory input from proprioceptor, visual, and vestibular mechanisms are all generally reduced in the elderly.[56] The cutaneous and proprioceptive receptors have a longer latency and a higher threshold in the elderly.[43] Other changes that affect ambulation in the elderly include fewer dendrites, reduced nerve conduction velocity, greater monosynaptic latency, decreased excit-

EVALUATION MODEL

PHYSICAL SYSTEMS

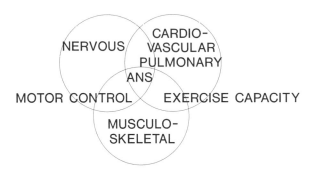

FIG 16–2.
Evaluation model depicting physical systems.

ability at the myoneural junction, decreased numbers of functional motor units,[28, 51] decreased reaction time, and a higher threshold for the H-reflex.[21, 39] All these changes result in an increased sensorimotor loop time.[39] These neural changes slow the generation of automatic motor programs,[9] increase the time required for peripheral feedback to be received centrally if the environmental conditions warrant movement alterations, and delay the transmission of efferent responses.

Musculoskeletal System

Changes in the musculoskeletal system with aging relevant to ambulation include less tightly packed muscle fibers, an increase in fat content between muscle fibers, an increase in fibrin deposits, a decrease in the number of type II fibers[28] and of functional motor units,[51] and loss of bone density. Clinically, a predominant finding in the elderly is a reduction in general flexibility.

Cardio-Vascular-Pulmonary System

Elders commonly exhibit an increased prevalence of coronary artery disease and hypertension. Cardiac structure and function in older individuals may demonstrate an increase in systolic blood pressure (BP); decreases in stroke volume, maximum heart rate, and coronary artery circulation; narrowing of the coronary vessels; and stenosis of the cardiac valves.[1, 41]

The pulmonary system shows a decrease in the compliance of the bony thorax, an increase in the compliance of lung tissue, and a decrease in diffusing capacity and efficiency in the work of breathing. In the peripheral vessels, there is an increase in the resistance to peripheral blood flow and a decrease in the elasticity of vessels and of the number of capillary beds in the muscles. Clinically, CVP changes may be manifested in the elderly as lowered aero-

bic capacity, diminished exercise tolerance, and positional hypotension.[1, 4]

All these changes can lead to a reduced ability to respond to the aerobic demand of functional activities and subsequently promote further decline in aerobic capacity.[4] Elders may be forced to decrease the speed of walking and stair climbing because they are unable to sustain the required output of energy resulting from the increased metabolic cost of these activities in a deconditioned state. The loss of speed, in turn, leads to an overall decrease in endurance for functional activities. For this reason, the 6-minute walk test, which measures the distance walked in the designated time, is a common tool used to assess endurance.

Motor Control and the Capacity to Sustain Movement

The quality and quantity of ambulation are related to the interaction of the nervous, musculoskeletal, and CVP systems, which control and sustain movement. Impairments in the nervous and musculoskeletal systems can lead to alterations in the programming, planning, or execution of ambulation. Impairments within the the CVP and musculoskeletal systems limit the individual's capacity to sustain ambulation.

Motor Control

Postural control and ambulation are the outcomes of complex interactions between the nervous and musculoskeletal systems and include automatic, reflexive, and volitional levels of control.[9, 40] The automatic level of control relies on central mechanisms to interpret the position of body segments, implement common movements, judge disturbances accurately, and respond with the appropriate timing, sequence, and force in order to maintain a posture or respond to previously encountered or minor changes in the external environment.[55] Central feedforward mechanisms, which may be involved in ambulation patterns, rely on automatic responses to known situations. Because the total system for the control of movement in the elderly individual may be slowed and the ability to respond to novel environmental conditions impaired, these automatic programs may not be adequate in some elderly individuals.

The reflexive level of control involves peripheral sensorimotor links consisting of proprioceptive and stretch receptor mechanisms in the periphery and higher-center reflexes such as the vestibulo-ocular reflex, all of which are elicited during movement. Volitional control requires conscious attention to the activity. Such attention is required if the environmental conditions are unusual, as when walking in darkness, or if the ability to monitor conditions has been altered internally in the individual, for example, diminished distal sensation in persons with diabetes.

Some of the motor control problems elders have in ambulation can be analyzed according to three conditions for purposeful movement. The present position of the body must be known, the target position or goal to be achieved must be accurately identified, and the correct combination of muscle forces in the correct sequence must be generated to move from the present position to the goal position.

The combination of feedforward and feedback mechanisms and the sensory input contributing to movement control normally allow movement to occur from the present body position toward a subsequent target position in a coordinated fashion.[9] Programs within the central nervous system (CNS) underlying the automatic nature of ambulation are altered with aging through changes in both peripheral and central inputs. Visual, vestibular, and proprioceptive mechanisms that monitor conditions internal to the body, such as limb position and muscle length-tension ratios, as well as the environmental conditions external to the individual, change with aging.[2, 35, 56] If the sensitivity of these modalities is reduced, it can be difficult for the individual to integrate the necessary afferent information into the motor plan to be executed by the musculoskeletal system.[55]

Equally relevant to ambulation, the ability to generate sufficient motor force[27, 31, 53] in the proper sequence is diminished in the elderly. Since the speed of walking is influenced by the intensity of lower extremity muscle activation,[9] the decreased walking speed of elders may be an accommodation to the decreased ability to generate sufficient force in the required time frame. The decreased number of motor units in the muscles will lead also to decreased force production,[14] further limiting the ability of the elderly individual to respond to changes in postural and environmental conditions.

Changes in the linkages between the nervous and musculoskeletal system that hinder ambulation may stem from other factors. Common chronic diseases, such as diabetes, may also contribute to neuromotor deficits in the elderly. In the older person with diabetes, the ability to perceive present body position or identify environmental conditions accurately may be diminished as a result of abnormal visual acuity and diminished proprioception. The ability to generate motor responses using the correct combination, sequence, and force for ambulation, especially during rapid movements, thus is likely to be impaired. It is not known whether the altered motor response is due to decreased muscle force, delayed nerve conduction velocity, diminished sensory awareness, processing of altered or limited sensory data in the CNS, or a combination of all these factors. It is evident, however, that these factors do

contribute to decreased ambulation in elders, creating a cycle in which reduced ambulation leads to lowered capacity to sustain movement, which in turn further limits ambulation.

Exercise Capacity

Functional limitations in ambulation due to changes in the CVP and musculoskeletal systems are the result of inefficient oxygen consumption and lowered capacity to sustain activity.[4] Various changes alter the normal linkage between the CVP and musculoskeletal systems.[47] A decline in cardiac output, decreased maximum heart rate, reduced vital capacity, increased residual volume, decreased oxygen saturation, increased resistance to peripheral blood flow, diminished blood flow to the muscles, and decreased ability to extract oxygen from the blood.[4, 14] can all affect the interdependent relationship between the CVP and musculoskeletal systems.

Differentiating among impairments resulting from aging, from pathologies, such as diabetes, or from a sedentary life-style is difficult.[50] For example, persons who fall tend to be weaker.[53] However, it is not clear which of these problems occurs first. What is evident is that if a fall occurs, many elders, even those who have been quite active, may reduce their activity level because of anxiety or fear of falling.[38] Intervention has been shown to be effective in altering the changes that accompany aging and result from a sedentary existence.[1] Improved strength, flexibility, and exercise capacity have occurred from a therapeutic exercise program in a wide range of elderly persons.[6, 15, 30, 36, 48] What has not yet been determined is the focus of treatment. Should the intervention concentrate on changing the individual by remediating the impairments; on teaching compensatory strategies, assuming the deficits are irreversible or the individual cannot respond to the intervention in a realistic period of time; or should it be focused on decreasing the demand made upon the individual performing the task by modifying the environment?

As knowledge of the relationships between pathology, impairments, functional limitations, and disability[19, 52] is expanded and differentiation between changes that accompany aging and those changes that occur as a result of a sedentary lifestyle made, interventions can be more specifically targeted to the underlying cause. Physical therapy intervention is commonly directed toward the individual. Physical therapists working with the elderly patients may also look to improve the functional abilities of elders by "social" interventions.[11] When changes cannot be effected in the individual,[13] or when many individuals share a common impairment, such as reduced speed of ambulation,[32] decreased extremity ROM, and decreased postural stability, a more efficient way to effect change may be to modify the environment. This may mean decreasing the step height in public places, having chairs of varying heights, altering the step height on buses, raising the height of toilet seats, prolonging the walk time at crossing lights, installing stall showers with grab bars and introducing lever doorknobs in homes for the elderly.

INTERVENTION

The intervention model proposed in this chapter is three dimensional, composed of factors that influence the difficulty of motor control, the capacity to sustain exercise and movement, and the level of postures and movements that are prerequisite to the functional outcomes of ambulation (Fig 16–3). The principles upon which this model has been developed have been integrated from a variety of sources. The practice models that have been developed to guide treatment of patients with musculoskeletal or neurologic involvement have provided one basis.[20, 40] The stages of control come from Stockmeyer's interpretation of Rood.[44] These stages were incorporated into the proprioceptive neuromuscular facilitation (PNF) therapeutic exercise approach by Sullivan et al.[45, 46] The treatment techniques and modalities that are classified within the stages represent the major physical therapy interventions including exercise, joint mobilization,[34] and physical agents. The sequencing of the difficulty of treatment postures and movements is derived from biomechanical and kinesiologic principles.[42] The exercise parameters are taken from

the protocols of altering exercise stress in patients with cardiovascular involvement,[4, 23] the concepts of progressive resistive exercise and principles of motor learning.

The physical therapy intervention is directed by the functional outcome desired by both the patient and the physical therapist. Ambulation with sufficient motor control and exercise capacity to be safe at a speed that allows functional independence with or without an assistive device on a variety of surfaces is the functional outcome we will consider here. Although our focus is toward improved ambulation, the person's ability to perform activities of daily living (ADL) skills and communicate would be included in the complete rehabilitation plan.

The functional outcome of intervention can be characterized as being performed with normal control or with compensatory strategies. Normal control that occurs in an individual with no physical impairments assumes a normal timing and sequencing of movement with an appropriate amount of force. When normal control is not possible— for example, when impairments limit function—using compensatory strategies to ambulate, perform ADL, or communicate occurs. Normal movement is efficient and requires the least amount of energy. Compensatory movements, although sometimes necessary, commonly require more energy. When determining functional outcomes and treatment goals for elders, the changes that occur as part of the aging process must be kept in mind.

The patient's functional capability, the impairments related to the limitations in ambulation, and the patient's potential for change are determined during the evaluation. The next step in the clinical decision-making process is to translate these evaluative findings into a plan for intervention. To do so the impairments that limit the patient's function are categorized within the context of the physical therapy intervention.

The patient's impairments are then translated into treatment goals (Fig 16–4). Generally, these could include to increase ROM, to increase the time that standing can be maintained without assistance, and to improve the ability to assume standing from sitting. These goals are based on the realistic assessment of what can be changed in the individual. If changes in the individual cannot be anticipated, the goals can reflect the teaching of compensatory movements and modifications in the environment that are directed toward the same functional outcomes.

For each treatment goal, specific procedures are designed to improve the impairments contributing to the limitation. These procedures include (1) postures associated with the desired functional activity, (2) techniques and elements to achieve the required stages of control, and (3) parameters to alter the duration, frequency, and intensity of the exercise. Each aspect of the procedure can be changed to alter the difficulty and stress of the procedure. The postures associated with ambulation include those re-

INTERVENTION MODEL

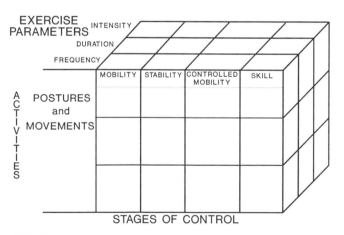

FIG 16–3.
Intervention model with three parameters to modify treatment difficulty: *activities*—changing posture and movement; *stages of control*—varying the muscular contraction and sensory input; and *exercise parameters*—altering the frequency, duration, and intensity.

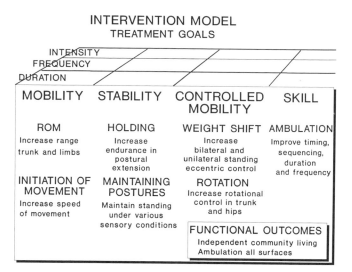

INTERVENTION MODEL
TREATMENT GOALS

INTENSITY
FREQUENCY
DURATION

MOBILITY	STABILITY	CONTROLLED MOBILITY	SKILL
ROM	HOLDING	WEIGHT SHIFT	AMBULATION
Increase range trunk and limbs	Increase endurance in postural extension	Increase bilateral and unilateral standing eccentric control	Improve timing, sequencing, duration and frequency
INITIATION OF MOVEMENT	MAINTAINING POSTURES	ROTATION	
Increase speed of movement	Maintain standing under various sensory conditions	Increase rotational control in trunk and hips	

FUNCTIONAL OUTCOMES
Independent community living
Ambulation all surfaces

FIG 16–4.
Treatment goals and functional outcomes sequenced according to the stages of control.

quired for the assumption of standing and those in which specific motor abilities can be practiced and achieved. The postures of supine, sideling, sitting, and standing represent the postural sequence to assume standing. In addition, the control of the lower trunk and lower extremities required for the assumption of standing and for ambulation can be enhanced in the hookling, bridging, and modified plantigrade positions. In addition to focusing on ambulatory control, these postures are included in treatment to increase weight-bearing stress.[26, 37, 41] For this reason, procedures in the quadruped position may be included in the treatment plan. The treatment techniques employed may include those that increase ROM, improve the ability to maintain a posture, and enhance the ability to move within or between postures.

The exercise parameters that can be altered with each of the treatment procedures are the frequency, duration, and intensity of the procedure. These parameters are varied according to the patient's learning ability, CVP status, or acuity of the dysfunction. In patients who demonstrate a deficit in learning, the practice schedule, the type of feedback provided, and the environmental conditions can be varied. As a result of neural damage, learning for some individuals may not be possible. Compensatory strategies or changes in the environment must be made to allow safe, independent function. Other patients who are limited by exercise capacity deficits and involvement of the CVP system may require modifications in the exercise parameters so that the appropriate stress occurs during the procedures.[4, 23] Heart rate, BP, and energy expenditure during the intervention program should be monitored in such circumstances. If involvement includes recovery from a musculoskeletal injury or surgery, exercise parameters should be adjusted according to the tissues' reactivity or ability to

respond to varying amounts of intensity or frequency of exercise. Elders may recover more slowly, manifest different responses to internal and external stress, and are more affected by the deleterious results of bed rest.[41, 47]

Stages of Control

Our understanding of the acquisition and execution of motor control has been based within anatomic, neurophysiologic, and learning theory. However, these theories must be translated into an applied intervention perspective in order to be clinically useful to physical therapists. One model that guides practice is the sequencing of the difficulty of motor tasks according to stages of control.[44, 46] In this model, the levels of difficulty, or stages of control, are mobility, stability, controlled mobility, and skill (Table 16–1).

When a patient's functional limitations can be attributed to impairments in motor control, the impairments are classified within these stages. Treatment techniques appropriate to the particular impairments are then determined. Imagine, for example, a patient with functional limitations of moving from sitting to standing and of climbing stairs. These functions are limited due to impairments of reduced ROM in the hip secondary to arthritic changes. The changes in the muscular and capsular tissue that limit range are classified within the stage of mobility. The patient's range is compared with that required for the activities of moving from sitting to standing, and flexing the lower extremity during stair climbing. The duration of the impairment is also assessed. Where the limitation is in soft tissue and has been of short duration, then the assumption can be made that change can occur and range can be increased. In this instance, techniques such as massage, hold-relax, and joint mobilization are indicated. If the impairment is chronic or if bone limits ROM, then tissue changes are unlikely to be possible. In such cases, treatment aimed at compensation would be indicated and might be directed toward altering the environment by raising the seat height and lowering stair height. Referral for surgical intervention might also be considered.

Mobility
Passive ROM and the Ability to Initiate Movement.—Range-of-motion deficits that impede ambulation are due to decreased flexibility; increased stiffness; or shortening of the skin, connective tissue, muscle, ligament, and capsule in the trunk, hip, knee, and ankle. During ambulation, these impairments of range may limit trunk counter-rotation, pelvic rotation, step length, and both dorsiflexion and plantarflexion motions during stance and swing.[38, 53] For example, decreased range into lumbar extension combined with tight hip flexors and plantarflexors may reduce terminal stance and step length.

TABLE 16–1.

Description of the Stages of Control

Mobility	Stability	Controlled Mobility	Static-Dynamic	Skill
ROM passive extensibility of the contractile and noncontractile tissues	Holding an isometric contraction of the extensors in shortened ranges	Weight shifting in weight-bearing postures	Weight bearing altering the base of support	Function ambulation, manipulation, communication
Initiate movement initiate and sustain movement in gravity-eliminated positions (2+/5)	Maintaining midline and weight-bearing postures	Trunk log rolling	Trunk segmental rotation	Trunk counter-rotation

Patients with decreased range in the trunk and lower extremity may alter the manner in which they move to standing from sitting and may need to climb stairs one at a time.[22] Normally, the first phase of assuming standing requires upper body and hip flexion, and as the feet move under the chair, flexion occurs at the knees and ankles. If these joints or surrounding tissues are stiff, then these initial flexion movements will be difficult. In addition, following prolonged sitting, erect standing may be difficult. Stair climbing may be limited by range deficits in the ankle, knee, or hip.

Abnormal range in the thoracic and cervical spine also can influence posture and gait. Typically, an elder will demonstrate an increase in thoracic kyphosis, flexion in the lower cervical region, and upper cervical extension, which moves the upper body's center of gravity anteriorly.[32, 54] Altered muscular activity to maintain postures, to move in sitting and standing, and to control postural responses may be required to offset this change in the center of gravity. In addition to altering posture and the pattern of ambulation, decreased range in the hip, knee, and ankle has been associated with the incidence of falling.[18]

Techniques.—If specific joint motions are limited from capsular or ligamentous tightness or from chronic joint effusion, then *joint mobilization* and measures to reduce edema should be incorporated. If specific muscle tightness is noted, *hold-relax* (HR) to increase contractile tissue extensibility would be performed. In this technique, a low-intensity isometric contraction is performed, followed by muscular relaxation and active movement into the new range. Heat, superficial or deep, depending on the involved tissue, or active warm-up activities may be useful before these ROM procedures. *Self-stretching* has the advantage that it can be performed independently, although it is not specific to any one tissue. During self-stretching, the movements and instructions should be sufficiently specific to direct the stretch toward the involved area while not increasing range in already mobile joints. Whether individual or group exercise is performed, it is essential that care be taken with persons who are osteoporotic or osteopenic.

Initiation of Movement.—Initiation is the most basic of active movement abilities and involves the capacity to initiate and sustain an active contraction throughout range.[46] It is equivalent to a 2+/5 (MMT) grade. In addition to muscle testing, initiation of movement has been measured by recording response times in a variety of tasks. In elders, especially those who are sedentary, response times are delayed, the delay being attributed to changes in the nervous and musculoskeletal systems.[43] When initiation of movement is slow or weak, postural reactions[21] and automatic movements in standing or during ambulation may not occur with sufficient speed to compensate for environmental changes or to allow for an appropriate rate of walking.[9, 27, 35] For example, if ankle proprioception is diminished and if the tissues around the ankle are stiff, the dorsiflexors may not be activated in a timely manner and also have to overcome internal resistance to flex the ankle during postural disturbances,[55] ambulation, and stair climbing. A slowed response also can be due to inattention and decreased visual and vestibular acuity.[56]

During active movement the patient with less-than-normal muscle strength may not be able to overcome the internal resistance of stiff tissues. If, for example, the hip extensors are weak, the patient may have difficulty overcoming the tightness in the hip flexor and anterior capsule following prolonged sitting and therefore may experience difficulty while coming to standing or achieving hip extension during terminal stance. Conversely, if the hip's posterior structures are shortened, the patient may have difficulty moving against this tightness when bending forward in sitting. Further research will need to be undertaken to determine if the weakness that reduces the ability to initiate movement can be attributed to a sedentary life-style, decreased flexibility, a decreased number of type II fibers, or a combination of these.

Techniques.—If the patient has difficulty initiating movement in the presence of increased tone as, for example, an individual with hemiplegia, then *rhythmic initiation* (RI) is chosen to enhance a more normal tone base before facilitating active movement. RI begins with passive, slow, rhythmic movement through small ranges. When the patient begins to relax, the challenge to the patient is increased by altering the parameters of the technique. The range, speed, and active participation are gradually increased. If the patient has weakness in the postural extensors, then *hold-relax-active motion* (HRAM) is performed to improve the holding ability in shortened ranges and initiation from the lengthened range. If weakness in the flexor muscles is evident, the technique of *repeated contractions* (RC) will promote increased activity by superimposing a reflexive onto a voluntary contraction. In this technique, as the patient's active response begins to diminish, a gentle stretch is provided to enhance the active contraction. By stimulating muscle spindle activity, these techniques also may enhance peripheral proprioceptive input. Electrical stimulation may augment voluntary contractions.

Stability

Holding a body segment in the shortened range of extension, maintaining midline and weight-bearing positions, and static control in upright postures are included at this stage.

Holding in Shortened Ranges.— This component of the stage of stability is also termed *tonic holding*. It is the ability of the postural extensor muscles to perform isometric contractions in the shortened range against gravitational or manual resistance. In relation to postural control and ambulation, key muscles are those of the lower trunk, hip, knee, and ankle extensors[53, 54] and the hip abductors. If these muscles are less than a grade of 3/5, and if an isometric contraction cannot be maintained for at least 10 seconds, this stage is considered to be deficient.

The ability to maintain a contraction against the resistance of gravity normally requires no more than about 40% effort and is performed primarily by type I muscle fibers. In elders with decreased strength and a decreased circulatory muscle bed, this ability may require proportionally more effort and become anaerobic more rapidly. The prolonged sitting of sedentary persons[8] in which the postural extensors are maintained in lengthened ranges may contribute to the findings of weakness. Although in elders type I motor units do not appear to be lost to the extent that type II motor units are,[51] many clinical findings suggest a decreased holding ability. These include fatigue, poor postural stability, and the decreased ability to maintain erect, upright postures.[33] Older persons tend to loose aerobic capacity which is dependent on type I motor units. The tonic holding level of stability provides the prerequisite control in the trunk, hip, knee and ankle extensors to maintain the upright position during gait.

Technique.— The technique of a *shortened held resisted contraction* (SHRC) is used to improve the ability of a postural extensor muscle to maintain the shortened range. This is a prerequisite ability for maintaining body weight in an upright posture. In this technique, the extensor muscle in or near its shortened range maintains an isometric contraction for 5 or more seconds. Increasing the duration of the contraction is the primary means of progression. Gravity, the weight of the limb, can be the resistive force, or manual and mechanical resistance can be applied, particularly if gravity is assisting. The intensity of the contraction needs to be considered carefully if the CVP system is involved. The contractions should not be more than about 40% of maximum, so the slow twitch fibers predominate. The progression is to increase the duration of the contraction, not the intensity. The individual should be able to breath comfortably during the exercise. Heart rate and BP should be monitored.

Maintaining Weight-Bearing Postures.—*Cocontraction, static postural control, static balance,* and *static stability* are terms that are commonly used to describe this component of stability. Maintaining any posture is included at this level of stability. From a functional perspective, an individual usually must stand before he can walk, and maintaining sitting and standing is inherently important. Particular to ambulation is maintaining upright postures, such as sitting and standing, and postures emphasizing specific muscular control. However, the muscular activity and kinetics for maintaining the standing position and walking are different.[54] In bilateral or unilateral standing, a person must maintain the position and keep the center of mass within the base of support. During walking, the center of mass continually moves within a changing base of support.

Techniques.— Maintaining the position requires muscle cocontraction. To promote stability with manual resistance, *alternating isometrics* (AI) and *rhythmic stabilization* (RS) are chosen. Additional resistance from weights or other media can be employed. Resistance is first applied slowly, consistent with the patient's ability. To achieve the goal of increasing the rate of response time, the speed of resistance is gradually increased. As this change is made, the intensity of the contraction is reduced. Initially, the resistance is rhythmic and anticipated, so the patient can learn the responses. These parameters are gradually altered. Also, the sensory stimuli available to the patient can be changed by asking the patient to balance without vision or to stand on foam. During these conditions the patient may be cued to focus on foot and ankle sensations.

Controlled Mobility

Weight shifting in a weight-bearing posture and trunk rotation are encompassed in this stage. Many of the impairments classified at this stage result from deficits at the previous stages of mobility and stability. However, some studies have noted that during weight-shifting tasks older persons have less ability to control the outer limits of sway even though they may be able to maintain a static posture.[2, 56] It is not clear whether the weight-shifting deficit is related to the range required during movement, to decreased sensory awareness, or to the diminished motor ability to modify and increase force production as the center of mass moves. Eccentric contractions that require less exercise capacity and force but may require more control than concentric contractions are essential to self-controlled weight-shifting activities.

The trunk rotation component of controlled mobility, demonstrated by reduced pelvic rotation during gait, commonly is limited.[32] Analyses of trunk motion, however, have not differentiated between the available passive movement and the active ability to control that movement. Functionally, it is apparent that older persons tend to rotate the body less and have difficulty isolating neck rotation from the rest of body movement.

Techniques.—Weight shifting can be performed either in a concentric-eccentric reversal of one muscle group, termed *agonistic reversal* (AR), or as a reversal of antagonists, termed *slow reversal hold* (SRH) or *slow reversal* (SR). In either condition, resistance can be applied manually or with weights. Progression is achieved by (1) increasing the range of the movement, which in turn requires an increase in the ability to control the center-of-gravity excursion; (2) moving the center of gravity over a fixed base of support, then moving the base of support under the center of gravity; (3) performing these movements on a stable surface, then on an unstable base; and (4) altering the sensory conditions. For example, in standing, weight shifting over the feet, as in a sway motion, is performed first before raising on the toes or heels, which decreases the size of the base. The patient can then stand on a balance board, maintaining a static position, then moving the board. Vision can be obscured, or the patient can stand on foam to challenge vestibular and proprioceptive mechanisms.

A deficit in eccentric control in the quadriceps and gluteals may be evaluated during the functional activities of descending stairs and moving from standing to sitting. To rectify this impairment, developing eccentric control of the quadriceps in the modified plantigrade position and the gluteals in bridging are emphasized. Proprioceptive feedback in the form of resistance may enhance the activity and increase motor unit activity. The treatment is progressed by withdrawing this input after sufficient strength has been achieved.

Static-Dynamic

An intermediate stage of control lying between the stages of controlled mobility and skill is described as the static-dynamic component, which encompasses unilateral stance and segmental trunk rotation. Within a posture in which the base of support is reduced, treatment can promote the static control required for unilateral stance and progress to dynamic control to simulate one step of the gait cycle. The static-dynamic level also encompasses the ability to move between postures, such as from supine, to sideling, to sitting, and to standing. This stage includes segmental trunk rotation.

Elders have difficulty with both unilateral weight bearing in standing and transitional movements. However, Winter et al. have found in elite elders that the relationship between static balance and ambulation is poor. During the unilateral stance phase of ambulation the center of gravity is not within the unilateral base of support but rather stays more central.[54] In contrast, during unilateral standing, the center of gravity must be within the base of support. The walking pattern of nonelite elderly people, however, is different. Many elderly have a longer stance time and more lateral sway. Thus, it could be argued that for some elders the relationship between unilateral stance and gait is similar. In addition, unilateral stance is important during other functional activities, such as climbing stairs and dressing.

In contrast to ambulation, the forces at the ankle and hip are in a mediolateral direction during unilateral standing. To balance in this position requires motion, position sense, and muscular control in the subtalar and hip joints. In elders, sensation and motor control of these joints are not commonly documented, no doubt a result of the difficulty in obtaining objective measures.

Elders are reported to fall during transitional movements from supine to sitting and to standing.[38] It is not clear if these problems result from the control of the transitional movement, including decreased range and weakness in the quadriceps and gluteals, or from the postural hypotension and dizziness related to the changing postures. In older patients, heart rate and BP should be measured after rising from supine to sitting and from sitting to standing to determine if hypotension is the problem. To diminish this problem, elders should maintain the new position for a few seconds before continuing with an activity. In addition, the strength of the lower extremity postural extensor muscles needs to be assessed, and if weakness exists, a strengthening program should be initiated.

Techniques.—The weight-bearing procedures can be performed independently with or without resistance. AI and RS can enhance the stability control of the supporting segments; SRH and SR, the dynamic control of the moving limbs. In the trunk, segmental upper and lower trunk motions can be initiated either in the upper or the lower body. For example, while sitting, the trunk segmental movements can be either the upper body moving on a fixed lower trunk or the lower trunk moving under a stabilized upper body. Although both movements are functionally important, upper-trunk weight shifting may first be easier because weight is borne on the lower trunk. In standing, trunk movements may be performed by either segment.

Skill

Locomotion, Manipulation (ADL), and Communication.—The functional outcome of intervention, ambulation, occurs at the skill stage of control. At this stage the normal timing and sequencing of movement are promoted to achieve a normal quality of ambulation.[24] Some patients having no physical impairments may have difficulty ambulating within their environment. In these cases the deficit may be with automatic movement, with difficulty learning and transferring functional abilities to other environmental conditions, or with reduced exercise capacity for movement. For example, some elders with primarily cognitive deficits may have difficulty walking, especially in a new environment because they cannot remember directions. The problem may be one of motor learning, of adapting to the environment, or of understanding the task, rather than of deficits of motor control or exercise capacity.

During the gait pattern of many elders, a slower ambulatory speed, longer stance time, and increased lateral sway in the upper body are observed.[32] These conditions may alter the center of mass to base of support relationship and muscular responses.[15] For example, in younger persons and in the fit elderly the muscular responses that control the mass of the upper body during ambulation occur primarily in the hip and back extensors and hip abductors.[55] In some elders, because of the more lateral projections of the gait pattern, an increase in abductor control may be required.

Practicing the functional task—whether it be walking, dressing, or feeding—is emphasized at this skill stage. When the patient has difficulty performing the task, the therapist determines the underlying reason and develops a program to rectify that impairment, as has been described. At the skill stage the activity itself is practiced under a variety of environmental conditions.

Techniques.—The techniques at the skill stage promote the timing and sequencing of responses. *Resisted progression* (RP) while the patient is walking is used to improve the sequencing of body segments. Manual contacts are commonly positioned on the pelvis to guide and direct the proper progression. Additional support may be provided by the parallel bars, an assistive device, or having the patient hold the therapist's shoulders. If the patient has difficulty activating the distal musculature at the initiation of movement, the technique of *normal timing* (NT) may be indicated. For example, at the beginning of the swing phase, a patient has difficulty initiating dorsiflexion even though there is sufficient strength at other points in the range. At the initiation of the limb movement, dorsi-

flexion is facilitated by repeated stretches added to the voluntary attempt. For patients who have more difficulty with the timing and control of proximal segments, the techniques of SR, SRH, and AR are used.

Strengthening

Strengthening inherent in aspects of motor control and exercise capacity, has eluded easy definition. From a motor control perspective, strength impairments may be a result of delayed or improper neural messages, leading to activation of an insufficient number of motor units, in an inappropriate sequence, and lacking the speed or endurance to produce an adequate response. From an exercise capacity perspective, the reduced ability to diffuse oxygen into the blood and the reduced capillary bed within the muscle may provide insufficient energy to support and maintain the muscular response.[4] Reduced aerobic power can be noted while performing many functional activities including walking and stair climbing. The physiologic changes that commonly occur with aging require that while promoting increased strength the frequency, duration, and intensity of the treatment procedures be carefully monitored to work within and improve the patient's exercise capacity.

Techniques.—To increase the strength of the response, RC and *timing for emphasis* (TE) are performed. In RC and TE, the active voluntary response is enhanced by superimposing a stretch reflexive response. The purpose of the stretch reflexive response is to increase motor unit recruitment, hypertrophy motor fibers, and reinforce motor learning. The technique of TE further enhances the response of the weak segment by adding overflow from stronger musculature. Other techniques such as AI, SRH, and AR can be performed with increased resistance to enhance isometric, isotonic, or eccentric responses and can be performed with additional repetitions to improve endurance.

In addition, endurance can be promoted by having the patient increase the frequency of the task as part of a home program, using elastic or weight resistance. Pulleys, weights, or isokinetic devices provide a useful adjunct to the strengthening and endurance program.

CASE STUDY APPLYING MODEL

Mrs. J is a 79-year-old who comes to your facility with increasing difficulty walking on uneven surfaces and complaints of unsteady gait. To evaluate her status, the environmental, social, and psychologic factors that may be influencing her ambulation are explored. Then the impairments related to the functional outcome of ambulation are determined by assessing the physical systems. These impairments are then sequenced within the stages of control with consideration of her exercise capacity. In the clinical decision-making process, the next step is to develop the intervention plan and to determine specific treatment procedures leading toward the anticipated outcome.

Mrs. J's functional limitations are decreased walking speed and poor ability to climb stairs, having to use a bannister and descend step to step. The environmental, psychologic, and medical factors that may positively or negatively influence her physical functioning include living in a second-floor walk-up, enjoying a close friendship circle with the local church group, having medical costs paid by Medicare, being an insulin-dependent diabetic, having slight hypertension, showing some evidence of osteoarthritis (OA) of the knees by radiograph, and presently being satisfied with life but concerned about a sick spouse. Measurements of the physical systems have noted reduced range in the trunk into extension and rotation, stiffness near the ends of range in the lower extremities, diminished sensation including position sense in the feet and toes, minimal swelling around the ankles, decreased muscle strength of 4−/5 in the lower extremity extensors and 3/5 of the dorsiflexors, and decreased ability to maintain standing without vision. The patient has reduced aerobic capacity shown as increased heart rate, respiratory rate, and blood pressure while climbing one flight of stairs (Fig 16–5). Organizing the findings in the evaluation model will help the therapist differentiate problems from environmental vs. physical origin and then determine if the limitation is more easily rectified by modifying the environment, by teaching compensatory strategies, or by changing the person.

The evaluated impairments are classified into the in-

tervention model and according to their control or capacity characteristics. For example, the decreased trunk and limb range is *Mobility-ROM;* the decreased ability to maintain standing is related to the *Stability* stage. Diminished aerobic capacity during walking comes within the duration, frequency, and intensity of this skilled activity.

The functional outcome desired by the patient is multifaceted: to maintain independent community living, including ambulation on all surfaces and stairs; to improve safety; and to increase walking speed. The therapist determines which of the impairments need to be changed to achieve this outcome. The impairments that are amenable to change compared with those that may require compensatory strategies or modifications of the environment are determined. Considering these three alternatives, the degree of independence that can be achieved and the projected time required to accomplish both treatment goals and functional outcomes can then be projected.

The treatment goals sequenced within the model are stated as positive changes in the impairments. Some goals anticipate change in the individual and may include:

1. Increasing ROM in the hips, knees, and ankles, in the spine, and in the proximal upper extremities;
2. Improving the ability to initiate movement at a speed, frequency, and intensity necessary for static and dynamic postural responses and ambulation;
3. Improving static and dynamic stability of the postural muscles with the sequencing and duration needed for postural responses and for ambulation; and
4. Improving strength in the postural muscles during weight-bearing activities including concentric and eccentric contractions with the needed intensity, duration, and frequency for functional activities.

If change in the person is not realistic, then compensatory strategies and environmental change may be needed and may include:

1. Adding a half stair to reduce the ROM requirements of stair climbing; adding raised toilet seat and bars if decreased lower extremity range or strength requires this modification;
2. Additional assistive devices to improve stability and speed while ambulating;
3. Increasing the stability of and adding an additional bannister to provide external support while stair climbing; and
4. Improving patient shoe support and augmenting education regarding foot care.

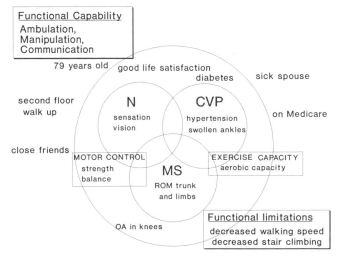

FIG 16–5.
Evaluation model with findings of Mrs. J.

Treatment Plan

During treatment, many stages of control can be achieved simultaneously, but the procedures usually begin at the mobility stage because the other stages cannot occur without range and the ability to initiate movement. In addition, this ensures a better chance of success. With Mrs. J, treatment would begin with improving the range in her trunk and lower extremities, enhancing the holding ability of her postural extensors, and improving her ability to maintain postures. The treatment procedures can be progressed by changing any of the three units of the procedure: the activity, the posture, and movement pattern; the stage of control and particular techniques; or the exercise parameters. For example, when range in the ankle and hips has shown some improvement and static standing balance is better, then promoting eccentric control of the ankle musculature and dynamic standing balance would be logical progressions. In addition, by varying the environmental conditions, such as the chair height, the floor surface, or the treatment location, the physical demands can be altered and the ability for Mrs. J to generalize to other situations enhanced. Her home program would include procedures that have been shown to be successful in the clinic—so are one stage less difficult than the procedures currently being performed by the therapist and can improve the endurance for exercise by increasing the duration and frequency of the program. Depending on the changes occurring in her physical status, her home environment would be modified as needed.

Specific Treatment Procedures

The suggestions made for the intervention sequence incorporate progressions of the activity, the postures chosen, and the stages of control beginning with the least difficult and moving to those requiring more skill. These treatment suggestions represent a general perspective that may need to be modified for individual patients. Many of these procedures can be performed as group activities, especially with persons functioning at high levels or those with similar impairments.[3, 30] Group activities, in addition to improving the physical parameters, may enhance socialization[29] and discussion about creative ways to overcome physical impairments. This exercise program might also be appropriate to prevent common impairments[26] and improve or maintain functional capability.

In all these procedures, the duration, frequency, and intensity must be monitored and individually adapted. If the program developed is too vigorous, the individual may complain of tissue soreness and be discouraged from participating, or the program may stress cardiopulmonary structures and excessive fatigue or other signs may result. Tissue changes that have occurred over a long time will take time to reverse. Many procedures are suggested so that the program can be varied and address many of the existing and anticipated problems.

The procedures are sequenced according to the difficulty of treatment activities, the postures, and movement patterns. This progression is chosen to decrease the need to move Mrs. J between postures during treatment. The stages of motor control are sequenced within each activity.

Procedures in *Supine*

In supine, upper trunk extension can be combined with scapula retraction and shoulder flexion, abduction, and external rotation. In the lower body, the movements that can be performed in supine include trunk flexion, extension, and rotation; hip flexion, extension, and rotation; and ankle movements.

Mobility.—*ROM*. Goals include improving or maintaining range and decreasing tissue stiffness, particularly in the trunk, hips, knees, and ankles. Techniques to achieve these goals include heat, massage, HR, and joint mobilization.

Mobility.—*Initiation of movement*. Goals include improving the ability to initiate and move through the range. Although Mrs. J is ambulatory and can initiate all movements, because her ankle musculature is weak and the timing of the contraction is slowed, the initiation of ankle dorsiflexion and plantarflexion is emphasized.[53, 55] HRAM, RC, and electrical stimulation are techniques which may be used to achieve these goals.

Stability.—*Holding in the shortened range*. Goals include holding an isometric contraction in the shortened range of the postural extensors. The duration of this low-intensity isometric contraction is gradually increased from 5 to 30 to 60 seconds. The level of intensity begins with gravitational resistance in spine; then external resistance may be added. In supine, the lower body extensors are resisted by placing a pillow under the knees and having Mrs. J perform quadriceps and gluteal sets by pushing into the pillow. At home, she increases the duration of the holding contraction, being careful to breathe smoothly during the exercise. The difficulty can be increased by altering the gravitational resistance and having Mrs. J roll into the prone position and hold with the postural extensors and scapula retractors. This position also is beneficial to stretch her tight hip flexors. By stretching hip flexors and strengthening trunk and hip extensors, she may be able to stand more erect and have a greater range into hip extension during gait. When positioning patients in prone, care must be taken to monitor heart rate and ease of respiration—common problems of those with hypertension. If CVP problems arise, an alternative posture in which to resist the upper trunk extensors, such as sitting, would be chosen.

Procedures in the *Hooklying Posture*

Mobility.—Although a pelvic tilt can be performed in this posture, range into lumbar flexion is not commonly a problem. To increase range of lumbar rotation, hooklying is an appropriate posture for the spine and is not weight bearing, a consideration in those with osteopenia. The technique to increase range of the muscular tissue would be HR. Once range is gained, the patient can maintain that range by performing rhythmic rotational movements to the end of range as part of the home program. The increased lower trunk rotation is desired for improved pelvic rotation and stride length during gait.

Stability.—Maintaining the posture and improving isometric ability of the lower abdominals and back extensors can be enhanced by AI with manual contacts on the knees. The patient can perform lower abdominal exercises by flattening the back and bringing one knee toward the chest. Most elders will not have sufficient abdominal control to maintain the lumbar spine position and bring the other leg toward the chest as well. To resist a hip abduction motion, an elastic strapping can be placed around the knees.

Procedures in the *Bridging Posture*

In bridging the lower trunk and hip extensors, and the hip abductors can be enhanced in their shortened ranges.

Mobility.—The patient needs to have sufficient range in the hip flexors and strength in the trunk and hip extensors (3/5) so the hips can be extended. If not, mobility is gained in non–weight-bearing postures such as supine or prone. If the hip extensors cannot overcome the resistance of gravity, their strength is increased in supine.

Stability.—As Mrs. J maintains the position for an increasing amount of time, the endurance of the back and hip extensors is increasing. The techniques of AI and RS with resistance provided at the hips, knees, or ankles can progressively increase the difficulty of the procedure. Improving the stance phase of gait and unilateral stance for stair climbing is the goal. As part of her home program, resistance provided by elastic material can be placed at the pelvis or knees to emphasize extensor or abductor control.

Controlled Mobility.—Pelvic lateral shifting and rotation can be performed independently by Mrs. J as part of her home program as well as with the SRH technique. The concentric-eccentric reversal of moving into and out of bridging is designed to help her ability to descend stairs.

Static-Dynamic.—Lifting one leg from the supporting surface increases the resistance to the supporting limb and focuses on the control needed for unilateral stance and single-limb support while descending stairs.

Procedures in the *Sitting* Posture

The movements that can be performed in sitting include upper trunk extension, trunk extension with rotation, lumbar spine extension and flexion, hip flexion, knee flexion and extension, and ankle dorsiflexion.

Mobility.—Range can be gained in the upper trunk and upper extremities, and into hip flexion, with the techniques of HR and joint mobilization. This range can be maintained by self-stretching movements.

Stability.—Holding in the shortened range of the upper trunk extensors and scapular retractors can be performed, with resistance provided manually, by pulleys, or by elastic material.

Controlled Mobility.—Weight shifting of the trunk on the hips will improve the control needed for assuming standing from sitting and the movements needed during dressing.

Skill.—Lower extremity movements can emphasize the quadriceps and dorsiflexor activity that is required for postural responses in standing and during the gait sequence. Many elders may lose their balance backward when reaching overhead or looking up. Improved dorsiflexor and quadriceps control may help to reduce this tendency. For many elders, weak quadriceps may limit stair climbing and moving between standing and sitting. Elastic band, isotonic, or isokinetic resistance may be appropriate to increase quadriceps strength.

Activities in the *Modified Plantigrade* Position

Modified plantigrade treatment can include exercises for the lower trunk, knee extensors, and ankle. Control around these joints can be emphasized in this posture, which is also easily incorporated into the home program.

Controlled Mobility.—Weight shifting and performing small-range knee extensor eccentric exercises are directed toward improving Mrs. J's ability to descend stairs. By positioning an elastic band around her knee and attaching it to an immovable object, such as the leg of a table, concentric-eccentric resistance can be given to quadriceps and hamstring contractions.

Static-Dynamic.—Lifting one upper or lower extremity can be performed with gradually increasing resistance provided by an elastic band or a weight. Improved control over unilateral stance and reduced fatigue of the trunk extensors are the goals.

Procedures in *Standing*

In standing, trunk, hip, knee, and ankle control can be enhanced. As these more difficult procedures are attempted, Mrs. J may require additional support such as the parallel bars or standing next to a stable surface.

Controlled Mobility and Static-Dynamic.—During both bilateral and unilateral standing, weight shifting can be performed rocking the body in various directions and then rocking up on toes and on the heels. Changing the surface to a balance board will further challenge responses. If enhanced proprioceptive awareness is desired, to improve her confidence in walking on uneven surfaces or when going to the bathroom at night, these balance tasks can be performed with the eyes closed. As this increased challenge is undertaken, to ensure safety the parallel bars or other supporting surfaces are used.

Skill.—Resisted progression can emphasize the sequencing of pelvic motions during gait. At this skill stage the activity itself is practiced to enhance learning and improve endurance. A treadmill may be useful for this. To improve CVP endurance, upper and lower body ergometers (bicycles) may be appropriate.

The *QUADRUPED posture* was not included in Mrs. J's treatment program because of her age, cardiac status, and arthritic knees. However, for others it may be very appropriate to increase upper extremity weight bearing and improve trunk stability.

SUMMARY

Primary functional goals of physical therapy with the elderly population are to maintain or improve walking speed and to ensure safety while walking and moving between postures. This therapeutic program has been designed to improve the components of movement associated with these functional activities.

In the illustrative case study, the patient's functional capability was evaluated considering the environmental, social, and medical factors as they might influence physical functioning. The physical systems were assessed, comparing the patient's findings to changes expected as part of the aging process and referring to the physical requirements of functional activities. The impairments related to the functional limitations were judged relative to the (1)

patient's ability to change; (2) need to develop compensatory activities; or (3) the need to make environmental modifications. To develop the treatment plan, the physical impairments were categorized within the intervention model, and the functional outcome and treatment goals were determined. The specific treatment procedures were incorporated into the stages of control, the appropriate postures, and movements, along with consideration of the exercise parameters. The group and home program complemented any individual therapy needed.

The framework of practice, with its evaluation and intervention models, provides a logical rationale for the development and sequencing of an intervention program. Therapists are guided in interpreting the anatomic and physiologic changes that occur with the aging process and connecting those to their specific patients' impairments. These are matched to possible interventions. This program has emphasized improving the prerequisite abilities to ambulation so that this functional task can occur in as automatic a fashion as possible.

REFERENCES

1. Ades PA, et al: Exercise conditioning in the elderly coronary patient. *J Am Geriatr Soc* 1987; 35:121–124.
2. Allum JHJ: Vestibular and proprioceptive control of sway stabilization, in Bless W, Brandt T (eds): *Disorders of Posture and Gait.* Amsterdam, Elsevier, 1986, pp 19–40.
3. Amundsen LR, DeVahl JM, Ellingham CT: Evaluation of a group exercise program for elderly women. *Phys Ther* 1989; 69:475–483.
4. Astrand I, Astrand PO, Hallback I, et al: Reduction in maximal oxygen uptake with age. *J Appl Physiol* 1973; 35:649–654.
5. Bellucci G, Hoyer WJ: Feedback effects on the performance and self reinforcing behavior of elderly and young adult women. *J Gerontol* 1975; 30:456–460.
6. Bendall MJ, Bassey EJ, Pearson MB: Factors affecting walking speed of elderly people. *Age Ageing* 1989; 18:327–332.
7. Blanke DJ, Hageman PA: Comparison of gait of young men and elderly men. *Phys Ther* 1989; 69:144–148.
8. Boyce WJ, Vessey MP: Habitual physical inertia and other factors in relation to risk of fracture of the proximal femur. *Age Ageing* 1988; 17:319–327.
9. Brooks VB: *The Neural Basis of Motor Control.* New York, Oxford University Press, 1986.
10. Brownlee MC, et al: Consideration of spacial orientation mechanisms as related to elderly fallers. *Gerontology* 1989; 35:323–331.
11. Caradoc-Davies TH, Dixon GS, Campbell AJ: Benefit from admission to a geriatric assessment and rehabilitation unit. *J Am Geriatr Soc* 1989; 37:25–28.
12. Chesworth BM, Vandervoot AA: Age and passive ankle stiffness in healthy women. *Phys Ther* 1989; 69:217–224.

13. Crilly RG, Willems DA, et al: Effect of exercise on postural sway in the elderly. *Gerontology* 1989; 35:137–143.

14. Fiatarone MA, Evans WJ: Exercise in the oldest old. *Top Geriatr Rehabil* 1990; 5:63–77.

15. Fiatarone MA, et al: High-intensity strength training in nonagenarians: effects on skeletal muscle. *JAMA* 1990; 263:3029–3032.

16. Finley FR, Cody KA, Finizie RV: Locomotion patterns in elderly women. *Phys Med Rehabil* 1969; 3:140–146.

17. Friedman PJ, Richmond DE, Baskett JJ: A prospective trial of serial gait speed as a measure of rehabilitation in the elderly. *Age Ageing* 1988; 17:227–235.

18. Gehlsen GM, Whaley MH: Falls in the elderly. Part II. Balance, strength and flexibility. *Arch Phys Med Rehabil* 1990; 71:739–741.

19. Guccione AA: Physical therapy diagnosis and the relationship between impairments and function. *Phys Ther* 1991; 71:449–504.

20. Harris BA, Dyreck DA: A model of orthopaedic dysfunction for clinical decision making in physical therapy practice. *Phys Ther* 1989; 69:548–553.

21. Hart BA: Fractionated myostatic reflex times in women by activity level and age. *Gerontology* 1986; 41:361–365.

22. Himann JF, et al: Age-related changes in speed of walking. *Med Sci Sports Exerc* 1988; 161–166.

23. Hirschberg GG, Ralston HJ: Energy cost of stair climbing in normal and hemiplegic subjects. *Am J Phys Med* 1965; 44:165–168.

24. Holden MK, Gill KM, Magliozzi MR: Gait assessment for neurologically impaired patients: Standards for outcome assessment. *Phys Ther* 1986; 66:1530–1539.

25. Jette AM, Harris BA, Cleary PD, et al: Functional recovery after hip fracture. *Arch Phys Med Rehabil* 1987; 68(10): 735-740.

26. Krolner B, Taft B, Nielsen SP, et al: Physical exercise a prophylaxis against involutional vetebral bone loss: A controlled trial. The Biochemical Society and the Medical Research Society. *Clin Sci* 1983; 64:541–546.

27. Larsson L, Grimby G, Karlsson J: Muscle strength and speed of movement in relation to age and muscle morphology. *J Appl Physiol* 1979; 46:451–456.

28. Lexell J, Taylor C, Sjostrumm M: What is the cause of the aging atrophy? *J Neurosci* 1988; 84:275–294.

29. Molloy DW, et al: Acute effects of exercise on neuropsychological function in elderly subjects. *J Am Geriatr Soc* 1988; 36:29–33.

30. Morey MC, et al: Evaluation of a supervised exercise program in a geriatric population. *J Am Geriatr Soc* 1989; 37:348–354.

31. Murray MP, et al: Age related differences in knee muscle strength in normal women. *J Gerontol* 1985; 40:275–280.

32. Murray MP, Kory RC, Clarkson BH: Walking patterns in healthy old men. *J Gerontol* 1969; 24:169–178.

33. Overstall PW, Exton-Smith AN, Imms FJ, et al: Falls in the elderly related to postural imbalance. *Br Med J* 1977; 1:261–264.

34. Paris SW: *Foundations of Clinical Orthopaedics*. St Augustine, Fla, Institute Press, 1989.

35. Pyykko I, et al: Postural control in elderly subjects. *Age Ageing* 1990; 19:215–221.

36. Rikli R, Busch S: Motor performance of women as a function of age and physical activity level. *J Gerontol* 1986; 51:645–649.

37. Rowe JW, Kahn RL: Human aging: Usual and successful. *Science* 1987; 237:143–149.

38. Rubinstein LZ, et al: Falls and instability in the elderly. *J Am Geriatr Soc* 1988; 36:266–278.

39. Sabbahi MA, Sedgwick EM: Age related changes in monosynaptic reflex excitability. *J Gerontol* 1982; 37:24–32.

40. Schenkman M, Butler RB: A model for multisystem evaluation, interpretation and treatment of individuals with neurologic dysfunction. *Phys Ther* 1989; 69:538–547.

41. Shephard RJ: The scientific basis of exercise prescribing for the very old. *J Am Geriatr Soc* 1990; 38:62–70.

42. Soderberg GL: *Kinesiology Application to Pathological Motion*. Baltimore, Williams & Wilkins, 1986.

43. Spirduso WW: Reaction and movement times as a function of age and physical activity level. *J Gerontol* 1975; 30:435–440.

44. Stockmeyer SA: An interpretation of the approach of Rood to the treatment of neuromuscular dysfunction. *Am J Phys Med* 1967; 46:900–954.

45. Sullivan PE, Markos PD: *Clinical Procedures in Therapeutic Exercise*. Norwalk, Conn, Appleton & Lange, 1986.

46. Sullivan PE, Markos PD, Minor MD: *An Integrated Approach to Therapeutic Exercise: Theory and Clinical Application*. Reston, Virginia, Reston Publishers, 1982.

47. Thompson RF, Crist DM, Marsh M: Effects of physical exercise for elderly patients with physical impairments. *J Am Geriatr Soc* 1988; 36:130–135.

48. Thompson RF, Crist DM, Osborn LA: Treadmill exercise electrocardiography in the elderly with physical impairments. *Gerontology* 1990; 36:112–118.

49. Tinetti ME: Performance-oriented assessments of mobility problems in elderly patients. *J Am Geriatr Soc* 1986; 34:119–126.

50. Tinetti ME: Factors associated with serious injury during falls by ambulatory nursing home residents. *J Am Geriatr Soc* 1987; 35:644–648.

51. Tomonage M: Histochemical and ultrastructural changes in senile human skeletal muscle. *J Am Geriatr Soc* 1977; 25:125–131.

52. Wade DT: Measurement in rehabilitation: Commentary. *Age Ageing* 1988; 17:289–292.

53. Whipple RH, Wolfson LI, Ameiman PM: The relationship of knee and ankle weakness to falls in nursing home residents: An isokinetic study. *J Am Geriatr Soc* 1987; 35:13–20.

54. Winter DA, Patia AE, Frank JS, et al: Biomechanical walking pattern changes in the fit and healthy elderly. *Phys Ther* 1990; 70:340–347.

55. Wolfson LI, Whipple R, Amerman RN, et al: Stressing the postural response. *J Am Geriatr Soc* 1986; 34:845–850.

56. Woollacott MH, Shumway-Cook A, Nashner LM: Aging and postural control: Changes in sensory organization and muscular coordination. *Int J Aging Hum Dev* 1986; 23:97–114.

Lower Extremity Orthotics in Geriatric Rehabilitation

Kenneth E. Perkins, M.S.P.T., P.T., C.O.

INTRODUCTION

The inherently complex interrelationship of biomechanics and neuromuscular capability that creates human locomotion, especially when coupled with the range of impairments often found in older persons, can be confusing even to an experienced physical therapist. Multiple medical conditions in the elderly can also precipitate alterations in ambulation patterns that increase energy consumption and further tax the weakened physical systems that underlie movement. Ultimately, these factors can result in less functional gait patterns and contribute to an overall decrease in ambulation. If allowed to persist, nonambulatory function can have profound effects on the length and quality of life.

Orthotics can be constructed to address a multitude of problems. Persistent rehabilitation problems in the lower extremity such as weakness, instability, abnormal tone, impaired tissue integrity, bony deformities, joint range limitations, muscle imbalances, and pain are some conditions that can be positively influenced through the skillful design and application of orthotics. Through the use of various materials such as plastics, metals, foams, cork, and crepe, orthotic intervention is essentially an application of pressure to specific areas for the purpose of creating a force system. These force systems remediate or accommodate structural deficits or painful problem areas that interfere with the function of normal ambulation.

Proper orthotic and therapeutic intervention is often a team venture. The basis of clinical reasoning in the fields of both physical therapy and orthotics lies in the therapeutic principles that are common to both. Applications of these principles in physical therapy take the form of "hands-on" intervention such as therapeutic exercises and adjunctive modalities based on the therapist's evaluation. In orthotics, a definitive object, the orthosis, is the end product of the evaluative process. The reasoning process used to make orthotic decisions is elusive to many physical therapists. The goal of this chapter is to expose the clinical physical therapist to a thought process to strategize an orthotic plan and achieve an optimal orthotic outcome with an older adult patient. A systematic approach for problem solving is especially warranted to meet the challenges in this population.

TEAMWORK

The complexities of using orthotics as a part of the rehabilitation program are amplified by the variety of devices currently available. Regional and personal preferences often underlie choices in design and materials. As a result, the device, and not the patient's needs, becomes the point of focus of discussions between therapist and orthotist—a situation potentially serious for the patient if the device does not fully meet biomechanical needs. The use of orthotics must be integrated with the appropriate therapeutic plan. In this way, attention is directed not so much toward the device itself but toward identifying the needs of the individual, correctly matching the device to these needs, and instituting a treatment program that achieves the goals of rehabilitation.

The responsibility of the physical therapist is to identify abnormal positions and movements that occur during standing and ambulation and to use this functional information to determine the location of the primary biomechanical problem area. This established primary problem area represents a strategic starting point for orthotic and therapeutic intervention. The responsibility of the orthotist is to use the clinical data on movement dysfunction provided by the physical therapist's assessment of the primary problem area to fabricate an orthotic system that effectively enhances ambulation by addressing the need to support, accommodate, assist, or protect structural problems of the primary problem area. Establishing communication is the first step that team members must take in order to help make appropriate orthotic decisions.

Terminology

Problems with communication among team members, stemming from a lack in understanding of the basic terminology of each other's fields, affect all levels of team interaction. A generic identification system has been developed that names each orthotic appliance according to the anatomic area that it controls or encompasses, for example, foot orthosis, FO, or ankle-foot orthosis, AFO. The entire body can be outlined in this fashion: cervical (C), thoracic (T), lumber (L), sacral (S), hip (H), knee (K), ankle (A), and foot (F).

Lack of knowledge, overprotection of professional boundaries, personal fears of incompetence, and the need "to know everything and to be right" are just a few of the factors that hinder discussion among professionals and between patients and practitioners. Unfortunately, this can affect team interaction to the extent that appropriate systems, programs, and goals are never fully established or achieved. To prevent this situation from developing, it is helpful to understand that it is not essential for a therapist to know all the exact names, designs, components, and materials used in the many orthotics that are currently available or being developed. It is important, however, to communicate accurately in general terms to provide the orthotist with an accurate description of the area of movement dysfunction. The focus of communication should be on information that is pertinent to both the physical therapist and the orthotist. Once the problem is identified and the overall goals of treatment are communicated, team members can work on how to address the causes underlying the movement dysfunction. Discussion is then related to the specific impairments that influence the creation of the functional problem and how multiple problem areas act to alter a patient's normal structure-function relationships during the gait cycle, increasing energy expenditure in ambulation. Based on the functional goals agreed upon by the patient, the physical therapist, and the orthotist, the orthotic system is developed and integrated into the therapeutic plan of care to promote low energy consumption during ambulation.

IDENTIFYING PRIMARY PROBLEM AREAS

The objective of observational gait analysis is to identify deviations in the determinants of gait from the anticipated "normal" pattern of joint excursions that normally occur throughout the trunk and upper and lower extremities. When movement dysfunction or abnormal use of the trunk or limbs is noted from a biomechanical point of view, the therapist must use these observations to decide where the primary problem areas are and establish how they may be contributing to the observed pattern of gait deviations. Is the primary problem in the structures of the foot, or rather the foot and ankle complex? Is dysfunctional movement the result of a structural rotation such as bony deformity of the tibia? Is the gait abnormality a single problem at the knee, the hip, or the spinal area, or is it really a combination of problems in all these areas? These changes in observed function occur when the functional demands on the primary joints or muscle groups exceed their structural capabilities, and the normal structure-function relationship is altered. The individual then compensates for an altered structure-function relationship in the lower extremity by using other joints or muscle groups to perform the activity. Therefore, it is essential that the primary problem is distinguished from other compensatory movements that must also occur in order for the individual to accomplish the activity of walking.

The challenge of a physical therapy evaluation lies in sorting out the primary problem area from the compensatory movements that are its sequelae. Consider, for example, a primary problem area at the ankle that presents clinically as restricted ankle dorsiflexion. Decreased range of motion (ROM) could be due to many reasons, for example, acute joint trauma or chronic soft tissue contracture. The patient with limited dorsiflexion often externally rotates the lower extremity on the affected side. This compensation effectively overcomes the impediment to ambulation posed by the lost ROM at the ankle and contributes

to reducing the increased energy expenditure that the impaired structure triggers. Prolonged ambulation in this abnormal manner can foster the creation of secondary problems such as increased tightness and muscle length shortening of the external rotators on that side. Although external rotation may appear to be the patient's problem, the therapist must be able to discern that it is not just a compensatory movement in response to another impairment. Evaluation and treatment plans should first focus on evaluating and treating the primary impairment and then proceed to identify any other remaining difficulties, once these fundamental problems have been adequately addressed.

Objective kinematic observation of abnormal function, such as excessive external rotation, alone will not provide sufficient information to fully determine the primary impairment nor provide enough information on which one can establish an appropriate orthotic or therapeutic plan. Observing and listing aberrations in movement only serve to direct the attention of the therapist to potential areas of concern. The therapist must perform further assessments, such as strength and ROM, at all the involved joints of the lower extremity to propose a kinetic sequence of events that explains the observed pattern of movement. At the conclusion of this sequential analysis, the therapist will identify the primary problem toward which therapeutic intervention will first be directed.

The common foundation that weds orthotic and therapeutic interventions rests on the evidence that has established the relationship between the determinants of gait and energy expenditure. This relationship essentially states that normal structure promotes normal function, and normal ambulatory function occurs at low-energy expenditure levels. Orthotic and therapeutic intervention then is established as a procedure that uses the relationship between structure and function to promote low energy.

THE DETERMINANTS OF GAIT

Studies on human ambulation have generally indicated that human locomotion has evolved in a way that minimizes the energy requirements of ambulation.[2] When a person ambulates normally, the determinants of gait, which include pelvic rotation, pelvic tilt, lateral pelvic displacement, knee flexion, walking-base width, and cadence, combine to restrict the excursion of a person's center of gravity during ambulation. As a result of controlling excessive joint motion and limiting muscle recruitment and use, the energy requirements of ambulation are reduced. Any deviation that affects any of the determinants of gait also represents a change in energy efficiency. Therefore, the overall goal of all orthotic management in the elderly is to remedy structural changes that impede ambulation and, in combination with therapeutic intervention, restore energy-efficient gait patterns.

In stance, the foot and ankle function to absorb the shock of impact, adjust to uneven surfaces, and provide stability as a person moves from heel contact through toe-off. The stance phase can be divided into an *initial contact phase,* in which the structures of the foot must be accommodative and flexible, that progresses into a *single-limb–support phase,* which requires structures that are stable, supportive, and more rigid. Dysfunctional movement, therefore, can be conceptualized as an alteration in the demands for flexibility during stance vs. the stability requirements of stance. If the structures are too rigid at the initial phase of stance, they do not allow appropriate shock absorption or accommodation to occur. Excessive rigidity could result in structural problems due to unabsorbed impact and predispose the individual to falls, twists, and sprains, resulting from an inability to accommodate to uneven support surfaces. Problems may arise in stance phase as a result of excessive flexibility or instability, when biomechanical support is needed, especially during single-limb support. If the demand for more dorsiflexion ROM is unmet as the lower limb moves over the ankle and foot, a compensatory pronation can occur that could result in the development of plantar fasciitis in a foot that was previously symptom free.

Since the foot and ankle work together to promote normal low-energy movement, any structural alteration in one area can have a profound effect on the other structures and therefore alter function in other areas. For example, a calcaneus in an excessive valgus position during mid- to terminal stance also alters the normal support surface position for the talus. As a result, forces created in weight bearing predispose the talus to move more medially on the surface of this altered support. This creates an abnormal increase in midfoot pronation. Under these conditions, the tibia, which is supported by the talus, is positioned in prolonged internal rotation through the latter portion of stance phase. As a result, this kinetic sequence of events contributes to excessive valgus stress at the knee at a time in stance when the quadriceps contract to pull the knee into extension. This results in the patella's being pulled more laterally toward the lateral femoral condyle. Over time, repeated stress could lead to the development of a laterally dislocating patella, chondromalacia, or symptoms of excessive stress to the medial collateral ligaments, which could be affected by the increased valgus position of the knee. Similarly, problems at the hip could be attributed to a tightened iliotibial band that was a functional response to problems at the knee, which themselves may have originated from primary problems in the foot. Problems in the thoracic region can also create excessive demands on the structures of the foot. If the patient adopts a position of excessive trunk flexion, compensations must occur at the hip, knee, and ankle.

Once the source of the functional difficulties is identified, it is necessary to explain why the primary problem exists in the first place. This necessitates the evaluation of the muscular, skeletal, and nervous systems for impairments that could be implicated in creating pain or other conditions that alter normal function. The information gathered by the physical therapist's assessment has a direct effect on decisions regarding orthotic choice, material, and design. For example, consider impairment of the muscular system that effectively prevents normal dorsiflexion movement during the swing phase of gait. Using a dorsiflexion-assist AFO, which compensates for lost active dorsiflexion by placing the foot and ankle in the appropriate position during swing, would be an appropriate orthotic choice for this problem to enhance function.

Movement dysfunction at the ankle may also result from impairments of the nervous system. An abnormal response to stretch may elicit clonus or an extension pattern promoting plantarflexion. In this case, selection of a dorsiflexion-assist AFO would not be appropriate. This would provide a quick stretch to the plantarflexors during swing and permit the person's body weight to stretch the plantarflexors during stance to further promote abnormal tone and an inappropriate motor response. This type of orthotic intervention only serves to create further deterioration of muscle and joint structure-function relationships. Here the primary problem at the ankle would be more appropriately addressed orthotically if material and design concerns focused on controlling and diminishing the characteristics that elicit abnormal tone from an impaired nervous system. In this case, an AFO that blocked ankle motion in swing and effectively inhibited motion while providing support in stance would be a more appropriate orthotic choice. In addition, a rocker-soled shoe could be used in this case to accommodate for the ankle motion lost by using the AFO as well as to approximate normal motion in terminal stance.

In summary, the existence of abnormal compensatory movements indicates that the normal structure-function relationships of the lower extremity during the gait cycle have been altered. Altered ambulatory function can be observed kinematically and is likely to initiate an increase in energy expenditure. When the therapist identifies and assesses those physical impairments that contribute to the primary problem, orthotic and therapeutic intervention can be effectively combined to promote more energy-efficient and symmetric gait in the elderly.

CONNECTING PHYSICAL THERAPY TO ORTHOTIC DESIGN

The purpose of the physical therapist's assessment, as described above, is to identify and evaluate primary problem areas in relationship to the body systems involved and provide an explanation for the dysfunctional gait pattern. Therapists must also consider the extent to which these problems will be improved by treating the contributing impairments through rehabilitation. This allows one to assess the degree to which orthotic intervention will be required and the difficulties that may be experienced in trying to remediate the primary problem area. In order to achieve these objectives, therapists may find it more useful to adopt a *systems approach*. By maintaining a therapist's focus on the interrelatedness of structural impairments that alter functional performance, an orthotic systems approach limits excessive concentration on the device or "thing" that will purportedly solve the problem before the problem has been adequately characterized. An orthotic systems approach addresses the initiating causes of the primary problem as well as all the other problem areas altering the normal relationship between structure and function. Focusing on the orthotic device tends to be a "dead end to thinking" and can leave many problem areas unaddressed. A systems approach is an effective means of integrating the perspectives of rehabilitation and orthotics to achieve the patient's goals.

Based on the degree to which rehabilitation procedures alone will be able to alter primary problems and promote more normal function, the orthotic goal is to design the most appropriate orthotic system needed to compensate for these primary structural problems and any other remaining structural problems that continue to interfere with function. If, as in the previous example of the patient with an excessive external rotation of the lower extremity, the level of intervention was limited to providing "a thing"—for instance, a twister cable to derotate the limb, with no further involvement of either therapist or orthotist—the patient suffers the injustice of a less-than-thorough evaluation. A quick orthotic "fix" can have an immediate effect on the position of the limb, but the overall effect is to leave the primary problem, which *creates* the demand for the external rotation of the limb, unaddressed. Cost, time, pain, and further primary problem deterioration are all affected when shortcuts to proper intervention are practiced. The elderly, like all other patients, cannot afford this type of shortsighted intervention.

Interim or Definitive Approach

The potential for rehabilitation and the gap between the patient's clinical presentation and functional requirements define the quantity and quality of change that may be achieved in primary problem areas. If a therapist anticipates that the structure-function relationship will undergo large degrees of change, based on the rehabilitation potential of the impaired body systems, an interim approach is indicated to meet the changing needs of the patient. An AFO with a double-action ankle joint component (Fig 17–1) having two channels to address a variety of ankle position and strength needs is an example of an interim orthotic approach. In using these channels, the team may decide, for example, to use pins to stabilize and springs to assist, or to keep the channels free to allow motion as progress is made from flaccidity to the active stages of motor recovery, as in dealing with a patient recovering from a cerebrovascular accident (CVA). A definitive approach, however, is best used with a structure-function relationship that is basically stable. The smaller the degree of expected change in the patient's impairments, the more definitive the approach can be. Whichever approach is used, the decision must be based on the magnitude of deviation away from normal structure-function relationships and the potential for rehabilitation.

BASIC CONCEPTS OF DESIGN

Orthotic intervention can be at a variety of levels ranging from the simple to the complex. No matter what degree of intervention is considered, orthotic designs use basic principles of pressures and the development of force systems. The design and the materials selected also consider the degree of support or control, accommodation, assistance, or protection required once the problem areas have been fully evaluated. The principles of orthotic designs are presented below.

Immobilization and Support

The difference between orthoses that immobilize, or provide maximum control of motion, and those that provide support is simply in the degree to which movement is permitted. There are several basic principles and concepts that are used to design an orthosis to immobilize or support a weakened structure. These include leverage, extended lever arms, three-point pressure, and total contact concepts. All these concepts are used to create force systems that alter or control motion. To be successful they must do so in a comfortable manner that enhances energy-efficient function. Each is briefly described.

The concept of leverage is perhaps best illustrated by the playground teeter-totter. Equal pressure on both ends with the axis in the middle results in a force system in equilibrium. If the axis is moved in either direction (or the

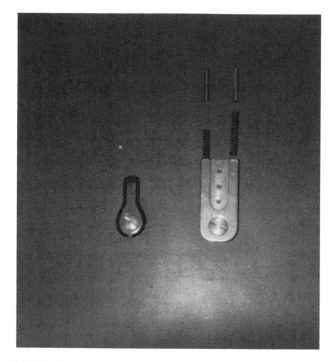

FIG 17–1.
A double-action ankle joint component has two channels for inserting pins to stabilize or springs to assist. The channels may also be kept open to allow free ankle motion.

lever arm is extended), more pressure is required on the shorter lever arm to achieve equilibrium. An effective orthotic system is biomechanically efficient and requires the patient to exert less force to accomplish the activity. By separating the points at which pressure is applied as much as possible (i.e., extending the lever arm), less force is required to counteract the opposing force created by the patient's body.

In a three-point pressure system, the configuration of the applied pressures can be used to create force systems that either immobilize or support. A patient with torn ligaments or weak quadriceps who is unable to stabilize the knee in stance is a common clinical problem. One three-point pressure system that addresses this problem utilizes two forces applied in a similar direction that are separated and opposed by a third force. Forces created in this way are used in knee orthoses (KOs) and knee-ankle-foot orthoses (KAFOs) to produce knee stability through immobilization during functional activities.

Another application of an alternative three-point pressure system is seen in an alternative KAFO design known as a floor-reaction orthosis (Fig 17–2). The three-point pressure system applied in this configuration results in a force system that works to inhibit knee buckling by opposing the rotational forces created at the ankle when the patient bears weight on the extremity. The solid ankle and long toe-plate design, which covers the ankle and extends the plastic the entire length of the foot, creates a force sys-

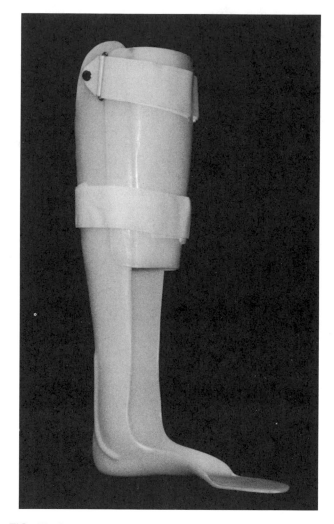

FIG 17–2.
A floor-reaction KAFO uses a three-point pressure system to prevent knee buckling.

tem that pushes the knee into extension the more the knee tries to move toward the ground. It should be noted, however, that the forces applied in this three-point pressure system are greater than those created by a simple knee immobilizer for the same knee problem. When the patient is unable to extend the knee at least actively against gravity, the patient can be observed to compensate by leaning forward and shifting the center of gravity anterior to the knee to provide the force required to prevent the knee from buckling during unassisted ambulation. In this case, material failure and patient discomfort constitute a more important factor in choice of an orthotic than the functional goal alone. In the end, the choice of the best and most comfortable three-point pressure system depends on criteria of residual strength, range of motion, the patient's height and weight, and other structural information as well as the desired functional goals.

The purpose of a total contact system is also to apply pressures in such a way as to provide controlled comfortable function. For example, an elder with a rigid cavus foot—a foot that has an excessively high arch that remains unchanged even with weight bearing—experiences excessive pressure due to the isolated areas of contact at the heel and forefoot. A total contact foot orthotic conforms to this exaggerated structural deviation and redistributes pressures throughout the entire plantar surface of the foot. As a result, high-pressure areas are reduced at the heel and forefoot, and the chances of experiencing skin breakdown and pain are reduced as well. Appropriate force systems, therefore, are those that apply pressures to stabilize, control, assist, or protect problems in a comfortable manner in the effort to enhance energy-efficient function.

Accommodation and Protection

The pressures created by maintained force systems applied to elderly patients have the potential to be uncomfortable and eventually destructive to tissue. *Pressure* is defined as the magnitude of the force applied divided by the size of the area of application ($P = F/A$). As can be easily deduced from this formula, the larger the area in relationship to the force applied, the smaller the resulting pressure will be. Orthotics themselves may be sources of abnormal pressure on the skin of elders. Pads that spread the application of the force over the widest possible area produce the least pressure and should be considered when designing the pad or appliance.

Pressure problems from increased force being applied to small surface areas are exacerbated in a geriatric population due to multiple problems that elders have, including ulceration from diabetic neuropathies, painful and enlarged bunion areas from prolonged wearing of ill-fitting shoes, and corn and callous formations over foot deformities that rub and press inside shoes. Soft cushions and relief areas from cutout pad designs along with extra depth or custom-molded shoes, which accommodate abnormal foot structure, can be used to protect and relieve pressure on these areas. This is especially important for areas undergoing repetitive stress where bony prominences or impaired circulation are involved. It is important to realize, however, that the relief of symptoms is not the only goal. These problems are usually an indication that a more thorough evaluation is called for to reveal the true cause for these pressure problems.

COMMON PROBLEMS

Evaluation of the patient to identify primary problems allows the therapist to explain the reasons for excessive pressure problems such as those seen in the above examples and to recommend an orthotic solution. Appropriate management may vary widely for what appears to be a simple problem area. For example, symptoms of discomfort under the first metatarsal head in an older person with diabetes may be remediated by several different orthotic solutions based on the therapist's findings on initial evaluation. For instance, a modified-donut foam pad with a soft transitional top cover can help to take pressure off a sensitive metatarsal area. This ring of foam redistributes pressure to the surrounding tissue areas. Using the top cover prevents the metatarsal head from sinking into the hole and having tissue constricted by the surrounding ring. This orthotic solution may provide protection and immediate pain relief, but it does not necessarily address the real underlying problem. Further evaluation may reveal excessive midfoot pronation that is structurally limited in its potential to be corrected. The flexor hallucis, in its attempt to use the first ray as a supportive strut or brace to block the effects of excessive pronation, may also have developed a contracture. If the excessively pronated foot position is a fixed problem unresponsive to therapeutic treatment, an accommodative soft foot orthotic would be appropriate to use. A soft insert can be added to accommodate and redistribute pressure and reduce shear forces to the metatarsal area in this case.

Shoe accommodations, such as a rocker-bottom shoe (Fig 17–3) or a metatarsal bar, are additional pressure-relieving measures that are generally considered to remediate forefoot pressure problems. The patient's gait pattern and how the person is actually functioning are paramount considerations in making these decisions effective. A gait pattern consisting of short shuffling steps that does not exhibit a heel-off or rollover from mid-to terminal stance would not necessarily benefit from a rocker-bottom shoe, since there is little weight shift to the forefoot with this type of gait pattern. This could potentially create instability problems in an elder since a rocker-bottom sole removes the distal support of the shoe itself and promotes rollover, which flexes the knee during stance phase. The patient in this example could fall from the loss of stability while lit-

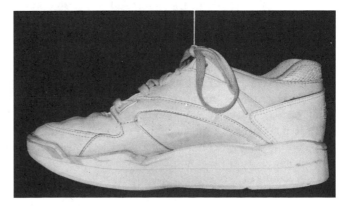

FIG 17–3.
A rocker bottom may be added to a shoe or sneaker to accommodate pressure problems in the forefoot.

tle has been done to reduce the pressures at the first metatarsal head. If bony or soft tissue structural problems contribute significantly to decreased ankle dorsiflexion ROM, this in turn would increase stress to the forefoot. The use of a metatarsal bar under these conditions would also be inappropriate. A metatarsal bar elevates the forefoot and requires more dorsiflexion range in standing and walking. In this case, the orthotist can consider an aggressive rocker bottom to relieve forefoot stress from heel-off through terminal stance. This allows the shoe to accommodate for the 10 to 15 degrees of missing dorsiflexion ROM that is required at the ankle to take a normal step in the stance phase of the gait cycle.

If excessive first metatarsal stress is a result of an inherently rigid non–shock-absorbing foot structure that is experiencing a fully correctable midfoot collapse, a semirigid orthotic approach could be used. A more resilient base material, such as Thermo Cork, provides control to modify midfoot pronation while at the same time absorbing stresses that are associated with bringing the foot back into its normal position, which in this case is a rigid conformation.

ORTHOTIC MATERIALS

Current principles of foot orthotic design suggest that, in general, rigid materials are not appropriate for rigid foot problems. More important, in making these decisions, evaluation of the degree of flexibility or rigidity in the primary problem area must be combined with the particular function to be performed and the stresses the device may create to deal with the functional problems. As in the previously described shuffling gait example, the patient does not ambulate with normal mid- and terminal stance. If the primary problem areas contributing to this gait deviation cannot be therapeutically enhanced, orthotic considerations must also be based on the actual structural demands of the functional activity as it is being performed. This means that the orthotist must choose materials that best suit a combination of biomechanical needs. For example, consider a patient with an inherently rigid foot bony configuration, who also experiences an excessive midfoot collapse. If the degree of collapse is sufficient to create forefoot shear stress that results in discomfort of the first metatarsal head, and the condition is fully correctable, the patient may benefit from a thermoforming polypropylene or subortholen rigid plastic material. These materials do have some give to them and actually have the capacity to act as compressive springs as a person's body weight stretches the plastic material during loading in stance. Furthermore, the benefit in using these more rigid materials is that they do not change their shape as much under repetitive loads to the degree that semirigid or soft foam materi-

als do. They will therefore act to redistribute plantar pressure and maintain more specific control to correct for mechanical deficiencies for a longer period of time.

Extremely rigid materials, such as acrylics and other thermosetting plastics, do not give, and as a result, they tend to transmit impact forces rather than absorb them as soft or semirigid materials. They also do not modify the force of impact as semirigid or thermoforming rigid plastic materials do. On the other hand, the benefit of these materials is that they do give an orthotic ultimate control. Evaluation of the degree of instability and the function being performed is important to consider along with minimizing the stress that the orthotic may be expected to tolerate. Consider, using the above example, the need to control excessive pronation instability in a person who is also tall and overweight and ambulates for short distances with a shuffling, nonjarring gait. In this case, a rigid orthotic that controls shear forces and has a protective metatarsal pad may be the best orthotic solution.

If excessive shear stress persists or the orthotic is uncomfortable due to the resistance required to control excessive pronation, then the patient may require the use of a plastic AFO (Fig 17–4). Blocking pronation with a force system that uses extended lever arms can provide more control for these problems as well as more comfort. If swelling is a problem, then a double-upright metal AFO with an appropriate shoe insert would be a more appropriate choice since plastic does not accommodate for changes in limb segment volume.

As these scenarios indicate, primary problem areas may develop for a variety of reasons, depending on the characteristics of the body systems involved. Generalizing from these examples to all kinds of orthotic intervention, it is clear that the evaluation of the primary problem areas must take into consideration all the factors contributing to the problem as well as how the specific function is being performed in order to fully determine how an orthotic can effectively meet the patient's needs.

EVALUATION AND TREATMENT

All the information presented here can be easily synthesized in an evaluation format that uses the SOAP (S = subjective data; O = objective data; A = assessment; P = plan) note as a foundation to organize and interpret functional problems in light of the relationship between energy expenditure and gait. Information on how to use this information in a SOAP format is presented below.

The S of SOAP

Biomechanically, pain can be a subjective response to excessive structural stress during functional activities. Mus-

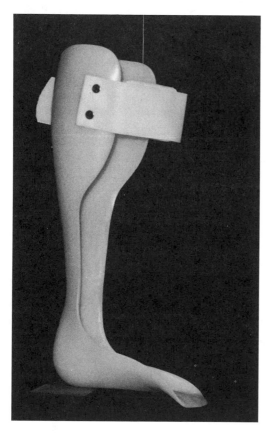

FIG 17–4.
A plastic AFO employs extended lever arms that can be used to prevent pronation as well as assist dorsiflexion. Note the height of the wall along the medial arch, which resists the forces pushing the forefoot into pronation.

cle contracture, muscle weakness, or bony deformities may all lead to dysfunctional movements such as asymmetric step lengths, steppage gaits, or excessively rotated limb positions and thereby also increase stress on anatomic structures. Individuals do vary in their abilities to deal with structural stress. A person with mild pronation, for example, may experience plantar fascia discomfort, whereas a person with moderate to severe pronation may not experience any discomfort at all. Abnormal function does not necessarily cause symptoms, although biomechanically induced symptoms are often a result of abnormal structure-function relationships.

It is also important to recognize that symptoms may be far removed from the primary structural problem area. Since limitations in one part of the kinetic chain can induce compensations in other parts of the chain in order to accomplish the activity, a painful symptom may be the end result of several compensatory movements.

Owing to the progressive nature of compensations, symptoms should be listed in their order of occurrence starting with the present time. This allows the therapist to relate current symptoms to previous ones and to track the

history of present alterations in structure-function relationships. It is the patient's *present* symptoms, however, that must be considered for appropriate development of specific treatment plans and goals.

The O of SOAP

A therapist must first learn to recognize deviations and compensatory movements as they occur during standing and walking. To begin, a static evaluation of posture and body part positions should be performed. It is often helpful for the therapist to split the body visually into right and left halves and then evaluate for any abnormalities or asymmetries when viewing the patient from anterior, posterior, and lateral standing positions. One can work from the ground up and include any asymmetric toe positions or problems; foot problems such as excessive pronation and valgus heel positions; leg problems such as rotational deviations; valgus or varus knee positions; hip positions and height; trunk, arm, and shoulder positions; and head and neck positions. Any abnormal or asymmetric observed positions are listed.

An observational analysis of movement can then be performed once the static evaluation has been completed. Again, the therapist, using the same format as above, simply lists what is observed to be abnormal or asymmetric as the patient ambulates. These observations include step lengths; walking-base widths; asymmetric stance times; excessive toe movements; any abnormal or asymmetric heel rise, whips, or positions; excessive hip and trunk rotations; asymmetric arm swinging; and any head and neck abnormalities. In performing the evaluation, it is important for the therapist to note if any assistance is required or any assistive device is being used for ambulation.

The problem list of gait deviations is a summary statement of the positions and movements required by the patient to stand and ambulate while overcoming structural problems. It is also important that the therapist does not make any hasty judgments or assumptions regarding what has been observed. Coming to a presumptuous conclusion may alter observations or result in an early conclusion of the assessment while the true primary problem waits to be discovered.

The kinematic problem list directs the therapist to where the non–weight-bearing part of the evaluation should begin. The non–weight-bearing part of the assessment includes ROM, muscle strength, tone, bony abnormalities, leg length, and callous patterns and locations. As the therapist gathers data, each finding is considered with respect to its possible contribution to the observed gait deviations. For example, if the therapist observed excessive right hip and knee flexion, shortened right stance phase, prolonged right swing phase, and a plantarflexed right foot in swing—for example, a typical steppage gait—the

ROM and strength of the right lower leg, especially at the foot and ankle, are evaluated to ascertain the presence of impairments that might cause the patient to walk in this way.

The non-weight–bearing portion of the objective section should also include subtalar neutral (STN) findings. The STN position is found just before heel-off in normal gait. Although a complete discussion of the concept of STN is beyond the scope of this chapter, its importance cannot be overstressed. Briefly, the therapist evaluates the foot and ankle in a non–weight-bearing position while the heel essentially looks to be in a "vertical" position. By relating hindfoot to forefoot positions in reference to the "vertical" heel, judgments can be made regarding foot and ankle function during weight bearing. Explanations for abnormal toe positions, callous formations, and knee and leg discomforts due to excessive or restricted rotational forces can often be derived from a thorough understanding of the biomechanics of the STN position.

The A of SOAP

The assessment section of a SOAP format is created by interpreting the structural limitations of the non–weight-bearing objective section and relating this information to the functional problems observed in standing and walking. By linking these observations together, the therapist is able to create a hierarchy of problem areas and from this suggest that the overall movement pattern is the result of specific impairments. This is the goal of the assessment section. The revelation of the specific impairments creating the overall pattern of abnormal movements establishes the primary problem area. The sequence of orthotic and therapeutic intervention begins here. This approach allows the therapist to categorize the fixed or changeable nature of the problem area. This approach also promotes more efficient treatment programs. Starting treatment at primary problem areas will often cause many of the other observed compensations and symptoms to simply disappear or resolve. Thus, the management of other compensations may be greatly eased.

In assessing compensations in the kinetic chain, it is important to remember that compensatory movements can create secondary problems. Biomechanical structural problems create stresses during function, which, in turn, have the potential to create additional structural problems. A patient with an asymmetric flat foot is a case in point. This asymmetry can create a functional leg length discrepancy that would tend to alter pelvic symmetry. This can lead to an asymmetric low back strain, which in turn alters posture and leads to even other problems. An excessive flat foot can also contribute to excessive plantar soft tissue strain, which can result in inflammation and pain that result in an antalgic gait or can create excessive stress to

posterior leg extrinsic foot musculature. These conditions can result in reduction of ankle ROM, which could affect function at the hip and knee. What this example illustrates is the importance of finding the primary problem that exists at the beginning of the kinetic chain of compensations. Characterizing the sequence of kinetic events to identify the source of the dysfunctional gait pattern is the essence of the therapist's assessment.

The P of SOAP

Therapeutically, decisions must be made on the rehabilitation potential of the primary problem areas. Orthotically, decisions must be made on how to support, accommodate, assist, or protect these problem areas. The overall plan should promote comfortable, energy-efficient, and symptom-free functional ambulation without dysfunctional compensatory motions. The closer the plan allows the primary problem area to approximate its normal structure-function relationship, the more successful the therapist will be in promoting more kinematically normal ambulation.

ORTHOTICS FOR THE GERIATRIC PATIENT

Is there an answer to the questions: What are the most appropriate orthotic devices or components available for use with the geriatric patient? Is plastic better than metal? Should an AFO or a KAFO be used? An energy study by Corcoran and associates concluded that plastic or metal AFOs has no significant effect on energy consumption or speed of gait. Another study by Lehneis, et al. found that orthotic designs that more closely complied with normal locomotor patterns, and that were also of lighter weight, did show a significant improvement in performance and also demonstrated lowered energy costs during ambulation.[3] These seemingly contradictory findings underscore a very important point: primary focus on the device can be misleading from the point of view of energy expenditure. It is more important to assess how the orthotic contributes to symmetric gait. Excessive structural instability resulting in abnormal pronation, for example, can be unaddressed with the use of a metal AFO attached to a shoe that does not have a supportive foot orthotic or supportive ankle valgus control strap, or a firm enough sole to help control this excessive motion, just as poorly as through the use of a plastic AFO in which the foot plate design does not reinforce and support the contours of a subtalar neutrally positioned foot. As the second study indicates and as this chapter strongly supports, orthotic designs that more closely comply with normal locomotor patterns produce the most energy-efficient ambulation. When this concept is used in evaluating a patient's structural primary problem areas, the most effective therapeutic and orthotic intervention will result in producing the most comfortable, energy-efficient gait possible for that patient. Using this information in assessing geriatric functional problems enhances the development of the most appropriate orthotic systems for the often complicated problems of the geriatric population. Some common orthotic scenarios that reinforce the need for thorough evaluation and treatment planning are presented below.

In dealing with foot, ankle, knee, hip, and low back problems related to excessive bilateral pronation, several concerns should be addressed. As previously mentioned, thermoforming or thermosetting plastics can be used to control instabilities resulting from excessive pronation. Choice of material is related to the degree of control needed, the patient's height and weight, and the functional level and activities performed. When imposing biomechanical control on unstable structures of the foot and ankle of the elderly, it is very important in the elderly to check true ankle ROM while maintaining an STN position, the position to be achieved by the foot orthotic. Recently, in our clinic, we evaluated a 68-year-old patient for excessive pronation and complaints of knee and low back pain. We recommended a polypropylene (University of California Berkeley Laboratory [UCBL]) shell (Fig 17–5), which is a thin, rigid plastic orthotic that cups the heel and extends raised borders along the medial and lateral sides of the foot, and heel lifts to accommodate for lost ankle ROM in standing. We also instituted an aggressive ROM program with the hopes of reducing and removing the entire heel lift supports as quickly as possible. Experimentally, we have found that using the UCBL without the accommodating heel lifts produced even more pronation than seen using no orthotic at all. The patient also experienced

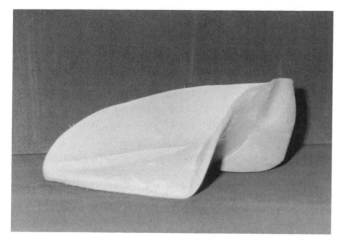

FIG 17–5.
A UCBL shell.

extreme discomfort along the longitudinal arch and lateral wall of the UCBL. We related this clinical finding to the structural problem of − 10 degrees of ankle dorsiflexion. As the patient stands and walks without his UCBLs, decreased ankle ROM is compensated by talonavicular collapse. Since this compensation is prevented by the UCBL, excessive pressure is generated when the patient walks and causes the patient's foot to ride up over the orthotic and eventually fall off its medial support. When this occurred, the patient exhibited a more uncontrolled and exaggerated degree of pronation in terminal stance. The appropriate heel accommodation resulted in a more normal comfortable ambulation and also relieved excess stress between therapeutic sessions. This allows a quicker return to neutral ankle dorsiflexion in standing since ROM gains are not lost through structural stresses created by remaining abnormal range in function.

In another case, unilateral heel pain was related to an asymmetric excessively pronating foot accompanied by a more mild pronating contralateral foot. The evaluation revealed a structural leg length increase of about 0.75 in. on the excessively pronating side. A unilateral increase in pronation can be attributed to structural-functional changes that occur to effectively modify the effects of a significant leg length discrepancy. The extra stress of pronation, however, can strain plantar soft tissue structures and result in heel pain. A common intervention seen for heel pain is to provide a soft pad for the heel. In this situation, a pad would result in further increasing the leg length discrepancy, exacerbating the cause of the excessive pronation on that side. Instead, we designed an orthotic system using bilateral subortholen foot orthotics combined with an appropriate heel and sole lift to the short side. In considering the use of accommodative lifts, if we chose to use an aggressive heel lift, rather than a heel and sole lift, the talus would plantarflex out of the stabilizing ankle mortise, resulting in increased pronation and instability. The resulting increase in pressure required to support this situation could make the orthotic uncomfortable and less effective as well. It is also important to note that heel lifts alone have a height limitation due to the sheer forces created in the sagittal plane. Clinically, we have found that the foot slides on the orthotic if we attempt to use heel lifts to accommodate angles greater than 15 degrees of plantarflexion.

Similar considerations must be made when designing AFO and KAFO systems as well. In practice, a metal AFO provides general leg and foot stability in the sagittal and coronal planes. If the therapist is also dealing with problems of excessive tone, a shoe insert that accommodates excessive midfoot pronation is equally important to minimize tone. If swelling is not an issue, a lightweight plastic system would be an alternative. Solid ankle designs prevent normal ankle motion. While eliminating stretching that elicits an increase in tone, these orthotics can also hinder normal function during the stance phase. Terminal rockers can be added to the shoes if needed, assuming that they will not contribute to any problem with instability in standing and walking.

In order to recommend a floor-reaction KAFO (Fig 17–2), the evaluation should reveal a grade 3 or better quadriceps strength and no ROM difficulties, since contracture can prevent the appropriate function of this force system. It is also important to consider if the patient functions with the affected extremity placed in excessive external rotation during ambulation. Even if the patient's strength and ROM are acceptable, a floor-reaction system will not be effective if the long toe plate lever arm is moved out of its normal position into external rotation. If the external rotation is not correctable, another KAFO system should be used.

Lightweight plastic KAFO systems have several advantages over metal systems. Plastic has the distinct advantage of conforming to body contours, which distributes pressure over larger areas than a metal system. Furthermore, it does not need to attach to the patient's shoe, which is more convenient for the patient. After a prolonged time of use, which is customarily the case among elders, the therapist should check the orthotic's mediolateral and circumferential fit for changes due to atrophy. Excessive movement within the orthosis can contribute to increasing levels of instability through the extended lever arms of the device.

CASE STUDIES

In the following case studies, treatment plans are based on the goal of obtaining a comfortable and symmetric gait pattern. In reviewing these cases, it is important to note that the objective list does not contain every position or kinematic compensation that a patient may have exhibited. It is essential only to obtain enough data that allow the therapist to identify the kinetic sequence of events and determine the primary problem area. Once the hierarchy of structural problems that alter function is created, the primary problem area, which resides at the base of the established pattern of movement, becomes the focus of attention for initiating orthotic and therapeutic intervention. Orthotically, consideration is given to the primary problem area's need for support, accommodation, assistance, or protection.

Case 1

Mrs. Q is a 91-year-old woman with a 35-year history of osteoarthritis whose radiographs indicate a bilateral col-

lapsed talonavicular area. She presently has a Baker's cyst behind the right knee.

S

Mrs. Q's pain started in the right knee, followed by right knee swelling. Pain and swelling developed next in the right foot and ankle. Pain developed in the extensor neck muscle groups after onset of right ankle and foot swelling.

O: Standing position

Mrs. Q's right lower extremity is always positioned ahead of the left lower extremity. Excessive knee, hip, and trunk flexion are noted. The cervical spine is held in extension. She exhibits severe pronation and valgus heels bilaterally. Her third, fourth, and fifth toes are clawed bilaterally.

She ambulates with a walker. She uses a step-to gait with the right lower extremity always positioned in front of the left. There is no heel strike on the right. The left lower extremity is held in an externally rotated position.

O: Non–weight-bearing

Her right knee lacks 15 degrees of extension. Her true ankle dorsiflexion is −10 degrees bilaterally.

A

The Baker's cyst prevents full knee extension and contributes to the step-to gait as well as to the need to position the right lower extremity ahead of the left. Bilateral pronation and valgus heel pose an instability problem that places excess stress on the posterior leg muscle groups. This contributes to a decrease in ankle dorsiflexion through excessive strain and tightness of the posterior muscles of the lower leg. This, in turn, requires more midfoot pronation and heel valgus to compensate for the lack of true ankle dorsiflexion ROM. Externally rotating the left lower extremity assists movement by compensating for the limited ankle ROM. Muscle shortening also explains the clawed toe positions in standing. Excess pronation and external rotation create a floor-reaction stress in terminal stance that promotes the development of the valgus positions of the great toes. The increase in knee flexion due to the development of the Baker's cyst forces the already compromised foot and ankle structure into more dorsiflexion. This excess strain may explain ankle swelling, which would be relieved by the forward positioning of the right lower extremity. In light of postural changes at the knee and hip, the patient must keep the neck in extension to see.

P

1. Refer patient for removal of the Baker's cyst.
2. Stretch or serial cast ankle to increase ankle ROM as much as possible.

3. Accommodate residual limitations in dorsiflexion with appropriate heel lifts.
4. Support the talonavicular joint in its established location relative to STN position with an accommodative soft orthotic.
5. Add a rocker to distal toe of shoes to promote rollover in terminal stance.

Case 2

Mr. F is a 60-year-old male.

S

Patient complains of 3 years of calf pain, experienced during running; he usually runs 10 to 15 miles per week. He does a soleus stretch, which helps relieve the discomfort. Pain is located in the lateral proximal calf at this time. He also states that it alternates between right and left calves. He also experiences Achilles discomfort.

O: Standing position

Clawing of the second, third, and fourth right and left toes is noted. The great toes are in valgus bilaterally. The great toes dorsiflex 45 degrees bilaterally without pain at the end of range. The fifth ray lateral border is prominent; rubbing is noted on the lateral sides of the fifth toes. A lateral view of standing posture shows an increase in thoracic kyphosis and lumbar lordosis. The right shoulder blade is prominent.

Increased valgus and pronation, left greater than the right, is noted during ambulation. Right arm swing is also reduced compared with the left.

O: Non–weight-bearing

Active dorsiflexion is approximately 5 to 10 degrees on the right and 5 degrees on the left. Right forefoot varus is seen in the STN position. The first ray of the right foot tends to move easily toward dorsiflexion. Left forefoot varus is noted in the STN position. The first ray on the left is plantarflexed.

Insole wear of the left insole shows that the area of the first metatarsal head and the distal tip of the first great toe have excessive wear. The right insole shows more wear at the distal tip of the great toe.

A

Mr. F's primary problem areas result in an increase in instability, demonstrated by an increased heel valgus and pronation seen on the left side more than the right during ambulation. This is most likely due to the right and left forefoot varus seen in a non–weight-bearing STN position. During weight bearing, the patient demonstrates a compensation of pronation and heel valgus as the forefoot

spins around to approach the ground during ambulation. The excessive strain of pronation also produces toe clawing as extra strains are placed on all muscle groups that cross under the arch. As the midfoot moves medially, an increase in the laterally directed shear forces of the forefoot is anticipated. This expectation is confirmed by the rubbing of the lateral fifth toe as it moves against the inside of the shoe.

The floor-reaction force tends to push both great toes into the valgus position as a response to the pronated position of the foot, especially during terminal stance. The position of the first ray of the right foot shows a tendency to move toward dorsiflexion, whereas the left first ray shows a plantarflexed position. This suggests a difference in function for right and left lower extremities. The left shows more instability, in terms of heel valgus and pronation. As a result, muscle groups on the left try to control this instability. The right side, however, appears to compensate by altering posture and movement patterns, as seen by a reduction of the right arm swing and a retraction of the right shoulder. Finally, we would expect the left insole wear to be more prominent on the left side, owing to increased tightness and plantar flexed first ray. On the right, we see more wear of the distal tip, since the first ray tends to be hypermobile into dorsiflexion and moves out of the way until the last phase of terminal stance.

Due to the excessive strain of all the leg posterior muscle groups, Mr. F has a tendency to shift his center of gravity posteriorly. When this occurs, a compensatory postural response could be expected, as seen in this patient's increase in lordosis and kyphosis. The primary problem areas indicate mostly a lack of stability and need support. Areas of tightness need to be addressed through an active stretching program.

P

1. Construct bilateral subortholen foot orthotics to modify pronation and heel valgus, allowing a break-in period of 2 to 3 weeks.
2. Stretch tight muscles in the leg and in the foot.
3. Mobilize the forefoot into a neutral position.

Case 3

Ms. W is a 72-year-old woman with a diagnosis of right spastic equinovarus.

S

Ms. W currently complains of pain in the right hip and leg and that she cannot walk "right" even with use of her present AFO.

O: Standing position

Her right foot demonstrates a varus heel when bearing weight on the lateral border of the foot. When the foot is manually placed into a foot-flat position by the therapist, the right hip and knee are forced into an internally rotated position. Her right knee is held in 15 degrees of flexion. When actively straightened, she notes a "pulling" on the lateral aspect of the right hip. In general, her weight is shifted onto the left lower extremity. The right shoulder is retracted.

Ms. W ambulates using crutches. A strong varus position of the foot at heel strike and midstance is demonstrated on the right. She also exhibits rollover in terminal stance with medial heel whip. Time in single-limb support on the left is longer than on the right lower extremity.

O: Non–weight-bearing

The right ankle lacks dorsiflexion (–10 degrees in plantarflexion).

A

The primary problem area is the maintained position of plantarflexion caused by spasticity. Spasticity in the posterior leg muscles, especially the gastrocnemius, contributes to the flexed position of the knee as well. A shortened gastrocnemius is further demonstrated in the medial heel whip at terminal stance. Efforts to stabilize the flexed knee and bring the equinovarus foot into contact with the floor result in internal rotation of the lower extremity. Weight shift onto the left lower extremity and the longer stance phase on the left are compensations for the impaired right extremity. Right shoulder retraction may be an attempt to relieve strain to the right lower extremity by shifting weight away from this area.

P

1. Serial casting or manual stretching to the right lower extremity.
2. Soft tissue mobilization and adjunctive modalities to increase ROM and decrease pain.
3. Cast for a plastic AFO in a position that accommodates ankle and knee positions that do not attain normal range after therapeutic intervention.
4. Balance with appropriate accommodative heel lifts on both lower extremities.

SUMMARY

The most appropriate geriatric orthotic intervention can be achieved by assessing primary problem areas in relationship to the physical impairments that contribute to them. This chapter emphasizes that a focused team approach will be a more successful approach rather than merely designing a "thing" that is poorly integrated into the overall treatment plan. This will result in a more appropriate orthotic and therapeutic intervention—one that meets the various needs of any patient population and one that is particularly pertinent to the variety of challenges presented by the geriatric population.

REFERENCES

1. Corcoran PJ, et al: Effects of plastic and metal leg braces on speed and energy cost of hemiparetic ambulation. *Arch Phys Med Rehabil* 1970; 51:69–77.
2. Fisher SF, Gullickson G: Energy cost of ambulation in health and disability: A literature review. *Arch Phys Med Rehabil* 1978; 59:124–133.
3. Lehneis HR, Bergofsky MD, Frisina W: Energy expenditure with advanced lower limb orthoses and with conventional braces. *Arch Phys Med Rehabil* 1976; 57:20–24.

ADDITIONAL READINGS

1. Corcoran PJ: Energy expenditure during ambulation, in Downey JA, Darling RD (eds): *Physiological Basis of Rehabilitation Medicine*. Philadelphia, WB Saunders, 1971.
2. Donatelli R: *The Biomechanics of the Foot and Ankle*. Philadelphia, FA Davis, 1990.
3. Gould JA (ed): *Orthopaedic and Sports Physical Therapy,* ed 2. St Louis, CV Mosby, 1990.
4. Hunt GC (ed): *Physical Therapy of the Foot and Ankle*. New York, Churchill Livingstone, 1988.

Conservative Pain Management of the Older Patient

John O. Barr, Ph.D., P.T.

INTRODUCTION

Interest in the management of pain experienced by elderly individuals has grown dramatically in recent years.* Although pain has been recognized to be the most common symptom for which health care is sought by the general population in the United States,[17] this observation may be even more applicable to the elderly. The validity of this premise, however, is based on a number of factors including predisposing physical and mental conditions, and on the elderly individual's willingness to report pain and to seek health care. This chapter focuses on conservative management of the older patient with pain. Noninvasive, nonsurgical, and nonpharmacologic approaches to patient care will be emphasized.

INCIDENCE OF PAIN

It has been estimated that over 85% of older adults have at least one chronic disease that may result in a range of discomforts, including pain.[23] Arthritis, which has a high rate of occurrence across older age-groups, is likely the most common cause of pain.[109] Other physical conditions that commonly result in chronic pain for the elderly include cancer, osteoporosis with compression fracture, degenerative disk disease, diabetic neuropathy, postherpetic and trigeminal neuralgias, and residual neurologic deficits.[68, 130] Acute postoperative pain is becoming a major concern as an increasing number of elderly individuals are undergoing surgery.[130] Pain associated with athletic injuries will become more common as a growing number of older persons pursue active recreational interests.[14]

Instances of atypical presentation of clinical pain have contributed to the controversy about the general occurrence of pain in the elderly. Acute myocardial infarction often occurs without significant pain in elderly persons. Appendicitis, gangrene of the bowel, peptic ulcer disease, and pneumonia may produce only mild discomfort. However, these conditions can contribute to behavioral changes (e.g., confusion) and nonspecific symptoms (e.g., fatigue). Although headaches are less common in the elderly, their presence may be associated with serious medical problems such as temporal arteritis or stroke.[23] Signs of inflammation, including redness, pain, elevated temperature, and swelling, may be much less marked in older individuals.[37] Information from major medical centers suggests that only 7% to 10% of pain clinic patients are over age 65.[51] It is important to recognize that data obtained through pain clinics may be skewed by large numbers of

*References 21, 39, 53, 54, 68, 98, 134, 138.

younger patients or by individuals with complex social and psychologic problems.[134]

The actual occurrence of pain in the elderly has been demonstrated using a number of approaches. Perhaps most relevant are surveys and interviews of elderly persons at different levels of functional independence. Nearly 70% of the 205 healthy elderly surveyed by Roy and Thomas reported some type of pain problem.[109] However, no significant differences were seen in social and physical/recreational activities when compared to respondents without pain. Lavsky-Shulan and associates interviewed 3,097 elderly living in rural settings and found 22% to have had low back pain in the prior year, with 15% to 42% experiencing some type of functional limitation.[71] In contrast, a survey of 132 elderly nursing home residents and day program participants by Roy and Thomas revealed 83% to have pain-related problems and 74% to claim that pain interfered with daily activities.[108] Although 50% of these individuals noted moderate to high levels of pain, analgesics were the only type of treatment reported. Surprisingly, 16% of respondents were not treated for their pain. Weekly interviews were employed by Brody and Kleban to document physical and mental health symptoms for 120 elderly people having at least one chronic condition and a range of cognitive capabilities (i.e., normal mental function, functional mental disturbance, and senile dementia).[19] Pain was reported at least once by 73% of all participants, although it was noted by significantly more subjects diagnosed with functional mental disturbance than by those with normal mental function (83% vs. 63%). Most frequently reported, pain accounted for 38% of symptoms overall, and it was the greatest cause of activity disturbances. From these few studies, it can be appreciated that pain is experienced with significant frequency by elderly persons. A trend also begins to emerge which implies that those older individuals who have less functional independence are more incapacitated by pain-related problems. Such a relationship requires further clarification through epidemiologic research.

ASSESSMENT OF CLINICAL PAIN

Concern for comprehensive assessment of pain experienced by the older patient is becoming more apparent.[51, 53, 54] It is critical that an accurate assessment be made of clinical pain. The assessment represents a synthesis of information derived from the patient's history, subjective interview, objective physical examination, and special tests (e.g., blood chemistry, roentgenograms, computerized tomographs, electrodiagnostic studies, etc.). Other references should be consulted for information concerning comprehensive patient evaluation, including physical, psychologic/psychiatric, and special testing procedures related to pain.[31, 41, 83, 119] The assessment should clarify the underlying basis for the pain, guide appropriate therapeutic interventions, and provide baseline information needed to determine the effectiveness of treatment. Ongoing re-evaluation of pain is necessary to disclose a change in the patient's physical status and to document response to treatment.

Pain has been defined as an unpleasant sensory and emotional experience associated with actual or potential tissue damage, or described in terms of such damage.[88] More simply, pain has been defined as a hurt that we feel.[117] Unfortunately, the assessment of pain is confounded by its private and subjective character.[26] The way in which an individual reports pain is related to a number of factors including age, gender, personality, ethnic/cultural heritage, behavioral needs, and past pain experiences.[84, 117] Elderly persons often believe that pain is an inevitable consequence of aging that must be endured without complaint. The presence of pain may be denied out of fear of medical procedures and expenses, loss of autonomy, and possible institutionalization. Conversely, pain complaints may be used to conceal or rationalize other functional impairments. Boredom and loneliness may contribute to increased perception and complaints of pain.[54]

The patient's history should include information about concurrent medical problems and present medications. Elderly persons consume nearly 25% of all prescription medications used in the United States.[67] One study found that analgesics were the third most frequent prescription drug and the most frequent nonprescription drug used by a community sample of nearly 3,500 persons 65 years of age and older.[52] Interestingly, another study demonstrated that older postsurgical patients had less analgesic medication both prescribed and administered.[36] Although these latter findings may have been related to concern by physicians and nurses for the physical status of older surgery patients with more concurrent illnesses, adequacy of pain management must be questioned. Dramatic pain relief may be attained by pharmacologic means in the elderly, as with the treatment of temporal arteritis using high doses of steroids. However, the hazards of medication use by the elderly are well known. These include multiple drug use, drug interactions, adverse drug reactions, medication errors, and the narrowing of the margin of safety between therapeutic and toxic doses.[67, 68, 93, 129] Thus, one goal of conservative treatment for the elderly is the appropriate reduction of medication usage.

Information concerning past remedies or treatments that have been both successful and unsuccessful in managing pain should also be included in the history. Through such inquiry, it may be possible to learn about patient biases for or against certain interventions, and also to gain further insight as to why a prior treatment was a success or a failure. Previous inadequate patient education may have contributed to a lack of enthusiasm for, and compliance with, a prior pain management program.

During the subjective interview, the patient should be given the opportunity to voluntarily verbalize complaints of pain and related symptoms (e.g., paresthesia, stiffness, joint warmth, etc.). The examiner should follow up with specific questions concerning the onset, occurrence, intensity (current vs. greatest vs. least), quality, distribution, and duration of pain. Pain at multiple sites, such as arthritic joints, may require that specific assessment tools be referenced to the worst or to multiple joints. Pain at rest should be distinguished from pain with movement.[15] A body diagram may be coded by the patient to document the quality and distribution of pain.[84] Factors that the patient believes to aggravate and relieve the pain should be identified (e.g., movements, postures, rest). Other indicators of pain such as facial expression, crying, and mood changes may be especially useful for documenting pain in patients with severely limited verbal abilities.

The objective examination typically focuses on physical signs or characteristics thought to be associated with a given pain problem. Sternbach has observed that patients with acute pain often present with increases in pulse rate, systolic blood pressure, and respiratory rate. Dilation of the pupils, perspiration, nausea and pallor of the skin may also be present.[117] Numerous physical criteria have been evaluated in relation to clinical pain problems, including duration of joint-loading time,[82] edema,[102] gait,[35] grip strength,[96] joint range of motion,[102] joint tenderness,[15] muscle strength and endurance,[113] posture,[139] pressure threshold and tolerance,[44] pulmonary functions,[107] skin temperature,[103] tissue compliance,[44] and tissue healing.[43] Portable automated timer systems have been used to measure functional aspects of patient movement such as "uptime"[110] and activity patterns.[46] It is important to note that lack of sensitivity to, or limited correlation with, pain has been noted for some of these criteria,[15] including some criteria that are more functional in character.[22, 59] Utilization of pain medications may be evaluated, with the type, amount, route, and frequency being documented. A standard "morphine equivalent" dose can be calculated, thus providing a basis for comparison among a range of pain medications.[101]

In the attempt to more objectively document patients' subjective pain experiences, a number of pain measurement tools have been developed.[86] A select sample of these tools that have particular relevance to the elderly will now be discussed.

Perhaps the simplest and most widely used evaluation

tool is the Verbal Rating Scale.[100] With this approach, patients are required to label their pain with a single word descriptor (e.g., no, mild, moderate, severe, or unbearable pain). Such adjectival scales may be preferred by patients who find them easy to understand, which may be associated with low scoring failure rates.[66] The major limitation of this approach is its lack of sensitivity in detecting changes based on a limited number of word categories.[59]

Using the Pain Estimate (also called the Numeric Rating Scale), patients rate the severity of their pain on a scale of 0 to 10, or 0 to 100. On this scale, 0 indicates no pain, and end points of 10 or 100 represent the worst possible pain that the patient could ever imagine.[120] It is critically important that the patient understand the definitions related to these end points. If, for example, the patient thought that a rating of 100 corresponded to "the worst pain I've ever had," pain that was even more severe the next day could not be properly rated. Primary advantages of this approach are that it is easy to understand and that patient ratings can be done verbally. The 0 to 10 format has less sensitivity than its 0 to 100 counterpart.

The Visual Analogue Pain Rating Scale consists of a 10-cm line with typical verbal anchors of "no pain" at the left and "pain as bad as it could be" at the right, when the scale is oriented horizontally (Fig 18–1, A).[111] Patients place a mark at one location on the line corresponding to the severity of their pain. This scale may also be used in a vertical orientation (Fig 18–1, B). A new unmarked scale is presented to the patient each time pain is to be rated, although there is controversy about showing the patient prior ratings.[15] It has been suggested that the scale should more appropriately be constructed to rate pain relief by employing anchors of "complete pain relief" and "no pain relief" (Fig 18–1, C).[57, 58] Such an approach, however, does not allow the documentation of worsened pain. Visual analogue scales have also been constructed to evaluate limitations in physical function that may be related to pain.[59] Unfortunately, visual analogue scales rely on vision and motor control, which may be compromised in the elderly patient. Although some studies have suggested that elderly individuals may have difficulty with abstract thought processes needed to understand and utilize visual analogue scales,[24, 60, 66] other studies with elderly patients have found these scales to be useful and reliable.[16] Vertical presentation of the scale in the format of a "pain thermometer" may be more effective with some elderly patients.[54]

The Graphic Rating Scale (Fig 18–1, D) consists of a visual analogue pain rating scale with additional word descriptors (e.g., mild, moderate, severe). Placement of these words without spacing along the line between anchors helps to improve the distribution of patient responses when using this type of scale.[111]

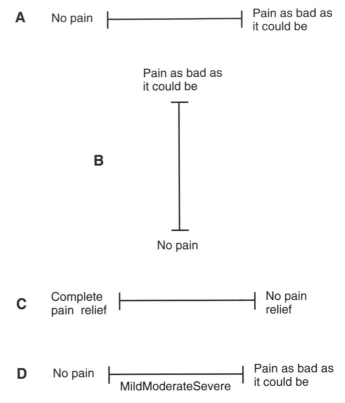

FIG 18–1.
Simple pain rating scales. **A,** Visual Analogue Pain Rating Scale (horizontal). **B,** Visual Analogue Pain Rating Scale (vertical). **C,** Visual Analogue Pain Relief Rating Scale. **D,** Graphic Rating Scale.

The McGill Pain Questionnaire is probably the best known of the comprehensive approaches to measurement of clinical pain.[85] The questionnaire includes a body diagram for information concerning the location of pain. Sensory, affective, and evaluative qualities of the pain experience are assessed via a pain rating index based on word descriptors. Pain intensity is measured with a five-category present pain intensity scale. A short-form version of the questionnaire has been developed in the attempt to reduce the amount of time needed to administer this tool to 2 to 5 minutes.[87] Although the short form may be less fatiguing for elderly patients who have problems with maintaining concentration, difficulty may still be encountered with complex word descriptors.[54]

A number of studies have compared these methods of rating pain,[34, 60, 100, 130] including some that have specifically examined elderly individuals with pain.[16, 53, 66] Helme and colleagues have recently suggested that appropriately screened patients over 70 years of age may actually be more reliable than younger individuals in reporting pain, mood, and activity using psychometric tools.[53] With the exception of the McGill Pain Questionnaire, the pain rating scales described above have been criticized for focusing primarily on the intensity of pain while excluding other qualitative characteristics. Controversy continues concerning appropriate mathematical and statistical analyses to be used with these scales.[26, 130, 131]

Recently, Herr and Mobily reviewed the complexities of clinical pain assessment with elderly persons and offered numerous practical suggestions.[54] A person's health status, severity of pain, and ability to cooperate will dictate the number and detail of evaluation sessions needed to adequately assess pain. It is critically important to establish good rapport and to avoid being rushed during evaluation sessions. Suspected impairments in vision, hearing, speech, and mental processes should be evaluated. Nursing home residents may have less formal education than elderly in the community. Pain measurement tools should be selected or modified to account for these factors that might limit the validity and reliability of testing procedures. The clinician should be assured that the patient understands and can successfully utilize a pain measurement tool, with supervision if necessary, if the tool is to be employed in the home setting.[15] Family members, friends, and other health care workers will provide useful information about changes in behavior or functioning.[54] Certain diagnoses associated with aging (e.g., Alzheimer's disease) may require the development, validation, and reliability testing of new measurement tools.

In rendering an assessment of clinical pain, the health care professional usually labels or further classifies pain experienced by the patient. Pain of less than 3 months' duration has been termed *acute,* whereas pain persisting for 3 or more months is referred to as *chronic.*[88] Acute pain occurs as a result of mechanical trauma, ischemia, or active inflammation. It is often associated with increased autonomic nervous system activity and anxiety. Chronic pain is not merely a time extension of acute pain. Indeed, chronic pain may lack a demonstrable physical basis. It is often associated with nonfunctional pain behaviors (i.e., attention-getting pain displays such as grimaces, guarded motion, or knee buckling) and depression in the general population.[117, 119, 129] The interdependence of chronic pain and depression has been noted to be even greater in the elderly.[129] Because of the higher occurrence of pain, chronic stress and depression are more likely in the elderly.[51] However, Middaugh and associates did not find depression to be more prevalent in older as compared with younger patients with chronic pain.[90]

Additional varieties of pain differ based on a number of characteristics including time frame, severity, quality, distribution, and likely basis. Acute recurrent pain is experienced when there is recurrent nociceptive stimulation associated with chronic pathology, as in rheumatoid and osteoarthritis. Acute ongoing pain occurs with continued nociceptive stimulation from uncontrolled malignancy.[129]

Subacute pain is often noted at 72 or more hours after trauma or inflammation. It may persist for 2 to 3 weeks.[77] It has been suggested that elderly patients have the tendency for pain to be referred from a site of origin to other regions of the body.[23] As discussion of other types of pain (e.g., radiating, myofascial, thalamic, phantom, etc.) is beyond the scope of this chapter, the reader should consult other sources.[83, 84, 88, 125]

THEORETICAL BASIS FOR PAIN

It has been widely proposed that pain is not simply a direct consequence of the normal aging process.[51, 69, 133] This position appears to be supported because of ambiguous results from psychophysical studies. These studies have induced pain by various means (e.g., heat, electrical shocks, mechanical pressure) while assessing behavioral responses (e.g., pain threshold, reaction, or tolerance) in human volunteers of different ages. On the balance, such studies of pain do not indicate age-specific changes in pain sensation.[51]

Mechanisms for modulating pain portrayed in Figure 18–2 are thought to be operational within the dorsal horn of the spinal cord.[47, 70, 128, 129, 140] Nociceptors attached to small-diameter afferents are activated by intense mechanical or thermal stimuli and by various chemical sensitizing or depolarizing agents liberated with trauma or inflammation (e.g., bradykinin, prostaglandin, histamine, substance P, lactic acid, potassium ions, etc.). Some of these agents may become concentrated in the vicinity of nociceptors due to circulatory impairment or to muscle spasm. Nociceptive excitation of small-diameter afferents (A delta and C fibers) results in the release of neurotransmitters that stimulate second-order neurons, ultimately resulting in the perception of pain at higher brain centers. Sensory input from large-diameter afferents associated with mechanoreceptors has an inhibitory effect on input from the smaller afferents conveying nociceptive input. Inhibitory descending control from the brain stem also can act to minimize the effect of nociceptive input. This descending inhibition is mediated by neurotransmitters such as norepinephrine (noradrenalin) and serotonin. Anatomic studies have demonstrated that nociceptors (i.e., free nerve endings) in the skin undergo little change with age.[25] Additional research is needed concerning possible changes in the small-diameter A delta and C afferent fibers associated with these nociceptors. Studies have shown age-related decreases in sensation of touch and vibration.[127] Age-associated decreases in the number of mechanoreceptors such as Merkel's, Meissner's, and pacinian corpuscles have been demonstrated. Structural changes have also been noted in these receptors and in their related large-diameter affer-

Dorsal Horn Chemistry

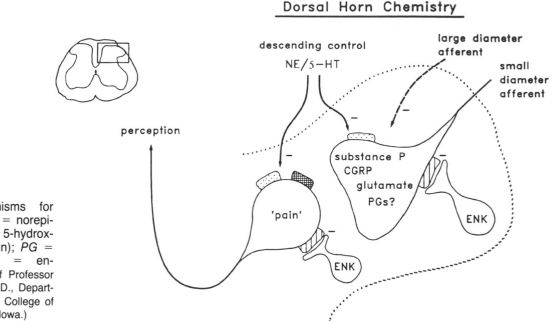

FIG 18–2.
Theoretical mechanisms for modulating pain. *NE* = norepinephrine; *5 HT* = 5-hydroxytryptamine (serotonin); *PG* = prostaglandin; *ENK* = enkephalin. (Courtesy of Professor Gerald F. Gebhart, Ph.D., Department of Pharmacology, College of Medicine, University of Iowa.)

ents.[25, 127] However, the confounding role of inactivity has not been ruled out as a basis for these changes.[25]

Oxidative deactivation of amines involved in descending inhibitory control is done by the enzyme monoamine oxidase (MAO). Interestingly, human hindbrain, plasma, and platelet MAO activity is increased after about 60 years of age.[106] The resultant age-related increase in the deactivation of key neurotransmitters might increase pain perception and affective disorders such as depression or mania.[51, 106] Endogenous opiate-like transmitters play a role in initiating one type of descending inhibition (via endorphins) and in local inhibition at the spinal cord level (via enkephalins). However, decreases in concentrations of endorphins and enkephalins, and a reduction of endogenous opiate receptors, have been noted in old age.[37, 129]

Thus, there are a number of anatomic and physiologic changes associated with aging that may actually predispose elderly individuals to both a greater incidence of clinical pain and to less effective pain relief with various conservative treatment interventions.

STRATEGIES FOR PAIN CONTROL

Pain management may be either the short- or long-term goal of a comprehensive treatment plan. Whenever possible, conditions underlying a clinical pain problem should be the focus of treatment. Those who care for elderly patients with pain have come to appreciate the importance of a comprehensive multidisciplinary approach to evaluation and treatment.[39, 56, 68, 90, 97, 104, 105] Such an approach may integrate the involvement of numerous health care professions including medicine, nursing, occupational therapy, orthotics and prosthetics, physical therapy, psychology, recreational therapy, social work, and so on. Middaugh and associates determined that patients 55 years of age and older benefited as much, if not more than, younger patients participating in a multidisciplinary chronic pain rehabilitation program.[90]

It has been noted that the selection of pain management strategies by health care professionals varies with the age of the patient.[21] Burke and Jerrett surveyed student nurses for their perceptions of the best interventions for acute pain.[21] Breathing and relaxation, imagery, and distraction techniques were selected less frequently for elderly persons as compared with younger adults. However, touch or massage, physical comfort approaches, verbal reassurance, and medication were more commonly selected for the elderly than for younger adults. Although these results were not analyzed statistically, different patterns of strategy selection were associated with patient age. Bartz Kvitek and colleagues determined that physical therapists given hypothetical patients were significantly less aggressive in goal setting for older patients.[12]

A wide array of conservative treatment approaches for pain control have been developed over the years. By way of an overview, Table 18–1 summarizes select conservative interventions used in pain management for the general population. Traditionally, these interventions have been used singly or in various combinations in the attempt to more completely treat factors underlying a clinical pain problem. Primary theoretical mechanisms of action are suggested relative to the mechanisms for modulating pain depicted in Figure 18–2. The reader is encouraged to con-

TABLE 18–1.

Primary Theoretical Mechanisms of Action for Conservative Treatment Interventions Used to Manage Pain.*

I. Decrease activity of nociceptors or their afferent nerve fibers.
  A. Limit mechanical stresses through:
    1. Prevention of acute edema formation with ice, compression, elevation, or electrical stimulation.
    2. Assistive gait device (e.g., cane, walker, and orthotics).
    3. Rest from stressful function.
    4. Limitation of the effects of gravity via hydrotherapy.
    5. Immobilization (e.g., orthotics, traction).
    6. Resorption of chronic edema via mild heat, massage, elevation and compression, or electrical stimulation.
    7. Elongation of restrictive connective tissue using vigorous heat (as with diathermy or ultrasound) and prolonged stretch.
    8. Restoration of normal joint arthrokinematics through joint mobilization, stretching or strengthening exercise, or biofeedback.
    9. Application of ergonomic principles.
  B. Limit effects of chemical depolarizing and sensitizing agents through:
    1. Enhanced local circulation produced with mild to moderate heat, massage, exercise, or electrical stimulation.
    2. Decreased local metabolic activity with cryotherapy (e.g., cold pack or ice massage).
    3. Decreased muscle spasm via select physical agents, massage, exercise, or biofeedback.
  C. Create local anesthetic or anti-inflammatory effects through:
    1. Iontophoresis (e.g., with Lidocaine or Dexamethasone).
    2. Phonophoresis (e.g., with hydrocortisone).
    3. Cryotherapy (e.g., cold pack or ice massage).
    4. TENS.
    5. Low-intensity laser.
II. Increase activity of mechanoreceptors or their afferent nerve fibers.
  A. Stimulate mechanoreceptors through:
    1. Passive and active joint range-of-motion exercise.
    2. Joint mobilization.
    3. Comfortable massage strokes (i.e., mild to moderate intensity).
    4. Voluntary (e.g., walking, swimming, bicycling) and electrically stimulated exercise.
  B. Directly stimulate large-diameter afferents from mechanoreceptors through:
    1. Comfortable low- to moderate-intensity TENS (e.g., "conventional," "pulse-burst," or "modulated" TENS modes).
    2. Comfortable submaximal intensity NMES.
III. Increase descending cortical or reticular formation inhibition.
  A. Reduce patient anxiety through:
    1. Progressive relaxation exercises.
    2. Inducing relaxation with biofeedback (e.g., EMG or thermal modes).
    3. Patient education concerning basis for pain and the plan for its successful treatment.
  B. Maximize a placebo effect.
  C. Increase physiologic and psychologic stress through use of uncomfortable "counterirritants" such as:
    1. Intense massage (e.g., strong friction, acupressure, connective tissue massage).
    2. Acupuncture or electroacupuncture.
    3. Uncomfortable but maximally tolerated NMES.
    4. Uncomfortable but maximally tolerated TENS (e.g., "strong low rate," "brief intense," "pulse-burst," or "hyperstimulation" modes).
    5. Uncomfortable brief ice massage.

*TENS = transcutaneous electrical nerve stimulation; NMES = neuromuscular electrical stimulation; EMG = electromyography.

sult other contemporary sources for detailed descriptions of specific treatment procedures.[3, 65, 83, 89, 98, 116, 123]

Recent review articles concerned with pain management for elderly individuals have most commonly recommended treatment strategies of assistive devices and orthotics, exercise, thermal agents (i.e., heat or cold), and transcutaneous electrical nerve stimulation (TENS).[39, 68, 95, 104, 105, 129, 137] These select conservative treatment approaches will be reviewed in relation to their application in pain control for the patient who is 55 years of age or older.

General Safety Precautions and Contraindications

Conservative treatment of elderly patients requires a number of general safety precautions. In general, the patient should have adequate sensation of temperature and pain in the area being treated in order to provide feedback to the clinician. A body region must also be sentient if peripheral sensory input is critical to a particular mechanism for pain relief. For example, sensation of light touch should be present where electrodes are applied for conventional low-intensity TENS. Potential for increased bleeding, hemorrhage, disruption of fragile tissues, fracture, spread of infection, cardiovascular or neurologic compromise, and enhanced growth or metastasis of cancer represent general contraindications for treatment. Special considerations are necessary in order to ensure safety of the elderly patient when using specific conservative treatment interventions.

Establishing Treatment Effectiveness

As discussed previously, age-associated changes may render the elderly person less responsive to treatment. It is important that clinicians and researchers appreciate that a patient's response to treatment will be based on a number of factors including the natural history of the underlying clinical problem, a placebo effect, and a specific treatment effect. Figure 18–3 illustrates these factors and emphasizes that in order for a treatment to be deemed "effective" its impact must be greater than that attributable to natural history and the placebo effect.[40] The periodic worsening and improvement of symptoms that reflect the natural history of some disease processes, such as rheumatoid arthritis, often present a confusing picture to the clinician attempting to assess the impact of a therapeutic intervention. Did the patient's status improve because of effective treatment or in spite of ineffective treatment?

It has been determined that approximately 30% to 70% of patients will obtain satisfactory pain relief from a placebo treatment.[13, 33, 40] Classically, placebo effects have been assessed in experimental research by randomly assigning patients to either active drug or sham drug (sugar

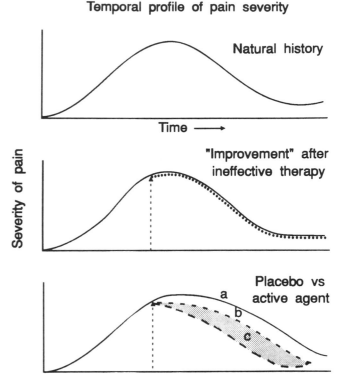

Temporal profile of pain severity

Severity of pain

Natural history

Time ⟶

"Improvement" after ineffective therapy

Placebo vs active agent

a

b

c

FIG 18–3.
Determination of treatment effectiveness. **A,** the natural history for the severity of pain associated with a clinical problem. **B,** "improvement" after an ineffective therapy is begun at the time indicated by the *arrow*. If it is not appreciated that a remission is expected to occur, the remission will be attributed to the therapy. **C,** the natural history of pain severity *(a)* is compared with results from placebo therapy *(b)* and somatically active therapy *(c)*. The analgesia attributable to active therapy (i.e., treatment effectiveness) is represented by the difference between *(b)* and *(c)*. The placebo component of the therapy is the difference between *(a)* and *(b)*. (Adapted from Fields HL, Levine JD: Placebo analgesia—a role for endorphins? in: *Trends in Neuroscience,* vol 7. Amsterdam, Elsevier Science Publishers, 1984, pp 371–273.)

pill placebo) groups under double-blind methodology. This methodology requires that neither the patient nor the clinician has knowledge of which treatment is being given. In some investigations it is impossible to disguise treatments so that the patient or researcher is unaware of which treatment is active or placebo. For this reason, noncrossover designs, where a subject receives only one experimental treatment intervention, have recently been favored.[70] Hamilton has suggested that under such conditions it may be most appropriate to ensure that the person doing patient assessments is not aware of the treatment given.[50] A placebo can be effective for anyone under the right conditions. It has been suggested, however, that older persons respond more frequently to placebos.[23] The placebo effect is not simply based on a reduction in a person's anxiety.

Larger placebo effects have been associated with patients having high anxiety, severe pain, or expectation of a good treatment outcome. The attitude of the health care worker, communicated by personal enthusiasm or skepticism about a treatment, can also influence the magnitude of a placebo response.[13, 40] In clinical practice the health care professional may choose to take advantage of the placebo effect as a means of maximizing pain relief. Controversy exists as to the effective duration of a given placebo effect.[33] Using a qualitative research paradigm for assessing clinical treatment effectiveness, Sternbach has implied that placebos do not work for longer than 1 to 2 weeks.[118] The physiologic basis for the placebo effect involves both endorphin and nonendorphin mechanisms.[69]

Unless involved in clinical research to establish the true effectiveness of a treatment intervention, practitioners will not consciously give sham treatments to their patients. Under clinical conditions, however, it is certainly desirable to establish the efficacy of a treatment in decreasing pain, improving limited function, and saving health care dollars. Valid and reliable testing procedures, including those discussed for the assessment of clinical pain, must be utilized at regular intervals during the course of patient treatment and follow-up examinations in order to establish the efficacy of an intervention.

Review of Select Treatment Strategies

In the following review of select treatment strategies for pain management, it will be valuable for the reader to consult Table 18–1 regarding theoretical mechanisms of action. Well-controlled studies done with individuals 55 years of age and older will be highlighted. It is important to recognize that investigators may inadvertently provide a suggestion of treatment effectiveness for a control or placebo treatment that is psychologically stronger than that given to an active treatment intervention. Such an influence might have occurred in the study by Deyo et al.[32] that reported TENS to be ineffective for chronic pain in the general population. The use of neutral or permissive instructions to all research subjects regardless of group assignment should help to minimize this problem.[6]

Assistive Devices and Orthotics

Ambulatory aids such as canes and walkers are probably the most common assistive devices used by the elderly with pain. Foot pain, knee pain, and leg pain were the most frequent complaints reported by 457 individuals over age 50 surveyed by Finsen.[42] A two-point cane gait (cane in hand opposite to involved hip) can reduce pain-inducing hip contact force by 36%.[18] Care must be taken, however, not to improperly overload the joints of the upper extrem-

ity when using these devices. Pressure on hip and knee joints during push-off may also be controlled through the use of raised seats on toilets and chairs. Appropriate shoe orthotics, including inserts and heel lifts, can be used to minimize foot, knee, and hip pain.[56, 80] Varying degrees of immobilization can be attained for neck and back pain with spinal orthoses. The limited temporary immobilization from a soft cervical collar may be appropriate for a patient with mild cervical spondylosis, whereas a patient with rheumatoid arthritis and atlantoaxial subluxation would benefit from a more rigid Philadelphia collar[95] or a sternal-occipitomandibular immobilizer (SOMI).[112] A thoracic lumbosacral orthosis (TLSO) may be used to manage compression fractures associated with spinal osteoporosis.[112] Finsen, however, has suggested that serious morbidity from back pain associated with osteoporotic fractures does not begin to occur until 80 years of age.[42]

Exercise

Exercise involves the performance of physical exertion for improvement of health. Various forms of exercise may be employed to modulate pain either directly or indirectly, as depicted in Table 18–1. A direct effect on pain may be achieved in some cases by increasing comfortable mechanoreceptor input to the central nervous system via active or passive exercise. Indirect effects of exercise on pain may be related to increased blood flow, which disperses chemical depolarizing/sensitizing agents; decreased edema; inhibition or fatigue of muscle spasm; enhanced range of motion, flexibility, strength, or endurance, which may improve biomechanical factors; and relaxation and reduction in anxiety. The importance of combining exercise with other therapeutic interventions (e.g., thermal agents) in order to attain significant clinical outcomes, including pain relief, is well recognized.[49, 65, 72]

Although it has been known for some time that elderly persons are capable of significant strength gains from voluntary resistive exercise,[94] published literature dealing with the effectiveness of exercise in controlling pain experienced by elderly persons is surprisingly sparse.

Minor and associates assessed the relative efficacy of three exercise protocols with patients having chronic rheumatoid arthritis or osteoarthritis.[92] The 120 subjects who entered the study had a mean age of 59 years. After baseline testing, subjects were stratified by diagnosis and randomly assigned to one of three groups: aerobic walking; aerobic aquatics; nonaerobic active range of motion (ROM) and relaxation exercise control. Subjects in all groups participated in exercises for flexibility and isometric strengthening. All exercise groups were supervised and met for 1 hour, three times per week, for 12 weeks. At the conclusion of this 12-week period, all subjects were consistently encouraged to continue exercise, including participation in community programs (aquatics, walking, and fitness). At the end of the 12-week period, the aerobics groups showed significant improvements over the nonaerobic group relative to aerobic capacity, 50-ft walking time, physical activity, anxiety, and depression. No significant between-group (aerobics vs. nonaerobic) difference was seen for pain. However, both the walking and nonaerobic groups demonstrated significant within-group improvements in pain. Three months later only aerobic capacity significantly differed between the groups. The nonaerobic group no longer had a significant improvement in pain. At the 9-month follow-up, no significant between-group differences were seen. Numerous significant within-group differences existed, including decreases in pain for the pool and nonaerobic groups. Significant changes in the intensity of medication regimens could not be disclosed at 12 weeks or 9 months. This study demonstrates that supervised exercise can successfully motivate elderly individuals to improve fitness and control pain without significantly exacerbating arthritic symptoms.

Most recently, Fisher and colleagues evaluated the effect of a muscle rehabilitation program on 15 men, mean age of 68 years, with knee osteoarthritis.[45] Testing was done initially, at 8 weeks (halfway through the rehabilitation program), at 16 weeks (at the end of the program), and at 4 and 8 months after the program. The 16-week supervised group rehabilitation program consisted of three 1-hour exercise sessions per week. The quadriceps muscles was exercised at combinations of three knee and four hip angles in a progressive program of active ROM, and isometric, isotonic, and endurance exercises. At the end of 16 weeks, significant increases averaging 25% were seen in knee extension strength, endurance, and speed. Walking time decreased 12%. Significant improvements in these parameters were sustained for up to 8 months later. As indicated by the Jette Functional Status Index, a significant decrease in pain was seen at 8 and 16 weeks of the program (averaging 10% and 28%, respectively), and this decrease was also seen at 4 and 8 months later (averaging 26% and 32%, respectively). Significant decreases in functional indices of dependence and difficulty were also seen at these time intervals.

Appropriate precautions should be followed when utilizing exercise with the elderly individual. Severe osteoporosis may even pose limitations for ROM exercises. Older hypertensive individuals who perform a Valsalva's maneuver during strenuous resistive exercise risk a dangerous elevation in blood pressure. Exercise-induced muscle damage and soreness occur especially after vigorous eccentric exercise in both young and old subjects. Although rates of tissue repair are similar for healthy active subjects, older subjects show significantly greater muscle shorten-

ing.[29] This may predispose the older individual to a greater short-term risk of further injury from exercise.

Therapeutic Thermal Agents

Traditionally, a wide range of thermal agents have been employed to treat painful conditions affecting the elderly. Thermal effects leading to the modulation of pain may be directly and/or reflexly mediated. It would thus seem important to know the effective depth of penetration into the body of the common thermal agents. Table 18–2 summarizes this information, as has been described by others.[48, 64, 65, 72, 77, 89, 135] A number of sources can be consulted for specific descriptions of thermal agent treatment procedures.[48, 64, 65, 72, 89]

Over the past 40 years a large number of studies have been concerned with establishing the efficacy and effectiveness of thermal agents in controlling pain and related clinical problems. Unfortunately, only a small number of published reports have specifically included elderly individuals as subjects. Representative studies that have included individuals 55 years of age or older are summarized in Table 18–3. Overall, treatment efficacy was demonstrated for the thermal agents utilized. However, significant treatment effectiveness—and that short term—was only shown in the studies by Wright[138] and Clarke.[28] As can be seen from Table 18–3, contrasting thermal agents (i.e., cold vs. heat) have been shown to have equivalent efficacy with some clinical pain problems.[49, 132] This may be related to separate but equally potent mechanisms of pain relief, which when combined with exercise act to further control pain and enhance function. It is important to recognize, however, that most studies have used small ex-

TABLE 18–2.

Depth of Effective Penetration Into the Body by Common Therapeutic Thermal Agents

Thermal Agent	Depth Into Soft Tissues
Cold pack	2 mm to 4 cm
Hot pack	2–5 mm
Hydrotherapy (warm)	2–5 mm
Paraffin	2–5 mm
Fluidotherapy	2–5 mm
Infrared	
Nonluminous	2–5 mm
Luminous	5 mm to 1 cm
Shortwave diathermy (27.12 MHz; subcutaneous fat < 2 cm thick)	1–3 cm
Microwave diathermy (2,450 MHz; nondirect contact applicator; subcutaneous fat < 0.5 cm thick)	1–5 cm
Ultrasound	
3 MHz	1–2 cm
1 MHz	1–5 cm

TABLE 18–3.

Published Studies Assessing Thermal Agents for the Elderly With Pain

Investigators	Subjects	Design	Treatment Protocol Details	Treatment Outcome

Aldes & Jadeson[2]	N = 233
	x̄ age = 62 yr
	Hypertrophic arthritis with chronic cervical or lumbosacral pain
		• Not blinded, sequential clinical trials of US
		• Not blinded, separate group same-age patients (N = 25) received sham US (unit off) in 1st treatment series
			• All patients had poor response to prior medical and PT treatments
			• 3 series of 8–12 treatments, 3–10 min duration, q 48 hr, at 10-day intervals
			• US: 0.8 + 1 MHz, at 1.3–11.9 W, direct coupling with oil or indirect with water, moving technique; US intensity and duration increased each series
			• 3rd series included infrared, hot pack, and hydrotherapy
			• Evaluated pre and 14-day post final series, q ≤ 3.5 mo to 1 yr post ("improvement" based on unspecified pain and ROM assessments)
				Descriptive results only:
				1. Sham-treated patients reported to show no improvement in 1st series; good response to active US in subsequent series
				2. At 12 mo post, 233 active US-treated patients:
				    44% = "apparently permanent improvement"
				    27% = "partial improvement"
				    29% = "questionable or no improvement"

Wright[138]	N = 38
	x̄ age = 62 yr
	Osteoarthritic knee
		• Not blinded, noncrossover
		• Randomized assignment to 1 of 3 treatments:
		  1. Placebo tablets
		  2. Placebo intra-articular injections (saline)
		  3. SWD
			• No patients had injections or SWD ≤ 6 mo prior
			• Treated as outpatient for 6 wk: placebo tablets B.I.D.; 4 placebo injections (1 q 2 wk); SWD 20 min 3 × wk
			• Evaluated pretreatment + q 2 wk (criteria: walking time, categorical evaluations of tenderness and pain; no. analgesic meds/day; "improvement" ≥ 2/4 criteria improved)
				1. Placebo injections: significantly better improvement than tablets
				2. Nonsignificant combined short (≤ 4 wk) and long-term (> 10 wk) differences placebo injections vs. SWD
				3. Better long-term improvement with SWD but not significant

Clarke et al.[28]	N = 45
	x̄ age = 61yr
	Chronic osteoarthrosis of knee
		• Non crossover ‡
		• Randomized assignment to 1 of 3 treatments:
		  1. Ice
		  2. SWD
		  3. Sham SWD (untuned)
			• Continued occasional med use
			• No injections or PT in prior year
			• Outpatient treatment ×3/wk for 3 wk
			• Specific treatment protocols "according to standard practice." Ice applied in bags above and below knee.
			• Evaluated pre and post treatment, and at 3 mo. (4 point verbal pain and stiffness rating scales)
				At conclusion of treatments:
				1. Significant improvement in pain for ice vs. SWD or sham SWD.
				2. Significant improvement in stiffness for ice vs. SWD or sham SWD.
				At 3 mo. post treatments:
				1. No significant difference between treatments.
				2. 82% of patients had improved pain, stiffness, knee ROM, walking time, and physician/patient assessments.

Hamer and Kirk[49]	N = 31 x̄ age = 59 yr Chronic frozen shoulder	• Noncrossover† • Prospective assignment of patients into cryotherapy or US groups	• Patients free to continue meds (except corticosteroids) • Treated 3×/wk • Cryotherapy: towels dipped in crushed ice	1. Both groups improved 2. No significant differences between groups for: Number of

Continued.

TABLE 18-3 (cont.).

Investigators	Subjects	Design	Treatment Protocol Details	Treatment Outcome
			and water to shoulder for 15 min • US: ?site for US 5–8 min continuous, at 0.5 W/cm^2 • All patients did passive and active exercise b.i.d., 10 min, for hospital and home programs • Patients discharged from outpatient therapy when pain relief attained • Evaluated pre- and post-treatment (pain assessment technique unspecified)	treatments (12.4 ice vs. 14.8 US), pain grade improvement (2.0 ice vs. 2.3 US), improvement in shoulder rotation (14.1 ice vs. 12.4 US)

Bulgen et al.[20]	N = 42
	x̄ age = 56 yrs
	Chronic frozen shoulder
		• Noncrossover†
		• Randomized assignment to 1 of 4 groups:
		  1. Ice packs and PNF
		  2. Maitland mobilization
		  3. Injection
		  4. Non-treatment
			• All got home pendulum exercise, non-ASA analgesics and diazepam (p.r.n. at night)
			• No specific details on ice packs, PNF, or mobilization
			• Injections of 20 mg methyl prednisone acetate and 1% lignocaine hydrochloride (0.5 mL to subacromial bursa, 0.5 mL to shoulder joint)
			• Groups no. 1 and 2 treated 3x/wk for 6 wk; no. 3 injected 1×/wk for 3 wk
			• Evaluated pretreatment, 1×/wk for 6 wk, and 1×/mo for 6 mo (pain assessed by visual analogue scale; ROM)
				1. Problems noted with use of visual analogue scale to assess pain; no data given, "majority pain free at 6 mo"
				2. ROM (cumulative) improvement: greatest for injection (no. 3), with significant between-group difference at wk 4; ice with best improvement at 6 mo but nonsignificant difference between groups

Williams et al.[132]	N = 18 x̄ age = 58 yr Rheumatoid arthritic shoulder	• "Single-blinded,"† noncrossover • Randomized assignment to hot pack or cold pack groups	• Patients free to continue meds (no steroid injection in prior 3 mo) • Treated 3 ×/wk for 3 wk • Hot pack: initially at 138° F; 8 layers of Turkish towel between pack and skin • Cold pack: crushed ice in Turkish towel, 4 layers between ice and skin • Both heat and cold done for 20 min, followed by supervised 20-min exercise program to cervical spine, both shoulders and upper extremities • Evaluated pre- and post-treatment (pain assessed with McGill Pain Questionnaire, parts 1 and 4)	1. Both groups improved, but no within-group statistics done 2. No significant differences between groups for: Pain rating index improvement: 5.7 heat vs. 6.9 cold Flexion ROM: 12.2 heat vs. 5.0 cold Abduction ROM: 26.1 heat vs. 22.8 cold

TABLE 18–3 (cont.).

Published Studies Assessing Thermal Agents for the Elderly With Pain

| Svarcova et al.[121] | N = 180
x̄ age = 63 yr
Osteoarthritis of hip or knee | • Not blinded, noncrossover
• Patients divided into 3 treatment groups:
1. US
2. Galvanic current
3. SWD
• Active and placebo medications given to one-half of subjects in each group | • US: moving 5 cm/sec, 3 fields, 5 min each
• Galvanic: 0.1 ma/cm², 20 min; SWD: pulsed at 46 MHz, 2 fields, 2 min each
• Active med: 400 mg ibuprofen
• US, galvanic current and SWD for 10 treatments, q 2 days, med B.I.D for 3 wk
• Evaluated at treatment sessions 5 and 10 (pain by visual analogue; 4 category "therapeutic effect" rating) | Between treatment comparisons only.
For pain relief (at treatment 10):
1. All treatments plus active med were significantly better than treatments alone
2. No significant differences between treatment groups
For "therapeutic effect":
1. No significant difference between groups
2. Overall, 89% of subjects rated treatments as "good" to "excellent" |

*PNF = proprioceptive neuromuscular facilitation; PT = physical therapy; ROM = range of motion; SWD = shortwave diathermy; US = ultrasound.
†Evaluator (blinded); separate therapist.

perimental group samples. This greatly contributes to the inability to statistically discern a difference between experimental treatment groups.[132] In addition, proposed theoretical mechanisms of action may not be supported by specific investigation. For example, Klemp and colleagues determined that ultrasound treatment of chronic fibromyotic upper trapezius muscles resulted in a significant *decrease* in muscle blood flow during treatment.[63]

Kauffman has reviewed factors related to the use of therapeutic heat and cold with the elderly.[62] Factors contributing to increased risk of thermal injury for the elderly include decreased reactivity of the hypothalamic thermoregulatory system; decreased autonomic and vasomotor responses; impairments of the circulatory system; loss of sweat glands; atrophy of skin, with reduction in circulation; lessened sensation of thirst; and decreased perception of thermal gradients. Common medications can further impair thermoregulatory control. Vasodilation in the skin may be hampered by diuretics, which limit volume expansion. Sweating in the skin may be inhibited by anticholinergic drugs. Various dermatologic conditions and spinal cord lesions may impair sweating as a mechanism of heat loss. Skin vasodilation associated with heating of a large body surface area may place hazardous demands on cardiac output.[62] Conversely, cold may produce a temporary increase in systolic and diastolic blood pressure, which poses a risk for hypertensive patients. It has been recommended that blood pressure be monitored and that treatment with cold be discontinued if blood pressure becomes elevated.[89] Increased mechanical stiffness of joints, aversion to cold, and cold intolerance may limit applications of cold with some older patients.[72, 89] Long-term use of steroids can produce fragile capillaries, which are easily damaged by thermal or mechanical agents.[89]

Precautions exist for electromagnetic energy generated by a number of therapeutic heating modalities (e.g., microwave and shortwave diathermy).[30, 61, 89] Of major concern for the elderly is the potential for interference with the functioning of cardiac pacemakers and other electromedical devices (e.g., urinary bladder stimulators, electrocardiographs, electromyographs, etc.). Jones reported on numerous cases of adverse physiologic dysfunction associated with electromagnetic field interference in patients having cardiac pacemakers. Significant interference occurred at distances of up to 15 ft.[61] Improvements in pacemaker design have eliminated this hazard for some pacemaker units.[89, 115] Based on electrocardiographic changes in experimental animals, it has been recommended that treatment be avoided over the heart with ultrasound, which is not an electromagnetic form of energy. Furthermore, cardiac pacemakers should not be directly exposed to ultrasound, which may interfere with electrical circuitry.[89] Metal components of objects external to (e.g., jewelry, clothing zippers or snaps, furniture, etc.) or implanted within patients (e.g., joint prostheses and surgical rods, plates, screws, etc.) act to focus electromagnetic energy in a manner that can produce burning of contiguous tissue. A similar focusing effect is produced by moisture on the skin, or in dressings and clothing. The patient's eyes, fluid-filled joints, inflamed tissues, and excessive adipose tissue should be avoided for similar reasons. Such problems are encountered most often with microwave and shortwave diathermy. Although therapeutic ultrasound does not produce dangerous heating of metal like the diathermies, it should not be applied over the eye. Further research on the effects of ultrasound on nonmetallic prosthetic joint components has been advocated.[89]

Specific precautions should be taken to prevent thermal injury of the older patient:[62, 72, 89]

1. Heating can act to increase the inflammatory process in acute, subacute, and chronic conditions. Deep heating of joints involved with certain pathologies (e.g., the arthritides) may contribute to temperature-sensitive enzymatic lysis of joint cartilage.[38] Superficial moist heating for less than 20 minutes, on the other hand, has been shown to result in a lowering of joint temperature.[55] Thus, it is critical that the most appropriate treatment modality be selected for a given clinical condition.

2. Operating temperatures for heating agents should be lowered, whereas those for cooling agents should be raised. For example, if a vigorous heating effect is needed to increase connective tissue extensibility in conjunction with prolonged stretch, targeted tissue should be heated to only 40°C as opposed to 45°C.[89] Typical modality intensity settings will need to be modified, and in some cases, thermostatic controls will need to be reset (e.g., for paraffin, hot pack, and cold pack units). Use of paraffin with a low melting point (104°F, as opposed to 124°F) has been recommended.[56] Both hot and cold packs may need to be better insulated with greater thicknesses of dry toweling, which the patient is not permitted to compress with body weight.

3. A slower rate of temperature change may be more desirable. Therapeutic ultrasound, which produces the most rapid deep-temperature elevation by easily penetrating subcutaneous fat, may need to be used with a modified technique (e.g., lower intensity, faster sound head movement, less overlap of sound head strokes).

4. Treatment times may need to be shortened. The customary 20- to 30-minute treatment time used with superficial heating agents may need to be limited to no longer than 20 minutes.[56, 89] More conservative treatment times for deeper-heating agents may also be appropriate (e.g., use of ultrasound for 5 minutes for each 150 cm² of skin surface[48] rather than for an area two to three times the size of the sound head.[89]

5. Reflex-based consensual vasodilation may be used to produce less pronounced increases in skin blood flow in body regions that cannot tolerate direct heating.[72] Consensual circulatory reactions for cold remain controversial.[65]

Although these modifications may improve the safety of various treatment interventions, further research is needed to determine if resultant therapeutic effects are lessened substantially.

A number of clinical factors should guide the health care professional in the selection and application of an appropriate thermal agent. Michlovitz has recently discussed key factors to consider when using thermal agents in the management of rheumatic diseases.[89] These factors, modified for a broader consideration of other pain-related diagnoses encountered with elderly patients, include:

1. The stage of the inflammatory/repair process is important to determine. Based on signs, symptoms, and physiologic characteristics, the acute inflammatory stage may last as long as 2 weeks. Cardinal signs of local pain, redness, increased temperature, swelling, and loss of function are common. Neutrophils predominate. The subacute stage of inflammation may continue for up to 1 month and is associated with a considerable lessening of cardinal signs. The chronic stage of inflammation occurs after 1 month and is associated with the presence of lymphocytes, monocytes, and macrophages, and with the proliferation of fibroblasts related to adhesion and scar formation.[89] Within the first 24 to 72 hours after trauma or onset of inflammation, heating agents are avoided to prevent aggravating changes in local permeability, circulation, and metabolism. Cooling the affected site results in decreased membrane permeability and vasoconstriction, which act to limit formation of edema. Local tissue metabolism is also lowered, which may also act to limit secondary hypoxic injury of adjacent tissues. Concurrent compression with an elastic wrap and elevation further act to control edema formation.[65] Beyond 72 hours, mild and then more vigorous local heating may be indicated. However, the patient is always monitored for signs and symptoms of aggravated inflammation. It should be appreciated that early vigorous cooling can also worsen inflammation.[89] In addition, cold may also be used to modulate pain in subacute and chronic stages.

2. The "target tissue" for the thermal agent must be determined. In the acute stage, cooling to the site of inflammation is desired. However, mild heating superficial to inflamed tissues may successfully relieve muscle spasm and related pain. In some chronic conditions, deep, vigorous heating combined with prolonged low-load stretch may be required to restore pain-free joint range of motion. However, it has been suggested that deep heating of subacute and chronic arthritic joints may promote cartilage destruction.[38]

3. The size of the body region (i.e., tissue volume) and number of joints involved present practical treatment considerations. The diathermies may more easily be used to heat large and relatively deep-body regions than ultrasound used on multiple fields. Unlike the diathermies, ultrasound will not dangerously heat subcutaneous fat. Hydrotherapy may be preferred to hotpacks or paraffin for superficial tissue heating when multiple joints or large body regions are involved.

4. The decision to continue treatment in the clinic or

via home program instruction may be guided in part by the suitability of appropriate treatment modalities. Some cooling agents (e.g., ice cubes in a plastic bag, or used for massage) and heating agents (e.g., moist towels microwaved in unsealed plastic bags, timer-controlled electric moist-heating pads, home paraffin units, etc.) may successfully be used in the home environment with proper patient education. All deep-heating agents (e.g., diathermies and ultrasound) require application by a health care professional in the clinic or home.

Transcutaneous Electrical Nerve Stimulation

The most common form of therapeutic electrical stimulation used for pain control is transcutaneous electrical nerve stimulation (TENS), which involves the stimulation of cutaneous and peripheral nerves via electrodes on the surface of the skin. Six types or "modes" of TENS have been most commonly discussed in the literature (i.e., conventional, strong low-rate, brief-intense, pulse-burst, modulated, and hyperstimulation TENS). Each mode employs unique electrical output characteristics and a variety of electrode site options. Different perceptual-motor qualities are associated with each mode as a result of nerve and/or muscle activation. Table 18–4 introduces key features of these common TENS modes, including typical stimulator characteristics, electrode sites, and desired perceptual-motor experience. In order to communicate effectively, it is important that

clinicians and researchers specify details of their methods rather than just relying on descriptive TENS mode labels. Other publications should be consulted for more detailed discussion of the theoretical bases for pain relief with TENS and associated clinical decision making.[7, 83]

Although a number of professional publications have suggested or recommended TENS for pain control with elderly patients,* a recent survey revealed that initiation of TENS treatment for the elderly by physical therapists was in reality quite low.[76] Despite the fact that hundreds of research papers have been published on TENS,[99] very few studies have been conducted with patients averaging ages in the mid-50s and above. Table 18–5 summarizes the handful of published studies that have assessed either the efficacy or effectiveness of TENS for elderly patients with acute and chronic pain. In addition, Levy and associates used TENS to treat experimental acute arthritis induced in rat knees.[78] A 5-minute TENS treatment resulted in a small but significant increase in temperature (largest mean value = 0.4°C) and a significant decrease in pressure measured intra-articularly. Synovial fluid volume and total leukocyte count were also significantly less than in the opposite nontreated knee.

We conducted a modified double-blind crossover study with elderly individuals (N = 22, mean age = 74 ± 10 years) having chronic musculoskeletal pain.[8] Although

*References 39, 56, 68, 73, 95, 104, 105, 122, 124, 126, 129, 137.

TABLE 18–4.
Common Modes of Transcutaneous Electrical Nerve Stimulation for Pain Control

Mode Classification	Typical Stimulator Output Characteristics	Typical Electrode Sites	Desired Perceptual-Motor Experience
Conventional (Barr et al.[10])	Frequency: 10–100 Hz Pulse duration: 50–100 μs Amplitude: low to medium*	At perimeter of painful area or over nerve to region; or at segmentally related area	Distinct paresthesia superimposed on painful area, or in segmentally related area
Strong low-rate (Andersson et al.[5])	Frequency: below 10 Hz Pulse duration: 100–300 μs Amplitude: high*	Over nerve related to muscle in or remote from painful area	Uncomfortable rhythmic muscle contractions at patient tolerance
Brief-intense (Leo et al.[75])	Frequency: 60–150 Hz Pulse duration: 50–250 μs Amplitude: high*	Over nerve related to muscle in or remote from painful area	Uncomfortable tetanic muscle contraction that fatigues, at patient tolerance
Pulse-burst (Mannheimer and Carlsson[82])	Frequency: high (60–100 Hz) modulated by low (0.5–4 Hz) Pulse duration: 50–200 μs Amplitude: low to high*	Over nerve related to muscle in or remote from painful area	Weak to strong intermittent tetanic muscle contraction and paresthesia
Modulated (Miller et al.[91])	Frequency, pulse duration, or amplitude modulated separately or together down 60% from preset values Amplitude: Low to high*	Any of these listed sites	Weak to strong sensation, with or without muscle contraction; may minimize perceptual accommodation
Hyperstimulation (= "noninvasive" electroacupuncture) (Leo[74])	Frequency: 1–100 Hz Pulse duration: up to 500 ms Amplitude: high*	Acupuncture points	Sharp burning sensation at tolerance; no muscle contraction

*Adequate to give desired perceptual-motor experience.

TABLE 18–5.
Published Studies Assessing TENS for the Elderly With Acute and Chronic Pain

Investigators	Subjects	Design	TENS Mode	Electrode Sites	Protocol Details	Treatment Outcome
Acute pain						
Smith et al.[114]	N = 50 (subject subset) $\bar{x}$age = 73 yr Total condylar–total knee replacement surgery	• Not blinded, noncrossover • Prospective division of patients into TENS and non-TENS groups	Unspecified (likely CONV or MR) "pleasant stimulation"	2 electrodes parallel to incision	• Preoperative TENS education • Patients adjusted TENS unit controls, with b.i.d. monitoring by PT • TENS continuous until discharge • All patients had PT (exercise and gait training)	Patients in TENS group had significantly fewer injections of Demerol, lower total Demerol dosage, fewer days until straight leg raise, shorter hospital stay; no significant difference in days until ambulation
Finsen et al.[43]	N = 51 $\bar{x}$age = 69 yr Lower extremity amputation due to diabetes or artherosclerosis	• Not blinded, noncrossover • Randomized postoperative assignment to: 1. Active TENS 2. Sham TENS (no stimulation) 3. Sham TENS and chlorpromazine	PB (90 µs impulses at 100 Hz; burst of 7 pulses 2×/sec; amplitude to discomfort)	2 electrodes over femoral nerve, 2 over sciatic nerve	• Treated 30 min 2×/day for 2 wk • TENS unit light on • Analgesic meds on demand • Pain assessment technique unspecified	1. Self-rated analgesic effect for all active TENS and 50% of sham TENS 2. Nonsignificant difference in analgesic use or phantom pain in first 4 wk 3. Active TENS had significantly more healing at 6 and 9 wk 4. Active TENS had significantly fewer cases of phantom pain at 16 wk (10%) than sham (36%) or sham plus chlorpromazine (58%); no difference ≥ 1 yr later
Chronic pain						
Abelson et al.[1]	N = 32 $\bar{x}$ age = 56 yr Rheumatoid arthritis with chronic wrist pain	• "Double-blind,"* noncrossover • Random assignment to active or placebo TENS (no stimulation) treatment	BI? (frequency = 70 Hz; high intensity)	Dorsal and ventral wrist	• Anti-inflammatory meds stopped 12 hr before treatment • Neutral statement on likely effects to both groups • Treated 15 min 1×/wk for 3 wk • TENS unit light on • Visual analogue pain relief rating pre- and post-treatment	Only within-group comparisons done: 1. Active TENS gave significant improvements in resting and grip pain, power and work 2. Placebo effect for pain averaged 17%; nonsignificant for all criteria

Study	Subjects	Design	Stimulation parameters	Electrode placement	Protocol	Results
Lewis et al.[79]	N = 28 Median age = 61 yr Osteoarthritis with chronic knee pain	• "Double-blind,"† crossover • Active and placebo TENS (no stimulation) treatment	CONV or BI? (frequency = 70 Hz)	4 electrodes at acupuncture points around knee	• Initial "washout" week, paracetamol only med (also available during TENS trials) • Home program: 30–60 min 3×/day for 3 wk of each treatment • TENS unit light on • Assessed weekly, including visual analogue pain relief rating	1. "> 50% pain relief" for 46% active, 43% placebo 2. Significant difference in median duration of pain relief: active (151 min) vs. placebo (110 min) 3. Significant improvement pain relief after 3 wk active, not placebo 4. Both groups had significant improvement in "pain index" based on knee ROM and weight bearing, and reduction in meds 5. Preferred treatment if continued > 3 wk: 43% active, 36% meds, 14% placebo
Langley et al.[70]	N = 33 x̄age = 54 yr Rheumatoid arthritis with chronic hand pain	• "Double-blind,"** noncrossover • Random assignment to group 1 or 2 active TENS or group 3 placebo TENS (no stimulation) treatments	1. BI? Frequency = 100 Hz; pulse duration = 200 μs 2. "Acupuncture-like" (PB?) Frequency = 100 Hz, on for 70 ms, pulsed 2/sec; both no. 1 and 2 at highest tolerated intensity, displayed on oscilloscope 3. Placebo = no current but given signal on oscilloscope	1 dorsal and 1 ventral, proximal to wrist	• Initial neutral instructions to all subjects • Strong suggestion given to placebo group • No meds < 24 hr prior • Treated once for 20 min • Pre- and post-treatment assessment each 15 min, including visual analogue pain rating	1. Overall "≥ 50% pain relief": 59% in group 1; 64% in 2, 55% in 3 2. Nonsignificant group differences, as all groups had significantly decreased resting and grip pain 3. Nonsignificant group differences for overall pain relief, total joint tenderness, or number of tender joints 4. No significant changes in power or work

*Patient blind to treatment; separate evaluator and therapist.
† Unable to determine adequacy of "double-blind" conditions.
BI = brief-intense; CONV = conventional; MR = modulated rate; PB = pulse-burst; PT = physical therapy; ROM = range of motion; TENS = transcutaneous electrical nerve stimulation.

all subjects were informed that TENS could possibly produce pain relief, this was done with neutral instructions. Each of three TENS treatments (conventional TENS: frequency = 60 Hz, 40 μs pulse duration, amplitude to distinct paresthesia; pulse-burst TENS: seven impulses each of 40 μs duration and frequency of 110 Hz, pulsed at two per second, amplitude producing maximum tolerated muscle contraction; sham control TENS: conventional TENS settings but stimulation on for only 10 seconds) was given to each subject for 30 minutes at 48-hour intervals over 1 week. Stimulation via two electrodes was perceived within the painful area. Pain and related functional limitations were assessed using separate visual analogue scales. Significantly less immediate pain relief was seen for the sham control treatment (19.5%, vs. 32.5% for true conventional and 33.9% for pulse-burst). When compared with the control treatment, both active TENS treatments produced significantly greater pain relief for up to 8 hours but had no significant effect on function as defined in this study.

Overall, these studies indicate both efficacy[114] and effectiveness of TENS in controlling a range of pain problems experienced by elderly individuals under controlled short-term conditions.[8, 43, 79] Only when strong suggestion was provided to a placebo TENS group was active TENS seen to be ineffective for older patients,[70] as has been the case for the general population.[32] Well-controlled studies assessing pain control with long-term TENS use (i.e., for greater than 1 month) in the elderly are sorely lacking.

Demand-type (synchronous) cardiac pacemakers represent the primary contraindication for electrical stimulators, including TENS devices. Although TENS has been safely used on the body close to older-style fixed-rate (synchronous) pacemakers and on regions remote from demand-type units, a wide range of hazardous electrical stimulation characteristics and electrode placements has yet to be fully investigated.[7] At this time it is probably safest to recommend that all patients with cardiac pacemakers be electrically monitored during both initial and extended trials of therapeutic electrical stimulation.[7, 27] If interference is noted, it may be possible to reprogram the pacemaker to a lower level of sensitivity.[27] It has also been suggested that electrical stimulation not be done on the anterior chest wall of patients with cardiac histories, over the carotid sinus, or close to the larynx.[83] The effects of TENS on patients with cerebral vascular accidents, transient ischemic attacks, epilepsy, and seizure disorders are not well established.

Dry skin associated with aging and cleansing of the skin with alcohol-based products act to increase the impedance under electrodes used for electrical stimulation. This will necessitate the use of higher-intensity stimulation, which may be uncomfortable and irritating to the skin. Skin impedance can be lowered by hydration of the skin with skin cream or nonabrasive electrode gel. Use of alternate electrode sites will prevent breakdown of fragile skin from cumulative effects of allergic, chemical, electrical, and mechanical irritation. Tape and self-adhering electrodes should be peeled back slowly while underlying skin is held down to prevent skin stripping.

Although clinical procedures involved in the application of TENS have been outlined elsewhere,[7, 83] factors related to successful pain control with TENS for the elderly merit specific discussion. Given that 60 TENS unit manufacturers are registered with the Food and Drug Administration (FDA),[134] the clinician is faced with a growing array of stimulators. Unfortunately, only a handful of publications have critically assessed specific brands and models of TENS units.[7] Equipment-related factors (e.g., reasonable cost; "user-friendly" instruction manuals and unit controls; durable unit components; independence between unit control settings and other unit output parameters; good battery life; electrical output limited to established safety standards) play an important role in the success or failure of treatment with TENS. The American National Standard for Transcutaneous Electrical Nerve Stimulators should be consulted for detailed safety guidelines.[4]

A guiding concept for the treatment of all patients with TENS, regardless of age, is a modification of the "KISS" principle (i.e., *k*eep *i*t *s*imple *s*timulation). Technology incorporated into some TENS units is inappropriately designed or too complex. Unit components are easily lost or misplaced by patients. Controls may be confusing and may be difficult to see or to adjust because of their small size. For this reason an older-style single-channel TENS unit with only one control dial (i.e., on/amplitude) may be superior to the latest subminiature multiprogrammable unit in some instances. Electrode systems need to be custom fit to each patient's needs and abilities. A patient with severe hand osteoarthritis may be unable to manipulate and secure traditional carbonized silicone rubber electrodes, conductive gel, and tape; only higher-priced reusable, self-adhering electrodes may be suitable. Health care professionals need to be familiar with options available in TENS units and components (e.g., lead wires, connectors, electrode styles, adhesive materials, battery packs, etc.) and be able to exercise reasonable freedom in selecting the optimal TENS setup for their patients.

Unfortunately, an adequate number of comparative studies have not been done to determine the best mode of TENS for treating specific types of pain. Wolf and colleagues have noted that some patients with peripheral nerve injuries benefit from higher-intensity stimulation.[136] Patients generally find conventional TENS and lower-amplitude versions of other modes (i.e., pulse-burst and modulated) to be most acceptable. We have found elderly patients with chronic pain to rate conventional low-intensity

TENS as being more comfortable than high-intensity pulse-burst TENS.[11] Although it has been recommended that initial treatment be done with conventional TENS (frequency at 60 Hz, short-pulse duration, and amplitude that gives distinct paresthesia in the painful region),[9, 10, 81] alternate TENS modes may need to be used in order to attain successful pain control.[7, 75, 83]

It is critically important that the patient and significant others be given adequate instruction in self-treatment and outcome documentation (e.g., via activity logs, pain and functional rating scales, etc.). The patient *must* attain successful pain control under the supervision of the health care professional before being released on a home program that has any hope of long-term success. Many insurance companies mandate at least a 1-month TENS unit rental period before purchase will be authorized.

CASE STUDIES

In order to more completely describe the application of conservative pain management principles, two case studies involving older patients are now presented.

Case 1

Mr. Jones is an 81-year-old retired electrical contractor, living alone, with severe degenerative joint disease. He was referred to the Physical Therapy Department as an outpatient on May 7, 1990, from the medical center Geriatric Evaluation Unit (GEU). His main complaint was right hip pain on weight bearing. Mr. Jones had tripped over a curb with his right foot 1 week prior, which had resulted in immediate hip pain. His related history included blindness; moderate bilateral hearing loss; no evidence of fracture by roentgenogram taken May 7, 1990; and a prescription for naproxen (375 mg, three times a day). The clinic physician felt that Mr. Jones should be assessed as a candidate for possible right total hip replacement by an orthopedist, but the patient was vigorously opposed to this idea. (Mr. Jones reported that a good friend had recently died as a result of complications associated with just such a surgery.) Evaluation in the Physical Therapy Department revealed moderately limited active and passive ROM, and 3/5 grade muscle strength of all right hip muscles (except abductors at 2/5) associated with pain. Strength at other right lower extremity joints and of other extremities and trunk was generally at 4/5. He was independently ambulatory with a slow antalgic gait using his sounding cane in the right hand. Mr. Jones noted only localized "deep" hip pain; his pain with weight bearing was rated 7/10; with active hip motion, 5/10; and at rest supine, 2/10 (by Pain Estimate Rating). It was the assessment of the physical ther-

apist that Mr. Jones had strained the muscles of his hip (principally the abductors) and was in a subacute stage. The initial treatment plan included patient education/recommendations for reduction of mechanical forces on muscles of right hip in order to decrease pain and promote healing; gentle active ROM exercises to maintain and later increase hip ROM in order to restore safe functional gait. It was recommended that weight-bearing activity be temporarily decreased, but he refused to be fitted for a standard straight cane. He was willing to limit ambulation, especially on stairs, for a period of "a couple weeks." He was instructed in an initial home program of gentle active ROM exercises for the right hip. Since he was planning to leave the community for the next few months to visit his children out of state, he was instructed to arrange for reevaluation upon his return.

Mr. Jones attended Physical Therapy after another GEU visit on Oct 8, 1990. The GEU physician had increased naproxen, 375 mg, to four times a day. Roentgenograms remained negative. On this occasion, he reported increased right hip pain extending to lateral mid thigh: rated 8/10 with weight bearing, 6/10 with active ROM, and 3/10 at rest supine. Patient exhibited marked tenderness to palpation at right greater trochanter only; while he was uncooperative for manual muscle testing of hip, no distal weakness was noted. Mr. Jones now accepted fitting and instruction in use of a straight cane, which he found to be safer using in the right hand. His home ROM exercise program was modified to self-assisted ROM in pain-free range only. A future trial of TENS for pain control was suggested to Mr. Jones.

A trial of TENS for pain control was begun on Oct 15, 1990. Pain rating prior to treatment was 8/10 during weight bearing of ambulation, even with cane on right. TENS was begun in the "conventional" mode (frequency = 60 Hz, phase width = 40 μs, amplitude adjusted to produce a "distinct electrical sensation overlying the area of pain"). One TENS unit channel was used, with one electrode over the greater trochanter, the other at midlateral thigh. At the end of stimulation for 20 minutes, Mr. Jones rated pain with weight bearing and ROM at 3/10, and pain at rest 0/10. With the TENS unit turned off, significant carryover of pain reduction was seen for approximately 2 hours. A second TENS trial was done on Oct 19, 1990, initial pain again at 8/10 with weight bearing. Within 20 minutes of stimulation, this pain was reduced to 4/10, with significant poststimulation carryover again for 2 hours. Mr. Jones was formally instructed in a home TENS program on Oct 22, 1990, to be done twice a day in conjunction with the self-assisted ROM program. Reusable self-adhering electrodes could be applied and cared for by Mr. Jones after detailed instruction and supervision. He also mastered TENS unit operations (including the battery recharging procedure and use of alternate electrode sites).

On Nov 15, 1990, Mr. Jones was admitted to the hospital with a small gastrointestinal bleed. Although taken off naproxen, he continued after discharge to regularly reduce his pain with weight bearing to 3/10 and had no pain at rest. Unfortunately, on Jan 1, 1991, he fractured his right hip while lifting heavy pails of water for his six dogs. However, he underwent a successful right total hip replacement on Jan 17, 1991, which included conventional postoperative physical therapy. At a return GEU visit on Oct 13, 1991, Mr. Jones demonstrated a symmetric pain-free gait without any assistive device. Strength of the right hip muscles was found to be 4–5/5, with full ROM throughout. Mr. Jones was continuing a home exercise program of resistive exercise and walking on a daily basis.

This case illustrates the practical implementation of conservative pain management strategies for a highly independent older individual. The physical therapy program involved extensive patient education and psychologic support. The program included the use of an assistive device, exercise, and TENS in a manner that helped both to control pain and to maintain functional independence during an 8-month period leading up to "dreaded" total joint replacement surgery.

Case 2

Mrs. Smith is a 61-year-old right-hand dominant female hospital clerk with a chief complaint of right shoulder pain. She was seen initially in the Physical Therapy Department on Aug 20, 1991. Her shoulder pain began suddenly on Aug 19, 1991, while tearing paper from a computer printer; pain at that time was recollected at 10/10. She was referred from the Orthopedics Department with a diagnosis of right subacromial bursitis and a prescription for topical 5% hydrocortisone. The patient was taking ibuprofen and acetaminophen as needed. Physical therapy evaluation revealed a "painful arc" of active right shoulder abduction ROM from 60 to 120 degrees in neutral rotation and from 90 to 120 degrees in full external rotation. A manual muscle test of the right deltoid and rotator cuff muscles was rated at 4/5 (with pain); elbow and wrist flexors/extensors and hand muscles were all 5/5. The patient noted sharp intermittent pain localized to the right subacromial area. Pain with active shoulder abduction was rated 7/10 and was relieved by rest and medications. Manual examination of the cervical spine did not reproduce shoulder pain. The patient reported not being allergic to cold or medications. Mrs. Smith was assessed to have acute onset right subacromial bursitis. Short-term treatment goals were to decrease inflammation and pain; the long-term goal was to restore pain-free ROM and shoulder strength. Physical

therapy treatment consisted of rest from repeated trauma in the workplace through temporary job task reassignment; instruction in home program (application of specific ergonomic principles in the workplace; ice massage for 7 to 10 minutes, twice a day for 1 week; gentle pain-free ROM exercise); outpatient treatment three times a week consisting of phonophoresis (using 5% hydrocortisone with continuous 1-MHz ultrasound, at 0.7 to 0.8 W/cm^2, moving technique for 7 minutes); and exercise (ROM; progressive resistive exercise when inflammation over).

At physical therapy re-evaluation on Aug 29, 1991, Mrs. Smith reported the right shoulder was generally feeling better. Examination disclosed a painful arc from 70 to 120 degrees in neutral and from 90 to 115 degrees in external rotation; manual muscle tests were unchanged; medication use was still as needed. Pain with active shoulder abduction was rated 6/10. On Sept 6, 1991, Mrs. Smith claimed that she was pleased with her progress on pain control but noted shoulder "weakness." Examination showed a painful arc of active shoulder abduction (in neutral rotation) at 90 to 110 degrees; pain was rated 4/10; muscle strength tests were unchanged. The patient claimed less frequent medication use. She was begun on gentle progressive resistive exercise for the right shoulder using a "yellow"-coded Theraband and was monitored closely for increased inflammation. At a clinic visit on Sept 13, 1991, phonophoresis was discontinued. A painful arc remained at 90 to 110 degrees, with pain rated at 4/10 and strength unchanged. Medication use was now infrequent. Mrs. Smith's exercise program progressed to "red"-coded Theraband.

Mrs. Smith was discharged from formal outpatient physical therapy on Sept 20, 1991, claiming to be pain free. The patient had resumed her original workload, with task modifications. No painful arc with active right shoulder abduction was present; thus, pain was rated 0/10. Manual muscle testing showed deltoid and rotator cuff muscles at 4+/5, without pain. Medications were being used infrequently for inflammation or pain. Mrs. Smith's home progressive resistive exercise program, using "green-" and then "blue"-coded Therabands with proprioceptive neuromuscular facilitation (PNF) patterns (D1 and D2 flexion), was reviewed, and she was determined to be independent in its application. She was assessed as having good progress with her program, which she continued at home and in the workplace. She appeared to understand that she was at risk for recurrence of this condition. A formal re-evaluation was to be done in 2 months.

This case illustrates the successful conservative management of an injured older employee. Specific outpatient physical therapy care was provided in the acute and subacute stages of her condition. A detailed home program was instituted for a 3-month period that actively involved the patient in her own recovery and set the stage for prevention of a recurrence. Clinical improvement by natural history of the healing process cannot be ruled out as a significant factor in this case. However, left untreated, it is very possible that this condition would have been exacerbated in the workplace and might have progressed to a chronic painful or frozen shoulder.

SUMMARY

A large proportion of older individuals experience significant physical pain as a result of the aging process and related acute and chronic illness. Fortunately, there is growing interest both in accurate assessment of clinical pain and in conservative pain management for the older patient. Conservative treatment strategies exist that have been demonstrated to be either efficacious or effective in the control of pain and associated problems for individuals aged 55 and older. However, given physiologic age-related changes, concerns for patient safety require further modifications in treatment protocols. Additional well-controlled studies of pain assessment tools and a wider range of conservative treatment interventions are warranted.

REFERENCES

1. Abelson K, Langley GB, Sheppeard H, et al: Transcutaneous electrical nerve stimulation in rheumatoid arthritis. *N Z Med J* 1983; 96:156–158.
2. Aldes JH, Jadeson WJ: Ultrasonic therapy in the treatment of hypertrophic arthritis in elderly patients. *Ann West M & S* 1952; 6:545–550.
3. Alon G, DeDomenico G: *High Voltage Stimulation: An Integrated Approach to Clinical Electrotherapy,* ed 1. Chattanooga, Tenn, Chattanooga Corporation, 1987.
4. *American National Standard for Transcutaneous Electrical Nerve Stimulators.* ANSI/AAMI NS4–1985. Arlington, Va, Association for the Advancement of Medical Instrumentation, 1986.
5. Andersson SA, Hansson G, Holmgren E, et al: Evaluation of the pain suppressive effect of different frequencies of peripheral electrical stimulation in chronic pain conditions. *Acta Orthop Scand* 1976; 47:149–157.
6. Barr JO: TENS for chronic low back pain (letter). *New Engl J Med* 1990; 323:1423–1424.
7. Barr JO: Transcutaneous electrical nerve stimulation for pain management, in Nelson RM, Currier DP (eds): *Clinical Electrotherapy,* ed 2. Norwalk, Conn, Appleton & Lange, 1991.
8. Barr JO, Forrest SE, Potratz PE, et al: Effectiveness of transcutaneous electrical nerve stimulation (TENS) for the elderly with chronic pain (abstract). *Phys Ther* 1989; 69:165.
9. Barr JO, Nielsen DH, Soderberg GL: Investigation of transcutaneous electrical nerve stimulation parameters for altering pain perception. *Phys Ther* 1986; 66:1515–1521.
10. Barr JO: The effect of transcutaneous electrical nerve stimulation parameters on experimentally induced acute pain (abstract). *Phys Ther* 1981; 61:582.
11. Barr JO, Weissenbuehler SA, Bandstra EJ, et al: Effectiveness and comfort level of transcutaneous electrical nerve stimulation (TENS) in elderly with chronic pain (abstract). *Phys Ther* 1987; 67:775.
12. Barta Kvitek SD, Shaver BJ, Blood H, et al: Age bias: Physical therapists and older patients. *J Gerontol* 1986; 41:706–709.
13. Beecher HK: The placebo effect as a nonspecific force surrounding disease and the treatment of disease, in Janzen R (ed): *Pain: Basic Principles, Pharmacology, Therapy.* Baltimore, Williams & Wilkins, 1972.
14. Bell AT: The older athlete, in Sanders B (ed): *Sports Physical Therapy.* Norwalk, Conn, Appleton & Lange, 1990.
15. Bird HA, Dixon JS: The measurement of pain. *Baillieres Clin Rheumatol* 1987; 1:71–89.
16. Boeckstyns MS, Backer M: Reliability and validity of the evaluation of pain in patients with total knee replacement. Pain 1989; 38:29–33.
17. Bonica JJ: Management of pain. Lecture as visiting professor, Department of Anesthesiology, College of Medicine, University of Iowa, Iowa City, Dec 7, 1988.
18. Brand RA, Crowinshield RD: The effect of cane use on hip contact force. *Clin Orthop* 1980; 147:181–184.
19. Brody E, Kleban M: Day-to-day mental and physical health symptoms of older people. A report on health logs. *Gerontologist* 1983; 23:75–85.
20. Bulgen DY, Binder AI, Hazelman BL, et al: Frozen shoulder: Prospective clinical study with an evaluation of three treatment regimens. *Ann Rheum Dis* 1984; 43:353–360.
21. Burke SO, Jerrett M: Pain management across age groups. *West J Nurs Res* 1989; 11:164–178.
22. Burton KE, Wright V: Functional assessment. *Br J Rheumatol* 1983; 22(suppl):44–47.
23. Butler R, Gastel B: Care of the aged: Perspectives on pain and discomfort, in Ng L, Bonica J (eds): *Pain, Discomfort and Humanitarian Care.* New York, Elsevier/North-Holland, 1980.
24. Carlsson A: Assessment of chronic pain. I. Aspects of the reliability and validity of the visual analogue scale. *Pain* 1983; 16:87–101.
25. Cauna N: The effects of aging on receptor organs of the human dermis, in Montogna W (ed): *Aging.* New York, Pergamon Press, 1965.
26. Chapman CR: Measurement of pain: Problems and issues, in Bonica JJ, Albe-Fessard D (eds): *Advances in Pain Research & Therapy,* vol. 1: New York, Raven Press, 1976, pp 345–353.
27. Chen D, Mersamma P, Puliyodil AP, et al: Cardiac pacemaker inhibition by transcutaneous electrical nerve stimulation. *Arch Phys Med Rehabil* 1990; 71:27–30.

28. Clarke GR, Willis LA, Stenners L, et al: Evaluation of physiotherapy in the treatment of osteoarthrosis of the knee. *Rheumatol Rehabil* 1974; 13:190–197.

29. Clarkson PM, Dedrick ME: Exercise-induced muscle damage, repair and adaptation in old and young subjects. *J Gerontol* 1988; 43:M91–96.

30. Cook TM, Barr JO: Instrumentation, in Nelson RM, Currier DP (eds): *Clinical Electrotherapy*, ed 2. Norwalk, Conn, Appleton & Lange, 1991.

31. Cyriax J: *Textbook of Orthopaedic Medicine: Diagnosis of Soft Tissue Lesions*, ed 6. Baltimore, Williams & Wilkins, 1975.

32. Deyo RA, Walsh NE, Martin DC, et al: A controlled trial of transcutaneous electrical nerve stimulation (TENS) and exercise for chronic low back pain. *New Engl J Med* 1990; 322:1627–1634.

33. Doongaji DR, Vahia VN, Zharucha MPE: On placebos, placebo responses and placebo responders. A review of psychological, psychopharmacological, and psychophysiological factors. II. Psychopharmacological and psychophysiological factors. *J Postgrad Med* 1978; 24:147–157.

34. Downie WW, Leatham PA, Rhind VM, et al: Studies with pain rating scales. *Ann Rheum Dis* 1978; 37:378–381.

35. Ducroquet R, Ducroquet J, Ducroquet P: *Walking and Limping: A Study of Normal and Pathological Walking.* Philadelphia, JB Lippincott, 1968.

36. Faherty BS, Grier MR: Analgesic medication for elderly people post-surgery. *Nurs Res* 1984; 33:369–372.

37. Falck I: Observations on altered patterns of response in old age. *Methods Find Exp Clin Pharmacol* 1987; 9:149–151.

38. Feibel A, Fast A: Deep heating of joints: A reconsideration. *Arch Phys Med Rehabil* 1976; 57:513–514.

39. Ferrell BR, Ferrell BA: Easing the pain. *Geriatr Nurs* 1990; 11:175–178.

40. Fields HL: *Pain.* New York, McGraw-Hill, 1987.

41. Finneson BE: *Low Back Pain*, ed 2. Philadelphia, JB Lippincott, 1980.

42. Finsen V: Osteoporosis and back pain among the elderly. *Acta Med Scand* 1988; 223:443–449.

43. Finsen V, Persen L, Lovlien M, et al: Transcutaneous electrical nerve stimulation after major amputation. *J Bone Joint Surg* 1988; 70B:109–112.

44. Fischer AA: Advances in documentation of pain and soft tissue pathology. *Med Times* 1983; 12:24–31.

45. Fisher NM, Pendergast DR, Gresham GE, et al: Muscle rehabilitation: Its effect on muscular and functional performance of patients with knee osteoarthritis. *Arch Phys Med Rehabil* 1991; 72:367–374.

46. Follick MJ, Ahern DK, Laser-Wolston N, et al: Chronic pain: Electromechanical recording device for measuring patients' activity patterns. *Arch Phys Med Rehabil* 1985; 66:75–79.

47. Gebhart GF: Personal communication, Department of Pharmacology, College of Medicine, University of Iowa, Jan 7, 1991.

48. Griffin JE, Karselis TC: *Physical Agents for Physical Therapists*, ed 2. Springfield, Ill, Charles C Thomas, 1982.

49. Hamer J, Kirk JA: Physiotherapy and the frozen shoulder: A comparative trial of ice and ultrasonic therapy, *N Z Med J* 1976; 83:191–192.

50. Hamilton M: *Lectures on the Methodology of Clinical Research*, ed 2. Edinburgh, Churchill Livingstone, 1974.

51. Harkins SW, Kwentus J, Price DD: Pain and the elderly, in Benedetti C, Chapman RC, Moricca G (eds): *Advances in Pain Research and Therapy*, vol 7. New York, Raven Press, 1984, pp 103–121.

52. Helling DK, Lemke JH, Semla TP, et al: Medication use characteristics in the elderly: The Iowa 65+ rural health study. *J Am Geriatr Soc* 1987; 35:4–12.

53. Helme RD, Katz B, Gibson S, et al: Can psychometric tools be used to analyze pain in a geriatric population? *Clin Exp Neurol* 1989; 26:113–117.

54. Herr KA, Mobily PR: Complexities of pain assessment in the elderly: Clinical considerations. *J Gerontol Nurs*, 1991; 17:12–19.

55. Horvath SM, Hollander JL: Intra-articular temperature as a measure of joint reaction. *J Clin Invest* 1949; 28:469–473.

56. Hunt TE: Management of chronic non-rheumatic pain in the elderly. *J Am Geriatr Soc* 1976; 24:402–406.

57. Huskisson EC: Measurement of pain. *Lancet*, 1974; 2(4889):1127–1131.

58. Huskisson EC: Visual analogue scales, in Melzack R (ed): *Pain Measurement and Assessment*. New York, Raven Press, 1983.

59. Huskisson EC, Jones J, Scott PJ: Application of visual analogue scales to the measurement of functional capacity. *Rheumatol Rehabil* 1976; 15:185–187.

60. Jensen MP, Karoly P, Braver S: The measurement of clinical pain intensity: A comparison of six methods. *Pain* 1986; 27:117–126.

61. Jones SL: Electromagnetic field interference and cardiac pacemakers. *Phys Ther* 1976; 56:1013–1018.

62. Kauffman T: Thermoregulation and use of heat and cold, in Littrup Jackson O (ed): *Therapeutic Considerations for the Elderly*. New York, Churchill Livingstone, 1987.

63. Klemp P, Staberg B, Korsgard J, et al: Reduced blood flow in fibromyotic muscles during ultrasound therapy. *Scand J Rehabil Med* 1982; 15:21–23.

64. Kloth L, Morrison MA, Ferguson BH: *Therapeutic Microwave and Shortwave Diathermy. A Review of Thermal Effectiveness, Safe Use, and State of the Art.* Rockville, Md, US Department of Health and Human Services, HHS Publication FDA 85-8237, 1984.

65. Knight KL: *Cryotherapy: Theory, Technique, and Physiology.* Chattanooga, Tenn, Chattanooga Corporation, 1985.

66. Kremer E, Atkinson JH, Ignelzi RJ: Measurement of pain: Patient preference does not confound pain measurement. *Pain* 1981; 10:241–248.

67. Krupa LR, Vener AM: Hazards of drug use among the elderly. *Gerontologist* 1979; 19:90–94.

68. Kwentus JA, Harkins SW, Lignon N, et al: Current concepts of geriatric pain and its treatment. *Geriatrics* 1985; 40:48–57.

69. Langley GB, Sheppeard H: Transcutaneous electrical nerve stimulation (TNS) and its relationship to placebo therapy: A review. *N Z Med J* 1987; 100:215–217.

70. Langley GB, Sheppeard H, Johnson M, et al: The analgesic effects of transcutaneous electrical nerve stimulation and placebo in chronic pain patients. A double blind non-crossover comparison. *Rheumatol Int* 1984; 4:119–123.

71. Lavsky-Shulan M, Wallace RB, Kohout FJ, et al: Prevalence and functional correlates of low back pain in the elderly: The Iowa 65+ rural health study. *J Am Geriatr Soc* 1985; 33:23–28.

72. Lehmann JF (ed): *Therapeutic Heat and Cold,* ed 3. Baltimore, Williams & Wilkins, 1982.

73. Leijon G, Boivie J: Central post-stroke pain—the effect of high and low frequency TENS. *Pain* 1989; 38:187–191.

74. Leo KC: Use of electrical stimulation at acupuncture points for the treatment of reflex sympathetic dystrophy in a child. A case report. *Phys Ther* 1983; 63:957–959.

75. Leo KC, Dostal WF, Bossen DG, et al: Effect of transcutaneous electrical nerve stimulation characteristics on clinical pain. *Phys Ther* 1986; 66:200–205.

76. Leseberg KA, Schunk C: TENS and geriatrics. *Clin Manage Phys Ther* 1990; 10:23–25.

77. Levi SJ, Maihafer GC: Traditional approaches to pain, in Echternach JL (ed): *Pain. Clinics in Physical Therapy,* vol 12. New York, Churchill Livingstone, 1987.

78. Levy A, Dalith M, Abramovici A, et al: Transcutaneous electrical nerve stimulation in experimental acute arthritis. *Arch Phys Med Rehabil* 1987; 68:75–78.

79. Lewis D, Lewis B, Sturrock RD: Transcutaneous electrical nerve stimulation in osteoarthritis: A therapeutic alternative. *Ann Rheum Dis* 1984; 43:47–49.

80. Liang MH, Fortin P: The management of osteoarthritis of the hip and knees (editorial). *New Engl J Med* 1991; 325:125–127.

81. Linzer M, Long DM: Transcutaneous neural stimulation for relief of pain. *IEEE Trans Biomed Eng* 1976; 23:341–344.

82. Mannheimer C, Carlsson CA: The analgesic effect of transcutaneous electrical nerve stimulation (TNS) in patients with rheumatoid arthritis. A comparative study of different pulse patterns. *Pain* 1979; 6:329–334.

83. Mannheimer JS, Lampe GN: *Clinical Transcutaneous Electrical Nerve Stimulation.* Philadelphia, FA Davis, 1984.

84. Melzack R: *The Puzzle of Pain.* New York, Basic Books, 1973.

85. Melzack R: The McGill pain questionnaire: Major properties and scoring methods. *Pain* 1975; 1:277–299.

86. Melzack R (ed): *Pain Measurement and Assessment.* New York, Raven Press, 1983.

87. Melzack R: The short form McGill pain questionnaire. *Pain* 1987; 30:191–197.

88. Merskey H (ed): Classification of chronic pain. Descriptions of chronic pain syndromes and definitions of pain terms. *Pain* 1986; (suppl 3): S1–S226.

89. Michlovitz SL: *Thermal Agents in Rehabilitation,* ed 2. Philadelphia, FA Davis, 1990.

90. Middaugh SJ, Levin RB, Kee WG, et al: Chronic pain: Its treatment in geriatric and younger patients. *Arch Phys Med Rehabil* 1988; 69:1021–1026.

91. Miller BA, Smith KB, Real JL, et al: A comparison of modulated-rate and conventional TENS (abstract). *Phys Ther* 1984; 64:744.

92. Minor MA, Hewitt JE, Webel RR, et al: Efficacy of physical conditioning exercise in patients with rheumatoid arthritis and osteoarthritis. *Arthritis Rheum* 1989; 32:1396–1405.

93. Morgan J, Furst DE: Implications of drug therapy in the elderly. *Clin Rheum Dis* 1986; 12:227–244.

94. Moritani T, deVries HA: Potential for gross muscle hypertrophy in older men. *J Gerontol* 1980; 35:672–682.

95. Moskovich R: Neck pain in the elderly: Common causes and management. *Geriatrics* 1988; 43:65–70, 77, 81–82, 85–90.

96. Myers DB, Grennan DM, Palmer DG: Hand grip function in patients with rheumatoid arthritis. *Arch Phys Med Rehabil* 1980; 61:369–373.

97. Nation EM, Warfield CA: Pain in the elderly. *Hosp Pract* 1989; 24:113, 117–118.

98. Nelson RM, Currier DP (eds): *Clinical Electrotherapy,* ed 2. Norwalk, Conn, Appleton & Lange, 1987.

99. Nolan MF: A chronological indexing of the clinical and basic science literature concerning transcutaneous electrical nerve stimulation (TENS) 1967–1987. Section on Clinical Electrophysiology, Alexandria, Va, American Physical Therapy Association, 1988.

100. Ohnhaus EE, Adler R: Methodological problems in the measurement of pain. A comparison between the verbal rating scale and the visual analogue scale. *Pain* 1975; 1:379–384.

101. Olin BR, Hunsaker LM, Covington TR, et al (eds): *Drug Facts and Comparisons.* St Louis, JB Lippincott, 1989.

102. Paris DL, Bayres F, Gucker B: Effects of the neuroprobe in the treatment of second-degree ankle inversion sprains. *Phys Ther* 1983; 63:35–40.

103. Pochaczevsky R: Assessment of back pain by contact thermography of extremity dermatomes. *Orthop Rev* 1983; 12:45–58.

104. Portenoy RK: Optimal pain control in elderly cancer patients. *Geriatrics* 1987; 42:33–41.

105. Portenoy RK, Farkash A: Practical management of nonmalignant pain in the elderly. *Geriatrics* 1988; 43:29–40, 44–47.

106. Robinson D, Davis J, Niles A, et al: Relation of sex and aging to monoamine oxidase activity of human brain plasma and platelets. *Arch Gen Psychiatry* 1971; 24:536–539.

107. Rooney SM, Jain S, McCornack P, et al: A comparison of pulmonary function tests for post-thoracotomy pain using

cryoanalgesia and transcutaneous nerve stimulation. *Ann Thorac Surg* 1986; 41:204–207.

108. Roy R, Thomas MR: A survey of chronic pain in an elderly population. *Can Fam Physician* 1986; 32:513–516.

109. Roy R, Thomas MR: Elderly persons with and without pain: A comparative study. *Clin J Pain* 1987; 3:102–106.

110. Sanders SH: Toward a practical system for the automatic measurement of "up time" in chronic pain patients. *Pain* 1980; 9:103–109.

111. Scott J, Huskisson EC: Graphic representation of pain. *Pain* 1976; 2:175–184.

112. Shurr DG, Cook TM: *Prosthetics and Orthotics*. Norwalk, Conn, Appleton & Lange, 1990.

113. Smidt GL, Herring T, Amundsen L, et al: Assessment of abdominal and back extensor function. A quantitative approach and results for chronic low-back pain patients. *Spine* 1983; 8:211–219.

114. Smith MJ, Hutchins RC, Hehenberger D: Transcutaneous neural stimulation use in postoperative knee rehabilitation. *Am J Sports Med* 1983; 11:75–82.

115. Smyth NPD, Parsonnet V, Escher DJW, et al: The pacemaker patient and the electromagnetic environment. *JAMA* 1974; 227:1412.

116. Snyder-Mackler L, Robinson AJ: *Clinical Electrophysiology: Electrotherapy and Electrophysiological Testing*. Baltimore, Williams & Wilkins, 1989.

117. Sternbach R: *Pain: A Psychophysiological Analysis*. New York, Academic Press, 1968.

118. Sternbach R: Evaluation of pain relief. *Surg Neurol* 1975; 4:199–201.

119. Sternbach RA: Psychophysiology of pain. *Int J Psychiatry Med* 1975; 6:63–73.

120. Sternbach RA, Murphy RW, Timmermans G, et al: Measuring the severity of clinical pain, in Bonica JJ (ed): *Advances in Neurology*, vol 4. New York, Raven Press, 1974.

121. Svarcova J, Trnasky K, Zvarova J: The influence of ultrasound, galvanic currents and shortwave diathermy on pain intensity in patients with osteoarthritis. *Scand J Rheumatol Suppl* 1988; 67:83–85.

122. Swezey R: Low back pain in the elderly: Practical management concerns. *Geriatrics* 1988; 43:39–44.

123. Tappan RM: *Healing Massage Techniques: Holistic, Classic, and Emerging Methods*, ed 2. Norwalk, Conn, Appleton & Lange, 1988.

124. Thorsteinsson G: *Chronic pain: Use of TENS in the elderly, Geriatrics* 1987; 42:75–77, 81–82.

125. Travel JG, Simons DG: *Myofascial Pain and Dysfunction. The Trigger Point Manual*. Baltimore, Williams & Wilkins, 1983.

126. Tyler E, Caldwell C, Ghia JN: Transcutaneous electrical nerve stimulation: An alternative approach to the management of postoperative pain. *Anesth Analg* 1982; 61:449–456.

127. Verrillo RT: Age related changes in the sensitivity to vibration. *J Gerontol* 1980; 35:185–193.

128. Wall PD: The gate control theory of pain mechanisms. A re-examination and re-statement. *Brain* 1978; 101:1–18.

129. Wall RT: Use of analgesics in the elderly. *Clin Geriatr Med* 1990; 6:345–364.

130. Walsh TD, Leber B: Measurement of chronic pain: Visual analog scales and McGill Melzack pain questionnaire compared, in Bonica JJ, Lindblom U, Iggo A, (eds): *Advances in Pain Research and Therapy*, vol 5. New York, Raven Press, 1983.

131. Wewers ME, Lowe NK: A critical review of visual analogue scales in the measurement of clinical phenomena. *Res Nurs Health* 1990; 13:227–236.

132. Williams J, Harvey J, Tannebaum H: Use of superficial heat vs ice for the rheumatoid arthritic shoulder: A pilot study. *Physiother Can* 1986; 38:8–13.

133. Witte M: Pain control. *J Gerontol Nurs* 1989; 15:32–37.

134. Witters D, Lapp A, Hinckley SM: A descriptive study of transcutaneous electrical nerve stimulation devices and their electrical output characteristics. *J Clin Electrophysiol* 1991; 3:9–16.

135. Wolf SL, Basmajian JV: Intramuscular temperature changes deep to localized cutaneous cold stimulation. *Phys Ther* 1973; 53:1284–1288.

136. Wolf SL, Gersh MR, Rao VR: Examination of electrode placements and stimulating parameters in treating chronic pain with conventional transcutaneous electrical nerve stimulation (TENS). *Pain* 1981; 11:37–47.

137. Workman BS, Ciccone V, Christophidis N: Pain management for the elderly. *Aust Fam Physician* 1989; 18:1515–1521, 1524–1525, 1527.

138. Wright V: Treatment of osteoarthritis of the knees. *Ann Rheum Dis* 1964; 23:389.

139. Zacharkow D: *Posture: Sitting, Standing, Chair Design and Exercise*. Springfield, Ill, Charles C Thomas, 1988.

140. Zimmerman M: Peripheral and central nervous mechanisms of nociception, pain and pain therapy, in Bonica JJ, Liebeskind JC, Albe-Fessard DG (eds): *Advances in Pain Research and Therapy*, vol 3. New York, Raven Press, 1979, pp 3–32.

Chronic Dermal Wounds in Older Adults

Rita A. Wong, M.S., P.T.

INTRODUCTION

Advanced Age and Chronic Dermal Wounds

Chronic dermal wounds occur most frequently in the older population. This higher prevalence in the elderly corresponds to a higher proportion of older adults who suffer from the health problems known to increase the risk of ulcer development and delayed wound healing (Table 19–1). These conditions include (1) circulatory diseases often leading to symptomatic arterial or venous insufficiency, (2) diabetes mellitus, and (3) hypertension. Additionally, frail elders, with multiple medical problems, may have numerous risk factors including nutritional inadequacies, anemia, decreased mobility, and muscle atrophy.

Normal age-related changes in skin alter the rate and quality of wound healing. Dermal wounds occurring in older adults are associated with a slower overall rate of wound healing and weaker, less supple wound scars.[49, 59, 67, 77, 85, 103] These age-related changes do not, however, predispose an older person to nonhealing ulcers. Therefore, the inability of an ulcer to heal represents pathology that warrants vigorous intervention and should not be considered a normal consequence of the aging process. Identification of the underlying cause of the initial ulceration, and delay in normal wound healing, is essential for effective intervention.

Normal Tissue-Healing Process

When a tissue is injured, the body's natural response is to activate the inflammatory process. This process guides each sequential step of tissue repair and protects the wound against invading microorganisms.[109] In young people the presence of blastema cells (the undifferentiated new cells that signal the beginning of tissue repair) becomes evident within about 12 hours of injury. In older people, these cells may not be evident for several days.[49]

Typically, the tissue moves into the proliferative phase within about 3 days in young people and 7 days in older people. In this stage, wound contraction and epithelialization occur. In the final stage of wound repair, the remodeling stage, the wound is no longer open. The connective tissue, which is usually laid down in a fairly random manner in the proliferative stage, becomes better aligned with the stresses put upon it, resulting in a strong, pliable scar. This process can take up to 1 year to complete. With advanced age, the scar is not as strong or pliable. Thus, the scar of an older person is in greater danger of reinjury than the scar of a younger person.[117]

Wound Classification

In general, chronic dermal wounds are classified according to the predominant underlying cause of their occurrence:

arterial insufficiency, venous insufficiency, excessive pressure (decubitus ulcer), and neuropathy (insensitivity). An ulcer can fit into more than one of these categories. Ulcers are also categorized according to their severity. Two different systems of classification are frequently used. The more general classification, often associated with pressure and venous insufficiency ulcers, assigns the ulcer to one of four stages dependent on the depth of the ulcer (Table 19–2). An alternative system, described by Wagner and often associated with neuropathic and arterial insufficiency ulcers, considers depth of the ulcer as well as the health of the surrounding tissues (Table 19–3).[125]

This chapter will discuss the epidemiology, etiology, and clinical signs and symptoms for each of the four general causes of chronic ulcers: arterial insufficiency, venous insufficiency, pressure induced, and neuropathy. Tests used to identify high-risk clients will be described as well as general treatment approaches and interventions.

Regardless of the underlying cause of the ulcer, the general treatment approach includes removal of risk factors that impede the normal healing process (see Table

TABLE 19–1.

Factors That May Delay Wound Healing

1. Inadequate blood supply to the wound
2. Wound infection
3. Inadequate nutrition
4. Adherent scab or eschar
5. Wound edema
6. Venous hypertension
7. Anemia
8. Cigarette smoking
9. Systemic hypertension
10. Decreased capillary membrane diffusion
11. Increased blood glucose levels
12. Medications—steroids, certain immunosuppressive drugs, high doses of antimicrobial agents (e.g., >0.001% povidone-iodine; >0.5% sodium hypochlorite)[51]

TABLE 19–2.

Traditional Classification of Ulcer Stages

Stage	Description
Stage 1	Skin is intact
	Localized erythema
	Redness lasting >50% of the time pressure was applied
Stage 2	Wound involving the epidermis and dermis
	Does *not* extend beyond the dermis
Stage 3	Wound involving epidermis, dermis, and subcutaneous tissue
	Does *not* extend into muscle
Stage 4	Wound involving epidermis, dermis, subcutaneous tissue, muscle, and possibly bone
	May appear small from the surface but could have a deep sinus tract into muscle or bone

TABLE 19–3.

Wagner Classification System of Ulcer Stages

Stage	Description
0	Intact skin
1	Superficial ulcer involving skin only
2	Deep ulcer involving muscle and, perhaps, bone and joint structures
3	Localized infection—may be abscess or osteomyelitis
4	Gangrene, limited to forefoot area
5	Gangrene of the majority of the foot

19–1), augmentation of normal wound healing, and prevention of injury recurrence.[42] The final section of the chapter will identify common interventions for the treatment of dermal wounds, review the rationale for their use, and discuss any special considerations when applying these modalities to older adults. The ultimate goal of intervention is complete closure of the wound with a strong, resilient scar.

Wound Evaluation

Treatment approach will be influenced by the wound characteristics. Therefore, the general appearance of the wound should be noted. Is the wound open or closed? If it is open, what color is the tissue? Is granulation tissue evident? Does the wound look clean and free of necrotic tissue and pus? Is there any drainage from the wound? If yes, is the drainage clear and thin, purulent and thick, or bloody? How much drainage is there? A wound culture should be taken from the deepest part of the wound, not simply from the surface tissue.

If the wound is covered, what is covering it? Is it covered by thick, crusty material; tightly adherent eschar; thick, purulent material; or healthy granulation tissue? Adherent eschar, purulent materials, and necrotic tissue need to be removed in order for wound healing to progress. Wound infection needs to be eliminated, and excessive fluid loss needs to be brought under control.

The external dimensions of the wound can be reliably traced by placing a material such as transparent sterile X-ray film against the wound and tracing its outline.[90] Graph paper can then be used to calculate the approximate size of the wound. The depth of the wound can be determined by placing a sterile, cotton-tipped probe into the wound and recording the depth of penetration of the probe.

The Health Care Team

Physical therapists working with patients with chronic dermal wounds are usually working as part of an interdisciplinary team. Each team member brings essential skills and

knowledge. The team may include, but is not limited to, a family practitioner or other physician, vascular surgeon, nurse, dietitian, physical therapist, occupational therapist, orthotist, and podiatrist.

The family practitioner will evaluate and treat the patient for general medical conditions that may impede the overall healing process. A vascular surgeon will determine the location and severity of vascular insufficiencies and the appropriateness of various surgical approaches for re-establishing more normal vascular hemodynamics (either arterial or venous) as well as the need for skin grafting to close the wound. Nursing will develop and implement a care plan to monitor the wound environment; minimize risk factors for delayed wound healing; and make dressing changes as needed to maintain a clean, healthy tissue environment supportive to healing. A dietitian should plan the specific dietary needs of the patient to ensure adequate nutritional support during the healing process. Other health professionals can be consulted as needed, depending on the patient's specific needs. For example, an orthotist may fabricate appropriate footwear for the client with an ulcer on the foot.

The role of physical therapy is usually adjunctive. Through the use of physical agents, gait modifications, selective exercise activities, and patient education, physical therapists provide important augmentation of the healing process. Our interdisciplinary team role must always be considered in our overall treatment planning. Both patient and care givers must become an integral part of the health care team, as the healing of a chronic dermal wound is a long-term process. Both care givers and patient need to understand the purpose of each intervention and recognize inappropriate treatment responses.

Good communication between all members of the team is essential. Each team member should understand the unique perspective of other members of the team and work to build a consistent, effective overall treatment approach. Since the purpose of this chapter is to address the specific role of physical therapy in wound management, the specific activities of other team members have only been mentioned briefly. This does not imply less value for the role of other team members but simply reflects the main focus of the chapter.

CHRONIC DERMAL WOUNDS FROM ARTERIAL INSUFFICIENCY

Epidemiology

Arteriosclerosis obliterans (ASO) represents about 90% to 95% of all cases of chronic occlusive arterial disease.[40, 93] ASO is also known as *atherosclerotic vascular disease* and *obliterative arteriosclerosis*.[40, 92] Most dermal ulcers associated with arterial insufficiency are secondary to ASO.[40]

Ulcers related to ASO indicate a severe compromise of local circulation and thus tissue nutrition. Typically, the distal foot, particularly the tips of the toes, is the first area to undergo ischemic damage.

ASO affects men more frequently than women, and prevalence increases with age. Paris et al., in a recent study of nursing home patients, found that 35% of the nursing home residents who were between 76 and 80 years of age had significant arterial disease.[104] This number gradually increased with increasing age. Approximately 65% of patients over 90 years of age had significant arterial disease. Petermans evaluated 261 elderly patients admitted to one acute care hospital in Belgium for medical problems not associated with vascular disease.[105] In this sample, with a mean age of 81, 58% were found to have ASO.

Etiology

The formation of atherosclerotic plaques begins in childhood with the laying down of fatty streaks within the intimal wall of the medium and large arteries. Over time, fibrous plaques develop. The progression to atherosclerotic vessel occlusion with onset of symptoms generally occurs very slowly over many decades.[40, 52] The body accommodates to this chronic, slowly progressive decrease in perfusion by producing collateral circulation in the area served by the occluded vessel and by decreasing peripheral vessel resistance so that blood can pass through the artery more easily. These adaptations delay the onset of ischemic symptoms until substantial narrowing of the lumen of the vessel occurs.[73, 93]

In the person with severe arterial insufficiency, minor trauma can result in a nonhealing ulcer. Tissue injury from a poorly fitting shoe, an ingrown toenail, or stubbing one's toe are examples of situations that can lead to dermal wounds in the person with ASO. In this individual, the increased oxygen demand that accompanies the normal inflammatory response to tissue injury may go unmet due to the inability to increase blood flow into the area. This unmet demand may lead to further tissue ischemia and, perhaps, cell death.

Risk factors for the development of ASO include cigarette smoking, diabetes mellitus, high intake of saturated fats, being a male, and sedentary life-style.[40, 63, 78, 104] Although the exact mechanism through which cigarette smoking exacerbates ASO is unknown, it is clear that individuals who smoke at least 20 cigarettes per day have much greater risk of developing symptomatic ASO than nonsmokers.[60, 78, 82, 93] The elimination of cigarette smoking is very important in controlling the progression of ASO.

Individuals with hypertension have a greater risk of complications from ASO than nonhypertensives.[40] Hyperglycemia related to diabetes mellitus has traditionally been believed to increase the risk of circulatory compromise and limb amputation. This increased amputation risk may relate more closely to the accelerated rate of development of peripheral neuropathies in people with diabetes mellitus who are hyperglycemic than to an accelerated circulatory compromise.[61, 82] Peripheral neuropathy is a major contributor to plantar ulcers—ulcers that often develop despite the presence of adequate circulation. Cigarette smoking has been closely associated with progression of arterial insufficiency and increased prevalence of amputation among patients with diabetes mellitus despite good conservative wound care of distal wounds.[82] It is imperative that individuals with arterial insufficiency stop smoking.

Clinical Signs and Symptoms of ASO in the Elderly

Elderly people, particularly those over age 70, may have atypical presentation of ASO. It is common in the elderly to have substantial pathology, even leading to gangrene of the part, without any complaints of intermittent claudication, one of the first and most commonly observed signs of ASO in the younger population.[63] Intermittent claudication stems from inadequate blood flow through the exercising muscle, usually occurring in the calf. The pain is first noted during ambulation and, characteristically, quickly disappears once the person sits down and stops contracting the calf muscles.

Elderly patients may complain that their legs feel heavy or cold, rather than painful. Characteristic changes in the skin below the level of circulatory compromise are frequently observed. Ulcers may develop on the toes (Fig 19–1).

Clinical Examination for Arterial Insufficiency

Halperin suggests that any elderly patient with trophic skin changes or risk factors for underlying arterial disease receive a simple bedside screening test for adequacy of arterial circulation.[63] More definitive testing should be done on any client with an abnormal response. During the first step in this procedure, the supine patient's legs are raised 60 to 75 degrees and maintained in this position. If the limb quickly becomes pale or cool, impaired systolic pressure is strongly suggested. The patient performs 20 to 30 repetitions of ankle pumps in this leg-elevated position. No substantial change in skin color and no drop in skin temperature suggest adequate perfusion pressure.

If the leg-elevated position proves symptomatic, then the severity of the insufficiency is evaluated next. The patient sits up and the legs are dangled off the side of the bed while the quality and time lag for color changes in the foot

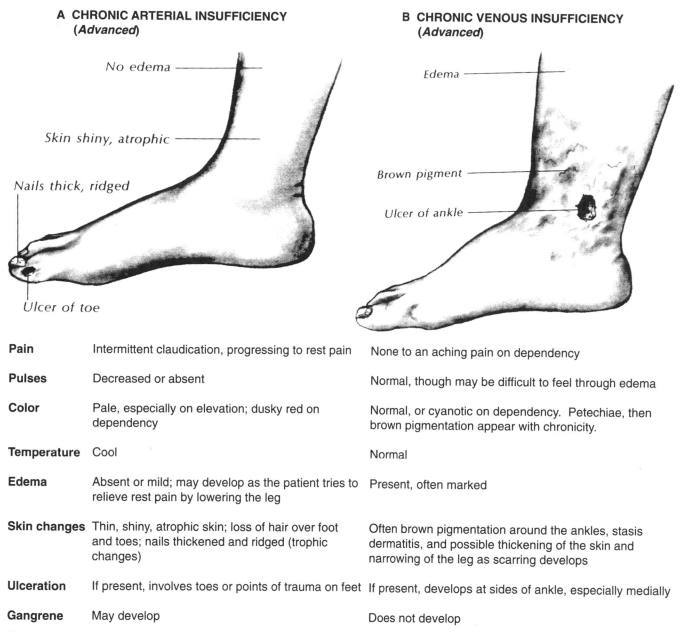

A CHRONIC ARTERIAL INSUFFICIENCY
(*Advanced*)

No edema

Skin shiny, atrophic

Nails thick, ridged

Ulcer of toe

B CHRONIC VENOUS INSUFFICIENCY
(*Advanced*)

Edema

Brown pigment

Ulcer of ankle

	A Chronic Arterial Insufficiency	B Chronic Venous Insufficiency
Pain	Intermittent claudication, progressing to rest pain	None to an aching pain on dependency
Pulses	Decreased or absent	Normal, though may be difficult to feel through edema
Color	Pale, especially on elevation; dusky red on dependency	Normal, or cyanotic on dependency. Petechiae, then brown pigmentation appear with chronicity.
Temperature	Cool	Normal
Edema	Absent or mild; may develop as the patient tries to relieve rest pain by lowering the leg	Present, often marked
Skin changes	Thin, shiny, atrophic skin; loss of hair over foot and toes; nails thickened and ridged (trophic changes)	Often brown pigmentation around the ankles, stasis dermatitis, and possible thickening of the skin and narrowing of the leg as scarring develops
Ulceration	If present, involves toes or points of trauma on feet	If present, develops at sides of ankle, especially medially
Gangrene	May develop	Does not develop

FIG 19–1.
Characteristics of chronic insufficiency of **(A)** arteries and **(B)** veins. (From Bates B: *Guide to Physical Examination and History Taking,* ed 4. Philadelphia, 1987, JB Lippincott, p 420. Used by permission.)

are observed and the time until the veins on the dorsum of the foot become distended is noted. Responses can be divided into three categories.

The patient is placed into category 1, a normal response, if color returns to the feet within 10 seconds and veins refill within 15 seconds. Category 2, a moderate obstruction, is suggested if the return of color to the feet requires 15 to 30 seconds and the venous refilling requires about 30 seconds. The client is placed into category 3, severe obstruction, if it takes more than 45 seconds for color

to return to the feet and for venous refilling to occur. In all three categories, venous filling time may not be reliable if the client has concurrent venous insufficiency.

Objective Tests for Arterial Insufficiency

Noninvasive hemodynamic assessment of blood flow can be done through flow-detecting Doppler ultrasound, volume-detecting plethysmography, or comparative assessment of ankle and arm systolic blood pressures. Doppler ultrasound is a simple, reliable, noninvasive test of arterial circulation. The frequency of the ultrasound unit is such that the pattern of soundwaves reflected from the moving blood provides a very sensitive indicator of blood flow in the area being sonated. The test is performed by first occluding blood flow to the lower leg with a blood pressure cuff. The ultrasound is applied as the cuff deflates, and the systolic pressure is recorded.[89]

Meaningful values are obtained by comparing the blood pressure response of the arm with that of the ankle, creating the ankle/arm, or the tibial/brachial, index. In young adults the ratio of ankle to arm pressure is 1:1, giving a pressure "index" of 1. In normal older adults the ankle pressure frequently exceeds the arm pressure, thus increasing the index to greater than 1. An ankle/arm index (A/A index) of less than 0.9 is suggestive of vascular disease.[92, 104] It is commonly believed that a value less than 0.7 or 0.75 confirms arterial disease.[33, 104] A value less than 0.5 indicates severe impairment. An ankle/arm index of greater than 0.45 is believed necessary for a foot ulcer to heal.[15]

Arteriography is the most invasive of the evaluative procedures and is usually reserved for patients for whom vascular reconstructive surgery is contemplated. Arteriography requires the injection of radiopaque dye into an artery with subsequent radiographic visualization of restrictions to the flow of dye through the arteries. This is considered to be a very reliable method of evaluating the specific location and severity of the vascular occlusions.

General Treatment Approaches

When the dermal wound is triggered by arterial insufficiency, improving arterial circulation as well as eliminating risk factors for delayed wound healing (Table 19–1) take priority. Arterial bypass surgery, endarterectomy, and transluminal angioplasty are frequently utilized. Arterially insufficient chronic dermal wounds do not usually occur until the occlusion is severe, potentially threatening limb viability. If the ankle/arm index is less than 0.45 or if substantial gangrene is present, the probability of wound healing with conservative intervention is low. Therefore, surgical intervention for the re-establishment of blood flow through the occluded segment usually takes precedence at this time. If the client has no substantial contraindications to surgery and the location of the occlusion is amenable to surgical intervention, this is the treatment of choice.[40] These procedures frequently provide at least temporary (1 to 3 years) circulatory patency. A sympathectomy is often used to inhibit vasorestrictive tone in the lower extremities if surgery is contraindicated or has proven unsuccessful.

Physical Therapy Intervention

A number of physical therapy interventions may be employed in the attainment of treatment goals (Table 19–4). Low-intensity electrical stimulation for tissue repair (ESTR) applied directly over the wound may augment normal healing and decrease wound infection. Whirlpool at neutral skin temperature will assist in wound cleaning and debridement. Hot packs placed over the low back may, reflexly, enhance blood flow to the feet. Also, patient and care-giver education in wound care and prevention of reinjury are essential components of any intervention.

CHRONIC DERMAL WOUNDS FROM VENOUS INSUFFICIENCY

Epidemiology

Fitzpatrick notes that "chronic venous insufficiency [CVI] of the legs is one of the most common medical problems in the elderly."[56] Coon et al. in a 1973 study found that CVI affected 7 million people in the United States and that over 500,000 of these individuals suffered from chronic ulcerations of their lower extremities.[35] Venous ulcers make up between 70% and 90% of all ulcers of the foot and lower leg.[65] Predisposing factors for the development of CVI are a history of thrombophlebitis, family history of venous insufficiency, and trauma.[6]

Unlike ulcers of arterial origin, venous ulcers rarely lead to limb amputation. However, venous ulcers tend to be very chronic problems, with a high incidence of recurrence. The ulcers are easy targets for infection. The decreased movement of blood through venous varicosities and incompetent valves increase the risk of acute thrombophlebitis with its potentially life-threatening consequences.

In a comprehensive study of the population of Göteborg, Sweden, 1,377 patients sought medical care for leg or foot ulcers in 1980.[65] At least 70% of these ulcers were believed to be of venous origin. The median age of the patients with ulcers was 73, and the majority were women. Men developed ulcers, on average, 5 to 10 years earlier than women. The incidence of ulcers increased rapidly with increasing age—1% of the 70-year-old population compared with 5% of the 90-year-old population. The Göteborg study also indicated that patients with ulcers had double the mortality rate of matched individuals without ulcers, primarily due to a higher-than-average rate of ischemic heart disease in these patients.

Etiology

In the lower extremities, the venous system is made up of deep, superficial, and communicating veins that connect

TABLE 19–4.

Summary of Physical Therapy Modalities for Wound Healing

Therapeutic Modality	Treatment Goals	Physiologic Effects of Modality	Expected Treatment Outcome			
			Arterial	Venous	Pressure	Neuropathic
Low-intensity electrical stimulation	Augment wound healing ↓ Wound infection	Stimulate endogenous bioelectric activity Bactericidal	+	+ +	+ +	?
Compression devices Dressings Elastic bandages Elastic stockings Pumps	↓ Wound and limb edema ↑ Wound nutrition	↑ Lymphatic and venous return ↓ Tissue colloid osmotic pressure Normalize fluid dynamics ↑ Fibrinolytic activity at wound margins	NI	+ +	+*	+†
Whirlpool	Clean wound and prepare for debridement Ease wound dressing removal	Water agitation helps remove debris, topical medications residue Softens necrotic, adherent tissue and bandages	+‡	+‡§	+	+
Nonthermal ultrasound	Augment wound healing	Accelerates or reactivates normal wound-healing process	?	+	+	?
Hyperbaric oxygen	↑ Wound nutrition	↑ O_2 saturation at the wound	+	+	+	?
Total contact casting/walking splint	↓ High plantar pressures to allow safe PWB gait Enhance wound healing	Redistributes plantar pressures to unload high-pressure areas Immobilizes irritated tissues to foster healing Minimizes deconditioning by allowing ambulation	NI	NI	NI	+ +
Consensual heating of low back	↑ Blood flow to feet	Induces reflex vasodilation of distal blood vessels by temperature of low back	+	NI	NI	NI
Patient/care giver education	Maximize wound healing Prevent wound recurrence	Client and/or care givers are able to take an active role in achieving wound healing and preventing wound recurrence	+ +	+ +	+ +	+ +

*Compression dressing if wound edema is present.
†Use compression devices if limb edema is present.
‡Use neutral water temperature.
§Avoid dependent limb position.
+ = some, but limited, evidence of positive outcomes; + + = substantial evidence of positive outcomes; ? = insufficient evidence to determine outcome; NI = modality is not indicated for this wound type; PWB = partial weight bearing.

the superficial and deep veins. In general, blood from the superficial veins returns to the heart by flowing through the communicating veins into the deep veins.

Unlike arteries, veins have very little smooth muscle. Therefore, active venous constriction is minimal. Veins also have a lower resistance to passive dilation from elevated local blood pressure than arteries. Movement of venous blood is dependent on blood flow pressure gradients and external compression of the deep veins by contraction of the calf muscles, particularly when the legs are in the dependent position. Competent venous valves control the direction of blood flow, only allowing movement toward the heart.

When the calf muscles contract, the deep veins are constricted, and the blood empties from them and moves toward the heart. Subsequent relaxation of the calf muscles with reopening of the deep veins provides a low-resistance pathway for blood to be drawn from superficial into deep veins.[24] During active calf muscle contraction, the blood pressure in the superficial veins drops from its normal value of 90 mm Hg with quiet standing to 20 to 30 mm Hg.[24] Damage to a venous valve may make this blood flow pattern ineffective, thus allowing blood to move in both directions.[94] This abnormal blood flow pattern results in unremitting hypertension in the affected superficial veins, which is believed to be the primary underlying cause of venous ulcers.[24] The traditional belief that venous ulcers result from inadequate oxygenation due to blood stagnation, although still taught, was proven incorrect many years ago.[17] Indeed, the blood flow in the area of a chronic venous wound is generally very good, but the diffusion of nutrients and waste products appears to be deficient.

Browse contends that ulcers occur because of changes in the microcirculation of the skin in response to superficial vein hypertension.[24] He presents strong evidence that unremitting hypertension in the superficial veins leads to a "stretching" of the interendothelial pores of the venules (Fig 19–2). With an increase in the size of these pores, larger molecules are allowed to diffuse out of the vein, changing the colloidal osmotic pressure gradients with resultant interstitial edema.

The diffusion of the large molecule fibrinogen into the interstitial space has been implicated in the delayed healing of venous ulcers.[6, 24, 25] In the presence of venous hypertension, normal fibrinolysis does not occur. A layer of fibrinogen gradually builds up around the involved capillaries. This excess of fibrin impedes diffusion across capillary membranes.

Clinical Examination for Venous Insufficiency

The signs and symptoms of CVI are outlined in Figure 19–1. The most common site of ulcer development is just

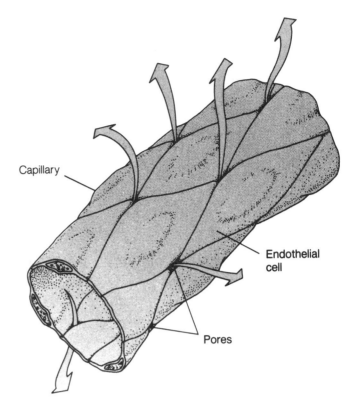

FIG 19–2.
Interendothelial pores of capillaries. As theorized by Browse, these pores can be stretched by prolonged, increased capillary pressure, thus allowing plasma proteins to escape into interstitial fluid. (From Sherwood L: *Fundamentals of Physiology: A Human Perspective.* St Paul, Minn, West Publishing, 1991, p 238. Used by permission.)

above the medial malleolus. Typically, the ulcer is shallow, irregularly shaped, and persistent and often becomes worse with prolonged walking or sitting with the legs dependent.

Tests for Venous Insufficiency

Strain gauge plethysmography and photoplethysmography, both noninvasive procedures, are traditional evaluation procedures for determining the competence of the venous valves.[108] With increasing frequency, Doppler ultrasound is being used to detect venous obstruction and incompetent valves. This form of diagnostic ultrasound is noninvasive and appears to be a very sensitive indicator of venous blood flow.

If surgical intervention is contemplated, then the more invasive venography is performed. The injection of radiopaque dye into the vein is followed by radiographic visualization of the vein. This technique outlines the exact locations of occlusions and valve incompetencies.

General Treatment Approaches

Decreasing the superficial venous hypertension is the key to preventing and healing venous ulcers. Queral and Dagher caution that "CVI of the lower extremities, leading to ulceration, is largely an incurable disease. However, treatment is possible and amelioration of the ulcer and the insufficiency is achievable."[108]

Conservative management of a CVI ulcer focuses on strategies to decrease limb edema. Complete bed rest with legs elevated will accomplish this goal, but this strategy is neither practical nor safe for most elderly clients.[62] The use of various external compression devices when legs are dependent are effective for many individuals. Surgical interventions to correct venous incompetency, such as vein ligation and stripping, are most successful when valve incompetence occurs in superficial veins and less successful with deep vein incompetence.[108] Successful treatment will be temporary, however, unless the patient complies with strategies to minimize lower extremity edema and hypertensive stress on a long-term basis.[45]

Physical Therapy Intervention

An array of treatment approaches, summarized in Table 19–4 and discussed in detail later in this chapter, are available to the physical therapist to meet the goals outlined above. Edema may be controlled through the long-term use of compression devices such as custom-fit or ready-made elastic stockings, standard or specialized elastic bandages, Unna's paste boots, and compression orthoses. In the presence of moderate or severe edema, the use of an intermittent, or sequential, compression pump may be warranted in addition to external compression garments or boots.[2] Use of these pumps is contraindicated in the presence of marked arterial insufficiency, local infection, acute thrombophlebitis, or lymph node infection.

Nonthermal ultrasound has been used to enhance the normal healing process. In selected cases, whirlpool may be beneficial to soften eschar prior to debridement or to clean the wound. Whirlpool should be used judiciously, however, to avoid increasing lower extremity edema and should not be continued once the wound is clean and debrided. Hyperbaric oxygen also has been used successfully to treat CVI ulcers.

Complete bed rest with limb elevation will foster wound healing, but this is neither practical nor safe for most elderly persons. The utilization of compression devices combined with frequent bouts of limb elevation is considered the hallmark of wound healing in CVI.

PRESSURE (DECUBITUS) ULCERS

Epidemiology

There is little doubt that pressure sores are a major problem confronting therapists and health practitioners in nearly every geriatric setting in the United States. Eighty-two percent of patients with decubitus ulcers are over 70 years of age.[124] Brandeis and colleagues have reported that prevalence estimates of pressure ulcers in the nursing home population have ranged from as low as 2.6% to as high as 24%.[20] In a study they conducted among 19,889 nursing home residents in 51 nursing homes, they found that 17.4% of the residents had pressure ulcers upon admission; 11.3% were classified as stage 2 or worse. This figure contrasts with an 8.9% prevalence of pressure sores among residents, which included 6.8% of residents with ulcers classified as stage 2 or worse. The presence of a pressure sore upon admission is an important clinical finding with grave implications. Berloz and Wilking found that patients who were admitted to a nursing home with a pressure sore were nearly twice as likely to die within 6 weeks of admission as patients who did not have a similar lesion upon admission.[11]

The magnitude of the problem is not merely confined to nursing homes. Allman and coworkers found that the prevalence of pressure sores among hospitalized patients was 4.7%.[4] Some have proposed that 10% to 25% of elderly patients admitted to a hospital will develop pressure sores, most often in the first 2 weeks.[36] There is some evidence to suggest that a number of factors influence the development of pressure sores in hospitalized elderly: fractures, fecal incontinence, hypoalbuminemia, and cognition.[4, 36] In a study of almost 5,000 nursing home residents, Spector et al. concluded that older age; being a male, nonwhite, or unable to bathe; needing help to transfer; being catheterized; experiencing fecal incontinence; being confined to bed; having been recently hospitalized; and having no rehabilitation potential were significantly related to having a pressure ulcer.[120]

Pressure ulcers can involve intensive therapeutic efforts by a multiplicity of professionals. The costs of total patient care for treatment of these lesions have ranged from $4,000 to $40,000, depending on the stage of the wound.[20]

Etiology

Prolonged pressure and shear forces, particularly over bony prominences, can impair blood flow, leading to tissue ischemia and ulcer formation.[10, 41] The duration of the pressure load, degree of accompanying shear forces, and general health status of the client have substantial impact on the amount of pressure needed to provoke ulcer formation.[10]

Normal capillary pressure ranges from 20 to 35 mm Hg.[10] Individuals with normal circulation can tolerate prolonged pressures much higher than 35 mm Hg without tissue damage. Part of the reason for this is that the pressure through the capillaries can increase up to diastolic levels in response to an outside pressure stress.[72] The skin, in particular, with its inherent ability to shunt blood, has a high tolerance for anoxia. Shearing forces cause a distortion of small blood vessels. Thus, the greater the shearing forces, the less external pressure is needed to occlude blood flow.[53] A very common source of shear force is lying in bed with the head of the bed elevated, particularly at an angle greater than 45 degrees (Fig 19–3). In this position, the skin overlying the ischium and sacrum stays in one position, and the underlying tissue moves in response to the forces of gravity and the weight of the body.

Deeper structures are more susceptible to ischemic damage in response to high shear forces than the skin.[10, 115] This often results in an ulcer that, although small in appearance, has a deep sinus tract. It is estimated that the typical pressures exerted by lying on a bony prominence will cause tissue damage within 2 to 6 hours.[112] Recent studies suggest that a normal individual without risk factors for pressure ulcers can probably withstand much longer periods of positioning-induced pressure without ulcer formation.[41, 112] For individuals with risk factors, the 2- to 6-hour time period is accurate.

Common risk factors for the development of pressure ulcers are identified in Table 19–5. Advanced age, per se,

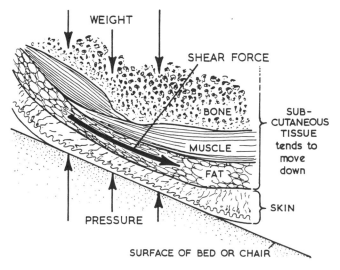

FIG 19–3.
Shear forces occurring when lying in bed with head of bed angled up. The skin overlying the trunk remains stationary as the body shifts downward, resulting in torsion of underlying tissue, including blood vessels. (From Fernandez S: *Physiotherapy* 1987; 73:451. Used by permission.)

TABLE 19–5.
Risk Factors for the Development of Pressure Ulcers

1. Immobility
2. Decreased sensation
3. Muscle atrophy
4. Decreased circulation
5. Positioning allowing high shear forces
6. Poor nutritional status
7. Incontinence
8. Site of a previous ulcer
9. Edema at the site of increased pressure
10. Anemia

does not increase one's risk of developing a pressure ulcer, but many chronic conditions common to old age frequently place older people in a high-risk category.[10, 95] Additionally, normal skin changes of advanced age such as decreased extensibility of the skin and decreased skin blood flow may compromise the tissue's ability to adapt to a compressing force.[39]

Recently, Schubert has implicated low systolic blood pressure, particularly prevalent in ill individuals over 70 years of age, as an additional risk factor for the development of pressure ulcers.[115, 116] He found that healthy adults, both young and old, demonstrate similar circulatory responses to pressure. Hospitalized ill elders, however, demonstrated relatively lower systolic blood pressures. In ill elders, lower systolic pressure was significantly correlated to low peak skin blood cell flux and a slower circulatory recovery postocclusion. This suggests that low blood pressure may be an important risk factor for the development of a decubitus ulcer in the frail elderly patient.

Clinical Signs and Symptoms of Decubitus Ulcer Formation

Pressure ulcers do not occur spontaneously. At least one and often multiple risk factors for pressure ulcers are present (Table 19–5). The patient who develops a decubitus ulcer is usually ill and probably has limited mobility, often including limited bed mobility. Sensory loss or decreased cognition may impair the patient's awareness of excessive pressure.

Skin redness over areas exposed to pressure, particularly bony prominences, may indicate damaging pressure levels. A transitory hyperemic response occurs any time pressure is removed from the skin. Normally, this redness should disappear within 50% to 75% of the time the pressure was applied.[83] Redness that lasts longer than this time period indicates a stage 1 decubitus ulcer formation (Table 19–2). Because of the tendency for damage to deep structures prior to superficial structures, the presence of prolonged hyperemia, even in the absence of observable tissue damage, should be taken very seriously. The potential damage beneath the skin may be very difficult to identify. Areas at greatest risk of pressure ulceration are illustrated in Figure 19–4.

Objective Evaluation of Decubitus Ulcer Risk

Few clinical tools are readily available to measure the effects of external pressure on blood flow through the involved tissue. Laser Doppler fluxmetry, which measures microcirculatory changes, may be of some value. This device measures the number of skin blood cells in a given portion of skin. *Skin blood cell flux* (SBF) is defined as "the product of the number of skin blood cells and their velocities within the measuring volume."[116] When applying this technique, blood flow is temporarily occluded, and when pressure is released, the rate of blood flow change is measured. This technique can identify individuals with sluggish postpressure responses and low occlusive pressures, which may help to identify high-risk patients. The limitation of this technique is that it only measures very superficial skin blood flow, and it is not readily available in clinical settings.

If arterial or venous insufficiency is suspected, the vascular tests identified in previous sections should be performed. No evaluation technique is clinically available to

reliably measure the shear forces that are strongly implicated in tissue breakdown, particularly at the sacrum and ischium.

General Treatment Approaches

The key to preventing decubitus ulcers and reversing the delayed wound healing associated with them is pressure relief. The patient, or the care givers, need to ensure frequent positioning changes and consistent use of the appropriate pressure-relieving cushions and mattresses prescribed for the patient. A summary of the various pressure-relieving devices, with discussion of the benefits and drawbacks of each, is discussed in detail elsewhere.[51]

As with other types of ulcers, the factors that may delay wound healing need to be addressed if a healthy wound environment is to be achieved (Table 19–1). If the client's medical condition will support involvement in a muscle-strengthening program, consequent increases in muscle mass may assist in decreasing the threat of decubitus formation as well as increasing mobility.

Physical Therapy Intervention

Patient and care-giver education are important primary interventions. Thorough instruction in proper positioning procedures to avoid excess time in one position and effective use of individualized pressure-relieving devices is essential. Since immobility is a major contributing factor to pressure ulcers, all clients who are capable should receive therapeutic exercise and functional training to maximize their ability to move, thus decreasing the time periods of sustained tissue pressure. Even small improvements, such as improving the client's ability to roll from side to side, can be very beneficial. Low-intensity electrical current or nonthermal ultrasound may be used to enhance wound healing. Whirlpool may be used for wound cleaning and debriding.

NEUROPATHIC PLANTAR ULCERS

Neuropathic plantar ulcers are a special category of pressure ulcer. These ulcers do not develop in response to prolonged periods of maintained pressure, as with decubitus ulcers. Rather, these ulcers develop in response to repetitive pressure stresses on weight-bearing surfaces of the foot in people with peripheral neuropathy.

Epidemiology

The vast majority of plantar ulcers occur in people with diabetes mellitus (DM).[64] The National Center for Health

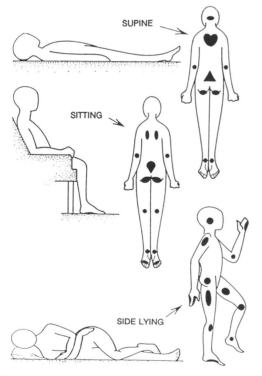

FIG 19–4.
Areas at greatest risk for pressure ulcer formation. (From Fernandez S: *Physiotherapy* 1987; 73:450. Used by permission.)

Statistics identifies diabetes mellitus as one of the five most common chronic diseases of people over age 65.[66] The incidence of DM gradually increases with increasing age until about 65 years of age when it levels off to 9.3% of the population.[66] The prevalence of DM in the elderly black and Hispanic population is, however, as high as 20% to 24%.

The increased prevalence of DM in the older population combined with the long period of time between onset of disease and onset of neuropathic changes increases the probability that plantar ulcers will be most evident in old age. Foot pathologies associated with DM are frequently responsible for long periods of inactivity, illness, hospitalization, and limb amputation.[66, 87, 117] One common diabetic foot pathology, peripheral neuropathy, is a major contributing factor to plantar ulcers in the person with DM. It is estimated that 25% of people with a 10-year history of DM and 50% of people with a 20-year history of DM have distal neuropathic changes.[117]

Etiology

Repetitive mechanical stress, not vascular insufficiency, is the primary precipitating factor in the development of plantar ulcers.[64, 118] A lack of protective sensation in the foot, common among people with diabetic neuropathy, impedes the individual from sensing potentially damaging intensities of plantar pressure. Over time, with continued ambulation, this repetitive stress can lead to overt tissue damage and ulcer formation.

Normal foot biomechanics allow considerable force to be safely placed across the foot because weight-bearing forces are distributed over a large surface area. In a normal upright posture the body's weight rests primarily on the heel and the five metatarsal bones, with the midfoot and great toe assuming a lesser amount of weight and the four smaller toes assuming very little weight.[29]

If biomechanical abnormalities exist, the weight-bearing surfaces may become malaligned, leading to abnormally large loads being carried over small surface areas. Individuals with intact sensation feel discomfort from these abnormal weight-bearing forces and alter their gait, or their footwear, to relieve this repetitive mechanical stress. However, the person who lacks protective sensation will, unknowingly, continue to submit the foot to these excessive stresses, thus placing the foot at risk for injury. Even minor biomechanical abnormalities can, over time, lead to substantial trauma in the person with neuropathy. The metatarsal heads and the great toe are frequent sites of increased plantar pressures and ulceration.[64, 118]

Foot deformities and biomechanical abnormalities are common in diabetic clients and may arise from many sources. Motor neuropathy may accompany sensory neuro-

pathy, leading to weakness in the intrinsic and extrinsic muscles of the foot.[37] Resultant muscle imbalances foster the development of such deformities as claw and hammer toes, both of which increase pressures under the metatarsal heads.[18, 19, 71, 97, 121] Foot deformities associated with age-related biomechanical dysfunction may also be present in this population, including hallux valgus, hammer toes, plantarflexed first ray, and pes planus.[50] These deformities are frequently associated with increased pressure over the metatarsal heads and the great toe.

Decreased range of motion (ROM) in the ankle is frequently observed in the elderly person with DM. Decreased joint flexibility will alter dynamic joint movement, possibly leading to abnormal weight-bearing pressures during gait. Hallux limitus has been associated with high pressures under the great toe and ulcers of the great toe.[13] Decreased dorsiflexion and subtalar joint movement has been implicated in increased forefoot pressures and history of plantar ulcers in patients with peripheral neuropathy.[98]

The risk of ulceration is further enhanced by changes in the forefoot fat pad. Foot deformities, such as claw and hammer toes, frequently result in distal slippage of the fat pad. Gooding et al. found that patients with DM have significantly thinner forefoot fat pads than age-matched subjects without diabetes.[58] These changes result in decreased cushioning over the metatarsal areas most likely to be exposed to high plantar pressures.

Autonomic neuropathy is also implicated in increased risk of ulceration. The patient with an autonomic neuropathy will lack natural skin hydration, resulting in skin that is very dry and easily fissured. The autonomically denervated limb will be unable to "deactivate" the arteriovenous shunting mechanism. This neuropathic change is believed to be the mechanism responsible for the fivefold increase in foot blood flow reported by Archer et al. in their study of people with nonpainful autonomic denervation of the foot.[7] Despite this high blood flow, the adequacy of local tissue nutrition is unclear because the blood is being shunted through the arteriovenous system and away from the nutritive capillaries.[7, 117] A secondary complication of this high blood flow is osteopenia, resulting in increased risk of neuropathic fracture at the foot. This is a very serious complication of autonomic neuropathy that greatly compromises the individual's ability to ambulate.

Blood flow compromise secondary to atherosclerotic occlusions may coexist with neuropathy, further complicating wound healing. People with DM have a risk of large-vessel occlusion similar to that of age-matched nondiabetics. However, atherosclerosis in medium-sized vessels, particularly the tibial and peroneal, occurs much more frequently in people with DM than nondiabetics.[71, 73, 117] In contrast to traditional teachings, blood flow compromise in the foot has not been found to be related to microcirculatory disease. An increased thickening of the basement membrane surrounding muscle capillaries is frequently observed in DM and has led to the hypothesis that this local change is a factor in delayed healing of skin wounds. However, no comparable lesion has been observed in skin of the foot.[87, 117] Circulatory compromise in the foot appears to stem primarily from compromised blood flow through the peroneal and tibial arteries, not from microcirculatory changes.[87]

Clinical Signs and Symptoms of Neuropathic Ulcer

Signs of high plantar pressure may include localized areas of increased warmth, redness, discoloration, hematoma, callous formation, or swelling, particularly if these changes occur on a weight-bearing surface. A traumatized area may have a "boggy" feeling to it. An overt ulcer may be superficial or deep and may or may not involve tissue necrosis. The ulcer may be open or covered with a scab, eschar, or thick callus. A large callus overlying the ulcer may mask underlying tissue damage. Removal of the callus is necessary to adequately evaluate the underlying tissue.[117] Wagner's six-stage classification system is often used to categorize the severity of plantar ulcers (Table 19–3). The client should also be evaluated for signs of autonomic dysfunction, including increased warmth and redness of the entire foot; very dry, cracked skin; and loss of sweating in the foot.

Tests for Neuropathy and High Plantar Pressure

The presence of protective sensation can be reliably measured using Semmes-Weinstein monofilaments.[64] These thin nylon filaments are calibrated according to the force necessary to cause them to buckle when they are briefly pressed against the skin at a right angle to the skin (Fig 19–5). The lower the monofilament number, the lower the force needed to induce buckling, thus the more sensitive the monofilament. Protective sensation in the foot is considered absent if an individual cannot feel the 5.07 monofilament.[15] Monofilament testing should be performed at several sites on the foot, with emphasis on areas exposed to high weight-bearing pressure (Fig 19–6).[15, 64]

Motor nerve conduction velocity testing, described in most basic electrotherapy texts, can provide important information regarding the state of innervation of the muscles of the foot and, therefore, the practicality of potential muscle-strengthening programs as well as risk of foot deformity. Muscle testing, range-of-motion testing, and biomechanical evaluation of the foot should all be included in the evaluation of the insensitive diabetic foot. If an ulcer is not present, then a careful gait analysis, both static and dynamic, should be performed. This evaluation should focus

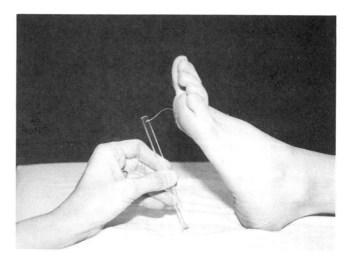

FIG 19–5.
Correct pressure to use for testing protective sensation using Semmes-Weinstein monofilaments. Note the "C" curve of the filament and the positioning of the filament perpendicular to the skin surface.

on identifying any gait abnormalities, subtle or obvious, that may predispose the patient to areas of high plantar pressures. If the client with an insensitive foot currently has a plantar ulcer, the gait evaluation must be deferred until the ulcer is healed or until an acceptable pressure-relieving device is in place.

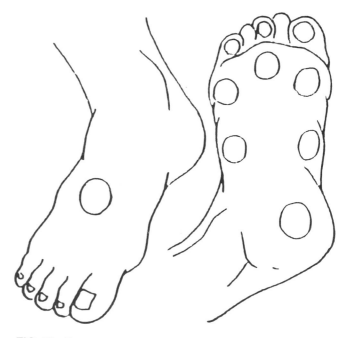

FIG 19–6.
Sites to test for protective sensation when using Semmes-Weinstein monofilaments. (From Birke J, Sims D: The insensitive foot, in Hunt G (ed): in *Physical Therapy of the Foot and Ankle.* New York, Churchill Livingstone, 1988, p 136. Used by permission.)

Qualitative assessment of high plantar pressure can be obtained with an inexpensive ink mat. An ink impression is obtained when the client stands on a three-layered mat. The top layer is dry and does not absorb any ink. The middle layer contains an even layer of ink. The lower layer is a clean paper surface onto which the ink impression is made. The greater the pressure, the darker the ink impression.

Presently, quantitative measurements of plantar pressures are performed primarily with research-focused, expensive equipment not readily available in most clinics. Microprocessor-controlled imaging systems are used to provide a computer-driven visual image of the forces a person places across an illumination plate, or force transducer, as the person stands or walks across the device.[19, 29]

If there is any indication of concurrent arterial or venous insufficiency, then vascular testing, as described in previous sections of this chapter, should also be obtained.

General Treatment Approaches

As with other ulcers, wound care is the first step in the care of a plantar ulcer. The wound must be clear of infection, necrotic tissue, and excessive callous formation in order for healing to progress. Plantar pressures must also be substantially decreased. This can be achieved by placing the client on complete bed rest, by allowing ambulation but with a strict non–weight-bearing (NWB) status, or by utilizing an external limb-support device (cast, walking splint, etc.).[12, 16, 62, 101] External support will substantially decrease the pressure over the ulcer site and decrease movement at the foot and ankle while allowing the patient to partial weight-bear on the foot.

Each approach has benefits and drawbacks. If the client complies with strict bed rest, the ulcer will usually heal and ulcer changes can be monitored easily.[32] However, the negative physiologic effects of bed rest are well documented, and elderly clients, in particular, are vulnerable to these negative effects.

Allowing ambulation but requiring a strict NWB status will also foster wound healing, allow the wound to be easily monitored, and eliminate the need for bed rest. However, even short periods of unprotected weight bearing may delay healing. If the client lacks the physical strength, balance, or determination to remain strictly non–weight bearing, this treatment approach may fail.

Total contact casting (TCC) is an effective wound-healing approach for many patients with neuropathic ulcers.[16] The primary drawback is the inability to inspect the ulcer visually at frequent intervals. A walking splint or a cutout shoe, which allows frequent inspection of the skin, may be more beneficial for clients with substantial circula-

tory compromise. The drawback of these latter devices is the higher risk of shearing and friction forces with weight bearing due to the less precise fit of the device.

Physical Therapy Intervention

Physical therapists are often involved in the evaluation for, and fabrication of, external pressure-relieving devices such as TCC, walking splints, and cutout shoes. The fabrication of these devices, particularly the TCC, requires a great deal of training and practice.[12] The entry-level physical therapy practitioner should understand the principles behind TCC, recognize appropriate clients for this approach, and effectively communicate this information to other members of the health care team. Fabricating TCC is an advanced clinical competency.

As with other types of ulcers, a team approach is needed to adequately treat these patients. Preventing infection, ensuring adequate nutrition for ulcer repair and control of diabetes, removal of calluses and adherent eschar, maximizing distal circulation, ensuring compliance with recommended weight-bearing status, providing patient education opportunities, prescribing and fabricating protective footwear and orthotics, and providing gait training will be a joint effort of many health professionals.

PHYSICAL THERAPY INTERVENTIONS TO AUGMENT WOUND HEALING

A wide variety of modalities are used by physical therapists to treat patients with chronic dermal wounds. Each modality is focused on one of two overall goals: (1) to directly amplify the body's natural healing process or (2) to eliminate factors that block the activity of the body's natural healing processes (e.g., wound infection, inadequate wound nutrition).

Electrical Stimulation of the Wound Site

For many years, low-intensity ESTR has been advocated for the augmentation of wound healing, regardless of the underlying cause of the ulcer. Several studies, each using slightly different pulse generators, have demonstrated the substantial benefit that accompanies this intervention.[3, 9, 28, 57, 74, 80, 128] Despite the effectiveness of ESTR, adoption of this technique by clinicians has been exceptionally slow. Physical therapists are the appropriate health care professionals to be introducing this technology to the health care community, which helps to establish the scientific credibility of the profession.

In Wolcott and coworkers' classic study, 20 elderly clients with ulcers from either arterial or venous insufficiency received ESTR.[128] For these 20 patients, the median decrease in ulcer size was 100% for the clients with venous insufficiency and 96% for those with arterial insufficiency. In both cases, these previously nonhealing ulcers healed at a rate of 14% per week, once the electrical stimulation was begun. Later researchers, using similar protocols, reported even more rapid healing rates.[28, 57, 80] Carley and Wainapel tested Wolcott's protocol using a matched-control design in which control subjects received sham electrical stimulation.[28] They found that the 35.6% per week healing rate of patients in the electrically stimulated group was twice that of patients in the sham treatment group. Kloth and Feedar, using a well-controlled design, demonstrated that high-voltage pulsed stimulation (HVPS), at very low output levels, can be used successfully to heal stage 4 decubitus ulcers.[80] In their study of 16 elderly patients, the wounds of patients in the electrical stimulation group healed completely within 7.3 weeks, at an average weekly healing rate of 45%. During this same time period, the wounds of subjects in the control group increased in size 29%. In all these studies, both experimental and control subjects received the same ulcer care. Kloth states that pressure was relieved from ulcer sites, a high-protein dietary supplement was utilized, wound tissue was debrided as needed, and the wounds were kept clean and free of infection.[80] All wounds were debrided before electrical stimulation was initiated, and elimination of any wound infection was the initial treatment priority.

Although it is clear that electrical stimulation can be very effective in wound healing, the ideal electrical stimulation parameters remain elusive. A variety of parameters have proven effective. One set of parameters, those used by Kloth and Feedar in their recent examination of wound healing with HVPS, is outlined in Table 19–6.[80] Most investigators have used unidirectional current, either pulsed or uninterrupted, both of which provide a means of controlling the polarity of each electrode. The polarity of the electrical current is implicated in both augmentation of wound healing and inhibition of infection. Placing the positive electrode over the wound is generally believed more effective in augmenting healing than placing the negative electrode over the wound. In contrast, the negative electrode over the wound may be more effective in inhibiting infection.[22, 23, 81]

The underlying rationale for enhanced tissue repair in response to ESTR is unknown, although many theories have been proposed. Increased adenosine triphosphate (ATP) production[30] as well as enhanced cellular migration at the wound site and increased collagen synthesis[5, 100] have been reported in skin wounds treated with electrical stimulation. Experimentally induced wounds treated with electrical stimulation have been found to have a greater tensile strength in addition to faster healing rates.[100]

Regardless of the underlying triggering mechanism, the effectiveness of the low-intensity current used with ESTR in reinitiating stalled wound healing is consistent with the Arndt-Schultz law of biologic response:

> Weak stimuli excite physiological activity, moderately strong stimuli favor it, strong stimuli retard physiological activity, and very strong stimuli arrest physiological activity.[38]

Compression Techniques

Control of edema is a major factor in attaining healing of chronic lower extremity ulcers complicated by insufficient venous function. In the presence of venous insufficiency, compression devices assist in decreasing interstitial fluid volumes. The pressure shift encourages the movement of fluids and proteins from the interstitial spaces into veins and lymphatics. Less venous reflux is noted, and the calf muscle pump can work more effectively.[91] This maintained external compression at the wound site has also been associated with increased fibrinolytic activity at the wound, thus improving wound nutrition.[26]

Many devices have been used to provide controlled compressive forces to the lower extremity. Among these are standard elastic bandages, ready-made elastic stock-

TABLE 19–6.

Protocol for ESTR Utilizing High-Voltage Pulsed Current*

Pulse rate	105 pulses per second
Intrapulse interval	50 μs
Amplitude	Sensory only; no muscle contraction
	If serous drainage after 1 hour of stimulation, increase amplitude
	If bloody drainage after 1 hour of stimulation, decrease amplitude
Duty cycle	Continuous
Treatment time	45 minutes, five times per week
Polarity	"+" over the wound for healing
	"−" over the wound if infected
	"Switch polarity" if healing plateau is reached

*Adapted from Kloth L, Feedar J: *Phys Ther* 1988; 68:503–508.

ings, custom-fit gradient-pressure elastic stockings, Unna's boots, legging orthoses, or intermittent pneumatic compression devices.[2, 31, 114, 123] The degree of compression needed, tolerance of the client, and activity level of the client dictate the specific device. Typically, the goal of compression devices is to provide sufficient compression to overcome the existing excessive outward capillary pressure gradients, thus stimulating fluid resorption.[114] Devices utilizing graded pressures, greater distally than proximally, enhance this movement of fluids.

The compression found in elastic compression stockings varies from about 8 to 50 mm Hg at the ankle. A pressure of 30 to 40 mm Hg at the ankle with a 15- to 20-mm Hg decrease proximally is common. A pressure of 40 to 50 mm Hg may occlude blood flow. Very light compression may be ineffective. If the edema and ulceration are limited to the distal extremity, a knee-high elastic stocking may suffice. If the edema extends above the knee, a full-length stocking will be required.

Standard elastic wraps and ready-made stockings are inexpensive and fairly easy to don but frequently do not provide appropriate levels of compression. Elastic bandages can be applied too loosely or tightly. These bandages frequently shift position with limb movement, resulting in inconsistent pressure application. Ready-made compression stockings usually come in three to four "standard" sizes—therefore having a limited range of clients for whom they are appropriate. However, they are much less expensive than custom-fit stockings.

In general, elastic compressive stockings should be put on before getting out of bed in the morning and taken off once in bed at the end of the day. This ensures that external compression is applied at all times when the legs are in a dependent position.

Custom-fit gradient-pressure stockings are often needed to obtain appropriate amount and placement of compression. Although these stockings provide a very precise fit, a frequent drawback of the snug fit is the inability of the individual to don the stockings independently. This is particularly common in older people who may require higher levels of external compression to counteract the venous hypertension.[119] Recently, increased availability of

custom-fit stockings in greater varieties of pressures and with zippers for easier donning has increased the practicality of this compression technique. If an ulcer is present, wound drainage may cause skin maceration. However, the development of very absorbent hydrophilic dressing materials that can be used under the stocking has decreased, but not eliminated, the risk of skin maceration.[110, 113]

Compression pumps are often needed in addition to gradient elastic stockings to enhance fluid resorption.[91] Two different types of inflation modes are commonly available, single- and multiple-chamber compression. The single-chamber unit inflates the entire chamber (distal and proximal portions) simultaneously. A newer variation, the multiple-chamber unit, inflates sequentially, beginning distally and moving proximally. Evidence suggests that the sequential mode of inflation results in more effective edema reduction in a shorter time period than the single-chamber method.[91] Typical parameters for compression pumps used to treat chronic venous insufficiency are listed in Table 19–7.

Total Contact Casting and Other Protected Weight-Bearing Devices

Unna's boot, TCC, and a variety of walking splints and shoes are available to allow selected clients with foot ulceration to remain ambulatory while fostering wound healing. Unna's boots are primarily used with clients with venous insufficiency ulcers who have intact sensation in the foot. The Unna's boot maximizes the muscle-pumping capability of the calf by providing an unyielding surface against which compressive forces on the interstitial tissues can develop. Thus, each muscle contraction promotes effective pumping of fluid into veins and lymphatics.

TCC is used primarily for the treatment of clients with Wagner's stage 1 and stage 2 neuropathic plantar ulcers (see Table 19–3). The goal of these devices is to redistribute the weight-bearing forces across the foot and immobilize inflamed tissues to allow healing to occur. The client's lack of sensation makes proper fit of these devices crucial.

Unna's boot, first described over 100 years ago, consists of a "nonstretchable, pliable, adhesive mold" that is

TABLE 19–7.

Compression Pump Parameters Frequently Utilized for Venous Insufficiency Wounds of the Lower Extremity

Parameter	Intermittent Pump	Sequential Pump
Compression	30–60 mm Hg (most often 30–40 mm Hg)	30–60 mm Hg (most often 30–40 mm Hg)
Duty cycle	90 sec "on"; 30 sec "off"	190 sec "on" with 60-sec sequential inflation of three areas: distal to proximal; 50 sec "off"
Treatment time	1–3 hr, two to three times daily	20 min–2 hr, two to three times daily

applied to the ulcered lower extremity somewhat like a cast.[86] These boots are left on for days or weeks, and patients are allowed to partial weight-bear on them. Contraindications to the use of Unna's boot include large amounts of wound drainage, wound infection, and arterial insufficiency. Unna's boot eliminates the need for daily donning and doffing of tightly fitting stockings and has been associated with more rapid ulcer healing than custom-fit gradient-pressure stockings.[70, 86] The major disadvantage is the inability to perform a daily visual check of the wound for signs of skin irritation or wound deterioration.

The TCC contours the foot much more precisely than the Unna's boot. Plaster is very carefully molded around the foot and lower leg to conform very closely to the contours of the limb, thus providing very even pressure distribution with minimal shearing or rubbing forces. A rocker-bottom heel is applied to the cast to minimize metatarsal pressure. This type of casting was introduced to this country by Brand in the 1960s for the treatment of plantar ulcers in patients with neuropathy related to Hanson's disease (leprosy). This intervention has since been expanded to include patients with diabetic neuropathy. The effectiveness of TCC in healing diabetic neuropathic plantar ulcers has been demonstrated by several researchers.[68, 84, 106, 118] In these studies, 73% to 100% of the ulcers treated with TCC healed completely within 5 to 6 weeks of initial casting. On average, these healed ulcers had been present from 9 to 14 months prior to initiation of TCC and had shown no evidence of healing prior to initiation of TCC. The lack of control groups weakens these studies slightly. However, the complete healing of ulcers of 9 to 14 months' duration within 5 to 6 weeks of the application of the TCC suggests that the intervention, not the passage of time, was the major influence in these successful outcomes. Mueller et al. recently reported on a controlled study that did provide support for the hypothesis that TCC is more effective than alternative conservative techniques in the treatment of plantar ulcers.[99] Helm et al. reported a low ulcer recurrence rate (19.3%) over a 2-year time period in clients treated with TCC and careful post-ulcer reinjury prevention training.[69] Nearly 50% of the ulcers that did recur were attributed to patients' nonadherence to the postulcer prevention plan.

The TCC is changed at least every 2 weeks. It is changed more frequently if loosening, large amounts of drainage, or damage to the cast is noted. For TCC to be effective, the cast must fit very precisely, and the client needs frequent follow-up and thorough training in care of the foot and cast. Birke et al. sum up the goals of TCC as follows: "The casts redistribute walking pressures, prevent direct trauma to the wound, reduce edema, and provide immobilization to joints and soft tissue."[12] A more de-

tailed description of the fabrication techniques for TCC are found in several publications.[12, 15, 32]

Total contact casting is contraindicated for individuals who have cellulitis, hypotrophic skin changes, infection, or severe arterial insufficiency (A/A index <0.45). Individuals classified by Wagner as having stage 3, 4, or 5 ulcers need medical or surgical intervention before TCC should be considered.[12] Efforts should be made to decrease lower leg edema prior to the application of a TCC.

For the client for whom TCC is contraindicated, a custom-molded walking splint may be appropriate.[12, 16, 44] This splint follows the general principles of the TCC except that it can be removed easily to check on the condition of the skin. This advantage is tempered by the fact that the fit is not as snug as the TCC, allowing more shearing forces on the ulcer, which may impede healing.

Birke and coworkers also describe the use of a walking sandal for clients with ulcers on the weight-bearing surfaces of their toes. These sandals remove pressure and shear forces from the toes but are less successful in redistributing weight throughout the foot and in decreasing joint movement at the foot and ankle. For selected patients, however, these may be very valuable tools.

Any technique that allows the patient to continue walking while the ulcer is healing is of great benefit to the elderly client. The detrimental effects of bed rest can be devastating, particularly to an individual on the verge of frailty. The techniques of Brand, Birke, and Sims should be given strong consideration in the overall treatment of neuropathic plantar wounds.

Whirlpool

Whirlpool is commonly used to clean and debride wounds because its agitation and moisture are believed to loosen, debride, and soften adherent eschar. Wet to dry dressings, often used to facilitate the separation of eschar and thickened exudate, may be very painful to detach. Soaking the wound in the whirlpool prior to removal of dressings may greatly decrease this discomfort. Antimicrobial agents can be added to the water to help fight wound infection. Warm water is often used to increase blood flow, induce relaxation, and decrease pain. However, although widely used, almost no information exists on which to judge objectively the effectiveness of whirlpool for enhancing wound healing. Some precautions to the use of whirlpool with chronic wounds, however, are well delineated.

In patients with severe arterial insufficiency, the whirlpool temperature should not be raised above a neutral water temperature, 92° F to 96° F (33.5° C to 35.5° C).[126] One must remember that any modality that increases tissue temperature also increases tissue metabolism, which increases the tissue's need for oxygen. Typically, the body meets this increased oxygen demand by vasodilation, thus increasing blood flow through the tissue. People with severe arterial insufficiency have inadequate blood flow at neutral tissue temperatures and are unlikely to be able to meet this increased demand for blood as tissue temperature rises. Thus, this increased metabolic demand may result in further tissue necrosis rather than healing. In addition, the arterially insufficient limb will allow greater local heat buildup than normally perfused tissue because of the lack of sufficient blood flow to conduct heat away from the local tissue.

Whirlpool also needs to be used cautiously for people with venous insufficiency. Placing a leg with chronic venous hypertension into the dependent position, then inducing vasodilation by circulating warm water around it, does not make any sense physiologically. This activity will simply promote further engorgement of the veins. For this same reason, Birke and Sims discourage the use of whirlpool for neuropathic ulcers.[15] In very limited situations, use of a large whirlpool or Hubbard tank may be appropriate. However, patient positioning in the tank should eliminate the dependent position, and a neutral water temperature should be used. If the wound is not infected and not in need of vigorous debridement, then whirlpool has no place.[93] Readers are referred to entry-level physical agents' texts for detailed descriptions of whirlpool application techniques.[96]

Nonthermal Ultrasound

Several researchers have found nonthermal ultrasound more effective than sham ultrasound in enhancing wound healing, particularly ulcers of venous origin.[27, 48, 111] In general, however, ultrasound appears to be less effective than several alternative treatment approaches. Three separate studies each reported a 33% to 35% decrease in wound size during a 4-week trial of 3-MHz, pulsed, nonthermal ultrasound at an intensity of 0.2 to 1 W/cm^2 delivered to the periphery of the wound for 5 to 10 minutes, one to three times weekly. However, within the same time frame, other studies of the effects of TCC, ESTR, Unna's boot, and compression garments plus compression pumps all report much greater wound healing.

The 3-MHz, rather than the standard 1-MHz, ultrasound is purported by Dyson to be the most effective frequency for dermal wounds because more energy is absorbed in superficial tissues.[47, 48] Indeed, one recent study that concluded that ultrasound was ineffective for wound healing used a 1-MHz frequency.[88] Parameters frequently identified as effective for wound healing are listed in Table 19–8.

Ultrasound seems to enhance the patient's ability to move through the inflammatory stage of repair. It does not

TABLE 19–8.

Ultrasound Parameters Frequently Utilized for Chronic Dermal Wounds

Frequency	3 MHz for stage 2 ulcers
	1 MHz for stage 3 or 4 ulcers
Intensity	0.2–1.0 W/cm^2
Duty cycle	20% pulsed
Treatment time	1–2 min per area 1½ times the size of the soundhead; three times weekly
Treatment location	Around the edges of the wound or Directly over the wound with water-based occlusive dressing as conducting medium

interfere with the inflammatory stage, which Dyson reminds us is the body's natural mechanism for stimulating and guiding the tissue repair process, but rather it enhances the body's ability to utilize the inflammatory stage to stimulate repair.[47, 48] In patients with normal wound hemodynamics, the use of nonthermal ultrasound has been associated with a stronger, more resilient wound scar.[48] The exact mechanism by which this occurs, however, remains elusive.

Despite the fact that the impact of ultrasound on wound healing may be less pronounced than with some other modalities, there are advantages to this modality. The treatment time is very short (about 10 minutes), and treatment frequency may be as low as one to three times per week. This technique does not require enclosing the leg in a cast or boot for long periods of time. It does not require advanced skills to apply the modality competently, and most patients find the modality very comfortable. Systematic study needs to be undertaken to evaluate the possibility of combining nonthermal ultrasound with other modalities to further enhance wound healing—for example, using custom-gradient elastic stockings and intermittent compression devices daily plus ultrasound three times per week for the client with chronic venous insufficiency ulcers.

Much remains unknown about the effectiveness of ultrasound for wound healing. The few studies to date have all examined venous insufficiency ulcers. No reason was given in any of these studies for the exclusion of ulcers from other pathologies. Except for the recognition that very low intensities of current are preferable, very little information is given to justify the arbitrary parameters used for treatment. Much further work is needed to determine if these are the "best" parameters.

Hyperbaric Oxygen

Hyperbaric oxygen (HBO) has been used successfully to treat venous insufficiency ulcers and decubitus ulcers.[43, 54, 55, 102] It has a lowe success rate, however, with arterially insufficient ulcers.[43, 54, 55, 122] With this technique, the ulcerated limb is placed in a pressurized chamber, and pure oxygen is circulated within the chamber at a rate of 4 to 8 L/min. The pressure within the chamber is either held steady at 1.03 atm of pressure (22 mm Hg) or varies cyclically from 1 atm of pressure up to 3 atm (810 mm Hg). Pressures above 22 mm Hg may occlude capillaries; therefore, any pressures above this level must be cyclic. The majority of studies of HBO have used the constant 22 mm Hg pressure. Large increases in the partial pressure of oxygen (Po_2) have been noted during HBO treatment.

It is unclear if the increased Po_2 values, the external compression, inpatient nursing care, or an interaction of these factors were the keys to its success. The effectiveness of Unna's boots, compression pumps, and other compression devices has been well documented. It may be that the 1.03 atm of pressure that was applied for several hours daily was the salient feature of successful ulcer healing, not the increased atmospheric oxygen. Also, in the majority of studies reviewed, patients were admitted as hospital inpatients for 2 to 8 weeks to receive HBO. The inpatient setting alone, with its ready access to high-quality, frequent wound care and the increased potential for longer periods of bed rest and decreased limb dependency, probably contributed to wound healing. The relative benefits of increased oxygen tensions, the unique aspect of HBO, cannot be ascertained from these studies. Will compression devices, bed rest, and good, frequent wound care be just as effective as HBO? Will a home program be just as effective? Much more research needs to be done to identify the comparative role of this modality in the treatment of ulcers.

Treating the Low Back for Vasodilation of the Feet

In the 1960s, the use of superficial heat to the low back was suggested as an effective adjunct to the treatment of peripheral vascular disease because of observations made by Abrahmson and Wessman that heating of the low back resulted in a reflex vasodilation of the skin vessels of the feet.[1, 127] No further evaluation of the effectiveness of this method of consensual heating for patients with PVD has been found in the literature. Further evaluation of this simple and safe technique is warranted.

Another indirect approach to increasing blood flow to the feet is through epidural electrical stimulation at the T10 spinal cord level using standard transcutaneous electrical nerve stimulation (TENS) parameters. This modality requires a surgical procedure to implant electrodes into the epidural space. Once implanted, the stimulation is given for many hours daily and has been found to be very effective in decreasing pain and avoiding limb amputations in

clients with severe arterial insufficiency. Owing to the implanted nature of the electrodes, physical therapists are not currently involved in this form of indirect stimulation.[8, 21, 34, 75, 76]

SUMMARY

Healthy elders have little risk of developing nonhealing ulcers. Ill and frail elders, however, are at a much higher risk, as all four leading causes of dermal wounds (arterial insufficiency, venous insufficiency, pressure, neuropathy) are closely associated with illnesses that are most prevalent in the older population.

Effective treatment of chronic dermal ulcers requires careful evaluation and individualized treatment approach based on team collaboration and involvement. The underlying cause of initial ulceration needs to be determined as well as the factors that are currently impeding the healing process. The health care team needs to develop a coordinated treatment approach that focuses first on removing the factors that are contributing to the nonhealing status (infection, eschar, poor nutrition, etc.) and then utilize interventions that will foster healing. The intervention is modified, as needed, to ensure continual movement toward healing. Once healing is achieved, it is essential that the patient and care givers be fully educated in strategies to prevent wound recurrence.

In situations where the physiologic effects of the modality have been carefully matched with the physiologic needs of the wound, many physical therapy modalities have been found to be effective in fostering wound healing. Electrical stimulation for tissue repair, compression pumps, and external support devices such as total contact casts are examples of modalities with strong clinical and research support for their effectiveness. Nonthermal ultrasound and hyperbaric oxygen have shown some evidence of effectiveness, particularly for clients with venous insufficiency ulcers. However, the extent of their benefit seems less pronounced than some alternative modalities available to us.

Whirlpool, although widely used for chronic wounds, has almost no research data to support, or refute, its usefulness. Clinically, it is often the preferred modality for cleaning wounds and preparing them for debridement. The ability of whirlpool to stimulate healing or disperse medication into the wound is questionable.

Physical therapists have a great deal to contribute to the care of patients with chronic ulcers. It is essential, however, that the intervention chosen fits the specific physiologic needs of the client and blends well with the overarching treatment approach of the involved health care team.

REFERENCES

1. Abramson D, et al: Indirect vasodilatation in thermotherapy. *Arch Phys Med Rehabil* 1965; 46:412–420.

2. Airaksinen O, Kolari P: Intermittent pneumatic compression therapy. *Crit Rev Phys Rehabil Med* 1992; 3:219–237.

3. Akers T, Gabrielson A: The effect of high volt galvanic stimulation on the rate of healing of decubitus ulcers. *Biomed Sci Instrum* 1984; 20:99–100.

4. Allman RM, et al: Pressure sores among hospitalized patients. *Ann Intern Med* 1986; 105:337–342.

5. Alvarez O, et al: The healing of superficial skin wounds is stimulated by external electric current. *J Invest Dermatol* 1983; 81:144–148.

6. Angel M, et al: The causes of skin ulcerations associated with venous insufficiency: A unifying hypothesis. *Plast Reconstr Surg* 1987; 79:289–297.

7. Archer A, Roberts V, Watkins P: Blood flow patterns in painful diabetic neuropathy. *Diabetologia* 1984; 27:563–567.

8. Augustinsson LE, et al: Epidural electrical stimulation in severe limb ischemia: Pain relief, increased blood flow, and a possible limb-saving effect. *Ann Surg* 1985; 202:104–110.

9. Barron J, Jacobson W, Tidd G: Treatment of decubitus ulcers: A new approach. *Minn Med* 1985; 68:103–106.

10. Bennett L, Lee B: Pressure versus shear in pressure sore causation, in Lee B (ed): *Chronic Ulcers of the Skin*. New York, McGraw-Hill, 1985, pp 39–56.

11. Berlowitz DR, Wilking SV: The short-term outcome of pressure sores. *J Am Geriatr Soc* 1990; 38:748–752.

12. Birke J, et al: Methods of treating plantar ulcers. *Phys Ther* 1991; 71:116–122.

13. Birke J, Cornwall M, Jackson M: Relationship between hallux limitus and ulceration of the great toe. *J Orthop Sports Phys Ther* 1988; 10:172–176.

14. Birke J, Sims D: Plantar sensory threshold in the ulcerative foot. *Lepr Rev* 1986; 57:261–267.

15. Birke J, Sims D: The insensitive foot, in Hunt G (ed): *Physical Therapy of the Foot and Ankle*. New York, Churchill Livingstone, 1988.

16. Birke J, Sims D, Buford W: Walking casts: Effect on plantar foot pressures. *J Rehabil Res Dev* 1985; 22:18–22.

17. Blalock A: Oxygen content of blood in patients with varicose veins. *Arch Surg* 1929; 19:898–905.

18. Boulton A, et al: Abnormalities of foot pressure in early diabetic neuropathy. *Diabetic Med* 1987; 4:225–228.

19. Boulton A, et al: Dynamic foot pressure and other studies as diagnostic and management aids in diabetic neuropathy. *Diabetes Care* 1983; 6:26–33.

20. Brandeis GH, et al: The epidemiology and natural history of pressure ulcers in elderly nursing home residents. *JAMA* 1990; 264:2905–2909.

21. Broseta J, et al: Spinal cord stimulation in peripheral arterial disease: A cooperative study. *J Neurosurg* 1986; 64:71–80.

22. Brown M, Gogia P: Effect of high voltage stimulation on cutaneous wound healing in rabbits. *Phys Ther* 1987; 67:662–667.

23. Brown M, McDonnell M, Menton D: Electrical stimulation effects of cutaneous wound healing in rabbits: A follow-up study. *Phys Ther* 1988; 68:955–960.

24. Browse N: The etiology of venous ulceration. *World J Surg* 1986; 10:938–943.

25. Browse NL, Burnand KG: Hypothesis: The cause of venous ulceration. *Lancet* 1982; 2(8292):243–245.

26. Burnand H, et al: Venous lipodermatosclerosis: Treatment by fibrinolytic enhancement and elastic compression. *Br Med J* 1980; 280:7–11.

27. Callam M, et al: A controlled study of weekly ultrasound therapy in chronic leg ulceration. *Lancet* 1987; 8552:204–206.

28. Carley P, Wainapel S: Electrotherapy for acceleration of wound healing: Low intensity direct current. *Arch Phys Med Rehabil* 1985; 66:443–446.

29. Cavanaugh P, Rodgers M, Liboshi A: Pressure distribution under symptom-free feet during barefoot standing. *Foot Ankle* 1987; 7:262–276.

30. Cheng H, et al: The effects of electric currents on ATP generation, protein synthesis and membrane transport in rat skin. *Clin Orthop* 1982; 171:264–272.

31. Christopoulos D, et al: Air-plethysmography and the effect of elastic compression on the venous hemodynamics of the leg. *J Vasc Surg* 1987; 5:148–189.

32. Coleman W, Brand P, Birke J: The total contact cast: A therapy for plantar ulceration on insensitive feet. *J Am Podiatr Assoc* 1984; 74:548–552.

33. Coni N: Posture and the arterial pressure in the ischaemic foot. *Age Ageing* 1983; 12:151–154.

34. Cook AW, et al: Vascular disease of extremities: electric stimulation of spinal cord and posterior roots. *N Y State J Med* 1976; 7B:366–368.

35. Coon WW, Willis PW, Keller JB: Venous thromboembolism and other venous diseases in the Tecumseh community health study. *Circulation* 1973; 48:839–846.

36. Cooney TG, Reuler JB: Pressure sores, in Cassel CK, et al (eds): *Geriatric Medicine*, ed 2. New York, Springer-Verlag, 1990.

37. Ctercteko G, et al: Vertical forces acting on the feet of diabetic patients with neuropathic ulceration. *Br J Surg* 1981; 68:608–614.

38. Cummings J: Role of light in wound healing, in Kloth LC, McCulloch JM, Feedar JA (eds): *Wound Healing: Alternatives in Management*. Philadelphia, FA Davis, 1990, p 290.

39. Czerniecki JM, et al: The effects of age and peripheral vascular disease on the circulatory and mechanical response of skin to loading. *Am J Phys Med Rehabil* 1990; 69:302–306.

40. Dagher FJ, Queral LA: Ischemic ulcers of the lower extremities, in Dagher FJ (ed): *Cutaneous Wounds*. New York, Futura Publishing, 1985.

41. Daniel RK, Priest DL, Wheatley DC: Etiological factors

in pressure sores: An experimental model. *Arch Phys Med Rehabil* 1981; 62:492–498.

42. Dayton P, Palladino S: Electrical stimulation of cutaneous ulcerations: A literature review. *J Am Podiatr Med Assoc* 1989; 79:318–321.

43. Diamond E, et al: The effect of hyperbaric oxygen on lower extremity ulceration. *J Am Podiatr Assoc* 1982; 72:180–185.

44. Diamond J, Sinacore D, Mueller M: Molded double rocker plaster shoe for healing a diabetic plantar ulcer: A case report. *Phys Ther* 1987; 67:1550–1552.

45. Dickey J: Stasis ulcers: The role of compliance in healing. *South Med J* 1991; 84:557–561.

46. Duckworth T, et al: Plantar pressure measurements and the prevention of ulceration in the diabetic foot. *J Bone Joint Surg* 1985; 67B:79–85.

47. Dyson M: Non-thermal cellular effects of ultrasound. *Br J Cancer Suppl* 1982; 45:165–171.

48. Dyson M: Stimulation of tissue repair by therapeutic ultrasound. *Infect Surg* 1982; 1:37–44

49. Eaglstein WH: Wound healing and aging. *Clin Geriatr Med* 1989; 5:183–188.

50. Edelstein J: Foot care for the aging. *Phys Ther* 1988; 68:1882–1886.

51. Feedar J, Kloth L: Conservative management of chronic wounds, in Kloth L, McCulloch J, Feedar J (eds): *Wound Healing: Alternatives in Management*. Philadelphia, FA Davis, 1990, pp 135–176.

52. Fell G, Strandness D: Management of vascular disease, in Kottke F, Stillwell G, Lehman J (eds): *Krusen's Handbook of Physical Medicine and Rehabilitation,* ed 3. Philadelphia, WB Saunders, 1982, pp 809–814.

53. Fernandez S: Physiotherapy prevention and treatment of pressure sores. *Physiotherapy* 1987; 73:450–454.

54. Fischer BH: Topical hyperbaric oxygen treatment of pressure sores and skin ulcers. *Lancet* 1969; 2: 405–409.

55. Fischer B: Treatment of ulcers on the leg with hyperbaric oxygen. *J Dermatol Surg* 1975; 1:55–58.

56. Fitzpatrick J: Stasis ulcers: Update on a common geriatric problem. *Geriatrics* 1989; 44:19–31.

57. Gault W, Gatens P: Use of low intensity direct current in management of ischemic skin ulcers. *Phys Ther* 1976; 56:265–268.

58. Gooding G, et al: Sonography of the sole of the foot: Evidence for loss of foot pad thickness in diabetes and its relationship to ulceration of the foot. *Invest Radiol* 1986; 21:45–48.

59. Goodson WH, Hunt TK: Wound healing and aging. *J Invest Dermatol* 1979; 73:88–91.

60. Gordon T, Kannel WR: Predisposition to atherosclerosis in the head, heart, and leg: The Framingham study. *JAMA* 1972; 221:661–666.

61. Greene D, Lattimer S, Sima A: Sorbitol, phosphoinositides, and sodium-potassium-ATPase in the pathogenesis of diabetic complications. *N Engl J Med* 1987; 316:599–606.

62. Gupta P, Saunders W: Chronic leg ulcers in the elderly treated with absolute bedrest. *Practitioner* 1982; 226:1611–1612.

63. Halperin JL: Peripheral vascular disease: Medical evaluation and treatment. *Geriatrics* 1987; 42:47–61.

64. Hampton G, Birke J: Treatment of wounds caused by pressure and insensitivity, in Kloth L, McCulloch J, Feedar J (eds): *Wound Healing: Alternatives in Management*. Philadelphia, FA Davis, 1990, pp 196–220.

65. Hansson C: Studies on leg and foot ulcers. *Acta Derm Venereol Suppl (Stockh)* 1988; 136:1–45.

66. Harris M: Epidemiology of DM among the elderly in the United States. *Clin Geriatr Med* 1990; 6:703–719.

67. Heikkinen E, et al: Age factor in the formation and metabolism of experimental granulation tissue. *J Gerontol* 1971; 26:294–298.

68. Helm P, Walker S: Total contact casting in diabetic patients with neuropathic foot ulceration. *Arch Phys Med Rehabil* 1984; 65:691–693.

69. Helm P, Walker S, Pullium G: Recurrence of neuropathic ulceration following healing in a total contact cast. *Arch Phys Med Rehabil* 1991; 72:967–970.

70. Hendricks W, Swallow R: Management of stasis leg ulcers with Unna's boots versus elastic support stockings. *J Am Acad Dermatol* 1985; 12:90–98.

71. Holewski J, et al: Prevalence of foot pathology and lower extremity complications in a diabetic outpatient clinic. *J Rehabil Res Dev* 1989; 26:35–44.

72. Holstein P, Nielson P, Barras J: Blood flow cessation at external pressure in the skin of normal limbs. *Microvasc Res* 1979; 17:71–79.

73. Husn EA: Skin ulcers secondary to arterial and venous disease, in Lee BK (ed): *Chronic Ulcers of the Skin*. New York, McGraw-Hill, 1985.

74. Ieran M, et al: Effect of low frequency pulsing electromagnetic fields on skin ulcers of venous origin in humans: A double-blind study. *J Orthop Res* 1990; 8:276–282.

75. Jacobs MJ, et al: Foot salvage and improvement of microvascular blood flow as a result of epidural spinal cord electrical stimulation. *J Vasc Surg* 1990; 12:354–360.

76. Jacobs MJ, et al: Epidural spinal cord microvascular blood flow in severe limb ischemia. *Ann Surg* 1988; 207:179–183.

77. Jarvinen M, Aho AJ, Toivonen H: Age dependent repair of muscle rupture. *Acta Orthop Scand* 1983; 54:64–74.

78. Juergens J, Barker N, Hines E: Arteriosclerosis obliterans: Review of 520 cases with special reference to pathogenic and prognostic factors. *Circulation* 1960; 21:188–195.

79. Kisner C, Colby LA: *Therapeutic Exercise: Foundation and Technique,* ed 2. Philadelphia, FA Davis, 1990, pp 409–420.

80. Kloth L, Feedar J: Acceleration of wound healing with high voltage monophasic pulsed current. *Phys Ther* 1988; 68:503–508.

81. Kloth L, Feedar J: Electrical stimulation in tissue repair, in Kloth LC, McCulloch JM, Feedar JA (eds): *Wound Healing: Alternatives in Management*. Philadelphia, FA Davis, 1990.

82. Knighton DR, et al: Amputation prevention in an independently reviewed at-risk diabetic population using a comprehensive wound care protocol. *Am J Surg* 1990; 160:466–472.

83. Kosiak M: Prevention and rehabilitation of ischemic ulcers, in Kottke F, Stillwell G, Lehman J (eds): *Krusen's Handbook of Physical Medicine and Rehabilitation,* ed 3. Philadelphia, WB Saunders, 1982, pp 881–888.

84. Laing P, Cogley D, Kenerman L: Neuropathic foot ulceration treated by total contact casting. *J Bone Joint Surg* 1991; 74B:133–136.

85. Leaming DB: The influence of age on wound healing. *J Surg Res* [Br] 1963; 3:43–47.

86. Lippman H, Briere J: Physical basis of external supports in chronic venous insufficiency. *Arch Phys Med Rehabil* 1971; 52:555–559.

87. Lipsky B, Pecoraro R, Ahroni J: Foot ulceration and infections in elderly diabetics. *Clin Geriatr Med* 1990; 6:747–769.

88. Lundeberg T, et al: Pulsed ultrasound does not improve healing of venous ulcers. *Scand J Rehabil Med* 1990; 22:195–197.

89. MacKinnon J: Doppler ultrasound assessment in peripheral vascular disease, in Kloth L, McCulloch J, Feedar J (eds): *Wound Healing: Alternatives in Management.* Philadelphia, FA Davis, 1990, pp 119–132.

90. Majeske C: Reliability of wound surface area measurements. *Phys Ther* 1992; 72:138–141.

91. Mayberry J, et al: Fifteen-year results of ambulatory compression therapy for chronic venous ulcers. *Surgery* 1991; 109:575–581.

92. McCulloch J: Peripheral vascular disease, in O'Sullivan S, Schmitz TJ (eds): *Physical Rehabilitation: Assessment and Treatment,* ed 2. Philadelphia, FA Davis, 1988.

93. McCulloch J, Hovde J: Treatment of wounds due to vascular problems, in Kloth L, McCulloch J, Feedar J (eds): *Wound Healing: Alternatives in Management.* Philadelphia, FA Davis, 1990, pp 177–195.

94. McEnroe C, O'Donnell T, Mackey W: Correlation of clinical findings with venous hemodynamics in 386 patients with chronic venous insufficiency. *Am J Surg* 1988; 156:148–152.

95. Meijer JH, et al: Method for the measurement of susceptibility to decubitus ulcer formation. *Med Biol Eng Comput* 1989; 27:502–506.

96. Michlovitz SL (ed): *Thermal Agents in Rehabilitation,* ed 2. Philadelphia, FA Davis, 1990.

97. Mueller M, et al: Relationship of foot deformity to ulcer location in patients with diabetes mellitus. *Phys Ther* 1990; 70:356–362.

98. Mueller MJ, et al: Insensitivity, limited joint mobility, and plantar ulcers in patients with diabetes mellitus. *Phys Ther* 1989; 69:453–462.

99. Mueller M, et al: Total contact casting in treatment of diabetic plantar ulcers: A controlled clinical trial. *Diabetes Care* 1989; 12:384–388.

100. Nessler J, Mass D: Direct-current electrical stimulation of tendon healing in vitro. *Clin Orthop* 1987; 217:303.

101. Novick A, et al: Effect of a walking splint and total contact cast on plantar forces. *J Prosthet Orthot* 1991; 3:168–178.

102. Olejniczak S, Zielinski A: Low hyperbaric therapy in the management of leg ulcers. *Mich Med* 1975; 74:707.

103. Olerud JE, et al: An assessment of human epidermal repair in elderly normal subjects using immunohistochemical methods. *J Invest Dermatol* 1988; 90:845–850.

104. Paris BE, et al: The prevalence and one-year outcome of limb arterial obstructive disease in a nursing home population. *J Am Geriatr Soc* 1988; 36:607–612.

105. Petermans J: Prevalence of disease of the large arteries in an elderly Belgian population: Relationship with some metabolic factors. *Acta Cardiol* 1984; 39:365–372.

106. Pollard J, LeQuesne L: Method of healing diabetic forefoot ulcers. *Br Med J* 1983; 286:437–438.

107. Pollard J, LeQuesne L, Tappin J: Forces under the foot. *J Biomed Eng* 1983; 5:37–40.

108. Queral L, Dagher F: Venous ulceration of the lower extremities, in Dagher F (ed): *Cutaneous Wounds.* New York, Futura Publishing, 1985.

109. Reed B, Zarro V: Inflammation and repair and the use of thermal agents, in Michlovitz S (ed): *Thermal Agents in Rehabilitation,* ed 2. Philadelphia, FA Davis, 1990, pp 3–17.

110. Rijswijk R, et al: Multicenter clinical evaluation of a hydrocolloid dressing for leg ulcers. *Cutis* 1985; 35:173–176.

111. Roche C, West J: A controlled trial investigating the effect of ultrasound on venous ulcers referred from general practitioners. *Physiotherapy* 1984; 70:475.

112. Romanus M: Microcirculatory reactions to local pressure induced ischemia: Vital microscopic study in hamster cheek pouch and pilot study in man. *Acta Chir Scand* 1977; 479(suppl):1–30.

113. Romasz R, Barnhart B, Schinagel E: Application of dextranomer beads (Debrisan) in the treatment of exudating skin lesions: Results of a cooperative study. *Angiology* 1982; 29:675–682.

114. Sayegh A: Intermittent pneumatic compression: Past, present and future. *Clin Rehabil* 1987; 1:59–64.

115. Schubert V: Hypotension as a risk factor for the development of pressure sores in elderly subjects. *Age Ageing* 1991; 20:255–261.

116. Schubert V, Fagrell B: Evaluation of the dynamic cutaneous post-ischemic hyperaemia and thermal response in elderly subjects and in an area at risk for pressure sores. *Clin Physiol* 1991; 11:169–182.

117. Sims DS, Cavanagh PR, Ulbrecht JS: Risk factors in the diabetic foot: Recognition and management. *Phys Ther* 1988; 68:1887–1902.

118. Sinacore DR, et al: Diabetic plantar ulcers treated by total contact casting: A clinical report. *Phys Ther* 1987; 67:1543–1557.

119. Smith P, et al: Sequential gradient pneumatic compression enhances venous ulcer healing: A randomized trial. *Surgery* 1990; 108:871–875.

120. Spector WD, et al: Factors associated with presence of decubitus ulcers at admission to nursing homes. *Gerontologist* 1988; 28:830–834.

121. Stokes I, Faris I, Hutton W: The neuropathic ulcer and loads on the foot in diabetic patients. *Acta Orthop Scand* 1975; 46:839–847.

122. Upson A: Topical hyperbaric oxygen in the treatment of recalcitrant open wounds: A clinical report. *Phys Ther* 1986; 66:1408–1412.

123. Vernick S, Shapiro D, Shaw F: Legging orthosis for venous and lymphatic insufficiency. *Arch Phys Med Rehabil* 1987; 68:459–461.

124. Versluysen M: Pressure sores in elderly patients: The epidemiology related to hip operations. *J Bone Joint Surg [Br]* 1985; 67:10–13.

125. Wagner F: The dysvascular foot: A system for diagnosis and treatment. *Foot Ankle* 1981; 2:64–122.

126. Walsh M: Hydrotherapy: The use of water as a therapeutic agent, in Michlovitz S (ed): *Thermal Agents in Rehabilitation,* ed 2. Philadelphia, FA Davis,1990, pp 109–132.

127. Wessman H, Kottke F: The effect of indirect heating on peripheral blood flow, pulse rate, blood pressure, and temperature. *Arch Phys Med Rehabil* 1967; 48:567–576.

128. Wolcott LE, et al: Accelerated healing of skin ulcers by electrotherapy: Preliminary clinical results. *South Med J* 1969; 62:795–801.

Patient Education as a Treatment Modality

Dale L. Avers, M.S. Ed., P.T.
Davis L. Gardner, M.A.

INTRODUCTION

Imparting information to a patient is one of the most frequently utilized modalities a physical therapist uses. However, it is often the least addressed in physical therapy schools and the least understood as far as effective methodology. Rehabilitation professionals often do not perceive themselves as educators in spite of the fact that the therapist spends much of any treatment session instructing patients in new techniques or home programs or facilitating relearning of motor skills. Utilizing appropriate education strategies grounded in sound theory and research may make the difference between the patient's success or failure in achieving rehabilitation goals. In this chapter, patient education and the physical therapist's role as a patient educator are emphasized in terms of a practical yet philosophically based experience that can influence older patients' self-direction in prescribed treatment regimens. A review of learning theories will be presented, followed by a philosophical approach to learning and patient education. Characteristics of older adult learners and some common barriers to their learning also will be summarized. The role of the care giver and teaching strategies to enhance this role will be discussed, and selected assessment methods will be presented. The chapter concludes with three typical patient education scenarios that illustrate some of the concepts presented relative to patient education as a treatment modality.

CHAPTER OBJECTIVES

As a result of studying this chapter, you should be able to:

1. Identify the characteristics of older adult learners that influence the planning and implementation of your patient education sessions
2. Identify typical obstacles to effective patient education interaction with older adults
3. Apply instructional strategies to improve your interaction with older adult learners in patient education settings
4. Develop and apply a patient education philosophy

LEARNING THEORIES

Learning by its very nature defies easy definition and simple theorizing. The concepts of behavioral change and experience are central to learning theories. In general, we have defined *learning* as a change, or potential for change, in behavior. Learning as a process, rather than an end product, focuses on what happens as learning takes place.

Explanations of this process are called *learning theories*. It is necessary to understand the components of how learning occurs in order to effectively address specific learning situations. We will adopt the organization schema of Merriam and Caffarella[22] to explore the development and application of learning theories through four learning orientations: behaviorist, cognitive, humanist, and social.

Behaviorist Orientation

Behaviorism is a familiar theory credited to John B. Watson (1878–1958) but that loosely also encompasses a number of researchers such as Thorndike, Tolman, Guthrie, Hull, and Skinner.[26] Important concepts of learning that are derived from a behaviorist orientation are Thorndike's Law of Exercise and Law of Readiness. The Law of Exercise asserts that the repetition of a meaningful connection between a situation and a response results in substantial learning when simultaneous reinforcement is present. Sheer repetition on its own does not strengthen learning. The Law of Readiness states that if the learner is ready for the connection, learning is enhanced; if not, learning is inhibited.

Behaviorist theories concentrate on observable behavior shaped by environmental forces. Behavioral theorists believe the teacher's role is to design an environment that elicits desired behavior and to extinguish behavior that is not desirable. The systematic design of instruction, behavioral objectives, notions of the instructor's accountability, programmed instruction, computer-assisted instruction, and competency-based education are strongly grounded in behavioral learning theory. An example in physical therapy patient education is verbally reinforcing a correct transfer technique as it is being performed while ignoring the behavior when the transfer technique is done incorrectly.

Cognitive Orientation

Piaget[22] conceptualized the process of cognition and thought development in developmental stages. He believed that the behavior of the human organism starts with the organization of sensorimotor reactions and becomes more intelligent as coordination between the reactions to objects becomes progressively more interrelated and complex. Thinking becomes possible after language develops—and with it, a new mental organization.

Bruner,[7] also interested in the process of intellectual growth, developed a theory about the act of learning involving the following four simultaneous processes: (1) ability to use specific skills in acquiring knowledge; (2) developing an attitude toward learning that involves a "sense of discovery" of relationships and a "need to know" feeling; (3) transformation, or the process of manipulating knowledge to make it fit new tasks; and (4) evaluation, or checking whether the way information is manipulated is adequate to the task. These acts of learning principles became the foundation for an instructional theory with the following tenets: (1) implanting a desire to learn; (2) organizing the body of knowledge to be taught; (3) sequencing the presentation of materials to be learned; and (4) specifying the nature and spacing of rewards and punishments. Each learner has a unique sequence preference based on past learning, stage of development, the nature of the material, and individual differences.

Gagne and Briggs[12] developed a model of "learning to learn" from which three aspects relevant to older adult learners can be discerned: learner needs, personal learning style, and the organized learning activity. These three aspects affect the ability to learn effectively in any learning situation.

Cognitive theories emphasize the internal mental processes that are within the learner's control and deal with the mental processing of information. Cognitive learning theories focus on how to facilitate understanding (cognition); how information is processed, stored, and retrieved; and meaningful learning rather than seeking general laws for controlling and predicting behavior. A concern of a cognitive researcher would be how aging affects an adult's ability to process and retrieve information and how it affects an adult's internal mental structures. An example of applied cognitive theory in geriatric physical therapy is in how the therapist would organize a treatment session when the goal is instructing the patient how to weight shift preparatory to ambulation. The therapist would build on the simple to complex tasks of supine and then sitting weight shifting before going to standing weight shifting. Then the progression would be from bipedal weight shifting to unilateral weight shifting to advancing a foot forward. Concern for the proper pacing of instruction would be addressed throughout the treatment session.

Humanist Orientation

Humanist theories consider learning from the perspective of the human potential for growth. From a learning theory perspective, humanism emphasizes that a person's perceptions are centered in experience, as well as the freedom and responsibility to become what one is capable of becoming. These tenets underlie much of adult learning theory that stresses the self-directedness of adults and the value of experience in the learning process. Two psychologists who have contributed much to our understanding of learning from this perspective are Abraham Maslow and Carl Rogers.

Maslow interpreted the goal of learning to be self-ac-

tualization or the full use of talents, capacities, and potentialities. Carl Rogers described his philosophy of learning and teaching in his book *Freedom to Learn for the 80's*.[25] He defined the elements of learning as a "quality of personal involvement"—with both feeling and cognitive aspects being part of the learning event. Learning is self-initiated so that even when the impetus or stimulus comes from an external source, the sense of discovery, of reaching out, of grasping and comprehending, comes from within. Learning is so pervasive that behavior, attitudes, and perhaps even the personality of the learner are affected. Learning is evaluated by the learner. The learner knows whether the instruction is meeting a need and is leading toward a goal.[25] Rogers states that significant learning combines the logical and the intuitive, the intellect and the feelings, the concept and the experience, the idea and the meaning.

Perceptual Theory

The perceptual theory suggests that views or perceptions of people, objects, and events in the individual's environment will have much to do with behavior. Adults who have lived in the world for a given number of years have had the opportunity to gain many perceptions of their environment and all the objects and events in it. Five concepts that affect an individual's perception of environment are beliefs, values, needs, attitudes, and self-experience.

Beliefs are what adults perceive to be true, whether these take the form of faith, knowledge, assumption, or superstition. Beliefs are reality to individuals, and individuals behave as if the beliefs are true. *Values* identify people's feelings about what is important to them and could be related to ideas, a way of life, material things, or people. *Needs* are what individuals require to maintain or enhance themselves. According to this concept, needs can be divided into two kinds: (1) physiologic needs, such as food, water, air, shelter; and (2) social needs, such as need for approval and acceptance, status, prestige, or power. *Attitudes* reflect an emotionalized belief about the degree of worth of someone or something. *Self-experience* (self-concept) is how people see themselves, how they feel about being that person, how they think others see them, how they see other people, and how they feel about this.

People are most threatened when they are forced to change the ways in which they seek to maintain or enhance their concept of self. Threat then causes defensive behavior and a narrowing and constricting of the perceptual field. When threatened, people are resistant and seek to maintain themselves instead of seeking growth or enhancement of self-concept. Rogers advocated that external threats should be kept to a minimum when learning is perceived as threatening to the self. A corollary is that self-evaluation and self-criticism are more acceptable to adults than evaluation by others. Humanist orientation emphasizes the individual's choice, responsibility, and internal motivation (locus of control). For example, the patient's desire to become independent following a severe stroke becomes the internal motivation for going through intense rehabilitation and discomfort. This motivation coupled with self-evaluation may lead the patient to develop new ways of doing things independent of the therapist.

Social Learning Theory

Social learning theory is a system of thought based on imitation or modeling. Bandura[5] postulated that one can learn from observation without having to imitate what was observed. He further explored self-directed behaviors. In order for people to regulate their own behavior, well-defined objectives or goals must be selected; contractual agreements are negotiated in order to further increase goal commitment; objective records of behavioral changes are utilized as additional sources of reinforcement for their self-controlling behavior; and the stimulus condition under which the behavior customarily occurs is altered. For example, for the older adult who has difficulty adhering to his diabetic diet, removing the source of temptation or storing the forbidden food in a different place would alter stimulus conditions. The progressive narrowing of stimulus control, for example, may initiate change over a period of time instead of creating a total change at one time.

The term *locus of control* is used to explain which behavior in the individual's repertoire will occur in a given situation. Typically, people with an internal locus of control will adhere more consistently and longer than those with an external locus of control, which requires external motivation such as praise and material rewards. Social learning theories provide us with an additional factor in how adults learn by acknowledging the importance of context and the learner's interaction with the environment to explain behavior.

Adult Learning Orientation

Andragogy is a term popularized by Knowles[19] to explain a philosophical orientation for adult education. His four main assumptions of changes in self-concept, role of experience, readiness to learn, and orientation to learning lay the foundation for the instruction of older adults.

Changes in self-concept occur as individuals grow and mature. Their self-concept moves from one of total dependency (as is the reality of an infant) to one of increasing self-directedness. Any experience that adults perceive as putting them in a position of being treated as a child will interfere with their learning, commonly resulting in expressions of resentment and resistance.

Role of experience defines the role of lifetime experiences. As individuals mature, they accumulate an expanding reservoir of experience, causing them to become an increasingly rich resource for learning and providing them with a broadening base to which to relate new learnings. Any situation in which adults' experiences are perceived to be devalued or ignored may be perceived as rejecting their experience and even their person.

The concept of *readiness to learn* explains the shift from an external stimulus to an internal stimulus. As individuals mature, their readiness to learn is decreasingly the product of biologic development and academic pressure and is increasingly the product of the developmental tasks required for the performance of evolving social roles. Learning experiences must be timed to coincide with the learners' developmental tasks. For example, a geriatric patient may need to attempt ambulation before comprehending the importance of general strengthening or balance activities.

Orientation to learning reflects the adult's purpose for learning. Adults tend to have a problem-centered orientation to learning. Real-life problems are the purpose for seeking educational opportunities. The immediate application of information learned is a primary need of the adult learner.[19]

In conclusion, the following principles developed by Darkenwald and Merriam[9] summarize the tenets applicable to patient education as a treatment modality:

1. Adults' readiness to learn depends on their previous learning.
2. Intrinsic motivation produces more pervasive and permanent learning.
3. Positive reinforcement is effective.
4. Material to be learned should be presented in an organized fashion.
5. Learning is enhanced by repetition.
6. Tasks and materials that are meaningful are more fully and easily learned.
7. Active participation in learning improves retention.
8. Environmental factors affect learning.
9. Adults learn throughout their lifetime.
10. Adults exhibit learning styles that illustrate various learning theories such as:
    a. Having personal strategies for coding information.
    b. Perceiving in different ways — cognitive procedures.
    c. Perceiving learning activities to be problem centered and relevant to life.
    d. Desiring some immediate appreciation.
    e. Having a concept of themselves as learners.
    f. Being self-directed.

PSYCHOLOGIC FACTORS OF THE LEARNING SITUATION

In order to develop a philosophic approach to patient education, physical therapists must understand their own motivations and biases toward their role as the helper, their attitudes toward their patients, and their attitudes toward the information they are sharing. It is also important to understand the older adult's perceptions of self and of learning as it affects the learning situation. This section will discuss factors contributing to the therapist's and patient's attitudes toward teaching and learning.

Therapist's Perception of the Patient Educator

The primary motivation for entering the health care field is to help people. This avowed motive is sincere in most cases. People become helpers because they really enjoy helping others and want to impact their lives positively. Although the motive to help others focuses on the needs of the patient, the needs of the "helper" must be acknowledged as a philosophy of patient education is developed. The helper's need to be needed and the helper's needs as a person both exist, that is: "I want to be needed and wanted but not to be completely responsible for a person." Another common but deeper, less obvious thought that can shape the physical therapist's attitudes is the "There but for the grace of God go I" reaction when the patient becomes a disturbing mirror image of the helper's real or potential suffering. Asserting authority is often the helper's defense against this phenomenon.

Two less apparent reasons for entering a health field are the desire to learn about oneself and the desire to exert control. The desire to exert control, to be in charge and to have some noticeable impact on the world, is particularly relevant when attempting to "teach" a patient. This attitude of control can make the physical therapist the "high priest" of the learning situation, perhaps inhibiting the learning situation.

In order to understand the effect of this attitude of "control" or dominance, a common model that is prevalent in our health care system, Parsons' *sick role model,* will be discussed. This model often shapes therapists' initial attitudes toward their professional responsibilities.

The sick role model was described by Parsons in 1951 as made up of four aspects that permeate the attitudes and behaviors of both the patient and the health care professional. The first is that the sick person is relieved of normal social responsibilities; that is, they do not have to get dressed; they may need help to go to the bathroom or to be fed. The second is that the sick person must be taken care of and thus assumes a dependent role. The third is that the sick person should regard getting well as an obligation,

that is, to be motivated. And the fourth is that the sick person should seek out expert help and cooperate with the process of getting well.[23]

This model implies that the health care professional is in a position of authority and the patient is in a role of dependency, obligated to get well according to the methods and desires of the health care professional. The patient hands the problem over to the professional and becomes passive, whereas the professional takes charge of all aspects of that patient and whatever problems are present. When the acuity of the situation lessens, Parsons[23] and Silverstone[28] describe the sick role as evolving into a patient role characterized by conformity, dependency, and receptivity to care that excludes patient aggressiveness and attempts at self-reliance.

Older Adults' Perception of Self

Human beings are complex individuals whose behavior, attitudes, and conditioning are affected by multiple internal and external forces. Any number of these forces can affect how older adult patients respond to medical situations and their attitudes toward the learning situation. This section briefly presents several of these forces that affect the geriatric patient.

Self-concept and Self-esteem

The view one has of one's self is called *self-concept,* and the value placed on that self-concept is *self-esteem.* Life experiences, attitudes toward self and others, belief, and value systems all factor into the self-concept/self-esteem equation of the older adult. Multiple losses are common as one grows older and can reinforce any existing negative self-perception or may negatively affect a lifelong positive self-perception. Losses can include the death of a spouse, adult children, grandchildren, friends, and peers or loss of health or of one's home. Retirement from the work force may be viewed as the loss of a productive role when no valued activities exist to replace the former occupation or profession. In addition to any or all of these, the geriatric patient participating in rehabilitation has experienced some degree of trauma and may have serious self-doubts concerning the ability to function again in the home, community, or work environment.

Sensitivity to Failure

Many therapists treating older adults will be a significant number of years younger than their patients. An older adult's sensitivity to failure may be affected by the age difference and the perceived lack of effort the younger person exhibits in movement and performing complicated tasks. It is important to realize the patient may be comparing current performance with previous, normal performance, thus enhancing the perception of failure. A negative self-concept and the older adult's view of his own personal crisis—that is, disability, illness, or personal loss—may also accentuate the sensitivity to failure.

Resistance to Change

The geriatric patient may express total hopelessness for improved function and exhibit a resignation to accepting the present limitations. This attitude may be manifested in resistance to suggestions, change, or help. Skepticism and even some degree of fear may underlie resistance. Resistance can be a normal coping strategy to change and fear and should not be viewed as a rigidity of attitude or behavior and thus unamenable to change. Rogers stated resistance may be observed when the individual feels threatened.

In summary, the geriatric patient in treatment sessions is an individual with a complex psychosocial profile that will influence the degree of willingness to learn. The therapist also has complex attitudes and beliefs regarding the role of the health care professional that affect the tone, manner, and flexibility of the therapist in the learning situation. Recognizing the underlying attitudes affecting the learning situation is the initial step in becoming an effective patient educator.

MOTIVATION AND LEARNING

When the underlying attitudes and values of both the older patient and the therapist are recognized and accepted, the therapist must develop strategies for facilitating and affecting the desired learning from a psychologic perspective. This section will discuss the role of motivation and choice as well as specific techniques to deal with the psychologic attitudes of both the older adult and therapist that were discussed in the preceding section.

Eliciting patient compliance is often a perceived goal of patient education. The lack of compliance or motivation is also a common reason to refer an older adult to psychologic services. The physical therapist often requests with a psychologic referral: "Increase their motivation so that they'll comply with my instructions" or concludes: "This patient isn't motivated because she isn't following my instructions on practicing transfer techniques." *Compliance* and *motivation* sometimes are used interchangeably, although they are very different concepts. It is important to understand the terms and implications of compliance and motivation in order to develop appropriate goals for patient education.

The term *compliance* implies that the older adult follows medical orders and does what the health care professional has instructed. Compliance is authoritarian in tone and implies that the patient must do as the therapist instructs in order for the patient education session to be successful. Compliance is a natural goal when operating under the sick role model because it implies the patient's subservience, dependence, and unquestioning obedience to authority.[10] The sick and patient role models foster the idea that the patient is dependent on the health professional in order to get better. This puts enormous responsibility on the therapist to make the patient better and may be one cause of therapist burnout.

Adherence, on the other hand, is a term that implies independent choice and action on the part of the patient. It implies a willingness to participate. Adherence can be defined as a consistent behavior that is accomplished through an internalization of learning, enhanced by independent coping and problem-solving skills.[2] *Motivation,* as used by Kemp,[18] is a complex attitude composed of wants, beliefs, and rewards vs. cost of the behavior. Motivation is not on a continuum of poor, average, or high. Rather, motivation is a characteristic of all adults that is manifested in behavior. Therapists incorrectly assess a patient's motivation as poor because the patient is not being "compliant" when, in fact, the patient might be "highly" motivated for another activity of greater value to the patient. The therapist who facilitates patient learning must discern the distinct differences in compliance and adherence and also must develop an understanding of these psychologic implications and attitudes.

Goals of Patient Education

D'Onofrio contends that the goals of education are to equip the learner with problem-solving skills whereby the learner can gain greater control over the directions of his own life.[10] Rogers goes further and suggests that the goal of education is to facilitate learning.[25] He states that instruction must develop the learner in order to decrease dependence on the instructor. Consistent with this philosophy, education is viewed as the process of facilitating the learner's problem-solving skills with the goal that the learner will gain control over any specific problem. Learning places the responsibility on the learner, the patient. To teach does not imply learning. Teaching is one-sided and asks nothing of the patient except that the patient must be present.

Payton asserts that only the patient can make the decision that a goal is worth working for.[24] Lindgren states that older patients should be viewed as individuals who are capable of making their own decisions—not as dependent recipients of medical care.[20] These two statements clearly convey the important message that older adults can and do exercise choice in whether or not they will participate in treatment sessions.

Rogers believes that it is impossible to "teach" anyone anything unless the learner wants to learn.[25] Think of the patient who sits through a detailed exercise program. A strong feeling is transmitted that the patient really is not listening to the therapist and is, in fact, in a hurry to leave. No matter how great a "facilitator of learning" the therapist is, if the patient does not want to learn, he will not.

Basically, one learns what one wants to learn. When one wants to learn, one is described as being "motivated," an internal phenomenon. Bille relates Maslow's needs hierarchy to patient motivation in an interesting and relevant manner.[6] Maslow theorized that one's basic physiologic needs (air, food, water, movement, sex, avoidance of pain) and safety and security needs (assurance that the world is regular and predictable; that death, destruction, or physical/social/emotional/economic harm is not imminent) must be met before affiliation and esteem needs can be met.

Bille applies this concept to the patient who has experienced physical trauma and whose current needs basically are physiologic and safety oriented. The patient may find it difficult to focus on adjusting to the trauma and the necessary rehabilitation and may not be able to envision managing the changes that may result from that trauma. Motivation will be enhanced, therefore, when instruction is centered on procedures that are, in the patient's perspective, physiologic and safety oriented, such as strength, mobility, ambulation, or activities of daily living (ADL). When these needs are met, self-esteem increases as progress is made.

Bille relates the need for esteem to the motivation to learn and states that as self-esteem increases, motivation to learn will increase. The therapist can foster the patient's self-esteem, and therefore motivation, when open, two-way communication exists. The patient needs to feel free and unthreatened in order to tell the therapist what has affected or lowered his self-esteem. The basic characteristics a teacher needs to exhibit in order to facilitate this open communication as described by Rogers[25] are realness or genuineness; prizing the learner; acceptance; trust; and empathic understanding. When the health care professional exhibits realness or genuineness, the façade is lifted, and the therapist comes into a direct personal encounter with the learner and meets the learner on a person-to-person basis, as peers or equals. There is no hiding behind an authoritarian role; there is no sterile façade. The physical therapist can express emotions and attitudes and becomes, to the patient, a real person, with convictions and feelings.

Rogers describes prizing the learner as valuing the learner's feelings, opinions, the person as a whole. Prizing is caring for the learner, accepting the learner as a separate person, appreciating the learner's differences as well as exhibiting a belief that the learner is fundamentally trustworthy. The physical therapist who exhibits this attitude can fully accept the fear and hesitation of the older adult as the older adult approaches his own personal crisis. This attitude allows the therapist to accept the "poor motivation" of the older adult and to make attempts to understand the factors contributing to the motivational problem. Empathic understanding is the therapist's ability to understand the patient's reactions from the patient's perspective and to have a sensitive awareness of the way the process of education and learning seems to the patient. The likelihood of significant learning is increased when these characteristics are exhibited by the therapist.[25]

In order to increase the patient's self-directedness, the therapist should provide opportunities for the patient to make decisions about treatment and to identify what is to be learned. Payton presents excellent examples of this process in his chapter the "Patient as Planner."[24] To increase the patient's motivation, the therapist should lead the patient to explore the range of concerns and then to identify the primary concern. Goal setting by the patient becomes a motivator because a greater degree of choice is exercised.

Payton also outlines four levels of patient participation in goal identification that range from the patient's free choice, with open-ended questions, to no choice, with the therapist prescribing and telling the patient what to do. The free-choice level is possible when the therapist does not suggest answers. This allows the patient autonomy, an important aspect of self-esteem and motivation. Payton uses the following as an example of the free-choice process:

Therapist:	What bothers you?
Patient:	I have a tingling on my left side.
Therapist:	Is there anything else bothering you?
Patient:	I have trouble using my left ankle.
Therapist:	Is there anything else?
Patient:	I can't move my toes.
Therapist:	What bothers you the most?
Patient:	It's hard for me to walk.[24]

By allowing the patient to explore several concerns, identification of the walking difficulty provided the basis for a goal statement that was generated by the patient. Therefore, the patient's motivational level was enhanced for treatment sessions because the therapist addressed the primary concern of the patient.

At the next level, the therapist asked questions and offered several options or suggestions, with permission to offer those options first being elicited from the patient. The resulting multiple-choice question still allowed the patient to exercise choice and control among the options. This level is in contrast with the lowest level when the question to the patient is followed by the therapist's immediate answer or recommendation. Thus, the patient's participation is excluded, self-esteem is questioned, and motivation is diminished.

Older adults may exhibit some resistance to becoming partners in treatment decisions and sessions. Anderson suggests that this reluctance may be based on their perceptions of health care professionals as "high priests" whose wisdom is all encompassing and whose decisions are not to be discussed or questioned.[1] This perception was described earlier in the discussion of the sick role model. Obviously in acute cases, this perception of the medical model may be the most appropriate one. However, in many situations the patient's progress will depend more on the helping process than on the sick role model of health care delivery.

In the sick role model, the patient has a more passive role in treatment sessions, whereas the therapist is the activist. In contrast, in the helping process, the patient is more active in identifying the problem, setting goals, exploring alternative solutions, and assessing the results. When the patient is active in the helping process, the patient's ability to appropriately cope with any problems that arise is strengthened. Coping may involve consulting with the therapist for opinions on the proposed solutions, but the intent is for the patient to become more of a partner than a passive recipient in the health care regimen.[1]

In summary, the helping process appears to be more congruent with the geriatric patient's need for self-esteem, autonomy, the exercise of choice, and the partnership Payton advocates. To be an effective patient educator requires an approach of empowering the patient rather than assuming an authoritarian role. An effective patient educator facilitates the learner's learning, appreciates the learner's differences, and helps the learner establish goals and responsibility for learning. A patient whose ideas, interests, concerns, and feelings have been heard and responded to by others is much more likely to enter into active, cooperative planning for necessary treatment. A patient who is actively involved in treatment planning is more likely to adhere to those cooperative plans and guarantee the success of treatment. The importance of self-esteem and choice relates closely to the geriatric patient's motivational level. Lasting gains are possible when the geriatric patient perceives the therapist as a supportive partner in treatment sessions. The therapist's degree of success when working with a geriatric patient is related to the perception of that patient as a person against a background of cognitive and psychosocial characteristics.

Strategies to Affect Learning

The therapist's actions and behaviors are keys in working with an older patient whose negative self-concept presents a significant obstacle to treatment progress. To attempt to counter these doubts and to modify the patient's perception of self to a positive rather than a negative view, the therapist should emphasize the successful experiences the patient has had as an adult in overcoming other difficult experiences. Other techniques can be to guide the patient to identify the reason(s) for any past failures and assist the patient to recognize that the reason(s) for failure may not be a factor in treatment. If, however, the reason(s) for past failure may be present in the therapeutic environment, the therapist should help the patient identify the factors that can be controlled at this time.[30] For example, consider the patient with previously treated low back pain who starts physical therapy. The patient's behavior indicates a reluctance to try the exercises. As the therapist explores this reluctance, the patient indicates, "No one really explained the previous exercises." The therapist indicates that doing an exercise incorrectly can cause increased pain. Extra care and a thorough explanation of the exercises are indicated in order to address the patient's history of perceived failure.

Creating a successful instructional environment and providing opportunities for successes, no matter how small they may be, are valuable tools. Any contributions the patient may make should be recognized, and establishing a partnership relationship in the treatment goals and sessions is helpful.[30] It should be remembered, however, that psychologic counseling is best done by counseling professionals.

During the treatment session, the therapist should provide tasks that the patient can do successfully. Focusing on relevant information in an organized clear manner, and providing adequate time for skill practice, can enhance successful performance. The therapist should sensitively give adequate, honest feedback and encouragement for correct responses and performance in order to diminish the chances for and perception of failure. It is necessary to stress the patient's positive contributions and correct performance of any tasks[30] and to be aware that depressed patients may demonstrate an increased sensitivity to failure and heightened self-criticism.

Accepting the patient's existing attitudes and recognizing that new attitudes, behaviors, and values cannot be forced on the geriatric patient may help temper any resistance to change of treatment. Creating constructive dialogue and reasoning instead of participating in arguments that tend to further entrench negative attitudes may help prevent these natural reactions of resistance and resignation. Discovering the source of patient motivation is paramount. Exploring the elements of Kemp's model for motivation described earlier may help the therapist address the patient's concerns or fears.[18]

The older adult's performance and learning can be affected by past experiences of mastering earlier developmental tasks. Havighurst succinctly identified six developmental tasks of old age: (1) adjusting to decreasing strength and health, (2) adjusting to retirement and reduced income, (3) adjusting to the death of a spouse, (4) establishing an explicit affiliation with members of one's own age-group, (5) meeting social and civic obligations, and (6) establishing satisfactory physical living arrangements.[16] Mastery of these six tasks for the older adult is dependent, to some degree, on how successfully the earlier developmental tasks through the childhood, adolescent, and young and middle adult years were mastered. Any deficits in mastery of earlier tasks or of these tasks for the older adult can affect the geriatric patient's motivation, learning, and performance.

Educational and Cultural Background

The number of years between earlier instructional activities and present instructional activities, previous level of education, and past experiences with learning are components of the geriatric patient's psychosocial profile. Instruction related to job and profession or participation in adult education and community education courses may be factors that will influence the patient's positive predisposition toward learning new tasks. However, if the patient primarily remembers negative experiences in earlier educational situations, these unpleasant memories may make it more difficult for the geriatric patient to be a cooperative and a willing participant in treatment sessions. The therapist should make every effort to ensure that the patient experiences success in the initial treatment sessions and to assist in the differentiation of any earlier negative experiences from present therapeutic procedures.

Many ethnic populations reside across the United States—the African-Americans, Native Americans, Asian-Americans and Pacific Islanders, and Hispanics being the standard four major groups. The therapist must remember that in addition to the patients' having lived many years, their ethnic environment will influence their predisposition toward, perception of, cooperation with, and follow-up of treatment. Traditional tribal and home treatment methods are influential in all four ethnic populations. *Illness* is not a word in some Pacific/Asian languages, and in others, *illness* is synonymous with acute conditions and death, and hospitals may be viewed with fear.[4]

Another consideration with ethnic geriatric patients is level of English proficiency and education. Language barriers are common for therapists working with the Pacific/Asian ethnic group, which is composed of 18 subgroups of Pacific Islanders and Asian-Americans. Using translators if the therapist—or another member of an interdisciplinary team—does not have bilingual-bicultural skills is very helpful. Although family members and friends may appear

to be the most logical choice for this important task, the recommended choice is an interpreter who has a background in medical terminology as well as in language and cultural expertise. Cultural differences must be translated in culturally appropriate terms. The same recommendation is made when selecting Hispanic translators. Many large institutions have employees who are willing to serve as translators. When working with an African-American elder, the therapist must remember the earlier segregation of health care facilities and must respect the black elder as a survivor of a health care system that was not accessible and perhaps was even hostile.[4]

Patient education materials for geriatric patients of ethnic groups must be designed with cultural diversity as one of several important considerations. The translator should examine the text carefully for any words or phrases that might be incorrectly interpreted. Illustrations should reflect ethnic customs when possible. Any number of reliable methods to test for appropriate reading level can be used. Field testing patient education materials using a sample of the intended audience before final production is recommended in order to determine the effectiveness of the material.

The extended family as care givers to the elderly is common among other cultures. A lack of familiarity with health care resources and the bureaucratic processes for access often results in underutilization by minorities. Among Hispanics, the use of formal health care services can be viewed as the family's failure to take care of its own. The health care an individual family member is allowed to receive may be subject to the approval or disapproval by the elder dominant family member.[4]

The norm for health care delivery in the United States evolved from the middle-class northern European models of care. The health care system in the United States will have increasing numbers of ethnic patients. Building a level of trust through demonstration of a sensitivity to their history and cultural view of illness and health care in order to negotiate successful treatment regimens with ethnic elders is effective.[4] The therapist should regard this interaction as an opportunity for learning and increasing cultural sensitivity and awareness.

THE OLDER ADULT AS A LEARNER

This section relates patient education as a treatment modality to the knowledge of the process by which older patients "learn." The statement "You can't teach old dogs new tricks" can be a negative influence on a new therapist who is beginning a career and who has not yet had enough experiences with older adults to recognize the fallacy of such a generalization. Older adults can and do learn. It is critical that a new therapist develop a dual role as a caring and competent therapist and as a skillful facilitative instructor in order to work with older adults successfully. This discussion will examine the cognitive and physical aspects that influence the ability and the predisposition of older adults to be effective and efficient learners in treatment sessions.

Cognitive Aspects

Cognition refers to intellectual processes, whereas *learning* generally is considered the acquisition of knowledge or skills achieved by study, instruction, practice, and experience. An individual's performance becomes the basis for inferring the level of learning that has been achieved. Two aspects must be considered in discussing cognitive learning—the end product and the process. Many research studies focus only on the end product. Therefore, when a person's performance improves in an intellectual or physical task, the inference is that learning has occurred. Failure in performance, however, does not infer that learning has not occurred or has been lost. Many factors affect an older adult's performance including motivation and physical and emotional states. The physical therapist must be sensitive to the fact that multiple variables affect the learning situation and avoid concluding that the older adult cannot learn.

Several areas relate to the cognitive abilities of older patients. Intelligence as measured by standard testing procedures has been shown to decline with increasing age. However, when adjusted for time—that is, when increased time (pacing) is allowed—no significant decline is observed.

Research generally concludes that memory does decline with age. However, this conclusion can be challenged because of methodologic considerations and multiple variables as well as the lack of a functional corollary with skills and tasks in everyday life. Studies that show declining memory changes in older adults may have utilized artificial tasks that were not relevant to the subject's everyday tasks. Babins states, therefore, that careful examination is needed of studies that show a decline in older adults' memory functions.[3] In other words, evidence exists to suggest that memory involving skills and tasks used frequently does not decline to the degree that infrequently used information declines. The adage "If you don't use it, you lose it" can be appropriately applied to cognition. Other research studies focus on the process, and results show that when new information can be related to older adults' existing knowledge, their new learning is facilitated.

Some factors involved in the cognition or intellectual processes can be accommodated by the physical therapist.

These factors are assessment of learning level, learning readiness, and learning styles.

Learning Level

Assessment of each patient's learning level is important for instructional planning, implementation, and patient education materials. Although the educational level of the older adult has been steadily increasing, one study reported about half of adults over age 65 did not complete high school. Within this group, women were more likely to have continued in school to junior high or high school, whereas men were more likely to have attended only some elementary grades.[13]

The patient history provides an excellent opportunity to gain information about the learning level already achieved by the patient. An estimate of learning level can be obtained by talking, in a conversational manner, about current or former employment positions. Duties and responsibilities at home, in the community, or in volunteer work and information on hobbies can give further assessment data on the cognitive functional level of the patient. Other indicators are the vocabulary used by the patient and the level of understanding demonstrated in response to questions and to the general conversation initiated to establish rapport with the patient. The physical therapist should utilize the assessment of the patient's learning and functional literacy level in patient education.

Learning Readiness

Learning readiness means that until basic skills are mastered, the mastery of more complex behavior is not possible. A number of factors can affect the patient's readiness to learn, some of which are closely related to the patient's motivational intensity discussed earlier.

Gage and Berliner reported studies conducted by Levinson and Reese with four age-groups—preschool, fifth graders, college freshmen, and the aged.[11] They found that in the older adult extensive practice was necessary to develop learning readiness. They also concluded that learning was less effective if practice was discontinued before the learner gained sufficient competence and confidence in the tasks. For older adults to process information into their first or primary memory store, application, practice, and rehearsal are essential.

To assess the patient's learning readiness for psychomotor activities, the therapist would determine the existing level of physical strength and skills in order to build from those points. To assess the patient's understanding of the reasons and need for therapy, determine the patient's level of understanding of the particular physical condition and prescribed treatment. The therapist should sequence instruction from simple skills and concepts to the more complex ones, with sufficient supervised practice to ensure the correctness of performance and to develop the patient's learning readiness to progress to more difficult and complex tasks.

Learning Styles and Information Processing

Learning style refers to how information is processed and is unique to each individual. An individual's learning style determines the consistent way the individual receives, retains, and retrieves information. Learning style also includes how an individual feels about and behaves in instructional experiences. An individual's learning style often is identified at one extreme or the other of any given learning style continuum, a classification that is probably too rigid to be realistic.

An individual's typical mode of perceiving, thinking, problem solving, remembering, selecting, and organizing information and educational experiences defines how that individual processes information. McLagan describes three primary dimensions of information processing as continua: content, initiative, and tactics—each of which has its own continuum. [21] She also emphasizes that a profile that responds to needed functions is more descriptive and realistic than labeling an individual at either fixed point of the three continua.

Content, the first dimension, ranges from a detail learner to a main idea learner. The detail learner will be attentive to the step-by-step explanation of a procedure but is less attentive to the overall goals of the therapy. The main idea learner will be eager to hear about the overall goals but may be less attentive to specific instructions and details. [21] For example, a detail learner will be more interested in the number of repetitions and appropriate time of day to perform the exercise, whereas a main idea learner will want to know the purposes and possible outcomes of the exercises.

Initiative, the second dimension, ranges from an active/aggressive/energetic learner to one who is passive in instructional sessions. The active/aggressive/energetic learner exerts a high degree of initiative and questions many aspects of the treatments, causes, and effects. However, conclusions may be reached erroneously. At the other extreme, the passive learner is one who exhibits little initiative and who must be encouraged to participate actively in treatment sessions. [21] A passive learner is a greater challenge to the instructor but does not indicate an unwillingness to learn.

The third dimension, *tactics,* refers to how information is processed in terms of organization and structure. The analytic learner processes best when structure is present and when step-by-step explanations and demonstrations are presented sequentially. The intuitive/creative learner, on the other hand, responds best to instruction that is less structured and more open-ended. Problem solving

and shared decision making in treatment sessions are more productive with the intuitive/creative information processor. [21]

In summary, Cassata condensed a number of findings related to cognitive aspects of the older adult learner:

1. Patients forget much of what the doctor tells them.
2. Instructions and advice are more likely to be forgotten than other information.
3. The more a patient is told, the greater the proportion he will forget.
4. Patients will remember (a) what they are told first and (b) what they consider most important.
5. Intelligent patients do not remember more than less intelligent patients.
6. Older patients remember just as much as younger ones.
7. Moderately anxious patients recall more of what they are told than highly anxious patients or patients who are not anxious.
8. The more medical knowledge a patient has, the more he will recall.
9. If the patient writes down what the doctor says, he will remember it just as well as if he only hears it. [8]

Physiologic Aspects

A number of changes occur with aging that can be accommodated by the therapist to facilitate the geriatric patient's learning. These changes may involve neurologic functions, vision and hearing impairment, and diminished motor dexterity. Worcester relates these physiologic changes to patient education. [31]

Neurologic Changes

Neurologic changes that may affect learning are slower nerve transmission, which affects pacing; decreased short-term memory; and a larger store of existing information that must be integrated into the treatment setting. Slower nerve transmission can slow the reception of information and reaction times of the patient and therefore will create the need for more time in the treatment session. Implications for instruction include sensitivity to the pacing of instruction and speech and frequently assessing the patient's level of understanding. [31]

Decreased short-term memory can cause difficulty in retaining new material and will necessitate repetition and adequate practice time. Short-term memory can be enhanced through multisensory approaches, that is, visuals, models, demonstrations, and patient education materials. The volume of information accumulated over a lifetime can interfere with learning when the new information is not congruent with prior information and experiences. Cognitive overload—too much information—also is a potential factor. Strategies for effective instruction can be to assess the patient's knowledge base about the particular physical condition, make connections between prior knowledge and new knowledge, clarify any misconceptions, and present less material in each treatment session.[31]

Visual Changes

Decreases in acuity, accommodation to dim lighting, and lens transparency are significant visual changes that may affect the patient's ability to learn effectively. The decreased sharpness of vision, or acuity, implies that details in print materials and illustrations are more difficult for the geriatric patient to see clearly. Therefore, illustrations in patient education materials need bold lines, a minimum of detail, and a plain print style. The use of larger, simple type styles and uppercase/lowercase letters for the text material is recommended strongly. In the same manner, decreased accommodation creates difficulty in the lens adjusting to different light intensities and to color differentiation. Bright overhead lights in the clinic may create accommodation difficulties for the geriatric patient, just as dim lights may make visual perception more difficult. The patient should not be placed in a position that faces any source of glare. For patient education materials, black ink on nonglare yellow paper for optimum acuity and accommodation should be used. Decreased lens transparency may be due to external as well as to internal causes. The therapist should make certain the patient's glasses are clean and should provide magnifying aids, if needed, when referring to patient education materials.[31]

Hearing Changes

High frequencies, such as the *c, ch, f, s, sh, t,* and *z* sounds, are more difficult for older adults to distinguish clearly. By asking the patient to repeat what was heard, the therapist can detect problems and correct errors. The therapist's pace of speech and clear enunciation are more important than volume because slow or loud speech does not necessarily increase reception. Background noises need to be controlled, as the geriatric patient may have difficulty screening sounds. Patient education materials that have illustrations and audio/videotapes with individual headsets can assist the hearing-impaired patient.[31]

Motor Changes

A number of changes in the musculoskeletal condition of the geriatric patient may affect the ability to respond to treatment. Adequate time must be provided to accommodate slower movement and responses, and adaptive equipment, as appropriate, should be available. The therapist

should plan to have the patient begin with simple tasks that can be accomplished, then build to more complex tasks.[31]

Implications for Patient Education Materials

This discussion of the cognitive aspects and physical changes has particular implications for patient education materials. The vocabulary level, sentence length, complexity, and organization of content should be examined carefully for comprehension. Reading level for print materials should approximate fourth- to sixth-grade level for ideal patient comprehension. Visual changes experienced by older adults dictate using clear, simple print styles. Black ink on nonglare paper and colors that are distinctly contrasting are recommended. Patient education materials should be tested with a representative sample of the audience for whom they are designed for clarity, comprehension, and readability before production—an instructional and cost-effective strategy.

In summary, the therapist ideally facilitates the older adult patient's moving toward self-direction. Therefore, consider the positive impact that occurs when learning style and information processing are investigated, assessed, and utilized. Awareness of the physical changes that occur in the older adult patient can enhance the learning experience when appropriate techniques are applied. Time spent in careful assessment of the many cognitive aspects of learning and the physical changes can create a more productive instructional time for each patient.

In summary, geriatric patients in treatment sessions will exhibit characteristics of older adult learners. The therapist who is aware of the cognitive and physiologic aspects discussed in this section is better prepared to work more effectively with geriatric patients and to facilitate their progress in treatment sessions.

THE CARE GIVER

Illness and disability present a serious crisis, not only for the patient but also for the family. Responses to illness will affect the current family interactions and establish new interactions with the health care team. A responsibility of the health care provider is to assist the patient and the family in responding to this crisis.

Assessment of the family should occur at the beginning of the rehabilitative process. Assessment will provide information on the individual dynamics of the family, identifying dysfunctions that may need special interventions. Observing interactions between key family members and the patient may reveal dependence issues, fear of the disability, or fatalism. Assessment also will reveal cultural or emotional issues that may be barriers to learning. The therapist must realize that the family will be experiencing grieving in similar ways to the patient.[17] The family may exhibit a resistance to instruction at this time. Often they feel powerless and worry excessively about the patient. This may be in part because of a lack of knowledge about the patient's future, current disability, or illness or about anticipated needs, resulting in fear and feelings of inadequacy.

Smith and Messikomer reported a study done on family care givers of 39 geriatric patients discharged from a rehabilitation center in Pennsylvania.[29] Of those who provided ADL support, half reported the tasks as burdensome. Giving baths and dealing with incontinence were particularly troublesome, with burden attributed to the amount of time required for the former and to the unpleasantness of the latter. The most prevalent problem expressed by care givers was fear about the impaired person's condition, followed by the uncertainty about the illness and its treatment, and the conflict between the needs of the care giver and the needs of the disabled individual.

The family's fears and apprehensions regarding care giving must be addressed as soon as they are recognized. Fear is a great source of stress for families. These fears identified by Hamberger and Tanner include the following:

- Accidentally injuring the patient
- Not knowing what to do in an emergency situation
- Receiving criticism from the patient and/or nursing staff
- Losing leisure or career time to become the care giver
- Accepting more responsibility than they can handle
- Causing adverse effects on the family as a unit[14]

These fears can be alleviated by teaching basic care-giving techniques utilizing the principles of andragogy. Studies have indicated providing thorough information about the disease or disability can significantly decrease stress in care giving. Providing the family with clear, necessary information in written format or media format such as a videotape provides the family with the needed information that can be absorbed in the care giver's own time and environment. Allowing time for the care giver to absorb the information presented will enhance learning. The family gains confidence as they participate in care giving (repetition) and eventually learn to carry out the treatments independently.

Modeling by the therapy staff can be a valuable teaching tool in order to instruct the family care giver in necessary care. Always approaching a stroke patient from the affected side in order to encourage the patient to look to that side is an example. Practicing hands-on training provides the care giver with active participation and the po-

tential for problem solving utilizing the professional's input. Often the care giver will verbalize that the professional therapists "perform the tasks easily" and "are more successful" with the patient. The therapist needs to acknowledge to the care giver that success is due to familiarity with, and repeated use of, the appropriate techniques. The care giver often may find a better way to perform the same task and share it with the therapist.

Hamberger and Tanner identify six educational objectives for the family:

1. Knowledge of illness
2. Knowledge of patient's functional potential
3. Knowledge of patient's functional limitations
4. Knowledge of needed treatments (theory, practical application, and complications)
5. Knowledge of prescribed medications
6. Knowledge of available resources[14]

The therapist's awareness of these six objectives can ensure that the family has adequate information relevant to the care-giving responsibilities.

Conflicts within the care giver can create internal stresses that conflict with the ideal environment needed to optimize the rehabilitation goals. Two stresses identified by Hasselkus relevant to patient education are (1) a sense of personal causation ("If only I had gotten to him quicker") and (2) a fear of inadequacy or "goofing up," which can make accompanying the patient to therapy sessions a frightening and threatening experience.[15] During the period prior to discharge, an attitude of "They know best" prevails with family members passively accepting the therapist's instructions and recommendations, despite fears and doubts about their own capabilities.

During the period immediately postdischarge to home care, the sense of failure on behalf of the family may shift from concern about long-term solutions to a focus on day-to-day problem solving. Some care givers describe this period in terms of "busy-ness" with multiple services being provided in the home, whereas other care givers describe these services as intrusive: "I was always waiting for someone" or "My days were never my own." While observation by the therapist of the care giver is an appropriate part of a treatment session, care givers may perceive such observation as threatening and respond with agitation and irritation.

The theme of managing can become predominant as care givers struggle to establish routines, to learn new tasks, and to bring a semblance of comfort to the new situation. During this period, learning behaviors can reflect tension between the previous pattern of "They know best" and an emerging pattern of critique and modification. Initial efforts to do what they were "supposed to do" are gradually, or sometimes quickly, modified to be compatible with what the care givers perceive to be their own capabilities and their sense of coping. For many care givers, their growing sense of special knowledge may provoke the need to "teach the professional how." An eagerness to share what is successful can prevail. This tension between the care giver's views and the therapist's views may derive from the professional's view of care giving. The perspective based in professional training and theoretical background and the care giver's view of the situation as a personal experience may be in conflict. Treatment may not succeed unless discrepancies are recognized and resolved. To minimize this clash of perspectives, focus on the family as the integrating agency and the primary source of help. According to Hasselkus, the therapist's role then becomes a facilitator, a supporter, and an assistant to the family as the family develops self-help strategies.[15] A specific strategy presented by Payton et al. is a learn-use-teach model whereby the care givers learn a skill, practice the skill, and then teach the skill to others.[24]

In summary, families as care givers have unique worries, concerns, fears, coping mechanisms, and experiences as a result of their care-giving responsibilities. The physical therapist would be remiss to ignore these concerns or the wealth of knowledge and experience that result from daily "hands-on" care. All experienced therapists probably have learned some of their most "functional" hints from a care giver or a patient. In understanding the characteristics of an older adult learner, the significance and importance of allowing the care giver to be self-directed are clear.

ASSESSMENT OF LEARNING

Patient education is only as effective as the results occurring from the education and learning experience. It cannot be assumed that learning has taken place because the instruction has occurred. Without evaluation, the instructor has no information on the success of the instructional activity. Successful evaluation not only indicates achievement but also reflects and provides information on the degree of instructional effectiveness.

For purposes of this section on assessment, *learning effectiveness* is defined as a change in behavior directed toward achieving the goals agreed upon in the initial patient session. The effectiveness of the educational experience can be evaluated many ways that vary from traditional tests. Variations of the question-and-answer format include learning contracts, self-report, interview, diaries, checklists, and return demonstration. Several will be described here.

Learning Contract

One of the most significant findings from research on adult learning is that when adults are internally motivated as contrasted with being taught something, they are highly self-directing. Learning that is engaged in for purely personal development can be independently planned and carried out completely by an individual on his own terms and with only a loose structure. Learning that has the purpose of improving one's competence to perform a given task or activity must take into account the needs and expectations of the learner, the therapist, the institution, and any medical or environmental concerns that may affect the activity. Learning contracts provide a means for negotiating a reconciliation between these external needs and expectations and the learner's internal needs and interests.

Knowles recommends that several steps be followed to develop a learning contract:

1. Identify the learning need
2. Specify the learning objectives
3. Specify learning resources and strategies
4. Specify evidence of accomplishment
5. Carry out the contract
6. Evaluate the learning[19]

The imposed environment and structure that inhibit the older adult's deep psychologic need to be self-directing may result in resistance, apathy, and withdrawal. Learning contracts provide a vehicle to make the planning of learning experiences a mutual undertaking between the physical therapist and the patient. By participation in goal setting, resource identification, strategy choice, and evaluation of the accomplishments, the patient develops a sense of ownership of, and commitment to, the plan. Furthermore, the basis for assessment of learning is evident.

Self-report

Self-report often is discounted as a reliable method of evaluation because of its subjective nature. However, self-report assessments of noncompliance have been found to be reliable, and patients often respond favorably to intervention techniques. Advantages of the self-report method of assessment are the speed and ease of administration and, if utilized correctly, its facilitation of the patient-therapist relationship. The supportive, empathic approach discussed earlier is recommended to obtain valid information and to develop a rapport with the patient so that inappropriate behaviors can be investigated and modified if indicated.

The issue of empowering the older adult and allowing him to be self-directing may entail giving the patient permission to be noncompliant. Acknowledging that adherence to a particular activity is difficult for the patient provides a supportive environment so that the patient feels comfortable in admitting any problems that may be occurring. Schunk states that self-report may lack some of the validity and objectivity of other methods in assessing adherence, but it can provide instant valuable information in the clinical setting.[27]

Checklist

A checklist can be used to assist in the evaluation of performance based on specific criteria. A checklist is an observational tool that allows for observing and recording the presence or absence of behaviors, characteristics, or events in specific learning situations. Activities on the checklist should be stated clearly and should reflect the most important components of the task. The more clearly the actions are described, the more accurate the learning assessment will be. The checklist can be used by family members in teaching each other specific tasks and care-giving responsibilities and also can be used as a reminder of important components within a treatment plan.

Return Demonstration

Return demonstration or checkout after instruction is usually some variation of "What did you hear me say?" or "Show me what you are going to do." The therapist checks for accuracy and completeness of what the patient understood from the instruction. A checkout is important not only immediately after instruction but also at a later date. By observing the patient perform the activity without cuing from the therapist, an accurate assessment of learning can be determined. Asking the patient to show how the home exercises are being done provides valuable information on the accuracy of the patient's understanding—without which adherence to the program is impossible. Care must be made to avoid a threatening or ridiculing atmosphere in order to allow the adult learner the choice to be self-directing or to be noncompliant.

Self-assessment Questions for the Therapist

The following questions, identified by Freedman and adapted by Gardner et al.,[13] may be helpful in a self-assessment of instruction and interaction.

1. *Have I correctly assessed what my patient knows?* What has been taught before, and how much does my patient remember? What technical terminology needs to be reviewed or clarified?
2. *Am I certain that I know what needs to be taught and what my patient should be able to do as a result of my instruction?* Do the objectives reflect our negotiated goals? Are they in the appropriate sequence?
3. *Have I planned an introduction to the instruction?* Have I planned how to communicate clearly what will be taught and what my expectations are in this session?
4. *Did I present the information clearly and give pertinent examples?* Did I confuse my patient in my instruction? Was my instruction in logical sequence, with pauses for my patient to assimilate the information and to ask questions? Were my directions clear? Were there clear-cut guidelines for my patient to follow?
5. *Did I present information and examples that were relevant to my patient?* Did I keep the instruction focused on the main points without cluttering my patient's information-processing mode with extraneous material? Were my examples clear and to the point?
6. *Did I prevent or avoid an information overload for my patient?* Did I present information appropriate for the time I had with my patient? Did I limit my instructional aids or handouts to those that emphasized the major points?
7. *Were my handouts and other instructional aids appropriate?* Were my handouts organized, clear, simple, and legible? Was the reading level appropriate for my patient? Did they accommodate any vision impairment?
8. *Did my patient have enough practice time?* Did I remember that older learners do not respond well under pressure or on timed tasks? Did I help my patient develop a sense of confidence in the task? Were my verbal and nonverbal feedback reinforcing?
9. *Did I help my patient by providing cues to proper performance?* Did I coach my patient during the practice period? Did I point out any specifics that my patient could monitor to determine correct or incorrect performance?
10. *Was I sensitive to my patient?* Was I aware of my patient's reaction to the information I presented? Did I try to see things from the patient's perspective?

The effectiveness of instruction is greatly enhanced by clear, concise, and direct verbal expression. The therapist's nonverbals of body language, voice tone, and eye contact should inspire confidence in the therapist without limiting interaction or intimidating the patient. The therapist's verbal and nonverbal behaviors can contribute significantly to creating a positive learning environment that is conducive to positive interaction between the patient and the therapist.

PATIENT EDUCATION SCENARIOS

The following three scenarios illustrate selected principles that have been presented in this chapter. As you read "The

Incident" and "The Dialogue" sections, make note of significant points that relate to the chapter's content. Then check to see if these points are included in the "Discussion" and "Summary" sections. You should identify more points than are included in those sections.

Scenario 1: The Inattentive Learner

The Incident

Mr. Smith, a 75-year-old white male, was admitted to a rehabilitation facility 3 weeks ago for stroke. Although he has been willing to work toward his goals in all previous sessions, today he is inattentive to the therapist, observed by his lack of eye contact, fidgeting, head movement, and other body language indicators. The therapist has to repeat instructions and, questions, and basically no progress is being made.

The Dialogue

Therapist:	Mr. Smith, you seem to be preoccupied today. What's on your mind?
Patient:	Well, as a matter of fact, I've got a problem I need to take care of at the bank, and I don't know how or when I can take care of it.
Therapist:	I can understand why you are preoccupied. Anytime my bank calls me, I get worried, too! What could we do to help you with this problem?
Patient:	Well, I really need to personally talk with my banker as soon as possible. But I just don't see how I can do it. *(Pause.)* Do you really mean that you can help?
Therapist:	The best we can do is to at least try. What do you need?
Patient:	I need a ride because I have to take care of this in person. But I don't know if I can get in and out of the car!
Therapist:	If I can arrange a car and driver for this afternoon, would you be willing this morning to work on how to get in and out of a car?
Patient:	Do you really think I can learn how to do that this morning?
Therapist:	Yes, I think you can with some hard work. You already have worked hard on improving your balance, and besides, you've been getting in and out of cars all your life. Let's go do it.

Discussion

The therapist recognized that the patient was distracted and preoccupied. The therapist provided an opportunity for the patient to say what factors were creating interference with this treatment session by asking an open-ended question that gave the patient the opportunity to state his need. The therapist further demonstrated realness and empathy with the patient's concern by stating that a call from his banker also would concern him.

With encouragement and another open-ended question, the therapist facilitated the patient's problem-solving skills, allowing the patient to maintain autonomy and self-empowerment, by determining how that need could be met. The therapist demonstrated prizing of the patient by addressing the patient's need and by referencing the patient's accomplishments in therapy as well as past experiences.

Summary

The therapist recognized that the patient's problem was primary to the patient and that the therapy was low on his priority list. Therefore, the patient was not ready to learn. By having the patient identify the reason for inattentiveness and then utilizing those needs and concerns, the therapist was able to negotiate the activity for this treatment session. Therefore, the patient's goals were accommodated and progress toward the discharge goals was made.

Scenario 2: Learned Helplessness

The Incident

Mrs. Bailey, a 69-year-old black female, has an above-knee amputation and has been referred to physical therapy for prosthetic training. She is accompanied by her husband who appears impatient and unwilling to let his wife attempt any task. She appears passive and willing for, if not expectant of, his assistance. During the evaluation, her passiveness and helplessness also appear to be her pattern of behavior in the home setting.

The Dialogue

Therapist:	Mrs. Bailey, what would you like to be able to do at home that you aren't doing now?
Patient:	Well, I'd like to be able to do things in my kitchen.
Therapist:	What kind of things do you want to do?
Patient:	I want to be able to cook dinner and do the dishes.
Therapist:	Is your husband doing those things now?
Husband:	Yeah. I cook and do the dishes because my wife can't stand up.
Therapist:	What would you like for your wife to be able to do?
Husband:	I'd like for her to be able to stay by herself so I can get out in the fields and do my work. But that would mean I'd have to leave her alone, and I just can't do that.
Therapist:	Mrs. Bailey, do you think that you could be able to stay by yourself?
Patient:	Well, my husband does everything for me now. I don't know if I can or not.

Therapist: Mr. Bailey, it is important to realize that your wife can learn to do a number of things for herself if she is given the opportunity. However, it means that you have to allow her enough time to perform a task in her way without interfering or taking over.

Husband: That's really hard to do. It is easier and quicker for me to do it for her. Besides, she was so sick that she really needed my help.

Therapist: I understand that. You obviously have done a terrific job, and lots of husbands would not have done as well as you have. However, she's progressing so well that she is ready to learn to walk on her artificial leg. For both of you to regain the independence you both want, she needs the opportunity, the time, and the encouragement to begin practicing those things that together we decide are the next steps in her treatment program.

Discussion

The therapist recognized that some social barriers prevented Mrs. Bailey's willingness to participate fully in a treatment program designed to promote her independence. Chief among these barriers was her husband's overt willingness to assist in her every movement. The therapist was sensitive that this level of care giving was required initially and positively acknowledged the husband's care giving.

The therapist recognized that in order to achieve the level of independence that both the Baileys desired, less assistance will be required from the husband and more initiative from Mrs. Bailey. The therapist achieved this in a supportive manner by focusing on both of their goals while describing the process in achieving those goals. In this way, goal negotiation is a mutual agreement rather than a unilateral decision by the therapist.

Summary

The therapist recognized the husband's care giving in a positive manner and then literally gave the husband permission to decrease the level of care giving as part of the treatment program, thus avoiding the exclusion the husband might feel as his wife worked toward greater independence. The therapist also made the wife aware that her physical condition now will safely accommodate increased activity and encouraged the patient's initiative by focusing on the patient's goal of being able to work in her kitchen.

Scenario 3: The Dominant Hurried Therapist

The Incident

Mrs. Miranda, an 80-year-old Hispanic female, checks in for her scheduled appointment at an outpatient clinic. She tells the receptionist in a thick accent that her granddaughter insisted she come and see about the pains in her right shoulder but that her granddaughter couldn't come with her. After a considerable period in the waiting room, she was shown to a treatment cubicle by the receptionist and was told to wait for the therapist. The therapist eventually rushed in to the cubicle and, without introduction, told the patient that he was here to "fix her shoulder."

The Dialogue

Therapist: So, honey, the receptionist tells me your left shoulder hurts. I think we can fix you up in a jiffy if you'll just do what I tell you to do.

Patient: *(Hesitantly with accent.)* Well, really, it's my—

Therapist: *(Interprets.)* Wudja say? Here, let's look at your shoulder.
(Therapist proceeds to examine left shoulder.)
I'm going to get a hot pack to put on your shoulder. Wait here.

Patient: Sí, sí.

Therapist: Wudja say?

Patient: Sí.

Therapist: Oh, well, whatever.
(Returns with the hot pack and places it on left shoulder.)
While the heat's on your shoulder, here's a sheet of exercises I wantcha to do. Eyeball these, and I'll be back in a flash.

Patient: *(Looks at the sheet, but her lack of proficiency in English impedes her understanding. Folds sheet and puts it in her lap.)*

Therapist: *(Returns and removes heat.)* Well, I know your little ole shoulder feels lots better now. Like I toldya, sweetie, you just do these exercises like it says, and I'll see ya next week.

Discussion

Mrs. Miranda represents an ethnic population whose knowledge of health care in the United States is sketchy at best. Her granddaughter, on the other hand, as a third-generation Hispanic, has become enculturated and recognized that her grandmother's traditional home remedies could be supplemented by professional care. Mrs. Miranda has some suspicion about people caring for her in an unfamiliar environment, but to please her granddaughter, she agreed to go to the clinic. In addition, Mrs. Miranda is aware of her limited English proficiency and her thick accent and is reluctant to speak when away from her community environment.

Often an older person has a greater comfort level with a nonauthoritarian person than with one who represents power and expertise. Mrs. Miranda told the receptionist and her granddaughter about her right shoulder pain; however, she did not persist in her attempt to correct the therapist when he placed the heat pack on the wrong shoulder. Further, she did not tell the therapist that she could not read the exercises on the paper that he gave her. No effort was made to determine her understanding or to demonstrate and practice the exercises.

This lack of communication occurred not only because of Mrs. Miranda's natural reluctance but also because of the therapist's dominant behaviors. The lack of an introduction, the ageist remarks, and no elicitation of the patient's needs or reasons for being at the clinic are examples of these behaviors. The therapist's body language also communicated to the patient that time was not available for attention to her situation. The numerous slang words used in the therapist's hurried speech only confounded Mrs. Miranda's difficulty with English. No directions were given concerning how she would make an appointment for next week.

Summary

This scenario attempts to present a negative role model for patient interaction that could result in, at the very least, ineffective treatment perhaps even to the wrong shoulder, and at the very most, the patient could actually be harmed if she didn't understand safety instructions. When communicating with an older person of an ethnic population, care must be given to adequately assess the level of English proficiency. The possibility that cultural perceptions of health care delivery can impede treatment necessitates the therapist's increased sensitivity. A willingness to assess the patient's understanding, the rate of speech, diction, attention to the patient's nonverbal reactions, and courtesy demonstrate this sensitivity.

SUMMARY

A therapist with competencies in the various treatment modalities can be successful with a geriatric patient only to the degree that the patient chooses to participate fully in the treatment regimen for the necessary time period. Given a therapist with the appropriate knowledge and skills in treatment techniques and modalities, the degree of success with a majority of geriatric patients will depend (1) on the patient's physical condition, level of motivation, care givers, and support systems and (2) on the therapist's skill as a patient educator.

A therapist who is a successful geriatric patient educator has developed the following:

1. A philosophy of patient education based on (a) some knowledge of learning theories from which a dominant orientation has evolved and (b) clarification of the therapist's approach as one of patient empowerment instead of authoritarian

2. An awareness of the characteristics of and sensitivity to the geriatric patient as an older adult learner
3. The ability to develop negotiated goals with patients
4. The ability to facilitate patients' learning
5. A willingness to regularly and honestly assess the quality and results of the instruction provided

Patient education as a treatment modality has a solid base in educational psychology and instructional theories as well as in everyday experience and practice. Geriatric patients need and deserve therapists who recognize the importance of this treatment modality and who will work to develop and enhance their competency as patient educators.

REFERENCES

1. Anderson T: An alternative frame of reference for rehabilitation: The helping process versus the medical model, in Marinelli RP, Orto AEO, (eds): *The Psychological and Social Impact of Physical Disability*. New York, Springer, 1977.
2. Avers D, Wharton MA: Improving exercise adherence: Instructional strategies. *Top Geriatr Rehabil* 1991; 6(3):62–73.
3. Babins L: Cognitive processes in the elderly: General factors to consider. *Gerontol Geriatr Educ* 1987–1988; 8:9–22.
4. Baker FM, et al: Rehabilitation in ethnic minority elders, in Brody SJ, Pawlson LG (eds): *Aging and Rehabilitation: The State of the Practice*. New York, Springer, 1990.
5. Bandura A: *Principle of Behavior Modification*. New York, Holt, Rinehart and Winston, 1969.
6. Bille DA: *Practical Approaches to Patient Teaching*. Boston, Little, Brown, 1981.
7. Bruner J: *Toward a Theory of Instruction*. Cambridge, Harvard University Press, 1966.
8. Cassata DA: Health communication theory and research: An overview of the communication specialist interface, in Nimmo D (ed): *Communication Yearbook II*. New York, ICA, 1978.
9. Darkenwald G, Merriam S: *Adult Education: Foundations of Practice*. New York, Harper & Row, 1982.
10. D'Onofrio CN: Patient compliance and patient education: Some fundamental issues, in Squires W (ed): *Patient Education, Inquiry Into the State of the Art*. New York, Springer-Verlag, 1980.
11. Gage NL, Berliner DC: *Educational Psychology*. Chicago, Rand-McNally College Publishing, 1975.
12. Gagne RM, Briggs LJ: *Principles of Instructional Design*. New York, Holt, Rinehart and Winston, 1979.
13. Gardner DL, Greenwell SC, Costich JF: Effective teaching of the older adult. *Top Geriatr Rehabil* 1991; 6(3):1–14.

14. Hamberger SG, Tanner RD: Nursing intervention with families of geriatric patients. *Top Geriatr Rehabil* 1988; 4(1):32–39.

15. Hasselkus BR: Rehabilitation: The family caregiver's view. *Top Geriatr Rehabil* 1988; 4(1):60–70.

16. Havighurst RJ: History of developmental psychology: Socialization and personality development through the lifespan, in Baltes PB, Schaie KW (eds); *Life Span Developmental Psychology*. New York, Academic Press, 1973.

17. Hibbard MR, et al: Cognitive therapy and the treatment of poststroke depression. *Top Geriatr Rehabil* 1990; 5(3):43–55.

18. Kemp BJ: Motivation, rehabilitation, and aging: A conceptual model. *Top Geriatr Rehabil* 1988; 3(3):41–51.

19. Knowles M: *The Adult Learner: A Neglected Species*. Houston, Gulf Publishing, 1978.

20. Lindgren CL: Understanding and promoting compliance in older patients. *The Older Patient* 1989; 3:28–30.

21. McLagan PA: *Helping Others Learn: Designing Programs for Adults*. Reading, Mass, Addison-Wesley, 1978.

22. Merriam SB, Caffarella RS: *Learning in Adulthood*. San Francisco, Jossey-Bass, 1991.

23. Parsons T: *The Social System*. New York, Free Press, 1951.

24. Payton OD, Nelson CE, Ozer MN: *Patient Participation in Program Planning: A Manual for Therapists*. Philadelphia, FA Davis, 1990.

25. Rogers C: *Freedom to Learn for the 80's*. Columbus, Charles E Merrill, 1983.

26. Sahakian WS: *Introduction to the Psychology of Learning*, ed 2. Itasca, Ill, Peacock Publishing, 1984.

27. Schunk C: Prediction and assessment of compliant behavior. *Top Geriatr Rehabil* 1988; 3(3):15–20.

28. Silverstone B: Social aspects of rehabilitation, in Williams TF (ed): *Rehabilitation in the Aging*. New York, Raven Press, 1984.

29. Smith V, Messikomer C: A role for the family in geriatric rehabilitation. *Top Geriatr Rehabil* 1988; 4(1):8–15.

30. Staropoli CJ, Waltz CF: *Developing and Evaluating Educational Programs for Health Care Providers*. Philadelphia, FA Davis, 1978.

31. Worcester MI: Tailoring teaching to the elderly in home care. *Home Health Q* 1990; 11:69–120.

The Social Context of Geriatric Care

Reimbursement Issues in Geriatric Physical Therapy

Jean Oulund Peteet, M.P.H., P.T.

INTRODUCTION

The preceding chapters have shown the wealth of technology, skill, knowledge, treatment, and programs available to the elderly to increase their function and enhance their lives. This chapter will provide a framework for understanding the current system of reimbursement for physical therapy services, discuss some of the issues involved in reimbursement, and challenge the reader to think about new models of delivery of care needed in order to continue to offer the services physical therapists are trained to provide.

INSURANCE PROGRAMS

The federal government provides some 80 programs to assist the elderly either directly or indirectly with long-term–care problems. There is no one program, however, designed to address all long-term–care problems in a comprehensive and coordinated manner. There is uniformity among states only in the Medicare program. Benefits in other insurance programs such as health maintenance organizations (HMOs) or indemnity plans (where coverage depends on a person's having an incident or medical problem) vary from state to state. An overview of the major programs that offer physical therapy services to the elderly will be discussed here.

Medicare

In 1965 the federal government became directly involved in health care in its enactment of Title 18 of the Social Security Act, known as the Medicare program, which provided for funding for acute medical care for people 65 years or older and certain people with disability. Medicare was not intended to be a program for long-term–care needs. Persons advocating national health insurance thought that a comprehensive system for our country would soon be developed. However, to date, such a system is not in place, and we are faced with working with the Medicare program as the major source of funding for all care for the elderly.

Medicare is administered by the federal government through an organization known as the Health Care Financing Administration (HCFA). The HCFA contracts with private insurance organizations called intermediaries and carriers to process claims and make Medicare payments. Medicare is a two-part program consisting of (1) Hospital Insurance (Part A), which helps to pay for inpatient hospital care, some care in a skilled nursing facility, home health care, and hospice care; and (2) Medical Insurance (Part B), which helps to pay for doctors' services, outpatient hospital services, durable medical equipment and some services not covered under Part A.[9]

Table 21–1 shows coverage of items most often needed by physical therapists for patients. Equipment is covered under Part B of Medicare. A physician's prescription is necessary for all items, but this alone will not ensure coverage by Medicare. Medical necessity must be documented, and often it is the physical therapist who is most able to address why the patient cannot function without a piece of equipment.

Generally, Part A Hospital Insurance coverage has deductibles and coinsurance, but most people over 65 do not pay premiums if they receive benefits under Social Security or the Railroad Retirement system. In addition, people under 65 can receive Part A benefits without paying premiums if they have been on Social Security or Railroad Retirement Board disability for more than 24 months.

Part B Medical Insurance has premiums, deductibles, and coinsurance amounts that the individual pays himself or through coverage by another insurance plan. Table 21–2 shows a comparison of benefits under Medicare Parts A and B.

The federal government pays groups of practicing physicians and other health care professionals to review the care given to Medicare patients. These groups are called Peer Review Organizations (PROs), and they have the authority to deny payments if care is deemed not medically necessary or has not been delivered in the most appropriate setting. PROs are also responsible for investigating beneficiary complaints about poor-quality care. Although such review of care should serve to improve quality and reduce costs, it also can have a significantly negative financial impact on health care providers. Medicare reviewers may determine retrospectively that a claim, that is, for physical therapy services, is in fact not medically necessary and deny payment to the therapist. If the therapist or facility has a large Medicare population and payment denials occur frequently, the therapist or facility may be unable to meet costs. Later in this chapter, suggestions for addressing this issue with patients and with Medicare will be discussed.

Costs have escalated in the Medicare program, making it imperative for the government to scrutinize closely the care being provided. An important change in reimbursement in the Medicare program occurred in 1983 when a Prospective Payment System (PPS) was enacted. Under this system, specific predetermined rates are set for each discharged patient. Diagnosis-related groups (DRGs) are the basis for this reimbursement system. The DRG system groups inpatients who are medically related in terms of diagnosis and treatment, and who are statistically similar in their length of hospital stay, in the same category.

TABLE 21-1.

Durable Medical Equipment (DME)

To be covered by Medicare, all the following conditions must be met. The equipment must be:
1. Prescribed by a physician
2. Rentable from a supplier (the method preferred by Medicare), returnable, and therefore, reusable by other patients
3. Used for a primarily medical purpose
4. Useful only to individuals who are sick or injured
5. Appropriate for use in the patient's home

Examples of equipment that may be covered:
   Walker, cane
   Wheelchair
   Prosthetic device for limb
   Prosthetic device for internal body organ
      Corrective lenses after cataract surgery
      Colostomy or ileostomy bags
      Breast prostheses
   Leg, back, neck brace
   Orthopedic shoes only if an integral part of a leg brace
   Surgical dressings, splints, casts
   Oxygen equipment

Examples of equipment never covered:
   Orthopedic shoes without a brace
   Dental devices

cohol and drug hospitals, and drug units within a general hospital. While the enactment of the PPS did not reduce benefits for Medicare recipients, there is the potential for decreased benefits and quality of care to patients as hospitals try to keep the length of stay of the elderly to a minimum in order to achieve maximum reimbursement from Medicare.

Medicare defines benefits under benefit periods. The first benefit period begins the first time a patient enters the hospital. It ends when the patient has been out of a hospital or other facility primarily providing skilled nursing or rehabilitation services for 60 days in a row. Ninety days of care is allowed in each benefit period. There is no limit to the number of benefit periods a patient can have for hospital and skilled nursing care. During 1991, Part A paid for

all but the first $628 of covered services for days 1 to 60 of a hospitalization. For days 61 to 90, Part A paid for all except $157 per day. If a patient goes beyond the 90 days of care in a benefit period, up to 60 lifetime reserve days can be applied toward care. Once lifetime days are used, there are no more.

Deductibles and coinsurance are a part of the Medicare plan. In 1991, the patient paid the first $100 annually for covered medical expenses under Part B. Generally, coinsurance was 20% of "approved" or "reasonable" charges. Medicare has specific guidelines on care they will approve and ceilings on the amount it considers "reasonable" as a charge. Additionally, there is a system of "assignment" whereby practitioners may choose or not choose to accept the amount Medicare will pay for a service.[9] The choice of assignment primarily applies to providers in outpatient settings, who may choose to accept or not accept assignment. If assignment is accepted, the provider agrees to accept as payment in full the amount the insurer (in this case, Medicare) will pay. If care is not provided on assignment, the patient is responsible for any amounts above the amounts approved by Medicare. An increasing number of providers have chosen to refuse to accept assignment in order to ensure themselves greater reimbursement. Physical therapists, usually only those in independent settings, may be able to reject assignment. Some things that might influence their decision are (1) the type of practice they have and whether the services they provide usually would be

TABLE 21-2.

Benefits Under Medicare

	Helps to Pay for:
Part A Hospital Insurance	
No premiums if benefits under Social Security	Inpatient hospital care
	Skilled nursing facility care
Must pay deductibles and coinsurance	Home health care
	Hospice care
Part B Medical Insurance	
Must pay premiums to receive it	Doctors' services
Must pay deductibles and coinsurance	Outpatient services
	Durable medical equipment

covered under Medicare and (2) the case mix of their patient population and their competition. If a practice wants to focus on care to elderly patients, it may be necessary to accept assignment in order to attract these patients to the practice. Patients, for financial reasons, will generally look for a provider who accepts assignment.

Despite attempts to control Medicare costs through the PPS and ongoing claims reviews, costs have rapidly increased, and this has prompted further federal legislation to address the problem. Ethical dilemmas are increasingly occurring as providers see that care is needed but will not be covered by Medicare and cannot be afforded by the patient.[11]

Supplemental Insurance

Medicare does not cover any long-term–care needs identified as "maintenance" care in any setting. *Maintenance care* is defined by Medicare as any care that does not significantly increase the patient's function but only maintains the condition of the patient.

The average cost of a year's stay in a nursing home in 1990 was about $30,000. Very little of this cost (about 1.5%) was covered by Medicare. This has prompted the need for supplemental insurance or "medigap" policies: policies underwritten by private insurance companies to cover such costs. Supplemental insurance, termed *Medex*, can also be purchased to cover the copayment of 20% that the elderly must pay under Medicare.

Long-term–care policies need to be reviewed carefully before purchase. There can be exclusions specifically for the care needed. For example, coverage might require the home-care provider to be state licensed or Medicare certified. Although this might first appear beneficial to the patient and no immediate barrier to services, many states do not license home health care providers. If a state does not license home care, benefits would be unavailable to the patient.

In evaluating any long-term–care policy, one should consider such things as whether there is a required hospital stay to receive benefits, guaranteed renewability, inflation coverage, coverage for home health care, and specific coverage of Alzheimer's and other organic-based mental illness. A good policy should pay benefits when the insured cannot perform basic activities of daily living (ADL). Who should buy these policies? Elderly who have exceptional financial resources and could afford to pay out of their pocket for a nursing home for several years usually do not need a policy. Elderly who have very little money usually cannot afford the policy premium. The policy most likely helps the people in the middle-income range. Individuals should be cautioned in purchasing policies as these policies are relatively new, and it is not clear, given the escalating costs of health care, whether insurance companies will be able to fulfill the obligations of the policy.

Prepaid Health Plans

There are some prepaid health plans such as HMOs that contract with Medicare to provide service to Medicare beneficiaries. Medicare pays these organizations directly for service.

The elderly can also choose to enroll in a prepaid health plan, if there is one available in their area, rather than receive benefits under Medicare's traditional fee-for-service system. These prepaid health plans charge the beneficiary fixed monthly premiums and minimal coinsurance payments. The benefits to the elderly are (1) there is minimal paperwork since they generally do not have to file any claims, and (2) many organizations offer additional services at minimal or no cost such as preventive care, dental care, hearing aids, and eyeglasses. In addition, in 1991, most HMOs that enrolled Medicare beneficiaries were required by the Medicare program to provide, at no additional charge, extended hospital and skilled nursing facility stays, expanded home health benefits, respite care, and coverage for certain drugs.[9]

A potential disadvantage for beneficiaries who choose an HMO is that they may have a limited choice in doctors, therapists, and hospitals. The HMO usually specifies which providers can be used in order to receive benefits. Since income received by the HMO is on a prepaid basis, there is increased incentive for the organization to minimize costs. A "gatekeeper," often a nurse or physician, may be used to control unnecessary use of services. HMOs ration physical therapy services by requiring physician authorization for a fixed number of visits. An elderly patient with a chronic problem requiring long-term physical therapy may find limited coverage authorized for a specific problem. This is more likely to occur in this setting than under a traditional indemnity, fee-for-service insurance plan.

Medicaid

The federal government became involved with health care for low-income individuals through the enactment of Title 19 of the Social Security Act by Congress in 1965. Financial assistance for low-income elderly is available through a joint federal and state program called Medicaid. In contrast with the Medicare program, Medicaid does support long-term services, principally nursing home care, but only for specified low-income persons or only after persons have exhausted their own resources. To qualify, annual income level must be at or below the national poverty level (1991 levels were set at $6,620 for one person and

$8,880 for a family of two), and the individual cannot have access to many financial resources such as bonds, stocks, or bank accounts. The state governments assist individuals by paying for health insurance premiums. Each state sets its own guidelines as to who qualifies for assistance. Physical therapists must know the specific requirements of each state in which they practice.

DOCUMENTATION REQUIREMENTS FOR REIMBURSEMENT

There are three important requirements for reimbursement to physical therapists under the Medicare program. First, services must be prescribed by a physician. Second, services must be "reasonable and necessary" to the individual's illness or injury and under accepted standards of medical practice; they must be of a level of complexity and sophistication such that only a licensed physical therapist can provide the service; and there must be the expectation that the condition will improve significantly in a reasonable period of time. Third, physician recertification is required every 30 days. Certification can be accomplished by written communication between the therapist and physician.[8]

On the face of it, these requirements might seem easily met even though the requirement for physician referral and continued authorization negates any direct access to physical therapy where allowed by state laws. In practice, documenting so that reimbursement is received for service not only requires a knowledge of Medicare guidelines but also additional help from therapists experienced in documentation and articles, such as those published in American Physical Therapy Association publications that address practical issues and offer "how-to" suggestions.

Examples of documentation that *would* support reimbursement for physical therapy for Medicare patients are the following:

1. Range of motion (ROM) measurements show loss of motion compared with the unaffected side.
2. Strength shows significant loss—in zero, trace, poor, fair range.
3. Type of exercise includes resistive exercises with weights or manually, muscle re-education, proprioceptive neuromuscular facilitation, and stretching.
4. Patient is treated for more than just pain, that is, loss of ROM and/or strength.
5. Evaluation is complete with measurement of ROM, strength, and functional assessment, and patient shows steady progress with objective evidence of improvement in baseline measures (strength, ROM, functional assessment).
6. Patient shows functional gains as a result of treatment.

An example follows of an initial evaluation summary that meets the requirements for Medicare reimbursement.

> This 70-year-old female patient suffered a fall 2 weeks ago, sustaining an eversion strain. She has rheumatoid arthritis, diagnosed 10 years ago, and has hypertension for which she is on daily medication. Patient presents in physical therapy with decreased ROM and strength on MMT (manual muscle test) (see details in initial evaluation) in the left ankle, decreased joint position sense in the left ankle, and a compensated gait pattern secondary to ligamentous instability of the LE (lower extremity). Patient was previously ambulating up to two blocks with a quad cane. She was able to take care of her own ADL (activities of daily living). She now requires a walker, and her endurance is 30 ft indoors. The goal of physical therapy is to return patient to previous level of functioning. It is anticipated that she will need physical therapy three times per week for 4 to 6 weeks consisting of therapeutic exercise including strengthening of the evertors, icing after treatment, and gait training.
>
> J. Jones, P.T.
> Oct 1, 1991

It is important to be specific as to the reason the patient has come to physical therapy. In the above example, the ankle sprain is the reason the patient needs physical therapy. The additional diagnosis of rheumatoid arthritis is important, however, to document, as it may provide help in explaining, if necessary, why progress might be slow.

Examples of documentation that *would not* support coverage of physical therapy services include:

1. Maintenance therapy that includes a program where expected improvement is insignificant in relation to the extent and duration of the service
2. General strengthening exercises that maintain strength and endurance
3. Hot packs and paraffin
4. Passive range of motion

Frequently, many elderly persons need maintenance services in order to prevent deterioration of their condition. Medicare does allow for a home health aide to provide such maintenance and for a nurse and physical therapist to review the status of the patient on a regular basis. An issue for physical therapists are those patients who require the skills of a physical therapist to "maintain" their condition because of the complexity of their medical/psychologic problems. Patients with problems such as multiple sclerosis or parkinsonism may have this need. Considerable documentation is required by all care givers to demonstrate that such care should be covered under Medicare in these instances.

It is important that physical therapists understand insurance regulations so that they can assist the patient and family in determining whether Medicare or another insurance might cover the needed therapy. Many other insurers follow Medicare guidelines for reimbursement because Medicare standards are the most stringent. It is not acceptable nor will reimbursement be made if the therapist argues, "The physician thought the patient needed therapy, so I thought the insurer would pay for it." The therapist cannot assume merely because a physician (or podiatrist or dentist) has requested physical therapy services that evaluation and treatment will be covered by Medicare or any other insurer.

METHODS OF REIMBURSEMENT IN DIFFERENT SETTINGS

Acute Care

Reimbursement for physical therapy services in acute care settings is included in the fixed payment assigned to the particular DRG under the PPS. Thus, whether a hospital provides physical therapy once a day or twice a day, 7 days a week, the reimbursement stays the same. It is therefore in the hospital's financial interest to determine the intensity of service that can reduce hospital length of stay and to provide no more than that minimum. Physical therapists in acute care settings must demonstrate their value in reducing hospital length of stay or risk potential cuts in positions. In some cases, hospitals are contracting the service out in order to try to provide service more efficiently and cost-effectively.

Rehabilitation

To date, rehabilitation hospitals are exempt from the PPS. Rehabilitation hospitals can increase intensity of physical therapy and other rehabilitation services as necessary and add programs, bill for such programs, and receive reimbursement. Rehabilitation does not have to be provided only in a rehabilitation hospital but may be provided in a unit within an acute care setting if the services and program provided meet Medicare requirements. This includes intensive, coordinated, multidisciplinary nursing and therapies. In addition, there must be documentation that the patient requires that level of intensity of service. There is discussion that at some future date a PPS will also be applied to rehabilitation hospitals. If and when that occurs, the intensity of service able to be provided will likely be monitored closely and may be reduced.

Skilled Nursing Facility

A skilled nursing facility (SNF) has staff and equipment to provide skilled nursing care or rehabilitation services and other health services. Most nursing homes are not SNFs, and many SNFs are not Medicare certified. If certified as a Medicare provider, the SNF provides care under the Part A coverage. Physical Therapists may provide care (meeting the already mentioned reimbursement criteria) either as employees of a facility or as independent contractors. The SNF receives a fixed hourly rate for physical therapy services based on a method termed *salary equivalency*. This method involves consideration of local hourly rates in the area for physical therapists and some expenses of providing care (e.g., billing, bookkeeping). A rate is set for each state, and that is the most the SNF may receive for physical therapy. In 1991, the hourly rate reimbursed by Medicare for physical therapy ranged from $27 to $43 per hour, depending on the state where therapy was provided.[3] This low rate can compromise the ability of the SNF to offer a practitioner a competitive salary or to develop a financially favorable contract with an independent physical therapist.

Outpatient

Medicare requires certification for any facility or independent practitioner who provides care to Medicare patients. These requirements include such areas as quality assurance, safety, nondiscrimination, and documentation standards. Medicare can withdraw certification from a facility or individual if standards are not met.

There are a number of issues that have to date not been resolved regarding differences in benefits to the patient and reimbursement to the provider that depend on where outpatient care is provided. One is that Medicare imposes a $750 cap on benefits per year for patients receiving outpatient care in an independent practice. This cap does not exist for hospital-based physical therapy services. A second issue is that independent practitioners are required to maintain an office with appropriate equipment.

In independent settings, therapists are generally reimbursed 80% of what Medicare defines as "reasonable charges." Reasonable charges can be based on four different considerations: the actual charge; a customary charge for similar service—that is, one charged by other practitioners in the area; the prevailing charge; and an inflation-indexed charge. Medicare will reimburse the least of these four amounts. This system will be eliminated as a "resource-based relative value system" is developed for both physical therapists and physicians in independent practice. This new system will include values for different types of work provided (e.g., a manual muscle test would be given a higher work value than administering a hot pack), overhead costs of the practice, and a value for malpractice. A concern is that this new system may have a bias toward reimbursement of treatments consisting of modalities.[4]

Home Health

Today, home health care is not only the provision of skilled care services such as nursing, physical therapy, home health assistance, and speech therapy. It also includes sophisticated services such as nutritional feeding via feeding tubes; intravenous, antibiotic, and pain therapy; and chemotherapy. Table 21–3 shows the services covered and not covered by the Medicare program. This has increased the level of complexity of the patients with whom physical therapists work.

Medicare will pay for covered home health service by a physical therapist who is employed by a participating home health agency or is an independent Medicare-certified physical therapist. Medicare currently has a requirement that an independently practicing therapist must maintain an office with equipment that is surveyed by Medicare before certification is issued. This is a disincentive to physical therapists who wish to have only home health patients as their population, as it adds an increased financial investment to meet the Medicare rule of an office. Private insurers that cover physical therapy in the home may only require that a therapist be licensed in that state.

Hospice Care

A hospice is a public or private organization that provides supportive services and pain relief to terminally ill patients in a home setting. Medicare Part A: Hospital Insurance helps to pay for these services when the following conditions are met: (1) a doctor certifies that a patient is terminally ill, (2) a patient chooses to receive care from a hospice instead of standard Medicare benefits for the terminal illness, and (3) care is provided by a Medicare-participating hospice program. Physical, occupational, and speech therapy are covered under Medicare, as are all other services, only when treatment is for pain relief and symptom management.[9]

Nursing Home, Chronic Care

As has been discussed above, the Medicare program only covers "skilled nursing care," requiring certification by the Medicare program for any facility wanting reimbursement from Medicare for such. The joint state-federal Medicaid program covers care in nursing homes that do not qualify for Medicare because they provide a lesser level of skilled service. In these settings, the physical therapist's role is usually to evaluate patients for their ability to make functional gains and to develop programs for nursing or physical therapy aides or assistants to carry out. The therapist may be an employee and receive a salary or, in a growing number of instances, provide service under a contractual agreement with the facility.

Retirement Communities

Retirement communities can be divided into two categories: they either (1) provide health services directly or indirectly or (2) provide no health services at all. Those that offer health services are becoming known as continuing care retirement communities. These communities may

---

TABLE 21–3.

Medicare Coverage of Home Health Services

Home Health Services Covered by Medicare
- Part-time or intermittent skilled nursing care
    This can include 8 hours of reasonable and necessary care per day for up to 21 consecutive days—or longer in certain circumstances
- Physical therapy
- Speech therapy

If intermittent skilled nursing care, or physical or speech therapy, is needed, Medicare also pays for:
- Occupational therapy
- Part-time or intermittent services of home health aides
- Medical social services
- Medical supplies
- Durable medical equipment (80% of approved amount)

Home Health Services Not Covered by Medicare
- 24-hour-a-day nursing care at home
- Drugs and biologicals
- Meals delivered to the home
- Homemaker services
- Blood transfusions

have long-term nursing care or only provide limited emergency care. They may finance these services through a rental fee, on a fee-for-service basis, or through an entrance fee. Similarly, the housing units may be rental, cooperative, condominium, or entrance-fee type.[5]

Coverage for specific problems for physical therapy would generally fall under the guidelines for service delivery in the patient's home. Some retirement communities, realizing the benefit to attract the elderly, offer preventive exercise programs. Reimbursement for this service, which might be provided by a variety of individuals including dance instructors, health club instructors, or physical therapists, would be by contractual arrangement with the retirement community. Physical therapists need to increase their involvement in these communities. It is here that preventive and wellness education and exercise can occur.

REIMBURSEMENT ISSUES

Complexity of Medicare Program

The Medicare program is complex and confusing, both for providers and patients. Documentation requirements are burdensome, costly, and frustrating as rules for reimbursement continue to be changed.

This frustration has led, in a number of instances, to resolving these issues in court. In the case *Fox* vs. *Bowen*,[1] senior citizens in Connecticut in 1977 sued the federal government for denying physical therapy coverage. Denial rate in Connecticut was in the 90th percentile at the time of the case. The court decided that the intermediary in Connecticut had inappropriately denied physical therapy to the elderly. An expert panel, which included physical therapists appointed by the judge, made a number of recommendations that it is hoped will have impact beyond this one state. These recommendations were (1) to request that Medicare intermediaries use only Medicare regulations and not interpretations and guidelines developed to make reviews easier for them but that resulted in contradictions between the law and interpretations, (2) to encourage evaluation by physical therapists (not nurses or doctors) in determining whether an elderly person would benefit from physical therapy, and (3) to educate physical therapists and intermediaries in appropriate documentation of physical therapy services. The third recommendation was based on the finding that a high percentage of physical therapy notes lacked sufficient documentation.[7] While adding documentation requirements may seem burdensome, it is, in effect, our only means of demonstrating the care that is given and also our only means of eliminating arbitrary decisions for coverage of care. Resorting to legal assistance to resolve disputes with insurers certainly cannot be the preferred method for creating change, but the decisions coming out of such cases can have positive impact on the practice of physical therapy across the country.

THE FUTURE IN LONG-TERM CARE REIMBURSEMENT

Federal Legislation

The federal government is seeking ways to decrease costs of health care as well as provide coverage for the many Americans who currently have no health care insurance. A major bill signed into law is the Omnibus Budget Reconciliation Act of 1990 (OBRA '90), which is designed to save $492 billion in Medicare and Medicaid costs over 5 years.[10] This savings is being achieved by reducing payments to providers as well as by increasing deductibles and premiums to consumers. This will have a direct effect on physical therapists' ability to treat patients and should challenge us to show that the services being provided are essential or in some cases to remind us to be increasingly efficient.

A major legislative change addressing nursing home needs is the Nursing Home Reform Amendments of OBRA '87, made effective in October 1990. This legislation focuses on a new philosophy whereby nursing homes are required to focus on each individual's highest potential for physical, mental, and psychosocial well-being by assessing these abilities and developing plans of care for individuals.[10] However, there is the argument that most of the needs of the elderly for long-term care are primarily for personal care and that a system of coverage through medical insurance alone—for example, by expanding Medicare—will not work. Reform of Medicare is needed apart from addressing long-term–care needs. Economists suggest that savings should come in part by encouraging more health maintenance organizations to control costs by setting a financial limit for each enrollee.[2] Expansion of HMOs and other developments force increased recognition of the need to be efficient in delivering care and makes us advocates for justifying continued care not initially allowed for patients.

Advocacy Role of Physical Therapists

Programs for populations such as the frail elderly, well elderly, older athletes, and adults with developmental disabilities are discussed in other chapters in this text. In our current health care system, components of these programs that address prevention and wellness are not covered as a rule by health insurers. These are programs that should be expanded if we are to prevent many injuries and subsequent illness from occurring.

Arguments are made supporting both the need to have

such programs covered under health insurance policies and the need to have some costs borne by the patient. Therapists cannot, however, wait until insurance companies cover a program to develop it. Active involvement is necessary through state and national organizations to convince insurers and patients of the value of our services. Many programs to the elderly can be provided at low cost, and supportive personnel can be used to assist in the program. We are being increasingly challenged to become more efficient in our delivery of care and to ensure insurers that we are providing care at the least possible cost. Therapists will need to be increasingly creative as to how to develop, market, and financially support programs that are vital to the elderly and require our knowledge and skills.

New Models

Many studies have been done to attempt to predict numbers of elderly who may need long-term care. A study by Kemper and Murtaugh predicts that of 2.2 million people who turned 65 in 1990, more than 900,000 (43%) are expected to need nursing homes. They also project that at least 9% of those elderly will spend at least 5 years in a nursing home.[6]

These predictions have major importance for medical care. If we merely build more nursing homes to accommodate this increase, we will fulfill that prediction. There may be more creative ways to accommodate the disabled elderly. We already know that our current structure has not been serving us well. Increasing the number of residentially based services and the flexibility of such services may offer the elderly more privacy and dignity.

New models for living situations are already being developed for the elderly. One model is that of a "full-service" life care retirement community where elderly can use the equity from a home purchased years ago, which is now too large, to purchase a smaller living unit in a complex offering meals, nursing care, activities, medical supervision, and transportation if needed. This can be ideal for a single person or even a couple where one partner is frail and may need ongoing nursing. It allows the elderly the independence of owning their own living quarters but having services readily available. Unfortunately, this approach does nothing for the poor who have never been able to purchase a home and have few resources to stay independent.

Physical therapists will increasingly need to be involved in the development of regulations, quality assurance, and reimbursement criteria for physical therapy as it is provided in all settings. Physical therapists will also need to further educate patients and insurers about what our profession can offer with more evidence that it is cost-effective. We will need to develop a better understanding of all needs of the elderly and a positive definition of "maintaining function" as we work with patients who have diseases that may span decades. It may be that our role as teachers increases and that that is where a substantial portion of the "skill" of our profession will lie.

Physical therapists have been pushed by escalating costs to critically review the care we provide. We are facing the opportunity to further define our profession and participate in developing effective systems of delivery of care.

SUMMARY

This chapter has provided the reader with a framework for understanding the planning and financing of long-term–care services and some of the issues surrounding the need for changes in reimbursement systems. This is an area that will continue to change as legislators, insurers, and health care providers work toward developing a comprehensive system for financing services for the elderly.

REFERENCES

1. *Fox* vs *Bowen,* 656 F Supp 1236 (DC Conn 1986).
2. Ginzberg E: The reform of Medicare—If I were king. *J Med Pract Manag* 1987; 3:151–153.
3. Harker C: Table of rates calculated for salary equivalency increases. *APTA Prog Rep* 1990; 19:9.
4. Hsiao W, et al: Results and policy implications of the resource-based relative-value study. *N Engl J Med* 1988; 319:881–888.
5. Jennings MC: Financing long-term care. *Top Health Care Financ* 1991; 17:49.
6. Kemper P, Murtaugh CM: Lifetime use of nursing home care. *N Engl J Med* 1991; 324:595–600.
7. Lewis CB: Fox vs Bowen: A landmark decision for physical therapy in geriatrics. *Whirlpool* 1987; 9:12–14.
8. *Medicare Home Health Care Agency Manual.* Washington, DC; US Department of Health and Human Services, Health Care Financing Administration, DHHS Publication No 11, 1990.
9. *The Medicare 1991 Handbook.* Baltimore, Md, US Department of Health and Human Services, Health Care Financing Administration, HCFA Publication No 10050, 1991.
10. Omnibus Budget Reconciliation Act of 1990, Summary. Washington, DC, American Physical Therapy Association, Governmental Affairs Committee, 1990.
11. Purtilo RB: Saying "no" to patients for cost-related reasons. *Phys Ther* 1988; 68:1243–1247.

ADDITIONAL READINGS

American Association of Retired Persons: *Knowing Your Rights.* Washington, DC, AARP, 1988.

Barry K: Status report: The continuing process of developing Medicare's outpatient PT screens. *Phys Ther Today* 1988; II (spring):18–22.

Carney K, Burns N, Brobst B: Hospice costs and Medicare reimbursement: An application of breakeven analysis. *Nurs Econ* 1989; 7:41–48.

Ellwood P: Shattuck lecture: Outcomes management, a technology of patient experience. *N Engl J Med* 1988; 318:1549–1556.

Entoven A: Consumer-choice health plan. *N Engl J Med* 1978; 298:650–658.

Freedman S, et al: Coverage of the uninsured and underinsured. *N Engl J Med* 1988; 318:843–847.

Gillick M: Long-term care options for the frail elderly. *J Am Geriatr Soc* 1989; 37:1198–1203.

Ginzberg E: The destabilization of health care. *N Engl J Med* 1986; 315:757–760.

Ginzberg E: For-profit medicine. *N Engl J Med* 1988; 319:757–761.

Harrington C: Public policy and the nursing home industry. *Int J Health Serv* 1984; 14:481–490.

Hillman A, et al: Managing the medical-industrial complex. *N Engl J Med* 1986; 315:511–513.

Himmelstein D, Woolhandler S: Cost without benefit. *N Engl J Med* 1986; 314:441–445.

Iglehart J: Second thoughts about HMOs for Medicare patients. *N Engl J Med* 1987; 316:1487–1492.

Kane R, Kane R: Long term care versus tender loving care, in Williams SJ, Torren PR (eds): *Introduction to Health Services*. New York, Wiley, 1984.

Kane R, Kane R: A nursing home in your future. *N Engl J Med* 1991; 324:627–629.

Kinzer D: The decline and fall of deregulation. *N Engl J Med* 1988; 318:112–116.

Magary J: The fundamental elements of Medicare documentation. *Phys Ther Today* 1988; II(spring):23–27.

Mechanic D: Approaches to controlling the costs of medical care: Short-range and long-range alternatives. *N Engl J Med* 1978; 298:249–254.

National Citizen's Coalition for Nursing Home Reform: Summary of nursing home amendments in the 1990 budget act (newsletter). Nov 2, 1990, pp 1–5.

O'Shaughnessy C: Financing and delivery of long-term care services for the elderly. Adapted from O'Shaughnessy C, et al: *Financing and Delivery of Long-term Care Services for the Elderly*. Library of Congress publication No 85–1033 EPW, Oct 17, 1985.

Ricker-Smith KL: A challenge for public policy: The chronically elderly and nursing homes. *Med Care* 1982; 20:1071–1079.

Roper W: Perspectives on physician-payment reform. *N Engl J Med* 1988; 319:865–867.

Roper W, et al: Effectiveness in health care. *N Engl J Med* 1988; 319:1197–1202.

Rowland M: The long term care quagmire. *New York Times*, Oct 4, 1990, p 16.

Weisset WG, et al: Models of adult day care: Findings from a national survey. *Gerontologist* 1989; 29:640–649.

Ethical and Legal Issues in Geriatric Physical Therapy

Andrew A. Guccione, Ph.D., P.T.
Deborah H. Shefrin, J.D., P.T.

INTRODUCTION

Not all the difficult decisions in physical therapy are related to choices about therapy. Sometimes the therapeutic choice appears quite simple, yet there arc other questions regarding the patient whose answers do not lie within the typical boundaries of physical therapy. These questions include:

1. When should the professional's opinion outweigh the concerns of the patient?
2. How do I decide how much time to give one patient and take away time from another?
3. What rights do patients have to control their care even when they are mentally incapacitated?
4. What do I do if I suspect someone has physically abused a patient?

Professional ethics and health care law provide the principal rules by which practitioners decide how they ought to act toward patients, other professionals, and one another as interdependent human beings. Specifically, ethics raises questions about the rightness or wrongness of actions on the basis of the self-chosen principles that an individual uses to guide conduct. The law deals with a smaller set of behaviors, including actions performed in a professional role, and judges their legal rightness or wrongness according to the rules agreed upon by specific legislative and judicial bodies. Often, law and ethics overlap, as their concerns are similar even if their scopes and processes are different. For instance, a legal proceeding may use the ethical standards of a professional group like the American Physical Therapy Association (APTA) or the opinions of expert practitioners to decide what standard of care applies to a case. Given the complexity of practitioner roles, health professionals simultaneously incur several kinds of obligations in providing care. When a person asks, "How ought I to behave? What do I owe as a professional obligation to my patient?" the questioner poses a broad ethical question whose answer may, in part, be already defined by the law.

It is always possible for the health practitioner to evaluate whether professional actions meet ethical and legal standards, even those activities that are routine behaviors. This chapter has two purposes. The first is to outline the ethical dimensions of professional practice and discuss the ethical issues that a physical therapist may confront as a practitioner to the elderly. The second is to identify the laws that have been passed and legal opinions that have been rendered to address these ethical issues from a legal perspective. These laws provide boundaries to the social context of geriatric care and place important constraints on professional actions.

PRINCIPLES OF ETHICS

There are situations in clinical practice that are so overwhelming in their consequences that no one doubts their ethical importance. Often, these cases are literally "life-and-death" issues, such as who can decide what medical care is appropriate for a terminally ill elder with senile dementia. While it is easy to assume that only unusual circumstances generate ethical problems, any professional action that a physical therapist might take toward another individual can be examined in light of its ethical impact. The day-to-day practice of physical therapy contains many instances in which physical therapists must consider what their ethical duties are and how they may act toward their patients. Because of the issues confronting elders, the need to make ethical decisions as part of one's clinical practice is particularly evident in geriatric physical therapy. The ethical obligations that may typically arise in any situation stem from five major concerns: respecting individual autonomy, avoiding negative consequences, promoting good consequences, maintaining professional fidelity, and ensuring justice.[11]

There are two ways in which we may understand autonomy as it relates to ethics.[1, 2] The first notion of autonomy comes from Immanuel Kant, whose view was that all individuals must always be treated as ends in themselves and never as means to an end. Kant believed that individuals are rational agents who freely impose upon themselves universalizable moral standards to which they will hold themselves accountable.[16] In comparison, John Stuart Mill developed the concept of autonomy from the perspective of freedom.[18] Mill thought that people should be limited in their actions only to the degree necessary to prevent harm to others and to allow everyone else a similar amount of freedom.

The second major category of ethical obligations draws attention to the probable consequences of an action and how these outcomes influence our decisions about what is the right thing to do. The primary consideration for physical therapists, as it is for all health professionals, is that the physical therapist do no harm (the principle of nonmaleficence). This cardinal rule of ethical health care is one that all health professionals cannot ethically and legally ignore. In its broadest form, *nonmaleficence* means: "Do no harm yourself, and protect individuals under your care from harming themselves or others."

In addition to avoiding harm, physical therapists are obliged to do as much good as they can (the principle of beneficence). Many individuals are initially attracted to physical therapy for the opportunity to do good by alleviating suffering and assisting patients to develop their fullest human potential. The promotion of well-being among individual elders extends the ethical dimensions of physical therapy to the societal level as the optimal health of all elders contributes to the common good of society.[26]

Next, there are general ethical obligations of fidelity that pertain to the professional-patient relationship. Commitment to truth telling and confidentiality, which are essential to good communication, provides a solid ethical foundation between a physical therapist and a patient. This relationship of trust assumes that the professional is committed to providing competent and compassionate care to all individuals. Although physical therapists can sort out the difference between being a professional care giver and being a friend to someone in need, elders who are lonely, and often very vulnerable when they are sick, may not make this distinction quite so easily. Therapists need to recognize that when an elder is sick, there may be a need for this person to feel safe among "friends." Even though professional care givers are "friendly" and honestly concerned about the patient's welfare, they are, in reality, not friends. For example, friends share their most troublesome problems with each other and derive support from each other. Professional care givers, on the other hand, would never burden a patient with their own personal problems or seek to have a patient provide emotional support for them.

It is not unusual for a therapist to develop a relationship with a patient in which many personal facts about the patient are shared openly with the therapist. This may include information about the elder's past or current medical history, personal relationships, and financial affairs. Family members and friends may seek to obtain information about the patient from the therapist, just as they would from any other member of the family or friend. Physical therapists are obligated to protect this information as a professional committed to confidentiality, divulging only essential information with only those who need to know such information and sharing personal information only with the prior explicit approval of the elder.

Finally, there is the principle of justice. The formal concern of justice is to ensure that individuals without relevant differences between them are treated equally. Rawls has argued for a concept of justice as fairness, whereby essential goods and services must be distributed equally unless an unequal distribution works in favor of the disadvantaged.[20] Physical therapists frequently concern themselves with issues of justice when they decide how to allocate resources to patients, including the time they spend with some individuals, which lessens the time they can spend with others. Considering only an individual's need for treatment, a therapist may opt to spend more time with a more therapeutically challenging patient who has the less overall potential, rather than the patient who actually needs less therapy to realize a greater rehabilitation potential. Given the shortage of physical therapy personnel in the United States, it is impractical to believe that each pa-

tient will receive an optimal amount of physical therapy based solely on the need for treatment. Physical therapists, especially those who work with elders, must increasingly consider the outcome of treatment in relationship to the investment of resources when choosing to provide more physical therapy resources to one patient than another.

THE CONCEPT OF RIGHTS

When a therapist needs to determine what ought to be done to act ethically in a particular situation, there is often a need to consider a patient's rights and their relevance to a decision about what to do. A *right* is a claim by one individual or group that can be made upon another person or group. Some rights are protected by law.

Rights and duties are correlative. If a person has a particular right or claim that can be made on someone else, then the person or group on whom that claim has been made has an obligation or duty to the person invoking that right. Rights take two forms: liberty rights and entitlement rights. The American notion of life, liberty, and the pursuit of happiness are well-known examples of liberty rights. Each person is free to engage in the exercise of these rights as long as an individual's actions do not infringe on the rights of others. The duty attached to a claim based on liberty rights requires that another party refrain from acting or interfering with the exercise of those rights.

Entitlement rights entail a different set of concerns. A claim made on another as an entitlement right requires that another party not only refrain from acting but also take positive actions to assist or enable another person to exercise that right. Social rights are often presented as entitlement rights. The debate over the right to health care has often hinged on the question of whether the government has a positive obligation to provide health care for all people. Some ethicists and politicians argue that the government has no such obligation to assist others in exercising their right to health care. Conceived as a liberty right, the right to health care obligates the government not to pass laws or allow regulations that prohibit individuals from receiving health care. Statutes against discrimination in the provision of health care on the basis of age, sex, race, creed, national or ethnic origin, or disability are an example of how a liberty right to health care corresponds to the government's duty to honor this claim made upon it. Presented as an entitlement right, the right to health care requires the government to do more than eliminate discrimination in order for a person to exercise the right to health care. One of the major barriers to receiving health care services, including physical therapy, is the ability to pay for these services. Therefore, some would argue that if an elder is unable to pay for health services, then the government must facilitate a person's entitlement right to health care by underwriting these services. To some extent, the government has already honored the right to health care as an entitlement by creating Medicare and Medicaid. These programs, however, do not allow all elders to receive all the services that might be recognized as "basic" to the health care of the elderly and essential for the humane treatment of our nation's elderly. The argument in the next few years over the right to health care as an entitlement will seek to establish a national consensus on what kinds and amounts of services constitute acceptable treatment of elders. Physical therapists who participate in this discussion and share their clinical expertise and experience can influence public policy in a way that will benefit everyone, including elders, through a just distribution of resources.

In health care the right to privacy may be conceived as both a liberty and an entitlement right. One has the right to have the details of one's medical care kept private, and therefore others must refrain from infringing on that privacy. Patients may also make a special claim on health care providers to maintain confidentiality. Conceived as an entitlement right, the right to privacy requires that professionals take appropriate actions to safeguard this entitlement in their record-keeping procedures and enable patients to exercise their right to privacy.

AUTONOMY AND PATERNALISM

Physical therapists have professional expertise that can promote good consequences for many individuals. The desire to do good and the knowledge of how to do it are strong motivations for physical therapists and a substantial consideration in their decisions about what they owe their patients. Therefore, physical therapists often refer to the principles of nonmaleficence and beneficence as justification for the actions that they may take to avoid negative consequences for their patients and promote their well-being. The desire to do good, however, often subtly encourages physical therapists to act paternalistically toward their patients. *Paternalism* has been defined as "interference with a person's liberty of action justified by reasons referring exclusively to the welfare, good, happiness, needs, interests or values of the person being coerced."[10] In short, paternalism denies the autonomy of the individual.

As described elsewhere in this text, physical therapists frequently experience situations in which patients ignore their home exercise programs or disregard safety instructions about how to use an assistive device. Sometimes, the physical therapist may believe that the patient should be "forced" into following the therapist's recommendations based on the reasoning that these suggestions were provided in the patient's best interests. Placing a professional's judgment of "what's best" for the individual ahead of

the expressed desires of the individual suggests that honoring a person's own choice (the principle of autonomy) should not count as much as the consequences that will follow (the principles of nonmaleficence and beneficence).

Autonomy cannot always be reconciled with the principles of nonmaleficence and beneficence in matters of health.[1] The consequences of some decisions that a patient might make may very well result in harm. For example, a patient's decision not to follow a physical therapy home program for range of motion might result in additional pain for the patient or further diminish function. Although this is distressing to the therapist, there is always the opportunity for the patient to reconsider. Sometimes, however, the exercise of autonomy may result in irreparable harm to the patient, or even death. For example, an elderly patient may refuse to take a cardiac medication that prevents a life-threatening arrythmia. A complete discussion of the complex ethical and legal issues surrounding this sort of situation is far beyond the scope of this chapter. It is, however, important to realize that a patient's mental status, mood, and outlook on life are essential data in such decisions. Therapists who have an ongoing, and often long-term, association with their geriatric patients may contribute much to understanding whether an elder is purposely choosing negative consequences, merely uneducated about the potentially harmful effects of not taking the medication, depressed to the point of contemplating suicide, or exhibiting signs of cognitive decline.

A physical therapist must then also consider whether interfering in an elder's autonomy is a temporary decision that will allow the individual increased autonomy in the future, or if the paternalistic act diminishes the person's autonomy on an ongoing basis for an unlimited period of time.[4, 5] For example, consider the ethical questions presented to the physical therapist in the case of Esther R. Esther R is an 84-year-old never-married female who has recently suffered a stroke and was transferred to a rehabilitation hospital within a week of the event. Although she generally cooperates with her therapist, she shows little interest in her program, and often states emphatically that she would rather "just go home to die." Should the therapist stop treatment and facilitate Ms. R's discharge home out of respect for her autonomy as an individual, or should the therapist continue to encourage her to participate as long as the patient offers no physical resistance to treatment in order for her to realize her full potential for rehabilitation?

The therapist may choose to act in a weakly paternalistic way and continue to coax and cajole Ms. R to receive treatment. On the grounds of preventing harm in the interim, the therapist might argue that the patient will be in a better position to make autonomous choices in the future when her depression is resolved and she has had sufficient time to adjust to the sudden changes in her life brought on by the stroke. On the other hand, at some later point in her rehabilitation, the therapist may also need to recognize that a patient's verbal request to be discharged from the hospital does represent the patient's own choice, regardless of the negative consequences that may ensue. In that instance, the therapist is obligated to communicate this fact to the rehabilitation team so that the appropriate discussions can take place and the discharge plan can be implemented, if necessary. Hospitals function to at least some degree, as the sociologist Erving Goffman put it, as "total institutions," controlling how the time of the individual will be spent, with whom, and under what conditions the "inmate" is free to leave.[14] Total control over all aspects of an elder's life may be even more predominant in the nursing home setting.[7] Once the patient has been taken into the system, time, energy, and money are invested in the process to make the person "better." It can be very difficult to reflect on what is happening to the patient, whether the patient has freely chosen to continue treatment, or perhaps to terminate treatment, when the patient still has rehabilitation potential. However, when members of the rehabilitation team forget to let the patient's own goals direct the team's efforts, the individual becomes a prisoner to the "good consequences" intended by others.

The conflict between the ethical principles of autonomy and the principles of nonmaleficence and beneficence in the case of Esther R underscores the nature of an ethical dilemma. An ethical dilemma exists whenever an individual is confronted with two or more mutually exclusive obligations in a single situation. Therapists confronted by an ethical dilemma find themselves proverbially "caught between a rock and a hard place." In fact, when a therapist weighs the alternatives, it is quite possible to find that no one alternative satisfies all ethical obligations at the same time. For example, one cannot always adhere to the principle of autonomy while simultaneously preventing all bad consequences from befalling a patient. In choosing what to do, one course of action will uphold one principle at the expense of another equally important and valued principle. Therefore, moral obligations, as specified by the general ethical principles outlined above, have come to be recognized as prima facie obligations, each needing to be recognized as relevant to the situation at hand on the first look.[21] None of these principles in itself, however, represents a final and absolute obligation. Otherwise, no decision in which a therapist weighted the importance of one ethical principle greater than another would be ethically defensible.

SOURCES OF ETHICAL CONFLICTS

Some situations with an ethical dimension require us to determine exactly where the ethical concern lies. Sometimes

a therapist may need to reconcile personal and professional beliefs. For example, although working with elders is a rewarding experience, this experience is not found with every elder. Try as one might, no physical therapist will be able to relate in a humanly meaningful way to every patient. However, every patient, regardless of the quality of the interaction for the therapist, deserves the best care that the therapist can render. The therapist in such a case must resolve the conflict between personal feelings and professional responsibilities.

Conflict can also occur between professionals or professional groups.[3] Other therapists, nurses, and physicians all have expectations of the physical therapist on the team. Some of these expectations facilitate a high level of performance among all the team members; other expectations are based on misinformation, misunderstanding, and mistrust. Such situations force us to consider what we owe our colleagues and what kinds of implicit promises have been made to each other by virtue of working together as a team.

Some ethical conflicts originate at the societal level. There is a wide difference of opinion within our society about how we ought to act toward elders, particularly in allocating health care resources. These differences are inevitable in a society that tolerates a range of political philosophies and also is composed of many cultures with different ideas about aging and the elderly. Some therapists, frustrated in their genuine desire to help their patients, may be tempted to do whatever is necessary on a case-by-case basis in order to achieve "justice" for each individual in their care. Just as laws do not resolve intra- or interpersonal conflicts, problems in the society at large must be addressed at the appropriate level and through the appropriate channels. Physical therapists who refrain from sharing their expertise delay recognition of unjust distributions of resources, where they exist, and perpetuate the conditions that hamper physical therapists in their efforts to allow all individuals to reach their full potential for rehabilitation.

PROFESSIONAL ETHICAL STANDARDS

Ethical analyses tend to focus only on the relationship between patient and professional and tend to divorce ethical problems from the larger social context in which they are found. As Beauchamp and Childress have commented:

> Moral principles . . . are not disembodied rules, cut off from their cultural setting. . . . "Morality," as we understand the term, emerges from shared experiences and social arrangements (tacit or otherwise).[2]

The professional community of physical therapists, the cultural setting of our ethical problems, has codified its shared experience and values in the APTA's Code of Ethics for the Physical Therapist and Standards of Conduct for the Physical Therapist Assistant. These two documents present the contextual framework for decision making by stating the behaviors to which all actions must conform. By endorsing a Code of Ethics, the physical therapy profession publicly states that certain ethical ideals should be implicit in every professional action committed by physical therapists. A patient reading the Code of Ethics or the Standards of Conduct can determine what ethical standards can be expected from physical therapy practitioners. For example, a patient who goes to any physical therapist can expect to be treated in a manner that supports personal dignity. Similarly, the Standards of Conduct indicate to the patient that physical therapist assistants are also ethically obligated to maintain confidentiality.

Although these documents do not provide specific answers to particular ethical problems, they do emphasize for the individual therapist or assistant those factors that the professional group believes are important to take into consideration when making an ethical decision. These ethical standards of the profession may also be used by others to formulate a legal decision as well. Failure to understand what is contained in these documents may adversely affect a physical therapist. The APTA's Code of Ethics ethically binds APTA members to its principles. Failure to meet these standards could result in sanctions such as being expelled from the association. The APTA's Code of Ethics can also affect nonmembers as well. Many state practice acts reference the Code of Ethics as the standard of ethical practice for all physical therapists licensed in that state, not just APTA members. Ignoring the Code of Ethics in these states may result in disciplinary action by a state board of licensure, which may even revoke a therapist's license. Official review of a therapist's actions by a licensing board may also look to the Patient's Bill of Rights to define what standard of care has been legally accepted.

LEGAL PROTECTION OF THE AUTONOMOUS INDIVIDUAL

Informed Consent

The essence of a clinical encounter between a physical therapist and a patient involves physically touching a patient for assessment and treatment. Although the physical therapist's "hands-on" actions are undeniably in the patient's best interests, a therapist may not touch a patient without that individual's permission to be touched. Touching without consent is known as battery, and a therapist may be sued when this occurs.[24] Most professional malpractice, however, does not involve touching without consent. Rather, allegations of malpractice tend to be made

when the patient has consented to being touched without having received enough information to give or refuse consent to the touching. When a therapist does not provide the patient with sufficient information to make a decision to receive or refuse treatment, the therapist may be held negligent for not allowing the patient to exercise the right to informed consent.

The term *informed consent* has been used in a legal context only for the last 35 years, when a California court ruled that a physician had a positive obligation to disclose any information regarding the risks and dangers of tests or treatments that was essential for an individual to make an informed decision.[22] The legal right to self-determination, however, was articulated earlier in the century when Judge Cardozo ruled that surgery performed on a mentally competent adult without the patient's consent was an assault for which the surgeon was liable.[23]

The legal concept of informed consent institutionalizes several of the ethical concepts described above and places particular legal obligations on the physical therapist. Respecting personal autonomy usually obliges a practitioner to assist an individual in the exercise of free choice by providing appropriate information and allowing the patient to develop sufficient understanding to make an informed decision.[2, 12, 13] From the moral point of view, informed consent is one way in which physical therapists respond to the principle of autonomy.[8] Although most actions that a physical therapist might take toward an elder are not as risky as those of a surgeon, every individual has a right to information that might lead the patient to reject the treatment, and the therapist has the correlative duty to furnish it. As Purtilo has noted, informed consent is a type of contract that is knowingly entered into by the physical therapist and the patient.[19] Under the law, contracts may only be made between equals and by those individuals who are legally free to enter into such binding agreements. Therefore, the physical therapist must share information with the patient to counteract the imbalance of knowledge between the two parties and legally ensure the patient's capacity for self-determination. Purtilo also identifies failure to inform an individual as a possible form of harm, which would be a violation of the principle of nonmaleficence. Furthermore, informed consent defines the patient's reasonable expectations to which the physical therapist must respond, a component of the principle of fidelity. Despite the legal recognition of these concepts, most patients do not understand the purpose of informed consent. In a now classic study, Cassileth and colleagues found that nearly 80% of 200 cancer patients believed that informed consent was a method of protecting physicians and not patients.[6]

As the term implies, informed consent involves two separate elements: information and consent. Legally, the information provided to the patient must satisfy four conditions. The information provided to the patient should outline the nature and the purpose of the treatment, alternatives to that particular treatment that the patient might choose instead, the risks and consequences of the proposed treatment, and the likelihood of success or failure of the treatment. Scott recommends that physical therapists provide patients with information checklists covering the most common physical therapy procedures or use them to guide discussion with a patient as a practical method of meeting the ethical and legal requirements of informed consent.[24]

In addition to the four conditions set on the information provided to the patient, the consent must be obtained from someone who is competent to consent, who clearly understands the information provided, and who agrees without coercion. In the case of the elderly individual, each of these three conditions may pose barriers to informed consent.[26] Elders suffer from the stereotype of declining mental competence. Present-day elders also often do not have the educational backgrounds of most members of society. Therefore, it is erroneously assumed that an older person is incapable of understanding complex information. Taking the time to explain to the patient is not merely educating the patient for therapeutic reasons. Ethically, it allows the individual to exercise autonomy, and legally to enter freely into a relationship with the therapist after an informed decision. Some elders are, in fact, mentally incapable of making decisions for themselves. This does not mean, however, that their rights to informed consent can be completely abrogated. Kapp stresses that there are degrees of mental incapacitation.[17] Even though an elder may be unable to make all decisions, there may be some decisions that are simple enough to be within the elder's grasp, particularly if environmental factors such as time of day or medications are controlled to present the decision to the patient during a period of lucidity.[17]

Living Wills

One of the areas of their lives over which most individuals wish to retain complete control is paradoxically enough the circumstances of one's death. The ability of technology to maintain the human body has created ethically troublesome questions of immense importance to most adults. Society has recognized that most of us wish to be able to tell our care givers how we want to be treated when we might otherwise be unable to communicate our choices. The Omnibus Budget Reconciliation Act of 1990 requires all health care facilities receiving Medicare or Medicaid funds to facilitate a patient's right to formulate advance directives about treatment in the event that the individual is no longer able to control the direction of treatment following loss of mental capacities. A Living Will is one type of advance directive that is recognized in most states. By executing a Living Will while still mentally competent, an individual indicates personal preferences for treatment; how treatment should be used to sustain life; and the conditions, if any, under which that person would find continuation of life unacceptable. Thus, elders have the opportunity to express how they wish to be treated, even if refusal of treatment may eventually lead to death if that is one's preference.

Durable Power of Attorney

Many health decisions do not concern prolonging life. These choices and decisions, some as simple as whether to participate in physical therapy or act as a research subject, also require the consent of the elder. Durable power of attorney is another method for ensuring that the patient retains a degree of autonomy, even though the patient's mental status prevents communication. A durable power of attorney is a legal document in which a person designates an agent who will act on the behalf of that person, should the individual become incapacitated. Durable power of attorney implies control over a broad array of decisions. Some states, therefore, specifically identify a durable power of attorney for health care decisions. This agent is not always the same person who has durable power of attorney over other matters, for example, handling finances.

Ideally, the surrogate is one who knows the individual very well, such as a spouse, child, or close friend, and can articulate what the incapacitated individual would say if able to do so. In comparison with Living Wills, durable power of attorney has the advantage of allowing the mentally compromised individual to direct all forms of medical treatment, not merely those related to death and dying. Unfortunately, even the closest spouse or friend may not have discussed every decision that might need to be made or know what the incapacitated person's views would have been on a particular issue. Doukas and McCullough recommend that elderly patients record their preferences through a values history, which establishes the general values that should underlie the decisions made on that individual's behalf by a proxy agent.[9]

ELDER ABUSE

One of the most distressing facts about the elderly is that they can be the victims of violence by criminals and abuse perpetrated by their care givers, including their family. Elder abuse may take many forms, but it generally involves some infliction of physical pain or mental anguish, unreasonable confinement, deprivation of services or articles that support an elder's physical or mental health, or financial exploitation.[25] The characteristics of an elder abuser are unclear. Sometimes the abusing spouse or child is continuing a tradition of family violence. The abuse may also stem from a care giver's own substance abuse problem, which predisposes to violence in stressful situations. Abusers may also have distinctly negative attitudes toward the elderly and unrealistic expectations of how much an elder can cooperate with the care giver. These negative attitudes are not limited to family members. Sometimes paid care givers with little training in geriatrics or appreciation for the elderly abuse patients. Physical therapists may assist the prevention of elder abuse by carefully guiding and educating all care givers in the proper treatment of the elder and establishing realistic expectations of an elder's dependency.

When a physical therapist suspects elder abuse, it should be reported to the appropriate authorities for investigation of the complaint and the initiation of adult protective services for the elder. These services will differ geographically. Each state has its own statutes that define who is responsible for reporting abuse and to which agency. Therefore, it is the responsibility of therapists to know the procedures specific to the states in which they practice.

The therapist may have learned of the abuse as part of confidential information or have been instructed by the patient not to reveal the situation. Although regulatory statutes that mandate reporting can be used to justify breaking the patient's confidentiality, such breaches of trust cannot be taken lightly.

Reporting abuse does not always lead to the consequences that the therapist might intend. One way in which an elder may be protected against further abuse is to be removed from the environment in which it occurs. Some elders will, however, refuse to leave their homes, even to escape violence. Elders may be reluctant to talk to investigators, fearing reprisals from the perpetrator of the abuse. Revelation of abusive conditions at home may unfortunately prompt additional abuse from the care giver who maltreated the elder in the first place.

The use of physical and chemical restraints has also come under intense ethical and legal scrutiny in recent years as a potential form of elder abuse. The Omnibus Budget Reconciliation Act of 1987 mandated several changes in nursing homes, including a prohibition on the use of physical and chemical restraints with nursing home residents except under certain conditions.[15] Physical restraints may never be used for discipline or the convenience of the nursing home staff, and a resident may refuse to be placed in a restraint. Restraints such as safety vests may be used to protect the patient or others from harm but should be as least restrictive as possible. A patient should be able to remove any physical restraint used as a safety reminder, such as a lap board on a wheelchair, without assistance from the staff. Proper record keeping is essential when restraints are used, as the professional applying the restraint may be held legally accountable if one is used without appropriate documentation and authorization. A physician's order to restrain the patient is required and must specify the purpose of the restraint, the type of restraint to be used, and the length of time it is required. If the patient is awake, a restraint must be released every 2 hours. While patient safety is a paramount consideration for every patient care provider, many professionals regard the attempt to reduce the use of physical and chemical restraints as a creative challenge that allows an elderly person an optimal amount of freedom of movement as well as protection from harm.

MAKING ETHICAL DECISIONS

Despite the intricacies of the issues that have been presented above, physical therapists do actually have to make difficult ethical decisions as part of their professional practice, just as they make difficult therapeutic choices. No matter how difficult this task may be, the need to decide can be inescapable. Fortunately, the overall process used to make choices about physical therapy procedures is the same as the process that is used to make other kinds of decisions in the clinic as well. In general, there are four steps to determine what is the ethically right thing to do: identifying the problem, formulating possible responses, weighing the alternatives, and choosing a course of action. The first step in the decision-making process requires us to determine what the facts of the case are. Specifically, it is essential to define just what the ethical problem is and what prima facie ethical principles are relevant to the situation. Often there are also additional facts about the context of the situation that are helpful to make a decision. Does the situation raise legal questions as well as ethical ones? It is quite possible that legal requirements prohibit or mandate certain actions by the therapist in response to the situation, as in the case of elder abuse discussed above. Identifying these in advance might decrease some of the uncertainty that accompanies many ethical judgments.

Because ethical problems can raise strong emotions very quickly, it is often thought that there is only one right thing to do. Physical therapists are fortunate in that most of the ethical decisions that they must make are not split-second life-or-death decisions. Although in some cases there is only one right thing to do, it sometimes happens that there are several equally acceptable and equally defensible things to do. The second step in ethical decision making is to list all the possible responses that may be made to a situation without prejudging the suitability of any one of them. Often the range of possible responses is much broader than originally thought, and careful consideration of all possible responses may yield an alternative plan that reflects more of the principles and values of the decision maker than the alternative that was conceived first. Once again, the law's constraints on professional behavior must also be considered.

Having set down the broadest array of responses, the decision maker must then proceed to weigh each of these options in light of the principles of ethics, the ideals of the professions, and the values of the individual therapist. In the case of a true dilemma, any option will compromise one principle while upholding the other.

Finally, one must settle on an alternative and implement a course of action. Resource constraints will rule some choices out of consideration. This is particularly true in matters of allocating scarce resources. For example, one way to provide physical therapy to every patient solely on the basis of need would be to hire as many therapists, physical therapist assistants, and aides as necessary in every physical therapy clinic. While this solution is ethically justifiable and obviates the need to ration resources, it is impossible to implement. In choosing to act, the therapist must be ready to take responsibility for acting. Although some ethical decisions are made with the same degree of uncertainty as other professional choices, following these four steps to make a decision can ensure that each therapist has made a reasonable and justifiable decision.

CASE: A DAY IN THE LIFE

Jennifer Radisson is the physical therapist assigned to the 18-bed geriatric rehabilitation unit at Village Falls Medical Center. She also covers a nursing home two blocks away from the hospital, which has contracted for services with Jennifer's physical therapy department of five therapists. Most of the patients on the geriatric unit are on active physical therapy programs. The therapists in this facility rarely have a slow day. Jennifer usually sees eight or nine patients at the nursing home for active therapy as well. Given her caseload, she is grateful for physical therapist assistants Bill Montoya, who works at the hospital, and Sabrina Jefferson, who works part-time at the nursing home. The nursing home has hired a physical therapy aide, Vivian Lesko, for a few hours each day to assist Jennifer, which has also helped her meet the needs of so many patients.

As Jennifer sits at the nurses' station at the hospital early one morning, sipping coffee and reviewing patient records, Dr. Virgilio stops by to inquire about the progress of Mrs. Godfrey, whose husband had been chief of medicine 30 years ago and was a major fund-raiser for the hospital's building campaign in the late 1960s. Although Jennifer is pleased with Mrs. Godfrey's progress, it has been slow. Dr. Virgilio reminds Jennifer how important the Godfreys have been to the medical center and suggests emphatically that Mrs. Godfrey's progress might be more substantial if Jennifer would increase the amount of time spent with her each day. Jennifer responds that she will do the best she can and makes a mental note to review Bill's caseload for openings.

Brian McSweeny, the head nurse on the unit, overhears the conversation and sits down next to Jennifer after Dr. Virgilio leaves. "Pushing for another donation, I bet," he whispers, "but don't give all your time away. There's a new patient in Room 1212, who was admitted last night. Seems like the poor guy lives alone with his son, who is known to the social worker down in detox. This new patient, whose last name is Gunther, is severely dehydrated, incontinent, and hasn't been out of bed for a week. The son says that he was fine until then."

"Thanks," Jennifer replies. "I'll put him right near the top of my priorities today."

Jennifer reviews her patient caseload. There is Mrs. Godfrey, the new patient Mr. Gunther, and two patients whose evaluations are still in progress. Jennifer is still not very clear about what their needs might be. In addition, Mrs. Reedy needs her discharge evaluation and referral, as she will be leaving the hospital for further rehabilitation closer to her daughter's home for her hip fracture. Mr. Stevenson and Ms. Sanborn are patients whose treatment goals and programs are well established. Jennifer cotreats Ms. Sanborn with Bill, the physical therapist assistant. She has used this opportunity to develop Bill's skills in treating neurologic patients. Bill has been carrying a full caseload of patients with diverse needs for the past 2 weeks.

As Jennifer is walking down the hall to meet the new patient, Mr. Gunther, she spies Mrs. Godfrey looking forlornly out the window.

"How are you doing today, Mrs. Godfrey?" she asks. "Is anything the matter?"

"Well, dear, I know my family is pushing everyone around here to wait on me hand and foot and to get me to therapy even more often than you do," Mrs. Godfrey replies. "But frankly, I don't even want to do what I'm doing now. Please don't take offense. You are a talented young woman, but I just really want to go home. I can afford to pay someone to help me."

Unsure of how to respond, Jennifer says, "Maybe we can talk about it later."

Jennifer introduces herself to Mr. Gunther, who is a thin, malnourished-looking man. As he responds to Jennifer's questions about his home life, Jennifer notices some small inconsistencies that suggest the need for a closer examination of his mental status. Given the number of other patients she has to see today, she decides to defer this issue until tomorrow.

As she is examining the skin on his lower extremities, she notices multiple cuts and several large areas of ecchymosis. "Did something happen to you recently?" she asks.

"Yeah, that lousy son of mine got stinking drunk and pushed me to the floor when he was supposed to be helping me," Mr. Gunther replies, almost with a laugh.

Jennifer is immediately unsure whether to believe him based on his questionable mental status. She concludes her examination and heads for the nurses' station to begin her note writing. When her beeper goes off, Jennifer responds immediately. The department secretary is transferring a call from Sabrina, the part-time physical therapist assistant at the nursing home.

Sabrina rapidly tells her that she was in a car accident on the way to work. "I'm shaken, but I'll be better by tomorrow. The car is the problem—it's a wreck. Look, I won't be in for the rest of the week. Maybe Vivian can do something with the patients. She really does know a lot about what I do with them," she says.

"Well, I agree," Jennifer says, "but I have to think about giving her so much responsibility, even if they really need the care."

As Jennifer heads toward the elevators and down to the department to discuss the situation with the department's chief physical therapist, she begins to review her predicament. She has a full caseload and now needs to cover for Sabrina or let an aide provide the care. She's not sure what to do about Mrs. Godfrey and Dr. Virgilio, nor what she should do with the information about Mr. Gunther's bruises. Bill cannot possibly increase his caseload without taking on a few patients whose problems exceed his expertise. As the elevator doors close in front of her, she wonders aloud, "What am I going to do now?"

If you were Jennifer, what would you do?

SUMMARY

Physical therapists in geriatric practice interact with patients, families, and coworkers in complex situations that can require careful ethical and legal analyses. A physical therapist is guided in the decision-making process by a concern to adhere to the ethical obligations of all health care practitioners and the rights of the patient. Specifically, with respect to the elderly patient, the therapist must seek solutions to ethical problems that conserve the individual's autonomy and promote well-being. Legally, autonomy is recognized through the requirements of informed consent. A strong commitment to ethical behavior and a sound knowledge of the laws governing professional

actions are essential components of a geriatric physical therapist's clinical practice.

REFERENCES

1. Appelbaum PA, Lidz CW, Meisel A: *Informed Consent: Legal Theory and Clinical Practice.* New York, Oxford University Press, 1987.
2. Beauchamp TL, Childress JF: *Principles of Biomedical Ethics,* ed 2. New York, Oxford University Press, 1983.
3. Bruckner J: Physical therapists as double agents: Ethical dilemmas of divided loyalties. *Phys Ther* 1987; 67:383–387.
4. Caplan AL: Informed consent and provider-patient relationships in rehabilitation medicine. *Arch Phys Med Rehabil* 1988; 69:312–317.
5. Caplan AL, Callahan D, Haas J: Ethical and policy issues in rehabilitation medicine. *Hastings Cent Rep* 1987; (special suppl):17(4):1–20.
6. Cassileth BR, et al: Informed consent—why its goals are imperfectly realized. *N Engl J Med* 1980; 302:896–900.
7. Collopy B, Boyle P, Jennings B: New directions in nursing home ethics. *Hastings Cent Rep* 1991; 21(suppl):1–15.
8. Coy JA: Autonomy-based informed consent: Ethical implications for patient non-compliance. *Phys Ther* 1989; 69:826–833..
9. Doukas DJ, McCullough LB: Assessing the values history of the elderly patient regarding critical and chronic care, in Gallo J, Reichel W, Anderson L (eds): *Handbook of Geriatric Assessment.* Rockville, Md, Aspen Publishers, 1988.
10. Dworkin G: Paternalism. *Monist* 1972; 56:64–84.
11. Francoeur RT: *Biomedical Ethics: A Guide to Decision Making.* New York, Wiley, 1983.
12. Gadow S: Advocacy: An ethical model for assisting patients with treatment decisions, in Wong CB, Swazey JP (eds): *Dilemmas of Dying: Policies and Procedures for Decisions Not to Treat.* Boston, GK Hall Medical Publishers, 1981.
13. Gadow S: A model for ethical decision making. *Oncol Nurs Forum* 1981; 7:44–47.
14. Goffman E: *Asylums.* Garden City, NY, Anchor Books, 1961.
15. Janelli LM, Scherer YK, Kanski GW, et al: What nursing staff members really know about physical restraints. *Rehabil Nurs* 1991; 16:345–348.
16. Kant I: *Foundations of the Metaphysics of Morals.* Indianapolis, Bobbs-Merrill, 1956.
17. Kapp MB: Medical treatment and the physician's legal duties, in Cassel CK, et al (eds): *Geriatric Medicine,* ed 2. New York, 1990; Springer-Verlag.
18. Mill JS: *On Liberty.* Indianapolis, Bobbs-Merrill, 1956.
19. Purtilo RB: Applying the principles of informed consent to patient care: Legal and ethical considerations for physical therapy. *Phys Ther* 1984; 64:934–937.
20. Rawls J: *A Theory of Justice.* Cambridge, Mass, Harvard University Press, 1971.

21. Ross WHD: *The Right and the Good*. Oxford, Clarendon Press, 1930.
22. *Salgo* vs *Leland Stanford, Jr, University Board of Trustees*. 154 Cal App 2d 560, 317 P 2nd 170 (1957).
23. *Schloendorff* vs *Society of New York Hospital*. 211 NY 127, 129, 105 NE 92, 93 (1914).
24. Scott RW: *Health Care Malpractice: A Primer on Legal Issues for Professionals*. Thorofare, NJ, Slack, 1990.
25. Staats DO, Koin D: Elder abuse, in Cassel CK, et al (eds): *Geriatric Medicine,* ed 2. New York, Springer-Verlag, 1990.
26. Wetle TL: Ethical aspects of decision making for and with the elderly, in Kapp MB, Pies HE, Doudera AE (eds): *Legal and Ethical Aspects of Health Care for the Elderly*. Ann Arbor, Health Administration Press, 1985.

Programs for Particular Populations

CHAPTER 23

The Frail and Institutionalized Elderly

Susan Neufeld Bloom, M.S., P.T.

INTRODUCTION

The growing elderly population provides a thriving market for the long-term–care industry. As the geriatric population increases, so does the need for rehabilitation services for these people. This chapter will focus on program development for the institutionalized frail elderly in the nursing home setting. The administrative aspects of working in this setting, from the standpoint of the physical therapist manager and the nursing home administrator, will be presented. Outpatient services for this population will also be discussed. It is hoped that the reader will gain insight into some of the challenges involved in initiating and providing rehabilitation services for the frail elderly so that one will be better prepared to meet these demands.

Profile of the Frail and Institutionalized Elderly

Burnside points out that "frailty is not exclusively defined by chronological age."[3] he further defines the frail elderly as "those vulnerable older persons who are dependent in one or more of the following areas: psychological, social, physical, cultural, or economic." By this definition, it should be evident that not all frail elderly are in institutions. Conversely, the majority of nursing home residents are frail because they do have needs in one or more of these areas.

Although less than 5% of persons over age 65 are in nursing homes and other institutions, this 5% will represent greater numbers with future growth of the elderly population.[4] The largest group of nursing home residents are aged 85 and older (45%), followed by those aged 74 to 85 years (39%), and 65 to 74 (16%).[6]

The typical nursing home resident is likely to be female and white and not currently married. The preponderance of women in the elderly population is due to the greater longevity of women than men. Female nursing home residents who were married are likely to be widows.[9] Only 6% are black.[6] Forty percent of nursing home residents are without a mental disorder such as chronic brain syndrome or dementia. However, 68% have one or more psychiatric symptoms that include, among other things, withdrawal, delusions, and hallucinations.[9] About half exhibit behavioral problems such as wandering, yelling, and hurting themselves physically.

According to 1985 statistics, most nursing home residents (91%) required assistance in the activities of daily living (ADL) of bathing, followed by 78% in dressing, 63% in toileting, and 40% in eating. Almost two thirds required assistance in transferring from bed to chair, and about the same percentage had walking difficulties.[6]

Medical necessity is a major reason for nursing home placement. Information exists on the incidence of chronic illness in the elderly, and there are morbidity statistics related to various diseases. However, there are no comprehensive data on the composition of nursing home residents with regard to prevalent illnesses and diseases. For those individuals with chronic illness or diseases, the nursing home setting is still the best option that our society has to provide at this time. Statistics have shown that there are two groups of patients entering a nursing home. There are the short-term (3 to 6 months) patients, who tend to be younger and more medically ill. And there are the long-term residents, who are older, generally confused, and often incontinent. Over half the persons admitted to a nursing home are no longer residents within 3 months. Many of these individuals have died in the nursing home, whereas many others have been discharged back to the hospital. About one third of nursing home discharges go back to the community.[8]

Risk Factors for Institutionalization

The degree of social support or lack of care givers is a contributing risk factor for institutionalization. Although 63% of residents have living children, these children may not live nearby or may not be capable of caring for their elderly parent. Studies have shown that elderly black persons are more likely to be cared for at home than their white counterparts and that they may have more "extended support systems" to care for them.[6] This is one of the main reasons for the small percentage of black people in nursing homes.

Another risk factor for institutionalization is believed to be the elderly individual's perception of his own health. There is some interesting evidence to suggest that perceived health correlates highly with mortality. Surveys have been conducted asking participants to evaluate their health, then correlated with mortality rates. They have found that self-assessed health can be a "sensitive and significant predictor of mortality even when the prior physical health status of the respondent is taken into account."[7]

A positive self-perception of health can also have an effect on physical functioning. One study involved a survey of frail elderly women, 85 years and older, residing in the community. Among other things, they looked at the respondents' abilities to perform ADL. The researchers found that positive health perception is related to two variables, level of independence and degree of social support available. These findings supported those of others that have shown that the elderly tend to equate functional independence with well-being.[14]

Medicare reimbursement also has had an effect on the types of patients being admitted to nursing homes. Skilled nursing facilities (SNFs) and intermediate care facilities (ICFs) have higher proportions of patients with ADL im-

Assessment of Balance / History of Falls.

Elements in the Assessment of Instability
I. Falls history.
    A. Onset - sudden vs gradual, frequency
    B. Activity at time of fall.
    C. Environmental Factors
    D. Presence of dizzyness, vertigo, lightheadness.
    E. Current meds, past meds
    F. Direction of falls.

II. Etiologic Assessment
    A. Sensory 1. vision → acuity, contrast, peripheral fields, depth perception, Bifocal
          2. Proprioception, vibration → distal to prox.   Ⓝ subtle mov't great toe.
          3. Vestibular → vestibuloocular fixation.
    B. Effector 1. Strength - prox. - isometric MMT, distal - isokinetic test
          2. ROM, flex. - ankle, knee, hip, trunk., C-sp.
          3. endurance. - 6 min. walk test
    C. Central processing 1. Feedback - postural stress test - manual.
          2. Feedforward - raising arms up, catching a ball.
          3. Response to changing conditions - reaction time.

III. Functional assessment
    A. Standing Reach
    B. Mobility Skills.
    C. Varied Conditions of performance.

IV. Environmental Assessment
    A. Functional home assessment.

pairments than retirement centers and other non–Medicare-certified facilities.[9] There were more functionally dependent residents in nursing homes in 1985 than in 1977, which is believed to be related to the Prospective Payment System (PPS).[9] This system classifies hospital patients according to diagnostic groups and assigns a specified number of patient days to each group. If patients are discharged before their length of stay is up, then the hospital recoups the monies for the unused days. Therefore, patients may not be medically stable or functionally independent when discharged from the hospital.

In summary, the factors that are often considered in studies that have looked at who is at risk for institutionalization are health status, social support, dependency in ADL, recent hospitalization, and prior living arrangements.

DEVELOPING THE REHABILITATION MENTALITY IN THE NURSING HOME SETTING

The nursing home industry is going through some very difficult changes at this time in adjusting to the reforms imposed by the Omnibus Budget Reconciliation Act (OBRA) of 1987. These mandated changes, known as the OBRA regulations, were enacted in 1989 and are ultimately intended to improve the quality of care being provided in nursing homes. However, in the meantime they will significantly affect the process of delivery of health care in the nursing home setting. The physical therapist who enters the nursing home to work must be sensitive to these changes and recognize that physical therapy may not be a priority in many nursing homes at this time. The physical therapist must also acknowledge that providing health care is a business, whether the facility is profit or nonprofit.

Rehabilitation and the Quality of Life

Sometimes, the newly hired or contracted physical therapist may even have to convince the administrator of the need for physical therapy. In these instances the physical therapist must develop some business panache and appeal to the administrator's sense of marketing. The therapist must foster the desire for physical therapy by creating the concept of rehabilitation for the administration and staff and making it an integral part of the nursing home itself. This is known as developing the "rehabilitation mentality."

One of the best ways to convince an administrator of the value of rehabilitation services is to explain how physical therapy can be a valuable selling point for the nursing home. Rehabilitation can be utilized to promote the facility as one that is concerned about the quality of life of its res-

idents. One can explain the term *rehabilitation* as the restoration of function or return to premorbid level of functioning. Implicit in this definition is that each individual is entitled to live at his optimal level of functioning, which is at the basis of the "quality-of-life" concept. Thus, the philosophy of rehabilitation is closely aligned with the philosophy of the nursing home, which is to provide residents with the opportunity to live the highest-quality life that they are able.

Rehabilitation, or restoration of function, also implies that improvement is possible. This should be especially emphasized because the older person has the ability to improve, despite the aging process. The geriatric population in the nursing home is not a homogeneous group, as was thought previously. Goals of rehabilitation should be developed for each individual and based on premorbid abilities, rather than goals that address the geriatric population in general.[4] The rehabilitation mentality emphasizes that the nursing home is a place where the elderly individual can improve functionally and not necessarily deteriorate or die. This gives the patient and family a sense of hope. It also allows families a means of allaying their guilt over having to place their loved ones in a nursing home. All of these elements promote the facility as a caring and hopeful environment.

Building the Rehabilitation Market

The growing elderly population provides a thriving market for the long-term–care industry. As the geriatric population increases, so does the need for rehabilitation services for this population. Despite the need for these services, the reimbursement climate for providing them is getting more restrictive, not only for rehabilitation but for all aspects of long-term care. Amidst this increasingly regulated environment, many administrators would prefer not to deal with Medicare reimbursement for rehabilitation services. This is because they may not be familiar or comfortable with the coverage requirements for skilled physical therapy under Medicare Part B or with the mechanics of billing for these services.

The simplistic breakdown of patients in a skilled nursing facility is into three primary payment groups. First is the private-pay patient who does not qualify for "skilled" physical therapy under the Medicare provisions. This individual pays for the nursing home stay entirely out of pocket. The second is the patient who qualifies for and requires either the skilled services of nursing or physical therapy. The third category is the Medical Assistance patient who may or may not require rehabilitation services. The state pays either a negotiated per diem rate or a flat-rate fee for these patients. The system and rate of payment vary from state to state.

From the beneficiary's standpoint, Medicare Part B will pay 80% of the physical therapy charge as long as the type and complexity of treatment meet the coverage criteria under Part B. The responsible party, either the patient or the individual who has power of attorney for the patient, pays the remaining 20% or copayment. However, there are private patients who are willing to pay the full cost for physical therapy if the services they require are not covered by Medicare Part B. This is where marketing and educating in regard to rehabilitation come into play, as will be discussed in more detail later.

For nursing homes that participate in the Medicare program as an SNF, the ability to provide physical therapy is required as a "condition of participation."[13] The extent of a nursing home administrator's knowledge about physical therapy reimbursement might be limited. They may know that the patient who requires "skilled" physical therapy must receive it 5 days a week. They might assume that a person with an admitting diagnosis of recent stroke or hip fracture will require this frequency of therapy and that Medicare will pay as long as the patient continues to demonstrate "reasonable" progress of some sort. They may also be aware that "specific" (as opposed to general) strengthening exercises and gait training for these types of patients are usually covered by Medicare.

Medicare requires only that the services of a registered or licensed physical therapist are available in the nursing home on a basis that is "adequate" to meet the needs of the types of patients who are admitted there. Space and equipment need only be "adequate" to treat these patients as well.[13] It does not stipulate the quality, quantity, and nature of services that are appropriate for these patients. So education in the rehabilitation mind-set is another area in which the physical therapist can benefit the administrator.

The nursing home administrator needs to know that the physical therapist does not only treat individuals with strokes and hip fractures, even though these are commonly the conditions most often thought of as requiring physical therapy. In educating the administrator concerning which patients may benefit from physical therapy, the emphasis should not be so much on particular diagnoses but on function. Administrators must know that physical therapy intervention can be beneficial for chronic conditions such as arthritis or cardiac disease and that the goals of treatment will focus on restoring the patient to a premorbid level of functioning. If there has been an exacerbation of a chronic illness or medical problems contributing to a temporary loss of function, then rehabilitation can be justified for coverage under Medicare Part B. This coverage always assumes that a return to previous functional abilities is the goal. Reimbursement also depends on whether these functional goals are realistic and appropriate to placement disposition, or where the person will be residing after discharge. For example, the ability to tolerate standing so that a meal can be prepared is not a reimbursable goal for a patient who will be residing permanently in the nursing home and will not be cooking. The same applies when judging the point to discontinue someone from therapy. According to common interpretation of Medicare regulations, the nursing home patient does not need to walk for extended distances. Progress in ambulation is usually covered for no more than 100 ft in the nursing home or as much as necessary to ambulate, for instance, to the dining room. Another appropriate functional goal in the nursing home would be ambulation to and from the patient's bathroom within the patient's own room. As limited as this scope of coverage is, such functional goals at least contribute to the patient's quality of life while in the nursing home.

These are the types of interventions that need to be stressed to the nursing home administrator when trying to expand knowledge of rehabilitation reimbursement. In all of the instances mentioned above, coverage would be under Medicare Part B. In the cases where therapy intervention cannot be justified on the basis of a temporary decline in function or medical exacerbation, some patients or families will want to pay privately for these types of functionally oriented activities that will improve their quality of life. Without elaborating on the details of Medicare coverage guidelines, which are covered elsewhere, a selling point to administrators is that there is a private-pay market for physical therapy. When there is an active rehabilitation service in the nursing home, families will not be as hesitant to place their loved one because they can still maintain hopes for that individual's improvement and possibility of returning home. This is the short-term philosophy of nursing home placement and one that helps to promote a positive marketing image.

Outpatient Physical Therapy

Another way of expanding this positive image to the community is to develop an outpatient physical therapy service based at the nursing home. Instead of the elderly's having to visit the busy hospital outpatient department, they can receive more personalized attention by therapists who specialize in treating the geriatric patient. This enables potential future patients to visit the nursing home on a nonthreatening basis and serves as an excellent marketing strategy for the nursing home.

A skilled nursing facility can obtain Medicare certification itself to provide outpatient physical therapy. There are also other routes to go if one wants to provide outpatient services out of the nursing home, which will be explored later when discussing program development. If the nursing home opts to provide outpatient therapy, it will involve an additional Medicare survey separate from the facility's survey. The survey is conducted on an annual basis and focuses particularly on the therapy department and the services provided. It also entails a closer look at clinical records and whether there are physician orders for physical therapy intervention and monthly recertifications for continuation of treatment. It also checks to see that the services provided were "adequate" to meet the rehabilitation needs of the patient and the established goals. It does not necessarily evaluate treatment outcomes and whether or not these goals were appropriate for the particular patient. Generally, it is more a paperwork process than a quality-assurance review.

Until recently, an SNF was only required to have the capability to provide physical therapy and speech-language pathology. The new OBRA regulations expanded the rehabilitation services definition to include occupational therapy as well.[10] The new regulations also scrutinize more closely whether or not residents are capable of carrying out ADL and maintaining that level of independence. The Medicare surveyors are usually instructed to investigate if resident functioning has declined since admission to the facility. The same applies to mobility, which includes ambulatory or wheelchair mobility and functional activities such as transferring. Facilities can be cited for patient care deficiencies contributing to declines in functional status. Even though Medicare guidelines are making justification for therapy coverage more difficult in some respects, these new survey requirements make rehabilitation intervention more crucial.

Determining Rehabilitation Potential on Admission

Nursing homes are also required to determine whether or not a patient has "rehabilitation potential" as part of the patient assessment on admission.[10] Use of an admission evaluation performed by the physical and occupational therapist can assist the nursing home in determining rehabilitation potential. It provides the nursing home with a detailed baseline for establishing functional abilities from the outset of a patient's stay. It also serves as a screening tool for patients who may benefit from a trial of physical therapy. When offered to all residents regardless of insurance status, it becomes an excellent marketing tool both for the nursing home and for the rehabilitation service. It gives the message to the public that the facility is concerned about the functioning of its residents and, again, highlights the potential for improvement in the elderly person.

The admissions counselor or a social worker can foster rehabilitation marketing efforts by making clients aware of the therapy services available at the facility. If the therapy personnel are on staff at the facility or there is a consistent contract arrangement, the following points can be emphasized:

1. Services available at least 5 days a week
2. Consistency of services with the same therapist
3. Team approach to patient care; available to coordinate treatment with rest of patient care team
4. Availability to interact on a regular basis with patients and family

It is important to keep in mind that the general public is not familiar with rehabilitation. Admissions counselors should also give a description of the different therapeutic disciplines. They can also assist you in screening patients for therapy and in establishing realistic treatment goals by obtaining information from the patient or family about premorbid or preadmission functioning. It is often helpful to prepare an admissions "script" to be used by whoever is responsible for the admissions process. An example of such a script is found in Table 23–1. It could also be included in an admissions information packet for the resident and family.

RESTORATIVE NURSING

Nursing Education and Training

The rehabilitation mentality is not just an approach to marketing; it is inherent in quality care. It must be instilled in all nursing home personnel. The largest group that needs to be influenced is the nursing staff. Above all other programs, a restorative nursing program needs to be developed first because it is the one that influences patient care the most. The nursing staff are the primary care givers, and these are the health care providers who are inevitably going to make the program work. They are instrumental in fostering an attitude of independence and self-sufficiency in patients, which is the keystone of a restorative program and the rehabilitation approach in the nursing home setting. Implementation of such a program may initially be viewed as a therapy project and not one in which nurses need to be involved. The nursing service needs to appreciate the importance of their role in the process and that it plays the key restorative role by encouraging independence in the residents. Nursing staff may also need to accept the idea that their jobs will be made easier by decreasing the residents' dependence on them. One of the best ways to achieve this realization is to let nurses see the influence of rehabilitation for themselves. As the residents begin to improve functionally and nurses see this carryover on the patient floors, they will see that it is easier to take care of the patients. Once this occurs, the effects can be cumulative. Nurses and aides will want to help the residents and each other, so that patients will become more functional sooner, and it will lessen their overburdened work loads.

Although one would think that the nursing staff would

TABLE 23–1.

Admissions Script for Admission Coordinators/Social Workers

- *What is rehab?*
   Rehabilitation is the process of providing services that will allow a person regardless of age or disability to achieve maximum physical, psychosocial, communicative, and vocational potential. The process also includes maintenance of improvement and prevention of regression.
- *What are the rehab disciplines?*
   Physical therapy. Focuses on physical functions that have been lost or impaired, such as the ability to walk or stand, and strength and balance deficits that may be the result of an illness or accident. Physical therapists use techniques of gait and balance training, manual skills, and therapeutic exercise. They also use physical agents or modalities as adjuncts to treatment, such as heat, cold, water, and electricity.
   Speech-language pathology. Deals with speech and language problems, which include communication skills (verbal and written) and the ability to read. It also assesses cognitive impairment and works with memory and comprehension.
   Occupational therapy. Concentrates in the nursing home on functional and self-care skills and training in ADL, which include dressing, feeding, and bathing. Occupational therapists fabricate assistive devices for self-care skills. They also work on fine motor control, perception, and cognitive skills.
- *What are the goals of the rehab effort?*
   To enhance quality of life for every resident. To allow residents to achieve their functional potential. To allow each and every resident to be as independent as possible and to live with self-esteem and dignity.
- *What are the benefits of rehab to the nursing home?*
   Enhances reputation of the facility by having quality rehabilitation services available. Gives families a sense of hope that their loved one's condition may be improved.
- *What is the Admissions Screening Evaluation?*
   This is a comprehensive assessment of an individual's physical functioning. It provides baseline information regarding strength and functional abilities to be maintained throughout the resident's stay. Also helps to identify those individuals in need of intervention by physical therapy, occupational therapy, or speech-language pathology.
- *Rehabilitation personnel evaluate the following:*
   Balance and stability for safety in walking; need for assistive devices to aid in walking, eating, or dressing; ability to transfer from bed to chair, wheelchair to toilet; strength and coordination as they relate to functional abilities and wheelchair mobility.

readily embrace the idea of making their jobs easier by making patients more independent, these changes can be difficult for some people. Whatever individuals are accustomed to doing is often perceived as the easiest, and learning a new way is always more difficult and energy consuming at first. The first time I conducted an in-service on transfer training for the nursing assistants provided an excellent learning experience of the obstacles faced by the physical therapist in this environment. Some of the staff had heard these lectures before, and it was obvious from their demeanor when they entered the room to attend the in-service that they believed there was nothing new I was going to tell them. However, by using a little humor and acknowledging their boredom, and also by presenting the material with a lot of enthusiasm, I was able to win a few of them over by the end of the in-service. One year later, after working hard with these individuals on restorative care throughout the year, I gave the same in-service. This time not only did most attendees stay attentive, but a few readily volunteered to demonstrate to the new staff some of the techniques that they had learned. For the benefit of

the old staff, I alluded to the in-service the year before, and we all recognized we had come a long way in developing a rehabilitation mentality.

One approach to dealing with these concerns is to convey that proper restorative care not only will lighten their work loads but will be safer for both the residents and staff. For example, proper transfer techniques and bed mobility have the potential of reducing the number of injuries for both patients and staff alike. Again, having the facts speak for themselves is often the best teaching approach. Gathering statistics or doing an ongoing study that looks at the number of resident-staff injuries can also be an excellent marketing tool for your restorative program and to present to the nursing home administrator. Medicare is increasingly holding nursing homes more accountable for risk management.

Another aspect to consider is how entrenched some nursing assistants are in the role of care givers. They may not be comfortable with the idea of patients trying to do for themselves, and they may foster a patient's dependency on them. Their sense of job security can also be threatened by the thought that increasing a patient's independence will lessen the necessity of their services. Some nursing assistants may become very emotionally attached to the patients they take care of, and it is not uncommon to hear a resident referred to as "my patient." In some ways, this is understandable because they spend a great deal of time with the residents. However, it should also be recognized that some of these attitudes toward care giving are not necessarily in the patient's best interests and should not be reinforced.

Program Goals

The primary goal of a restorative nursing program is to create an atmosphere in the facility that promotes the independence and self-sufficiency of each and every resident. Other goals of the program are to lessen the heavy work load on nursing personnel and to decrease the number of resident and staff injuries through instruction in the proper techniques of transfers, body mechanics, and self-care.

Training Program Curriculum

The facility-wide program should include an educational component and a consultative component, or a restorative screening procedure. First, there is the nursing education component. Prior to embarking on the program, it is imperative to meet with the director or assistant director of nursing, or the in-service coordinator (if the facility has one), to introduce the idea and to establish the educational needs of the nursing staff in regard to rehabilitation of the geriatric patient and restorative care. The most common components of restorative care include bed mobility, transfers, and gross mobility in ambulation. Other aspects of restorative care include proper bed and wheelchair positioning and basic range-of-motion (ROM) techniques. Another area that either a physical or occupational therapist should address is ADL and proper use of assistive devices. A suggested restorative care in-service curriculum is found in Table 23–2.

Training Approaches and Implementation

Obviously, giving a sample curriculum such as outlined in Table 23–2, in its entirety, entails a large time commitment from the nursing director and staff. The concept of giving such comprehensive training can be quite overwhelming to a facility that is accustomed to giving the one in-service per year required by Medicare. If this presents too much of an obstacle, then one might suggest targeting one of each of the six topics on an intermittent basis over the course of the year. However, if the facility makes the

TABLE 23–2.

Restorative Nursing In-Service Curriculum

I. Introduction.
   A. Principles of geriatric rehabilitation and restorative care.
   B. Goals of restorative program.
   C. Role of the restorative aide.
II. Positioning and bed mobility.
   A. Dangers of prolonged bed rest and immobility.
   B. Abnormal posturing in bed and chair.
   C. Positioning techniques and aides for proper positioning.
   D. Body mechanics for positioning and bed mobility.
III. Transfers.
   A. Body mechanics.
   B. Types of transfers (including use of Hoyer lift and emergency transfer techniques).
   C. Exercises to increase mobility in bed or chair.
IV. Exercise and ROM.*
   A. Definition of types of exercise.
   B. Principles of exercise and ROM.*
   C. Incorporating exercise into ADL.*
V. Ambulation and assistive devices.
   A. Preparation for ambulation.
   B. Guarding techniques for ambulation.
   C. Weight-bearing status and other precautions.
VI. Working as a rehabilitation team.
   A. Roles of occupational therapy and speech-language pathology.
   B. ADL techniques.

*ADL = activities of daily living; ROM = range of motion.

total commitment to a restorative care program, the entire six-lecture series can be presented. The preferred method is to present each lecture two or three times during the week, over a 6-week period. At the completion of the 6-week period, participants are given a certificate of completion or competence in the basic aspects of restorative care. This training program may also be given as part of the restorative nursing certificate program, which is now required for licensing of nursing assistants in many states. Lectures can be videotaped to be viewed on an individual basis or to be incorporated into a general nursing orientation.

Another approach to educating nursing staff concerning restorative care is the case study approach, using a patient for demonstration. Nursing personnel can identify a patient with restorative care needs in any of the areas mentioned above and allow the physical therapist to present this training at bedside or on the unit. The participants can also engage in discussion and hands-on practice of techniques.

The keys are consistency and repetition, whether lecture or practical is used as the approach. Restorative training needs to be an ongoing process throughout the year for the purpose of review and because of continual turnover of staff. The case study approach is a way of presenting a focus of information in a short amount of time, but it does not provide the comprehensive knowledge base that the lecture format does in the long run.

The Screening Assessment

The second major component of the restorative care program involves the physical therapist in the consultative role for screening patients in order to establish their restorative needs. The restorative screening assessment is generally a scaled-down version of the physical therapy evaluation. It often does not include the details of ROM measurement, manual muscle testing, sensation, and other neurologic testing that the full evaluation contains. Instead, the screening focuses on gross limitations in ROM and strength that would impair a patient's functional abilities in gross mobility and ADL. A screen should also succinctly identify for the nursing staff the degrees of assistance necessary for bed mobility, transfers, and ambulation. Those ADL for which the patient requires assistance or not are also documented. In addition, it may be appropriate to include a brief comment on cognition, communication abilities, and psychosocial status to give an overall picture of the patient. A sample screening form is pictured in Figure 23–1.

The primary purpose of the screening is to establish a restorative plan and to make recommendations to the nursing staff for the restorative care of the patient on the unit. The screening form is to serve as a quick reference tool for nursing. A copy of the plan should be kept in the medical record, and the director of nursing may be given a copy.

The restorative screening program should be a dynamic and ongoing one. Patients enter the program in one of two ways: (1) when discharged from an active course of therapy, and after having plateaued at a specified level of functioning; and (2) upon admission to the facility when not requiring a skilled course of therapy, or at any point in their stay at the facility when they are assessed by the physical therapist. Patients can be screened on a periodic basis (every 4 to 6 months) to assess whether any changes need to be made to the plan, or a nurse may request a screening evaluation if changes are identified on the unit. This periodic screening is not reimbursable unless a significant change in functional status is identified that requires physical therapy intervention on a skilled basis. If this is the case, a full physical therapy evaluation should be performed, which can be billed along with any justifiable charges for subsequent therapy.

Restorative Care and Carryover

Once the patient is screened and the restorative needs are identified, the challenge is to achieve carryover on the nursing unit. Again, the hope is that the nursing staff have bought into the concept of restorative care and will want to do it on their own volition. However, sometimes it is difficult to carry out this care on a regular basis. Many different approaches have been tried and many have failed. One of the best ways for a physical therapist to motivate the nursing staff is to act as a model and be seen out of the physical therapy department—and on the units! The physical therapist who stays in the department will be viewed as inaccessible and out of touch with the nursing needs and daily patient care struggles. Just lending an occasional helping hand can be most effective in gaining the cooperation of the nursing assistants. This does not have to be time-consuming and can be accomplished in a very casual manner. For example, it can be done when just passing by and seeing a need to reposition a patient in bed or in the wheelchair. Some of the best teaching on restorative care can be done on an informal basis such as this.

Some facilities will delegate one nursing assistant to serve as a "restorative aide." The role of this person is to assist nursing with keeping the residents mobile and with the functional aspects of patient care, such as dressing and getting the patient out of bed in the morning. This more likely works in a restorative or rehabilitative capacity than the nursing assistant who has been assigned to take care of the patient for the day. Aide duties involve ambulating patients who are not receiving active physical therapy. This individual also practices carryover on the floors in ambulation and functional activities with patients who are still on an active physical therapy program. This person is utilized on the patient floors and is under nursing supervision.

The position of a restorative aide can be helpful, but there is also a danger in having one such individual assigned to these tasks. When there is designated restorative aide, the tendency is that the other nursing assistants will expect the aide to handle all the maintenance ambulation and functional care of the patients on the unit. This defeats the ultimate goal of a restorative program, which is that each and every nursing assistant participates in carryover with functional activities on the unit.

The restorative aide is distinguished from a physical therapy aide or a rehabilitation technician as follows. According to the policy of the American Physical Therapy Association, the physical therapy aide performs "routine tasks related to the operation of a physical therapy service."[1] Furthermore, they "may function only with the continuous on-site supervision of the physical therapist or, where allowable by law and/or regulation, the physical therapist assistant."[1]

The verbal and written lines of communication must be clearly established in order for the restorative program to be successful. This includes the chain of command and supervisory control of the nursing assistants and the restorative aide. The nursing assistants need to know whom to

PHYSICAL THERAPY
PATIENT SCREENING EVALUATION

Name: _____ Date of Eval: _____ Date of Adm: _____

Database: _____

Range of Motion Limitations: _____

Strength Limitations: _____

Coordination: _____

Neurological: _____

	Intact	Altered	How
Sensation			
Respiratory			
Skin			
Cognition			
Communication			

Mobility	Ind	Suprv-Instr	Min Asst	Mod Asst	Max Asst	Unable	Comment
Rolling-Bed							
Sitting-Assume							
Sitting-Maintain							
Sit-Stand							
Stndg-Balance							
W/C							
Transfer							
Ambulation							

ADL _____

Psycho-Social: _____

Restorative Plan/Recommendations: _____

Therapist: _____ Date: _____

Pt. Name: _____ Physician: _____ File # _____

FIG 23-1.
A sample screening form for a restorative care program. (Courtesy of Mary T. Blackington, Meridian Health Care, Baltimore, Md.)

report to when they are having a problem with a patient, and the physical therapist needs to know whom to speak to when restorative care is not being properly carried out. Both nursing and physical therapy need to be accountable for their involvement, or the program will not work.

Information regarding restorative care can be relayed in patient care conferences or team meetings on the unit. The screening assessment provides the basis for written communication about the restorative care of the patients, but ongoing communication regarding functional progress or decline must also be relayed. Patient care flow sheets or an index card file for restorative care can be used for this and can also serve to document daily restorative care by nursing assistants. Diagrams on bulletin boards in the residents' rooms can also be helpful reminders of proper positioning or ROM techniques for individual patients. Another creative idea is "functional photography," or using a photograph of the resident involved in some functional activity to demonstrate abilities. This can be posted in the resident's room or on the door and serves as a means of identification for both staff and residents.[2]

The following points summarize the steps in embarking upon a facility-wide restorative program. The program should be planned in meetings with the director or assistant director of nursing. The first, and most important, thing is to elicit their cooperation and commitment.

1. Establish program goals with nursing
2. Define responsibilities of restorative care
3. Distinguish between restorative aide and rehabilitation aide
4. Establish responsibilities (job description) of restorative aide
5. Determine supervisory control, orientation, and training responsibilities
6. Establish lines of oral and written communication for relaying information about patient care and for accountability of nursing assistants in performing restorative care

REHABILITATION PROGRAM DEVELOPMENT

Once a solid commitment to restorative care has been established, one can begin to look at the development of other in-house rehabilitation programs that will further enhance the quality of life of the nursing home residents. When thinking about program ideas, it may help to do some brainstorming with the director of nursing. Once ideas are generated, prioritizing which programs to do first depends on patients' needs and which programs will benefit the largest number of residents. When designing programs, one should concentrate on programs that deal with gross mobility, functional activity, or ADL. Other large-scale needs may relate to restorative care, and any one of the aspects of restorative care could be made into a full-scale program.

Walking Program

A walking program is often the most obvious mobility need in terms of restorative care. The goal of such a program is to ensure that as many patients who are ambulatory walk each day on a regular basis and have the proper assistance to do so safely. This kind of program handles the large number of residents who are ambulatory but who are not attending physical therapy. If the nursing home does not employ a restorative aide, it is generally the responsibility of the nursing assistants to walk patients as part of the daily care plan. Most nursing homes work on a three-shift basis, with the two day shifts being 7 A.M. to 3 P.M. and 3 P.M. to 11 P.M. Because the morning care is usually tied up with bathing and dressing, it is not likely that the personnel are available to assist walking patients until later in the day. This usually occurs at the shift change, when the patient has been sitting most of the day and is likely to be too fatigued to participate fully in the activity. Once dinner is finished, it is generally time for the evening shift to prepare patients for bed. Therefore, the semiambulatory patient who needs some degree of assistance to ambulate may not have been offered assistance for more than one brief walk per day. This scenario illustrates the practical need for a formalized walking program.

One of the most informative guides for implementing a walking program in the nursing home is the *Maintenance Ambulation Program* by physical therapists Heim and Stoeckel.[5] Their instructional manual provides a comprehensive and systematic method for developing a workable walking program in the nursing home setting. It divides nursing home residents into three classifications as follows: those who require supervised or assisted ambulation on the unit by nursing staff; those who require supervised or assisted ambulation as above but who also continue on physical therapy; and those who have been discharged from an active physical therapy program but who still require skilled physical therapy to walk and who would decline if they did not receive ongoing skilled assistance to ambulate. The manual also includes flow sheets, descriptions and responsibilities of personnel involved, documentation guidelines, and forms for carrying out and maintaining the program on an ongoing basis. An exceptional design feature of this program is the way it shares the responsibility for the program between the physical therapy and the nursing staff. It puts the responsibility of maintaining the program on both disciplines because it allows entry into the system via either physical therapy or nursing.[5]

Turning and Positioning Program

Another way of encouraging gross mobility in the nursing home is through the TAP, or "turning and positioning," program. The way this program runs is that at certain times throughout the day a TAP announcement is made over the intercom system. At this announcement, all staff are supposed to drop whatever they are doing and interact with a resident in any way that encourages mobility. For bedbound patients, this would require that they are turned or repositioned. For those residents engaged in an activities class, this would be the time when the activities leader would ask all patients to stand or move about the room. For those residents sitting in a wheelchair in the hallway, this might be the time to get them to stand by their chair for the few minutes allotted to the TAP routine. This program is often nursing initiated, but if it does not exist in the facility, it is something that the physical therapist can help to get started.

Wheelchair Program

Another mobility-oriented activity is the wheelchair training program. The actual training of residents in wheelchair mobility can be accomplished in a class. However, more comprehensive assessment of proper wheelchair and fit would be better accomplished individually, if wheelchair adaptation is the goal. The physical therapist can also be helpful in taking an inventory of the types and physical condition of the wheelchairs in the facility. This input can be useful for administrators in helping them to determine their wheelchair needs when planning their capital budgets.

Once the residents have mastered use of the wheelchair, a resident wheelchair relay race is a particular way of demonstrating their accomplishment. This can be arranged with the Activities Department and is another opportunity to promote the team approach to patient care. Families of residents can be invited to attend, which is a good marketing event for the facility. Another idea for promoting public relations is to have a wheelchair marathon. Families and community members can participate in this event by sponsoring residents and contributing money according to how far they travel in the chair. In this way, funds can be raised for a particular community cause or national association. Not only will this be enjoyable for the residents, but it is an activity that will make them feel a part of the community and contribute to their feelings of self-worth.

Wound Care Program

Any program in which nursing and physical therapy can join forces to impact the quality of care of residents is one that is likely to meet with great success. A wound-healing program is such a program. Medicare has imposed stricter guidelines for reimbursement of chronic wound care such that nursing must explicitly document approaches to wound care in patients' care plans. Furthermore, there must be specific measurement of the wound on an ongoing basis that documents progress in treatment. Physical therapists can develop a hydrotherapy program in the nursing home and take part in debridement procedures in conjunction with nursing. Making recommendations to nursing regarding proper positioning is another important part of the program. We can also take a more active part in treatment by utilizing new advances in electrical stimulation. As described in another chapter of this book, physical therapy can provide nursing with a more aggressive approach to wound care than has been traditionally carried out in the nursing home.

Restorative Dining Program

An example functional program that deals with an ADL is a feeding or restorative dining program. This program illustrates the need for the physical therapist to be involved with other rehabilitation professionals. The expertise of an occupational therapist is critical to the success of feeding programs. Although physical therapists can adequately screen patients for the program in regard to the physical requirements of strength and coordination necessary for feeding, the training approaches and recommendations for assistive devices for restorative feeding are a particular competency of an occupational therapist.

Program Considerations

Regardless of the particular program, the basic elements of any program should include the following:

1. A method of screening either to evaluate functional abilities or to classify patients according to program requirements or guidelines.

2. A way of moving patients through, as well as in and out of, the system. New patients are continually admitted into the nursing home and others are discharged or die. Long-term residents demonstrate changes in functional status either as a result of improvement or deterioration. The system requires a means of entry either by physical therapy or by nursing, or other rehabilitation professionals, in order for it to be perpetuated.

3. A documentation/ communication system to con-

vey information about patients to all staff involved in the program on an ongoing basis and to ensure accountability.

4. A method of objectively evaluating the effectiveness of the program and determining if program goals have been met.

Program Costs

The primary cost in program development is the time it takes to plan, implement, and run these programs. Third-party payors do not reimburse providers for services other than for direct patient care. Once the programs are planned, it is appropriate (depending on the program) to get other nursing home personnel to run them on an ongoing basis. The payment options for the physical therapist in the nursing home situation are generally one of the following:

1. *Full-time employee of the nursing home.* Salary is paid by the nursing home, so that any time it takes to develop programs would need to be absorbed by the nursing home.

2. *Part-time employee or contract therapist.* Reimbursement is on an hourly basis, and any program time would need to be paid by the employer or contract.

3. *Employee or contracted physical therapist of a rehabilitation agency or other provider organization.* The provider bills the nursing home for services; so either the nursing home or the agency absorbs the costs of programs.

Third-party payors do not reimburse for group treatment. Some individuals may be willing to pay privately for a group program activity if the activity is considered important to the resident's well-being, and the charge is reasonable enough. Therefore, the ability to start programs depends largely on who is covering the development costs, and the viability of the programs is dependent on who is paying for the services.

NURSING HOME–BASED REHABILITATION EXPANSION

The Rehabilitation Agency

There are several alternative routes to providing outpatient services for the frail elderly. One avenue for expansion is to start a rehabilitation agency. This is a Medicare provider status for providing multidisciplinary care to people with physical disabilities. A rehabilitation agency must provide physical therapy, occupational therapy, or speech-language pathology and must have available social or vocational adjustment services.[12] If providing physical therapy, the facility must have at a minimum the equipment

necessary to provide the modalities of heat, cold, electrical stimulation, and hydrotherapy. The basic coverage guidelines for skilled physical therapy are the same as for any Medicare provider.

The administrative and financial management of the rehabilitation agency is more complicated than simply providing outpatient physical therapy at the nursing home. The annual financial cost report is more detailed in regard to administrative costs, and more statistics are required regarding the type and number of treatments provided. Administratively, a quarterly review of clinical records must be conducted.

The billing and clinical records are housed at one site that is considered the certified site, and extension units of the agency can operate at any number of other provider sites. Medicare Part B billing is done by the rehabilitation agency instead of by the individual nursing homes. This centralized system has a number of advantages over individualized provider services for each nursing home. It allows a large degree of control over the rehabilitation operations. In this respect, the quality of services provided can be better monitored through a home office. This structure lends itself well to nursing home chains because administrative overhead and other expenses can be shared throughout the system. The largest of these expenses is staffing. The system allows for better utilization of staff when different facilities have varying caseloads. Full-time staff can be utilized at a few sites, rather than hiring many part-time therapists to handle facilities where a full-time therapist cannot be justified on the basis of low or fluctuating patient loads.

As a rehabilitation agency, one can also provide services in the patient's home. The advantage to this is that the agency is not subject to the strict requirements of Medicare Part A, as it is when services are provided by a home health agency. The skilled requirements for coverage under Medicare Part A as a home health provider are more limited as to the types and degree of services provided to clients in the home than they would be as when provided on an outpatient basis. On the other hand, if the patient meets the Part A coverage requirements, then services would be totally covered if provided by home health. This is in contrast with a 20% copayment that is required if services are provided by the rehabilitation agency and is reimbursed under the Medicare Part B portion. This highlights the need for physical therapists to fully understand the intricacies of reimbursement that are detailed elsewhere.

The rehabilitation agency structure also enables contracting of services to other facilities and health care providers. Thus, it significantly broadens the market for rehabilitation services. One could contract with the local Department of Aging or senior citizen centers to provide consultation and direct care services to participants. Such centers sometimes have a small budget for consultation services for providing services to individual clients or for educational in-services to staff on patient management. Such lectures can include basics of gait training and proper use of assistive devices, or training in use of adaptive equipment for feeding and other ADL. The physical therapist's services may also be contracted to help develop, or to run, exercise or mobility classes at the senior center. If clients have Medicare Part B, ongoing physical therapy could be billed through the rehabilitation agency, or it could be billed privately.

Nursing home companies are building and entering into joint ventures with retirement centers and sharing the same grounds. With the growing elderly population and the increased longevity of the elderly, some retirement centers are finding increasing numbers of frail elderly as residents, rather than the more "well elderly" than were previously residing in these communities. The close proximity of such centers allows easy access to the nursing home when residents at the retirement centers become ill or disabled. This relationship can bring more rehabilitation patients into the nursing home and also affords the opportunity to provide outpatient services to residents of the retirement center. A rehabilitation agency based out of the nursing home would be able to treat other outpatients and to provide services at the retirement center.

Comprehensive Outpatient Rehabilitation Facility

A comprehensive outpatient rehabilitation facility or CORF, is the most recent development in Medicare outpatient certifications.[11] The concept of a CORF is to provide diagnostic, therapeutic (i.e., psychologic), and rehabilitation services all at one site. The focus of this type of facility does not necessarily have to be on rehabilitation, but it can be another way of providing these services if it suits the community's or organization's needs. A number of medical specialties and other services such as prosthetics and durable medical equipment can also be billed through a CORF structure. The major difference between a CORF and a rehabilitation agency is that all services at the CORF must be under the direction of a physician and must be provided on site. However, the physician's role in the CORF is more of a consultative and administrative one than a clinical one.

Outpatient Geriatric Assessment Clinics

Outpatient geriatric assessment clinics are an emerging trend for preventive care of the elderly. Although more well elderly will be utilizing these services, it is mentioned here because the frail elderly are likely to be identified through them. The scope and type of services provided by these clinics would depend on the medical needs of the community and the composition of the community's elderly population. These clinics provide another excellent opportunity for intervention by physical therapists as part of the multidisciplinary consultation team. They are also looking for resources in the community, such as rehabilitation or home health agencies, who will be able to provide the appropriate rehabilitation services to their clients. Although the intent of these outpatient assessment clinics is to prevent institutionalization, there are those clients who may be in need of nursing home placement.

SUMMARY

A variety of programs for the institutionalized frail elderly and service delivery options were discussed. It has been shown that there is much preliminary work to be done in preparing for the introduction of rehabilitation services. The key to a successful rehabilitation program in the nursing home is to develop a rehabilitation mentality in the facility's administration and the nursing home personnel. The rehabilitation mentality is reinforced through the restorative nursing program. The benefits of a successful inpatient program can produce an outpatient market and benefits for the facility. As our understanding of the health care needs of the geriatric population grows, so will the possibilities for our intervention as physical therapy practitioners and managers. It is the foresighted physical therapist who will take this clinical challenge and grow with it.

REFERENCES

1. American Physical Therapy Association: *Applicable House of Delegates Policies*. Alexandria, Va, American Physical Therapy Association, 1991.
2. Courtesy of Mary T Blackington. Meridian Health Care, Baltimore, Md.
3. Burnside I: *Nursing and the Aged: A Self-care Approach*, ed 3. St Louis, Mosby–Year Book, 1988.
4. Eliopoulos C: *Caring for the Elderly in Diverse Care Settings*. Philadelphia, JB Lippincott, 1990.
5. Heim M, Stoeckel L: *Maintenance Ambulation Program*. Jericho, NY, JHMCB Center for Nursing and Rehabilitation, 1985.
6. Hing E: Use of nursing homes by the elderly: Preliminary data from the 1985 National Nursing Home Survey. *Advance Data From Vital and Health Statistics, No 135*. Hyattsville, Md, Public Health Service, DHHS No (PHS) 87–1250, 1987.
7. Idler EL, Kasl SV, Lemke JH: Self-evaluated health and mortality among the elderly in New Haven, Connecticut,

and Iowa and Washington counties, Iowa, 1982–1986. *Am J Epidemiol* 1990; 131:91–103.

8. Kane R, Ouslander J, Abrass I: *Essentials of Geriatrics,* ed 2. New York, McGraw-Hill, 1989.

9. Lair TJ, Lefkowitz DC: Mental health and functional status of residents of nursing and personal care homes. *National Medical Expenditure Survey Research Findings 7.* Rockville, Md, Agency for Health Care Policy and Research, Public Health Service, DHHS Publication No (PHS) 90–3470, 1990.

10. *Medicare and Medicaid; Requirements for Long Term Care Facilities; Final Rule With Request for Comments.* US Department of Health and Human Services, Health Care Financing Administration, *Federal Register* 1989; 54:5316–5373.

11. *Medicare Program: Conditions of Participation and Conditions for Coverage: Specialized Providers.* US Department of Health and Human Services, Health Care Financing Administration, 42 CFR Chapter IV §485.50–485.74, 1990.

12. *Medicare Program: Conditions of Participation: Clinics, Rehabilitation Agencies, and Public Health Agencies as Providers of Outpatient Physical Therapy and/or Speech Pathology Services: Conditions of Coverage: Outpatient Physical Therapy Services Furnished by Physical Therapists in Independent Practice.* US Department of Health and Human Services, Health Care Financing Administration, 42 CFR, Chapter IV §405.1701–405.1805, 1990.

13. *Medicare Skilled Nursing Facility Manual.* Washington, DC, US Department of Health and Human Services, Health Care Financing Administration, HCFA No 12, 1990.

14. Schank MJ, Lough MA: Profile: Frail elderly women, maintaining independence. *J Adv Nurs* 1990; 15:674–682.

The Well Elderly

Marybeth Brown, Ph.D, P.T.

INTRODUCTION

The "graying" of America is a well-known fact. The burgeoning older adult population is a source of grave concern to federal planners, particularly those wondering about the viability of Medicare and Social Security into the 21st century.[8] Because of the increasingly higher percentages of men and women over age 65, projections indicate that the pool of available workers in industry—those able to shoulder the demands of physical occupations—is shrinking. Currently (and more so in the future), there is an increased demand on families for help as older adults are living longer, often with some form of physical disability. The current need for space in nursing homes and for older-adult living communities exceeds the availability of resources. Why this dismal scenario? Because those living beyond their 70s and 80s are experiencing considerable physical decline, to the extent that the majority of individuals over age 75 have some physical limitation. According to survey responses gathered by the US government from over 43,000 individuals randomly selected in the Northeast, 48% of those between the ages of 65 and 75 years have difficulty with one or more activities of daily living (ADL).[30] Those between the ages of 75 and 85 years have an even higher percentage of ADL difficulty—62%. The majority of people surveyed indicated that the biggest problem area was walking. Recent survey results indicate that women make up the greatest proportion of elders with physical limitation.[25]

How does all this fit into the well elderly? A substantial percentage of the physical difficulty experienced by today's older adult population can be prevented by adherence to a program of simple physical activity, prescribed and promoted by physical therapy. If exercise, in just about any capacity, could be incorporated into the daily routine, a shift to a healthier, more capable older adult population should and could occur.

What evidence is there to support this contention? First, European countries such as Switzerland and Sweden have a lower incidence of nursing home placement than the United States.[21] Slightly less than 3% of those over age 85 require placement compared with slightly over 5% in this country. What is the difference? Even after taking social and individual differences into account, one major factor is life-style. Most people in European countries walk to the store, to the library, and to visit friends and family. Fewer conveniences that limit physical participation (e.g., washing machines, dryers) are available. In other places of the world such as the republic of Georgia, longevity without physical infirmity is common.[28] Again, physical activity is the norm in this culture, and people of all ages are expected to participate in crop planting and gathering, tending of the animals, and so forth. Only

within the last century has the life-style of our country become so sedentary; exercise is an additive now in that activities such as farming, clothes washing, and heavy cleaning are no longer part of the normal way of life. Because exercise is an additive, many people choose not to do any.

Physical therapists are uniquely qualified to assist the older adult in maximizing physical function through exercise. It is the purpose of this chapter to provide the basic tools for evaluation and, to some extent, exercise prescription for those in the "young-old" (65 to 75 years) and the "older-old" (75 + years) categories.

What constitutes *well elderly?* Definitions vary, including only those without pathology (very few elders) to only those not currently in the hospital (nearly all elders).[20] For purposes of this chapter, *well elderly* is defined as those living in the community, accomplishing all or most ADL independently, without need for rehabilitation. Typically, the well elderly have some form of chronic disease (coronary artery disease, arthritis, diabetes), but disease does not preclude participation in physical activity.

THE NEED FOR EXERCISE IN THE WELL ELDERLY POPULATION

As indicated in other chapters of this text, changes occur in skeletal muscle with "normal" aging. Declines in strength have been reported for every muscle group that has been tested, averaging approximately 1% per year after the third decade.[3, 18] The rate of decline appears to vary from muscle group to muscle group, and from person to person, which makes characterizing the decline in strength with aging rather difficult. If disease, such as osteoarthritis, is present, the degree of strength change may be greater than that expected under average conditions. It should be noted that studies examining changes in strength with age have been conducted using typically sedentary but healthy subjects.[3, 18, 23]

Does muscle strength decrease in physically active individuals? The answer is unequivocally yes, but the magnitude of decline is far less than that seen in sedentary people. For example, in our clinic, master power lifters in their 60s generated 180 ft-lb of quadriceps torque, which was more than twice what age-matched sedentary men could accomplish. However, young power lifters (20 to 30 years) were capable of nearly twice as much torque as the master power lifters (312 vs. 180 ft-lb). It appears that continuous resistance exercise training markedly attenuates strength losses with aging but does not eliminate loss altogether.[9] What these data suggest is that a significant portion of the strength loss that occurs with age is due to disuse. A number of studies of humans and animals support the contention that a large portion of the change in strength and function with age is due to inactivity.[1, 2, 4, 9, 17, 23, 26]

Unfortunately, older men and women in our society expect to deteriorate, as the falsehood purporting the need to slow down with age is alive and well.

THE UTILITY OF EXERCISE FOR THE OLDER ADULT

During the past decade, particularly the last 5 years, a number of studies documenting the positive effects of exercise for the older adult have been published. These reports overwhelmingly confirm the "trainability" of the older adult for endurance, strength, and flexibility. It now appears that the older adult is as adaptable to exercise, on a relative basis, as a young man or woman. For example, Moritani and deVries found a 23% increase in elbow flexion strength following an 8-week weight-lifting program using dumbbells.[22] Improvements for the young men serving as controls, who performed the same type of strength training, averaged 19%. More recently, Frontera and associates trained men 60 to 72 years of age on a universal gym for 12 weeks. The training load was 80% of the individual's one-repetition maximum (1RM), and three sets of eight repetitions were performed three times a week. An enormous 109% increase in the 1RM was obtained.[14] Probably the most exciting study to date demonstrates that frail men *and* women can gain strength. Fiatarone et al. weight-trained ten long-term–care facility residents ranging in age from 86 to 96 years.[13] An 8-week program of three sets of eight repetitions of knee flexion and extension at 80% 1RM was performed three times per week. Initial quadriceps strength averaged 9 kg at the beginning of the study. The average strength gain at 8 weeks was 174%! Total muscle mass as determined by computerized tomography increased an average of 9% in the quadriceps. Furthermore, changes in functional mobility (e.g., time taken to rise from a chair) correlated with the improvements in muscle strength. The 174% improvement in strength compared with the 9% increase in muscle mass strongly suggests that disuse accounted for the major portion of the decline in strength. Results from our clinic indicate that healthy older men and women (60 to 71 years) can improve strength significantly with a program of relatively low-intensity stretching and strengthening.[10] In this instance, exercises were done in chairs, while standing, on all fours, and while lying on the floor, using the weight of the body part and gravity as resistance. These studies indicate that the potential to gain strength is present at all ages, using a variety of techniques.

It is important to note that all the subjects in the study by Fiatarone et al.[13] had medical problems: arthritis, coronary artery disease, osteoporosis, and hypertension. Yet high-intensity strength training was feasible in this population and was associated with remarkable gains in strength and an increase in functional ability. All subjects safely completed the protocol, even those with cardiovascular disease.

Flexibility is also amenable to change in the older adult. Range-of-motion (ROM) increases have been observed in the neck, shoulder, hip, and other joints as the result of an 8-week program of dance therapy,[19] a 10-week program of Feldenkrais exercises,[15] and with more traditional exercises emphasizing end range of motion.[10] Whether the increases in passive ROM translate to improvements in active range was not determined in any of these studies.

Cardiovascular adaptation to exercise has been observed in older adults between the ages of 60 and 79 years, even with programs of relatively low intensity (i.e., some percentage of maximal aerobic power [$\dot{V}O_2max$]). Seals et al. found that 11 men and women between the ages of 61 and 67 years increased their $\dot{V}O_2max$ an average of 30% in response to a 1-year endurance exercise program.[27] These investigators also observed that a program of walking at 40% of heart rate reserve increased $\dot{V}O_2max$ by 12%. Forty percent of heart rate reserve is well within the capability of most men and women above 60 years of age, even those with mild hypertension, pulmonary disease, arthritis, and other limitations. Recently, Hagberg demonstrated that 70- to 79-year-old men and women who trained three times per week for 26 weeks at 75% to 85% of $\dot{V}O_2max$ increased $\dot{V}O_2max$ an average of 22%.[16]

A few reports indicate the potential for an increase in standing balance in older men and women.[7, 10, 12] Fansler et al. reported that 12 subjects who engaged in the mental practice of balancing activities actually increased their static balancing times (one-legged standing) significantly.[12] Results from our clinic indicate that exercises for strength, balance, and flexibility had an effect on static balance in 60- to 70-year-old men and women with some degree of unsteadiness.[10] *Unsteadiness* was defined as an inability to stand on one leg with the eyes open for 50 seconds, even though standing for 60 seconds was requested. For the 33 of 60 individuals who were unsteady, one-legged standing times improved an average of 18 seconds after a 3-month low-intensity exercise program.[10] Pilot data from our clinic indicate that frail older men and women (mean age 79 years) with a history of falling can also improve performance on standing balancing tests such as the progressive Romberg and negotiating a three-stage obstacle course.[7]

Exercise can have an effect on an older person's ability to perform activities of daily living. Fiatarone et al. noted a marked improvement in time to rise from a seated position after an 8-week program of strengthening exercises for the quadriceps and knee flexors.[13] Our own pilot data suggest that walking, turning, rising from a chair, and willingness to engage in community activities also are improved with exercise.[7] Furthermore, anecdotal reports indicate that exercise has a positive effect on older people's fear of falling, sense of well-being, and personal confidence.

HOW TO GET STARTED

Observations

Appropriate exercise prescription for the well elderly is based, like all of physical therapy care, on information obtained from evaluation. Whether the desired outcome for exercise is improved flexibility, enhanced strength, or ability to run a marathon, evaluation is imperative.

An evaluation for an exercise program begins immediately with the introduction. The first 30 seconds of contact often provide the necessary information to get started at the proper level of evaluation. For example, if your client has difficulty rising from the waiting room chair, ambulates at a slow rate of speed to the evaluation area, and is puffing with the little bit of effort involved, it can be recognized immediately that strength, gait, and cardiovascular endurance must be examined at the start. Once lower extremity strength, gait, and cardiovascular endurance have been examined, other areas of evaluation need will be obvious—areas such as range of motion, balance, and other ADL capabilities. These observations will make it apparent to you if the client's desired exercise outcome is feasible. For example, if the aforementioned person desired to resume square dancing, you would have sufficient information to disabuse the client from attending dance classes immediately. Rather, a remedial program of strengthening activities with an emphasis on standing might better serve this individual as a first step. Perhaps the next step could be a course in ballroom dancing.

Your immediate observations can provide the majority of the information you need. Sharp observation skills are imperative, as is close attention to detail. Functional activities such as steps, rising from a chair, walking, and turning suggest strength and range deficits and limitations in balance. Any hesitancy in doing what is requested should be noted. It is important to note whether your client is lean, stout, tall, or disproportioned in some way and if posture is of concern. Other things to notice when meeting someone for the first time is whether they use an assistive device; have apparent swelling; wear clothes and shoes that were selected for ease of application; wear glasses; have appropriate skin color; or have obvious joint deformity. Again, this information serves as the basis for the remainder of the evaluation.

If older adults are simply coming into the clinic for exercise, the 30-second evaluation will provide adequate information to get started at an appropriate level of activity. For example, if most of the adults coming to the clinic use an assistive device, are slow to get started, and appear a little deficient in balance, exercises need to be done (at least initially) sitting or holding on to a chair or wall. If your client is robust, has a substantial quantity of muscle mass to work with, and is in good health, then a fairly rigorous program of exercise can be initiated, once baseline measures of heart rate and blood pressure are established.

History

Somewhere during the course of evaluation, some form of history taking is indicated. Over and above the usual information related to age, date, sex, and weight, some suggestions for inclusion are:

1. *Exercise history*. Is your client accustomed to physical activity or is this the first time they ever participated in exercise? Caution is indicated when progressing someone with no exercise background.

2. *Medical problems*. Are there conditions for which care must be taken, for example, heart disease, arthritis, diabetes, osteoporosis, or hypertension?

3. *Medications*. Is your client taking a medication that will alter exercise responses, for example, beta-blockers?

4. *Painful conditions*. Are there chronic conditions such as back or hip pain that require referral to a physician or accommodation in an exercise program?

5. *Recent injuries or surgeries*.

EVALUATION TOOLS

Flexibility

Most healthy young-old adults have ranges of motion within acceptable limits; the older-old are more likely to show deficits in range that limit functional performance. Thus, exercises for ROM enhancement are more important for those in the eighth and ninth decades. Regardless of age, ROM needs to be assessed functionally—during walking, getting up and down from a chair (preferably one that is lower than usual, like 16 in.), getting up and down from the floor (if appropriate), reaching for an object overhead, and reaching for something on the floor. If specific ranges are needed for billing purposes, a goniometric measurement can be made of those joints that were identified as deficient with functional assessment. For example, the author recently held exercise classes for a group of older (67 to 97 years) adults who were otherwise healthy but had a history of falling. Evaluation revealed that only 1 of the 17 participants had the ability to get off the floor once a fall had been sustained. In most instances, strength was not the problem; rather, knee flexion range of motion was inadequate to get the leg underneath the body.

Observations of numerous older adults over the years have revealed problem areas that are often gender specific. Women are more likely than men to have significant ROM deficits in ankle dorsiflexion, knee flexion, and shoulder elevation. Men are more likely than women to have deficits in the hip and trunk. Both men and women are likely to have major deficits in neck range (severe enough to make them unsafe for driving), hip extension, and trunk rotation.

If an older adult is a candidate for walking, fast walking, or jogging, two tests of flexibility are strongly recommended. They are the Thomas test for hip flexor tightness and a check of dorsiflexion range. More than 60% of our walking/jogging exercise participants experienced hip or back pain if hip flexor tightness was greater than 10 degrees. Once the tightness was reduced, pain subsided, suggesting a strong relationship between the two. The other possible limitation, dorsiflexion, is more often seen in women because of a long history of wearing high-heeled shoes. Unless dorsiflexion range is at least zero degrees (neutral), walking cannot be done comfortably. A good walking shoe can accommodate for the 10 degrees of dorsiflexion usually required during gait, but again, neutral ankle dorsiflexion is a minimum.

Strength

An imperative component of any physical examination is strength. An assessment of strength can be made in a multitude of ways, all of which have advantages and disadvantages: manual muscle testing MMT, isokinetic testing, speed of movement, gait, functional testing, hand-held dynamometry, force transducer tests, and 1RM.

Manual Muscle Testing

MMT has the major disadvantage of only identifying strength deficits when patients have lost 40% to 50% of pre-existing strength.[6] MMT is difficult in an older adult population, as some strength loss with aging is normal, but our methods are too crude to distinguish between age-associated strength losses and those sustained secondary to disuse and disease. MMT is rather static (assuming a break test is done), so whether patients can use their strength

during an activity requiring a large arc of motion cannot be discerned with this mode of testing.

Positive aspects of muscle testing include obtaining specific information about select muscle groups and getting some insight into functional loss. No other form of testing will give you knowledge about individual muscles (although for healthy older adults this information is not particularly useful). Selected muscle tests—for example, rising up onto the toes to test calf strength—will immediately indicate whether a client is likely to have difficulty with heel rise during gait.

There are three muscle test items recommended for inclusion in evaluation. The first, rising up on the toes 10 to 20 times (one leg at a time), is done to determine strength of the gastrocnemius-soleus group. If a grade of F+ or better cannot be achieved, the utility of a walking program is limited (i.e., strengthening must be done to bring clients into the F+ or better category). The second item examined is gluteus medius capability. Clients are asked to hold on to a chair or wall with one finger and then slowly lift a foot from the ground. If the pelvis drops, indicating gluteus medius weakness, remedial exercises are begun. Again, a walking program is not appropriate if the pelvis drops every time a step is taken. The final muscle test performed is for hip extension strength. The traditional prone posture is assumed, and clients are asked to raise the entire lower extremity against gravity through full ROM. Those with weakness of the hip extensors tend to walk with the trunk forward, which often results in back pain.

These muscle test items are offered as suggestions only. Strength can be determined in other ways that are equally effective but cannot provide a "grade," so to speak, which may be important for documentation purposes. For example, lack of heel rise during gait implicates the calf as being weak, but whether it falls in the trace, poor, or fair category cannot be determined by gait observation alone.

Isokinetic Testing

Isokinetic testing has the disadvantages of being nonfunctional and difficult for some older adults to learn, and results are hard to interpret as there are no age-appropriate norms available. There are two advantages to isokinetic testing, however, which are being able (1) to determine movement capability at different speeds and (2) to identify point of fatigue. Older adults often test reasonably well during a static form of muscle testing but perform poorly when speeds of 180 or 360 degrees/sec are requested. We use speeds of 300 degrees/sec routinely in our daily activities, and if a client is incapable of moving that fast, a significant deficit has been identified. The knee moves at 360 degrees/sec during normal velocity walking; the arm may move at 1,200 degrees/sec or more to throw a ball. Older men and women who cannot move quickly are at risk for falling. Thus, if isokinetic testing reveals inability to perform at faster speeds, exercise to correct this deficit should be instituted. For example, one client, age 79, with a history of falling, was found to have no protective reactions (arms or legs) when asked to perform a balance assessment. Isokinetic testing revealed a total inability to move the arm of the machine faster than 180 degrees/sec with either the upper or lower extremities. Exercises (using dance as the medium, as the client loved it) to emphasize control, balance, and speed were instituted.

Isokinetic dynamometry can be used to identify those who fatigue quickly. Protocols vary, but typically clients are asked to perform maximum contractions repetitively to look at the slope of decline after a certain number of contractions or maintain a certain proportion of output (e.g., 50% of a maximum isometric voluntary contraction for half a minute or so). Fatigue protocols are not appropriate for many clients, particularly those who are frail. Those elders with hypertension, joint deformity or pain, and cardiac compromise should also not be tested.

Speed of Movement

Another aspect of strength that needs to be evaluated is the speed with which the activity is accomplished. Some older adults have adequate passive ROM, but the speed with which they move within that range is unacceptable. Unless the arms can be raised in time to prevent a fall or the knees can be moved quickly through the normal 70-degree arc of motion during gait, strength is not adequate. Recognition of clients' willingness to use their strength in a dynamic, functional way is important.

Gait

Gait evaluation is useful for all kinds of evaluative purposes (strength, ROM, cardiovascular endurance, balance). Some strength deficits can be identified on the basis of deviations in the gait cycle. Lack of heel rise during terminal stance has already been identified as one indicator of inadequate calf strength. Other aspects of gait to note include pelvic drop, forward trunk lean, diminished or absent knee flexion during loading, and reduced knee flexion. Pelvic drop in the frontal plane indicates that muscles stabilizing the pelvis are not strong enough to do the job (gluteus medius, gluteus minimus, tensor fascia latea). Forward trunk lean frequently indicates inadequate hip extensors. Diminished or absent knee flexion right after heel strike suggests that the quadriceps are not strong enough to absorb the shock of loading (requires an F+ or better grade). Finally, reduced knee flexion during swing may indicate weakness of the gastrocnemius or hamstrings.

A proper gait evaluation should also include an assessment of velocity (strength deficits result in reduced gait speed), stride length, stride width, and variability in stride characteristics. Diminished stride and so forth may indicate reduced strength but also may be indicative of balance problems, sensory loss, or cardiovascular compromise.

Gait evaluation is quickly done (10 seconds of the 30-second examination) and reveals an enormous amount of information. Suspected strength deficits are identified, and follow-up testing on functional items such as rising from a chair or MMT can be done to confirm inadequate strength. Gait deficits do not provide much information regarding deficits in strength.

Functional Testing

Functional testing for strength purposes is important to do, more so if your client population falls into the older-old category. Functional testing for the lower extremities may include getting up and down from a seated position, sometimes from chairs of different heights. Some investigators advocate repeated bouts (five times) of rising and sitting back down.[29] Another functional test is walking up and down curbs of different heights. Testing may include curb heights of 4, 6, and 8 in. Walking devices are used if needed, and ability/inability is recorded appropriately, as is any loss of balance. Stair climbing is a third functional test that may be requested. Steps should be of normal height and include a handrail. Ability to negotiate steps, with or without rails or assistive devices, is noted. If appropriate, getting up and down from the floor may be included in the testing. Other options include picking an object up from the floor, stooping down into a cupboard, and walking up and down a ramp. Upper extremity tests may include putting on a sweatshirt (overhead, no buttons), reaching up into a cupboard, and picking up a weighted object and moving it a short distance.

The obvious advantage of functional testing is that it identifies ADL items that need remediation. A major disadvantage is that functional testing is nonspecific; strength deficits may be obscured by ROM or other problems, and none of the probable strength deficits identified on functional testing can be quantified. The experienced therapist can usually recognize what is balance, strength, or range limited, but a great deal of learning and expertise are required to reach that level of clinical competence.

Hand-Held Dynamometry

Hand-held dynamometry may be useful in that instant information is obtained regarding the capability of any major muscle group. Another advantage is that side-to-side differences can be discerned, and the process of data collection is time efficient. Disadvantages of dynamometry include the fact that some instruments are more reliable than others, the strength of the tester is vitally important (if the client is stronger than the therapist, the data are useless), and values reflect static strength only. Still, dynamometry can provide an index of client capability. For example, if quadriceps strength is less than 50% of body weight, some compensation or deviation is to be expected.

Force Transducer Tests

The advantages and disadvantages of using a force transducer are similar to those of using a hand-held dynamometer. Differences between the two are ease of application (positioning requirements for using a force transducer are cumbersome), number of muscle groups that can be tested (fewer with force transducer), and the nature of testing. The strength of the tester is not a factor when a force transducer is used.

One-Repetition Maximum

A 1RM test is tried and true but time-consuming to administer. Not all muscle groups can be evaluated this way, and many people need to be tested several times before a true 1RM is determined. If older adults are really deconditioned, the testing sometimes results in a lot of muscle soreness. Nonetheless, the 1RM test provides real data that may serve as a useful guide for improvement and can be correlated with changes in functional performance as well.

A number of options for strength testing have been presented, all of which have positive and negative aspects about them. What works best in your clinic will be based on mode of practice (is your clientele composed of average senior citizens, or are they master athletes?), the space available, machinery available, time you have to devote to the evaluation, how much real data you require, client expectation, and need for documentation.

Balance

Balance testing can be static or dynamic, and both have advantages and disadvantages. Examples of static testing that will be given are the stand on one leg test, the sharpened Romberg, the postural stress test, and the reach test. Dynamic tests include walking, walking through an obstacle course, and platform testing.

Static Balance

Standing on one leg with the eyes open (and closed if indicated) is an easy test to administer and provides a number value in less than a minute. Care must be taken not to allow the client to cheat by placing the swing leg on the stance leg, shifting position of the stance leg, or hopping. Several trials are required to make the client comfortable with the testing and to ensure reliable data. Whether someone can stand on one leg for 30 or 40 seconds is moot.

Whether a client can stand on one leg for less than 10 seconds is indicative of significant deficit. In our clinic, most of the adults tested are unable to stand on one leg with the eyes closed for more than 1 to 3 seconds. These values do not mean much in an absolute sense, but they at least indicate if the task can be accomplished at all. The eyes-closed test will give some insight as to whether the individual being tested should be counseled about walking around in the dark (e.g., going to the bathroom along a darkened corridor).

The sharpened Romberg is a popular test of static balance[5] with progressively difficult postures to maintain. The first segment of the six-part test is to stand with the feet together with the eyes open for 10 seconds. Grading is simple: able or not able to complete the requested task. The second segment requires the client to stand with feet together for 10 seconds but with the eyes closed. The third component of the test requires standing in the semitandem position (Fig 24–1) for 10 seconds, eyes open. The fourth component is standing in the semitandem position for 10 seconds with eyes closed. The fifth and last segments require the client to stand in the full tandem position (one foot immediately in front of the other, heel to toe—Fig 24–1), first with eyes open and then with eyes closed. This test is easy to administer and reasonably reliable and does not require much time to complete. One small problem with the test is that no instructions are provided as to how a client should be graded if the individual falls getting into the test position but then passes that particular segment of the test.

The postural stress test has been shown to be reliable and useful for identifying those with a predisposition to falling. This multistage examination requires the client to stand quietly (stage 1) at the beginning of the test and progress to the final stage of maintaining balance while a weight tied to the client's waist is dropped suddenly.[31] Obviously, this segment of the test is not performed if problems with safety are identified on simpler tasks.

The reach test has been found to be reliable and is

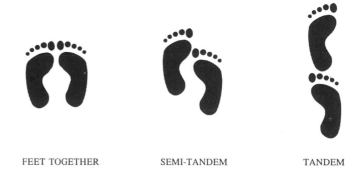

FEET TOGETHER   SEMI-TANDEM   TANDEM

FIG 24–1.
Foot placements for sharpened Romberg test.

simple to perform. Subjects stand comfortably and reach forward (not down) as far as they can along a yardstick that is placed on the wall next to them. Distance reached is recorded.[11]

Dynamic Balance

Examples of dynamic tests include movable platforms, the "get-up-and-go" test, walking an imaginary balance beam, and completing an obstacle course. None of these tests have norms, but the platform developed by the Nashner group[24] has been evaluated extensively. The platform, however, is extremely expensive and beyond the means of most clinics. Results apparently provide information that is no more useful in predicting falling behavior than the simple, no-cost one-legged stance test. The get-up-and-go test requires the client to rise from a chair and go toward a destination, as quickly as possible. Usually, turns are incorporated into the protocol. Trials are timed, and difficulties with doing the test are noted.

Similarities exist between the obstacle course, get-up-and-go test, and the imaginary balance beam. All are timed trials and challenge the client to operate within a discrete base of support. For example, the imaginary balance beam typically is a dark line painted on the floor. Trials are usually videotaped, and the number of times a client misses the "beam" is noted, as is time to complete the trial. Obstacle courses vary in difficulty but usually incorporate a number of functional tasks. The one we use has three levels of difficulty. The first task requires the client to rise from a chair, walk 10 ft, step up a 4-in. step, turn around, step down the step, return to the chair, and sit. Practice trials are permitted for safety's sake, although in real life no one gets two chances to prevent a fall. The second task requires standing from a seated position, walking forward, stepping over an obstacle (a 2×2 piece of wood), ascending a 6-in. step (no rail), turning, and repeating the process in reverse.

As with the other tests presented so far, what is selected to incorporate in the clinic will depend on time, money, the nature of the clientele, and how much information is needed. These tools will at least provide a start.

Activities of Daily Living

Any evaluation of the older adult must include some sort of ADL assessment. A number of options have been presented in Chapter 7 of this book and will not be elaborated here.

The assessment to be chosen will again depend on the client and the client's capabilities. For example, a 93-year-old woman who is barely getting by may be having difficulty with everything on the test sheet, but a healthy 65-year-old may simply have trouble taking the heavy gar-

bage cans to the curb. If your ADL assessment does not capture whatever difficulty the client is experiencing, make a notation in the record. Identifying the needs of your client is crucial.

Cardiovascular System

Another imperative for working with the older adult is some test of the cardiovascular system. Our facility does not have the means to do sophisticated stress testing, so we require all clients to have completed a stress test before the physical therapy evaluation. Most of the referring physicians are helpful in providing a safe or target heart rate range. During the other parts of the evaluation, blood pressure and heart rate are monitored to get some idea of how much challenge the cardiovascular system can tolerate.

Our clinic is not readily accessible, requiring clients to walk a considerable distance from the parking lot and ascend a flight of stairs just to get to the waiting room. If a 70-year-old client is sweating profusely by the time the individual arrives, has a heart rate of 130 beats per minute (bpm) and a blood pressure of 180/90, data suggest a walking program is probably more than adequate initially.

Even when a target heart rate or heart rate range is provided, it is hard to know where to start without some notion of what type of activity will generate such a heart rate response. Follow-up tests typically include normal speed walking, fast walking, or treadmill, and heart rate and blood pressure are monitored throughout. If a client wants a home exercise program for a specific piece of equipment, heart rate and blood pressure monitoring are done on that piece of equipment. A large number of people come to our clinic with exercise bikes, rowing machines, and so forth that are gathering dust in the basement. These items typically were gifts because "Uncle Harry needed to get some exercise." Now Uncle Harry needs proper guidelines on how to use his equipment appropriately.

To summarize, elsewhere in this text are specific exercise tests for examination of the cardiovascular system. Some type of follow-up may be indicated to determine how the heart will function during an actual exercise intervention. In other words, clients will probably need information related to how fast they should walk, whether to incorporate an incline on the treadmill, how much resistance to use on a bicycle, and how long to exercise. Supplemental information, over and above that gained from stress testing, typically is required.

Posture

In many instances, a detailed posture evaluation is not indicated. Paying attention to deviations from the norm is necessary, but this component of the evaluation can be taken care of during the initial 30-second sweep or at any other point in the examination. Items to note are hip asymmetry; genu valgus or varus; pronated or supinated feet; excessive lordosis, kyphosis, or scoliosis; and extremes of pelvic tilt. Postural faults that are likely to result in a painful condition must be accommodated. Someone with severe flat and painful feet, for example, is not likely to respond positively to a jogging program.

EXERCISE PRESCRIPTION

The information gathered during the evaluation needs to be integrated into a total picture from which an exercise plan will evolve. Successful exercise planning takes into account all the subtle and not-so-subtle changes that have occurred with aging, what goals the client has, chronic diseases (if present), physical capabilities, and painful conditions and is based on a common-sense approach. The following case histories are presented to illustrate these ideas.

CASE STUDIES

Mr. P

Mr. P is 67 years old, 5ft 10in., and weighs 267 lb. He is very sedentary. Physical evaluation revealed a forward head posture, 30 degrees of hip flexor tightness (Thomas test), bilateral iliotibial band tightness with knee pain, probable knee arthritis bilaterally, grade 3 flat feet. His gait was slow (48 m/min) with a foot flat approach at heel strike, no toe-off, and a bilateral pelvic drop during stance. Muscle testing revealed good strength throughout with the exception of plantar flexors (F+) and abdominals (P). Because the client weighed so much, he had difficulty getting out of chairs and up stairs. This man was very awkward, giving the impression of someone with little sense of body. Although Mr. P had had a nonremarkable stress test prior to coming in for evaluation, he was asked to walk on a treadmill so that heart rate (HR) and blood pressure (BP) responses could be determined. The client walked on the treadmill for 5 minutes (until fatigue) at a speed of 3.0 mph with no incline. HR increased to 134 bpm, which was estimated to be about 90% of his $\dot{V}o_2$max. Systolic blood pressure rose to over 200 mm Hg during the 3.0-mph test.

Mr. P came into the clinic for an exercise program at the behest of his wife, who had been urging him for months to "do something." His expectation was that a walking program would be prescribed, and he was not enthusiastic at the prospect. Thus, we had a client who was

rather unenthusiastic about the prospects of exercise, particularly walking, but he was aware of his need for activity. The week before the evaluation he had had extreme difficulty getting out of the seat of a theater, and this provided some motivation to seek care.

The client and therapist agreed on the following: for the first 2 to 3 months he would park in the lot farthest from our facility ($\frac{2}{10}$ mile) and walk in at a slightly faster-than-usual pace. Mr. P would participate three times per week in a flexibility and strengthening program aimed particularly at the trunk and lower extremities. Orthotics and good shoes would be obtained to accommodate for his flat feet and to decrease strain on the knees. The walking and exercise plan was designed to provide some cardiovascular stimulation and improved strength and ROM, respectively. At the end of 3 months, lower extremity strength and flexibility were adequate for the next phase of training. Walking more than a short distance really was not indicated for Mr. P, given his painful knees, excess weight, marginal strength, and lack of desire to do this type of exercise. Instead, a home bicycle program was chosen because the client had a bike, and he was interested in pursuing this form of activity.

A very modest program was begun consisting of biking at 100 W for 15 minutes. Over time the client progressed steadily, and program modifications were instituted once a month. He is currently biking for an hour using a 150-W protocol for 10 minutes as warm-up, a 300-W intensity for training, and a 15-minute cool-down at 100 W. The exercise bike is in front of the television, and the client barely notices that an hour has gone by. Mr. P performs his exercise regularly; he is very proud of himself and delighted with his ability to get from place to place without undue fatigue or difficulty.

Mrs. B

Mrs. B is 69 years old, 5 ft 4 in., and weighs 145 lb. Mrs. B described herself as very sedentary, and she had never exercised during her lifetime. She had no difficulty passing an exercise stress test; thus, there was no evidence of cardiovascular disease. Physical evaluation revealed nothing remarkable except that she was rather pigeon-toed during gait. The client had no history of painful joints, injuries, or recent surgeries. Standing balance was fine, and there were no problems with ADL. Strength and range were within normal limits.

Mrs. B's goal was to "become more active." Although she had no complaints of physical inability, she had just placed her mother in a nursing home because she was physically unable to live alone. Fear of having the same thing happen to her has motivated Mrs. B to seek help.

A 3-mph walk on the treadmill (no incline) provoked

a heart rate increase from 73 to 123 bpm. Blood pressure increased from 115/80 to 175/85 mm Hg. Walking was terminated after 6½ minutes secondary to fatigue.

Mrs. B did not believe she would exercise on her own, nor did she have any idea what she would enjoy doing. We agreed on an "in-house" program of general conditioning exercise classes that she would attend three to four times per week. This exercise program consists of six 15-minute segments, each progressively more difficult. Mrs. B joined the first three 15-minute segments initially and ultimately progressed to performing the last three 15-minute segments. Now Mrs. B usually comes in daily, exercises for 45 minutes, and then walks around the track at a brisk pace for 15 minutes. She actually wanted to try jogging, which was done, but the jarring associated with jogging provoked stress incontinence, and thus jogging was abandoned.

This client progressed to performing activities she never anticipated she was capable of doing. She would like to exercise even more intensely but realizes there are some limitations. She currently is trying a ski machine and has begun participating in community walks/runs to benefit charities. Exercise has resulted in increased socialization, as Mrs. B and other women in the exercise program now go out for dinner once a month.

Exercise in this case was successful because of the low-key nature of the program, at least initially; the social aspect of the exercise environment; the supervision provided; and a strong motivation to avoid further physical deterioration.

Mrs. M

Mrs. M is 72 years old, 5 ft 4 in., and weighs 96 lb. She is sedentary but active all day long, managing her own business. Her mother is in a nursing home because of osteoporosis and frailty. Mrs. M smokes a pack of cigarettes a day and has mild hypertension. She is cleared for exercise by her physician but is allowed a maximum heart rate of 110 bpm as long as her diastolic blood pressure does not rise beyond 90 mm Hg. Physical evaluation reveals a mild kyphosis but no other postural faults. Strength and range are good, and there are no gait or balance deficits. She was able to perform all ADL without difficulty. Mrs. M has a treadmill at home that she would like to use.

Treadmill walking was performed during the testing session to determine HR and BP responses. Treadmill speed was 2.0 mph initially and was increased by 0.5 mph every 2 minutes until an HR of 110 bpm was reached. Blood pressure was within acceptable limits. A walking program of 2.5 mph at a 2% incline for 20 minutes a day was begun. Within 6 weeks the client could walk at 3.0 mph, 2% incline, with the same HR and BP response. Ultimately, the amount of treadmill time was increased such that the client was walking 40 minutes a day. It should be mentioned that proper footwear was procured before the walking program began.

Four months into the program, Mrs. M broke her toe (unrelated to exercise), which did not heal for months because of low bone density and possibly her smoking. Once healing finally occurred, she resumed her program from the beginning. In addition, ten flights of stairs per day was added to provide loading through the long bones in an attempt to promote bone growth. Exercise seems to have checked the mild hypertension, and the client is now allowed a higher exercise intensity (125 bpm). Mrs. M exercises daily, but whether the program has affected bone density is unknown.

Mr. A

Mr. A is 79 years old, 5 ft 10 in., and weighs 165 lb. He is currently sedentary but has a 60-year history of climbing/hiking in the Alps. Mr. A is a member of a prestigious European Alpine club. Physical examination revealed a man with remarkable strength, agility, and no obvious physical deformities. Gait was purposeful, with a quick stride. Balance was surprisingly limited: 10 seconds of one-legged standing on the left, 15 seconds on the right. Mr. A's goal is to climb the Matterhorn on his 80th birthday, which is 6 months away.

Mr. A is sedentary because his wife became very ill and is now an invalid. Her condition has stabilized, and both have agreed that his climb is important, so training time will be set aside each day. Training will have to be done at home, however.

Stress testing confirmed the client to be without cardiovascular disease. Stress testing also revealed a man who has a higher $\dot{V}O_2$max than most men his age, but a lack of stamina was apparent.

Training initially consisted of 30 minutes of vigorous walking daily. Next, an obstacle course was set up in the yard consisting of rocks that had to be ascended or stepped around. This course had to be completed as quickly as possible but safely. The course had to be changed every other week so that familiarity did not become an issue. Thirty minutes of vigorous walking was increased to 1 hour of walking including a hill or two. At this point, hiking boots and a pack were added. As the weeks and months went by, greater distances, more weight in the pack, and more hills were added to tolerance. During weekends, excursions into higher altitudes were begun, and hikes of 15 to 20 miles were taken. Twenty-five to 30 flights of stairs were climbed daily. Mr. A is ready!

SUMMARY

The well elderly are fun and exciting to work with. They are extremely challenging because they are so diverse in their abilities. Exercise prescription for this population taxes the ingenuity of a physical therapist as no other group of clients or patients. The potential for change is tremendous, much more so than the change that may occur secondary to rehabilitation. Our ability to impact on the well-being of the older adult population is enormous. Exercise should be available for all seniors to prevent deterioration and to keep adults maximally capable, thereby eliminating the need for dependence on others. Physical therapists have the skill and knowledge to provide healthy older adults the best care possible.

REFERENCES

1. Aniansson A, Grimby G, Krotkiewska I, et al: Muscle strength and endurance in elderly people, with special reference to muscle morphology, in Asmussen E, Jorgensen K (eds): *Biomechanics VI-A*. Baltimore, University Park Press, 1978.
2. Aniansson A, Hedberg M, Henning GB, et al: Muscle morphology, enzymatic activity and muscle strength in elderly men: A follow-up study. *Muscle Nerve* 1986; 9:585–591.
3. Asmussen E, Freunsgaard K, Norgaard S: A follow-up study of selected physiologic functions in former physical education students—after 40 years. *J Am Geriatr Soc.* 1975; 23:442–450.
4. Asmussen E, Heeboll-Nielsen B: Isometric muscle strength of adult men and women. Communications From the Testing and Observation Institute of the Danish National Association for Infantile Paralysis, 1961.
5. Bannister R (ed): *Brain's Clinical Neurology,* ed 6, New York, Oxford University Press, 1985.
6. Beasley WC: Quantitative muscle testing: Principles and applications to research and clinical services. *Arch Phys Med Rehabil* 1961; 42:398–425.
7. Binder EF, Brown M, Birge S: Effects of a moderate intensity exercise program at reducing risk factors for falls in frail older adults (abstract). *Gerontologist* 1991; 31:219–220.
8. Brody JA, Brock DB: Epidemiologic and statistical characteristics of the United States elderly population, in Finch CE, Schneider EL (eds): *The Biology of Aging,* ed 2. New York, Van Nostrand Reinhold, 1985.
9. Brown M, Coggan A: Is muscle wasting inevitable with aging (abstract)? *Med Sci Sports Exerc* 1990; 22:434.
10. Brown M, Holloszy JO: Effects of a low intensity exercise program on selected physical performance characteristics of 60 to 71 year olds. *Aging* 1991; 3:129–139.
11. Duncan PW, Weiner DK, Chandler J, et al: Functional reach: A new clinical measure of balance. *J Gerontol* 1990; 45:M192–M197.
12. Fansler CC, Pott CC, Shepard KF: Effects of mental practice on balance in elderly women. *Phys Ther* 1985; 65:1332–1338.
13. Fiatarone MH, Mark SEC, Ryan WD, et al: High intensity strength training in nonagenarians. *JAMA* 1990; 263:3029–3034.
14. Frontera WR, Meredith CN, O'Reilly KP, et al: Strength conditioning in older men: Skeletal muscle hypertrophy and improved function. *J Appl Physiol* 1988; 64:1038–1044.
15. Gutman GM, Herbert CP, Brown SR: Feldenkrais versus conventional exercises for the elderly. *J Gerontol* 1977; 32:562–572.
16. Hagberg JM: Effect of training on the decline in $\dot{V}_{O_2}$max with aging. *Fed Proc* 1987; 46:1830–1833.
17. Kroll W, Clarkson PM: Age, isometric knee extension and fractionated resisted response time. *Exp Aging Res* 1978; 4:389–409.
18. Larsson L, Grimby G, Karlsson J: Muscle strength and speed of movement in relation to age and muscle morphology. *J Appl Physiol* 1979; 46:451–456.
19. Lesser M: The effects of rhythmic exercise on the range of motion in older adults. *Am Coll Ther J* 1978; 32:4–6.
20. Levenson SA: The physician, in Maguire GH (ed): *Care of the Elderly: A Health Team Approach*. Boston, Little, Brown, 1985, pp 95–112.
21. Mellstrom D, Rundgren A: Institutional care at the age of 79 in an urban population. *Aktuel Gerontol* 1983; 77:3769–3771.
22. Moritani T, deVries H: Potential for gross muscle hypertrophy in men. *J Gerontol* 1980; 35:672–682.
23. Murray MP, Gardner GM, Mollinger BS, et al: Strength of isometric and isokinetic contractions: Knee muscles of men aged 20 to 86. *Phys Ther* 1980; 60:412–419.
24. Nashner LM: Fixed patterns of rapid postural responses among leg muscles during stance. *Exp Brain Res* 1977; 26:59–72.
25. O'Brien SJ, Vertinsky PA: Unfit survivors: Exercise as a resource for aging women. *Gerontologist* 1991; 31:347–357.
26. Pearson MB, Bassey EJ, Bendall MJ: The effects of age on muscle strength and anthropometric indices within a group of elderly men and women. *Age Ageing* 1985; 14:230–234.
27. Seals DR, Hagberg JM, Hurley BF, et al: Endurance training in older men and women. I. Cardiovascular response to exercise. *J Appl Physiol* 1984; 57:1024–1029.
28. Shepard RJ: Demographic trends and goals for a geriatric society, in *Physical Activity and Aging,* ed 2. Rockville, MD, Aspen Publications, 1987, pp 255–276.
29. Tinetti M, Williams T, Mayewski R: Fall risk index for elderly patients based on number of chronic disabilities. *Am J Med* 1986; 80:429–434.
30. US Bureau of the Census. *Statistical Abstract of the United States,* ed 108. Washington, DC, Government Printing Office, 1988.
31. Wolfson L, Whipple R, Amernan P, et al: Stressing the postural response: A quantitative method for teaching balance. *J Am Geriatr Soc* 1986; 34:845–850.

The Older Athlete

Lynn Snyder-Mackler, Sc.D., P.T., S.C.S., A.T.C.
John F. Knarr, M.S., P.T., A.T.C.

INTRODUCTION

Individuals are living longer and staying physically active into old age. Moreover, the fitness craze of the 1970s and 1980s included people who came to athletics later in life. Continued or new exercise impacts an aging musculoskeletal system in many ways, not all of them positive. Certainly the demand for sports rehabilitation services for the geriatric patient will increase with the population and activity levels.

This chapter will define the geriatric athlete and describe typical musculoskeletal and cardiovascular characteristics found in these individuals. Common musculoskeletal problems will be discussed and the impact of aerobic conditioning on rehabilitation will be addressed. The role of comorbidity will also be considered. Designing exercise programs for the well elderly individual beginning an exercise program or cardiovascular conditioning will not be discussed. Practical considerations such as personnel, equipment, and marketing will be considered. Finally, case studies will be used to illustrate the interrelationship among the variables that affect treatment of the older athlete.

DEFINING THE POPULATION

Who is the geriatric athlete? Unless the population can be defined, identification of problems and potential solutions is difficult. It is actually easier to list who the geriatric athlete is not. The average well elderly person will not be discussed. The care of former athletes will not be reviewed unless they are still actively engaged in regular physical activity. There are three indistinct groups that make up this population of older athlete. Although there may be an overlap of problems, the groups have some apparent differences that influence their need for rehabilitation services. Each group will be dealt with in turn.

In the first group are former competitive athletes who have continued to exercise. For example, the football or field hockey team player could now be conditioning on a more individual basis using running, swimming, or cycling. (Former competitive athletes who no longer exercise are former athletes and will not be discussed in this chapter.) This group encompasses lifelong athletes who trained intensively for a period in their lives and may or may not be training at a relative intensity that is comparable with their earlier training levels. There are a wide variety of sports and training intensities included in this group. However, there are some similarities that necessitate this categorization. Virtually all the athletes who played team sports as competitive performers and who are still exercising are training at some other sport. For this group, previ-ous injury plays a large role in potential problems in old age.

The second group is composed of lifelong recreational athletes. Again, there is quite a spectrum of activities and training intensities included in this group. Most, however, are lifetime sports people. They play tennis or squash; they run or cycle. They may even participate in several different activities. Their involvement has been primarily in one sport or group of sports. This population may have a disproportionate amount of the overuse type of injury. For these individuals, athletic activity is as much a part of their routine as dressing or eating meals. They are reluctant to stop participating in an activity even in the face of significant pain or dysfunction.

The final group is made up of the nonathlete who began to exercise late in life (arbitrarily, after age 40). This is a smaller group but a significant one. These individuals present a unique set of problems related directly to beginning physical activity at an older age and indirectly to their reasons for beginning to exercise. In many instances, exercise has been prescribed (dictated) by a change in health status. Common examples of this type of individual may include the patient who has experienced coronary symptoms (or may be a prime candidate for them) that are the direct result of a number of controllable risk factors including improper diet (obese) and lack of exercise. In many cases, the physician has prescribed a progressive walking program as a beginning or introduction to exercise. The fact that a person's walking program was begun as a result of a heart attack does not protect him from musculoskeletal injury, but it may interfere with motivation for recovery.

The three groups described may differ in the quality of their exercise. Most older athletes are involved in racquet sports, running, walking, and low-impact sports like golf and bowling. All of these sports can be played in a highly competitive manner against an opponent, a score, or a time.[15] *Competitive* athletes can be found in any of the three categories of older athlete described above. Masters athletes are those who are 40 or older. There have been established competitive amateur Masters events for years. Swimming, weight lifting, road running, and track and field are some sports that have well-established Masters competitions. Professionally, the "Senior" Golf Tour and Masters runners are the most high profile. There was even an attempt to begin a "Senior" baseball league using professional baseball's spring training sites. The trend in population growth toward a larger number of elderly dictates that the number of events and competitors will continue to increase.

All the older athletes, regardless of the category in which they fall, have some generic age-related changes. Older athletes are generally less flexible,[15, 19, 23] and have smaller muscle masses,[9] lower aerobic capacities,[10, 18] and less well tuned thermoregulatory mechanisms[22] than they did at a younger age. They are likely to have osteoarthritis of the weight-bearing joints. These age-related changes impact training, injury, and treatment of the older athlete and must be considered when designing their rehabilitation program.

MUSCULOSKELETAL PROBLEMS

The older athlete, as the younger athlete, incurs acute or traumatic injury and overuse injury.[15] Unlike the younger athlete, however, these injuries are superimposed on an aging musculoskeletal system, and recovery may take longer. Prevention, therefore, takes on a much more important role in this population. Proper equipment selection and use (e.g., shoes, racquet) and stretching and training techniques must be encouraged in order to avoid such problems.

Acute, Traumatic Injury

Acute musculoskeletal trauma is different in the older athlete than in the younger. Since most older athletes no longer participate in collision sports, major contusions, fractures, and multiple ligament trauma rarely occur. However, when ligamentous sprains and muscle tears occur, these injuries can be devastating to the older athlete. Detraining or deconditioning occurs as a result of lack of exercise and takes much less time than training for persons of all ages. The rest required after ligamentous injury or muscle tear can mean the end of athletic activity for an older athlete because of this detraining effect. Fractures, when they occur, are often pathologic: osteoporosis and cancer are the most common causes. Fortunately, weight-bearing activity may serve a protective function for women in the case of bone loss and associated fractures, although the intensity and frequency of exercise necessary to achieve this effect are subject to conflicting information.[2]

Overuse Injury

Most serious athletes suffer from injuries that fall into the overuse category; older athletes are no exception. For the purposes of this chapter, we will operationally define *overuse injuries* as those injuries resulting from training but are not attributable to a single traumatic event. Older athletes may actually be more prone to this type of injury than younger athletes.[15] Several factors may contribute to this predisposition. First, they are less flexible than younger athletes.[15, 19, 23] Second, most have at least some arthritic changes in weight-bearing joints.[8] Third, muscle mass is reduced.[9]

Muscle soreness is common, especially when beginning an exercise program or adding new types of exercise to an existing program. This should not be a concern to the therapist. Muscle soreness is attributed to microscopic injury to muscle and connective tissue, which is a necessary prerequisite to muscle strengthening. A certain amount of soreness is expected. Delayed onset muscle soreness (DOMS) occurs in this population as well as in younger populations and occurs from 24 to 48 hours after exercise. Rest from exercise (a day off or exercise of uninvolved muscles) and, in some cases, the use of ice and aspirin or some other anti-inflammatory medication will take care of the problem, and the athlete will be ready to exercise again the next day. Eccentric exercise appears to be the biggest culprit for DOMS.[1, 3, 21] Prolonged muscle soreness (*significant* pain that lasts longer than 48 hours after exercise) should be evaluated. This could indicate muscle or tendon injury that may be the result of overtraining either by frequency, duration, or intensity.

Joint pain and associated effusion are also common in this population. Joint pain as a single symptom should be attended to when it occurs without an associated change in the type or intensity of the exercise or if there is sharp pain. Otherwise, transient joint pain should be watched and managed symptomatically. If joint effusion or other signs of inflammation occur (redness, warmth), the joint should be thoroughly evaluated, as it may be indicative of a more severe underlying problem such as arthritis, infection, fracture, or tumor.

Pain with specific movements or pain that occurs after certain activities that is not "joint pain" or DOMS can occur. These types of injuries are more like those "overuse" injuries that occur in younger athletes. They can usually be attributed to a specific set of circumstances or to structural abnormalities. For example, the athlete with medial knee pain may in fact have tendinitis of the pes anserine region. Other examples may include pain in the subacromial region as a result of impingement of the suprahumeral space, or plantar fasciitis, which may indicate a need for orthotic fabrication. They are approached as one approaches the problems in younger athletes. In our experience, older athletes respond well to treatment, but healing takes longer and may result in more residual dysfunction.

Prevention

Injury prevention has always been an integral part of sports medicine. Because even a minor injury can lead to the end of an older athlete's sports participation, prevention is extraordinarily important for the older athlete.

There is no substitute for an adequate warm-up prior

to exercise. Athletes who have always avoided this aspect of training find it essential as they age. The best warm-up for a specific activity is 10 minutes or so of low-intensity engagement in that activity. If tennis is the activity, then the players should begin by hitting balls across the net, slowly at first and then with increased velocity and movement. If running is the activity, the runner should begin the first mile at an easy jog and gradually pick up speed. This rule is easily generalized to other sports.

Warm-up is often confused with stretching. Although stretching may be a component of the warm-up for some athletes, stretching can be as much of a problem as it is a help. Improper or inconsistent stretching techniques (e.g., ballistic) can cause muscle strains and soreness. Stretching is often a prelude to activity. Although it may not be harmful, stretching a cold muscle is not a sensible idea. As a rule of thumb, we do not discourage athletes who have always stretched prior to exercise from doing so. We do, however, suggest that other athletes engage in more global activities to warm the muscles prior to stretching or even better to incorporate stretching into their cool-down routine. It seems logical to suggest stretching as a remedy for the flexibility changes that occur with aging. However, the reason for the loss of flexibility with aging may be less a result of soft tissue tightness and more a result of joint changes. Some changes include joint surface deterioration, breakdown of the collagen fibers, and a decrease in the viscosity of synovial fluid. In these cases, stretching may not be particularly helpful.

We strongly endorse the philosophy of "If it ain't broke, don't fix it" in sports rehabilitation. Others have suggested that abnormal physical findings such as increased Q angle, "tight hamstrings," and excessive pronation should be treated even in asymptomatic individuals. We do not advocate preventive orthotic fittings or other types of interventions to prevent injury. We do not interfere with an athlete's training regimen just because it *might* cause problems. Studies that have investigated predisposing factors for overuse injury have been remarkably unsuccessful in establishing a relationship between measurable variables (e.g., rear foot abnormalities, muscle strength and training regimens) and predisposition to injury.

CARDIOVASCULAR FUNCTION AND LIMITS TO PERFORMANCE

Longitudinal studies of cardiovascular fitness show a decline with increasing age. However, physically active individuals demonstrate less of a decline than sedentary individuals (Fig 25–1).[6, 16] Conventional wisdom about aerobic fitness and age is shattered almost weekly; the true limits to performance in the older athlete are largely unknown. Masters and age-group distance running, cycling, and swimming records are lowered at a staggering rate.[4] The Masters marathon record was shattered in 1990 when John Campbell (as a newly minted 40-year-old) finished among the top five runners of all age-groups, running a 2:11:04 in the Boston Marathon. Although the abil-

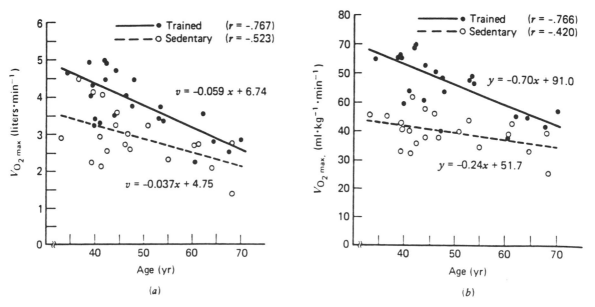

FIG 25–1.
Effects of age on $\dot{V}O_2$ max in trained and sedentary men. **A,** the y axis = $\dot{V}O_2$ max $1 \cdot min^{-1}$; **B,** the y axis = $\dot{V}O_2$ max mL $\cdot$ kg $\cdot$ min^{-1}. (From Brooks GA, Fahey TD (eds): *Exercise Physiology.* New York, Macmillan, 1985. Used by permission.)

ity to do work diminishes with increasing age, the limits are constantly being challenged.

COMORBIDITY

Systemic disease, degenerative disease, and previous injury can have a tremendous impact on athletic performance in the older adult and will likely influence choice of activity.

Systemic diseases whose incidence increases with age include cardiovascular disease and diabetes. Exercise has been shown to have a generally positive effect on these diseases.[5, 7, 11, 12] The therapist needs to be aware of the kinds of screening necessitated by the presence of systemic disease. For example, adults with diabetes should be carefully examined for signs of foot problems related to diminished peripheral sensation secondary to degeneration of myelin and a compromised vascular system due to arteriosclerosis. Other factors associated with diabetes mellitus include coronary complications, kidney failure, blindness, cataracts, and muscle weakness. Degenerative disease, most notably osteoarthritis, occurs in most older individuals.[8] However, the relationship of exercise to osteoarthritis is equivocal. Although athletes may have roentgenographic evidence of osteoarthritis, careful physical examination is essential before the osteoarthritis can be incriminated as the cause of exercise-related symptoms. Very often, the presence of osteoarthritis is sufficient for a physician or rehabilitation professional to attribute activity-related pain to arthritis, when in fact it may be merely coincidence that the patient's complaint is in the general area of a joint with osteoarthritis. Degenerative disk disease can also be a problem in the older athlete, but again, radiographic evidence is not sufficient to ascribe symptoms to its presence. Care should be taken to carefully evaluate other possible causes of pain like hypomobility, inflammation, and overuse.

PROGRAMMATIC CONSIDERATIONS

When we ask the question, "What do we know about athletic injuries in this population?" the answer is "Not much." Much of the literature is anecdotal. Few epidemiologic studies have been conducted. From the literature on sedentary individuals beginning low-to moderate-level exercise, we can conclude that injury rarely occurs. This, however, does not necessarily generalize to the older athlete. We would like to make some recommendations regarding personnel and facilities to rehabilitation professionals who would like to treat the older athlete.

Personnel

In our collective 30 years of practice of physical therapy and athletic training, we have treated many older athletes for musculoskeletal problems associated with their exercise. Once injuries occur, regardless of their incidence in the general population or other factors, the patient needs to be treated. Many of the aspects of treatment of the younger athlete can be generalized to the older athlete. But the differences inherent in an aging musculoskeletal system and other problems of aging are unique. Some of the changes affecting the skeletal system include deterioration of joint surfaces, breakdown of collagen fibers, and a decrease in the viscosity of synovial fluid, which can result in a loss of flexibility and an increase in joint stiffness. Changes affecting the muscular system include a decrease in the size, number, and type of muscle fibers. Individual motor units lose fibers, which results in a decrease in the force-generating ability of that muscle. There is an effective loss of type II fibers, which results in a higher percentage of type I fibers. Although this change in percentage may increase the muscle's ability to sustain performance during endurance activities, it may limit the muscle's ability to generate strength and power. Muscles experience a decrease in respiratory capacity and an increase in fat and connective tissues.

The rehabilitation professional who expects to treat the older athlete must have experience and a good working knowledge of the mechanisms of athletic injuries. The ideal individual would have firsthand experience with caring for athletes before, during, and after athletic participation and know both the physical and psychologic demands sports place on the participant. This medical care provider should be versed in a diversity of areas including anatomy, cardiovascular and muscle physiology, nutrition, biomechanics and kinesiology, physical training, flexibility and conditioning programs, protective/preventive taping and/or bracing, and rehabilitation. Understanding of age-related physiologic changes and their ramifications relating to physical exercise are vital to a safe and successful return to participation and, in some cases, competition. Knowledge of pathologic changes and their effects on the ability to participate in athletic activities is critical in the design and implementation of a rehabilitation program for the older athlete.

Facility

There is not much about a typical sports or orthopedic outpatient facility that needs to be changed to allow for treatment of the older athlete. Traditional physical therapy modalities (ice, electrical stimulation, ultrasound, and moist heat) are frequently used in the treatment of the older athlete. Exercise equipment used to treat this population may require some modifications such as the availability of lighter weights for exercise and slower velocities for instrumented treadmills. Electromechanical devices (which permit isokinetic, isotonic and isometric exercise, and passive motion exercise capabilities) and hydrotherapy are also helpful in the treatment of the older athlete.

Hydrotherapy is being used more frequently for large joint exercise and rehabilitation of athletic injuries involving all populations of athletes. Smaller exercise tanks have allowed many facilities without room for a therapeutic pool to incorporate much of pool therapy into a smaller area of practice. Its application is especially important when treating the older athlete since it reduces the weight-bearing effects imposed on joint surfaces. The use of this modality also allows the athlete to continue to train and maintain cardiovascular fitness while decreasing the amount of stress to pre-existing injuries.

The facility should allow for the treatment of different age athletes together. Interaction among athletes of various ages and sports is helpful to recovery from a motivational aspect. For this reason, a large open exercise area is preferable to small enclosed booths or cubicles. Although some privacy is lost, the effect of the interaction with other injured athletes is invaluable.

CASE STUDIES

Case 1

A 54-year-old left-handed college professor was referred to our clinic with right shoulder pain that was interfering with his exercise program. He had been a regular participant in an exercise program at the faculty fitness center for the past 5 years. His routine included aerobic exercise (on a treadmill or stair climber) that was unaffected by his pain, and weight lifting. He had some articular degeneration evident on X ray. He had been on nonsteroidal antiinflammatory medication for 2 weeks and noticed a marked improvement. His goal was to return to his weight-training program.

He had decreased passive range of motion in glenohumeral abduction, flexion, and external rotation. His right external rotation strength was 50% of that of the left as measured isokinetically at 120 degrees/sec. Otherwise, strength was equal in both extremities. All impingement tests were positive on the right.[17] He was tender to palpation of the tendon of the long head of the biceps, the supraspinatus tendon just proximal to its insertion, and the posterior joint capsule. Posterior and inferior glides of the glenohumeral joint were restricted.[17] Posterior glide was painful, and inferior glide reduced his symptoms.

Our hypothesis was that inflammation of the tendons and/or bursa in the suprahumeral space resulted in an impingement of these structures, causing pain during movement. The joint range of motion restriction and weakness resulted from the patient splinting and not using the arm fully.

The inflammation was being managed medically, and there had been an overall improvement since the patient began to take medication. Our treatment addressed the decreased range of motion and strength of the external rotators.

Treatment consisted of ultrasound (1.0 W/cm^2) to the posterior capsule, followed by inferior and posterior glides of the glenohumeral joint (Fig 25–2). Stretching using various techniques including contract-relax were used. Transverse friction massage was applied to the bicipital and supraspinatus tendons. Progressive resistive exercises included the use of dumbbells, Theraband, and proprioceptive neuromuscular facilitation techniques for strengthening.

The patient was advised to immediately return to those aspects of his athletic program that did not provoke pain in the right shoulder. He was treated twice a week for 4 weeks. We observed his upper extremity weight-lifting technique and made some suggestions to alter his mechanics (correcting his technique) to minimize his shoulder pain. The patient was encouraged to eliminate incline and military bench press, as these two exercises resulted in the most pain. His range of motion and strength returned to normal. He gradually resumed all his premorbid exercise activities, was weaned from the anti-inflammatory medication, and was discharged.

Case 2

A 73-year-old man was referred to our clinic with increasing left foot pain that was exacerbated by his running. The

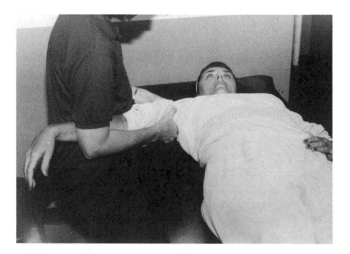

FIG 25–2.
Inferior and posterior glides of the glenohumeral joint can be used to improve range of motion.

patient stated that he experienced excruciating pain along the bottom of his foot when he stepped out of bed in the morning that gradually got better over the first hour he was awake. However, after his daily 6-mile run, his pain was much worse. His goal was to resume his running program.

He was tender to deep palpation along the plantar surfaces of both feet. Non–weight-bearing evaluation of his foot position showed normal rear foot and forefoot alignment bilaterally. However, in standing on the left foot as well as on videotaped walking and running on a treadmill, the midtarsal joint appeared to collapse during single-limb support. Accessory motion testing of the talonavicular joints revealed hypermobility bilaterally; calcaneocuboid joints had normal mobility.[17] Ankle range of motion did not appear to be affected. Toe flexor strength was decreased slightly on the left.

Our hypothesis was that midtarsal joint hypermobility was causing a severe plantar fasciitis on the left and a mild case on the right. We fitted him with orthoses for use during all activities including running. Other treatment included toe flexion exercises for strengthening and ultrasound to the plantar surfaces of both feet. He stopped running until the orthoses were fabricated. After 2 weeks, he was running 3 miles per day without discomfort. We treated him twice a week for 6 weeks, at which time he had stopped wearing the orthoses for all activities except running. At the time of discharge, he was again running 6 miles per day.

Case 3

A 65-year-old female golfer and cross-country skier tore her anterior cruciate ligament during her first downhill skiing experience 2 weeks prior to her referral to our clinic. She regularly played golf (three or four times per week from March through October) prior to her injury, and her major goal was to resume her golf schedule.

She had a positive Lachman's test on the right, with no end point.[17] She also had a positive lateral pivot shift.[17] Both test results were consistent with anterior cruciate instability. All other tests were negative. She complained that her knee would give out on her during level walking. Peak isometric torque of the right quadriceps was 60% of that of the left. Range of motion was 0 to 135 degrees, which was comparable with her left knee.

Our hypothesis was that strengthening her quadriceps would help to decrease the instability during walking and that she would be able to return to golfing. We treated her with weight-bearing and non–weight-bearing progressive resistive exercise, as well as neuromuscular electrical stimulation (NMES) to her quadriceps (Fig 25–3).[20] Although her right quadriceps strength increased to 90% of that of the left, she still had episodes of giving way during walking. She was fitted with a derotational brace and began to

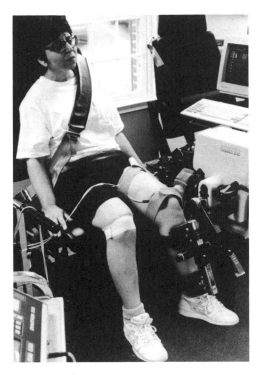

FIG 25–3.
Combination of neuromuscular electrical stimulation (NMES) and isokinetic exercise to improve the strength of the quadriceps.

golf. On her second day out, she heard a "pop" at the end of her swing, felt a sharp pain in her knee, and couldn't straighten it out.

She had torn her right medial meniscus and subsequently underwent a partial meniscectomy and an extra-articular reconstruction of her anterior cruciate ligament. Rehabilitation began in the second postoperative week with passive range of motion, weight-bearing quadriceps exercises including walking, limited-arc squats, stationary cycling, and NMES. After 3 months, she was back to all daily activities and had resumed playing golf wearing a brace.

Case 4

A 58-year-old female race walker was referred to our clinic with back pain. She had a 4-month history of left-sided low back pain with radiation into the left buttock and thigh. Prior to that time, she was a recreational race walker. She reported that "when it gets really bad," the pain extended to her knee. She had been treated at another clinic, where she received traction in the prone position and some joint mobilization treatment directed at her sacroiliac joint.

At the beginning of the examination, she had only slight discomfort in the left side of her back at about the L4 level. Posterior postural evaluation revealed no obvious asymmetry; no lateral deviations or pelvic asymmetry was noted. When she was asked to forward bend, she moved easily and symmetrically into flexion with normal sacroiliac mobility and excursion. However, most of her forward bending occurred in the upper back, as her lumbar spine remained quite fixed. Her movement into extension in standing was restricted but not painful. Repeated flexion in standing caused her back pain to begin to radiate into her left buttock. Repeated extension did not worsen or lessen these symptoms. Because her symptoms were exacerbated with flexion in standing, no supine flexion tests were performed. Prone extension was restricted but, again, had no effect on her symptoms.

Passive range of motion of the lumbar spine was examined in standing and side lying. She had very little motion into either flexion or extension as measured with inclinometers.[14] Passive intervertebral motion testing revealed significant restriction at both the L3–4 and L4–5 levels. The patient described a "stretching pain" during these tests that was unlike her typical symptoms and did not persist after the test. Neurologic examination of the lower extremities was negative.

Our hypothesis was that the patient had discogenic symptoms, which appeared to be resolving. She also had significant hypomobility of her lower lumbar spine. This case is a classic example of a "which came first?" dilemma. Did the joint restriction predispose her to the disk problem, or was the hypomobility a result of holding her back stiffly ("guarding") for the past few months? Pragmatically, we believed her disk problem could be treated symptomatically and that the mobility problems should be directly addressed using joint mobilization.

The patient was treated with exercise including prone lying, prone back extension, and eventually back flexion with the patient sitting (Fig 25–4). Intervertebral anterior glides and rotational mobilization techniques were also used. After 1 month, she began to walk at a slow speed on a treadmill. She gradually increased her speed to a comfortable race-walking pace on the treadmill. After 3 months her lumbar spine range of motion and intervertebral motion had improved. She was nearly pain free in all activities, and she had returned to race walking on the road/track without difficulty. As the patient's goal of pain-free activities of daily living (including race walking) was met, she was discharged.

Case 5

A 44-year-old Masters power lifter tore his right triceps brachii muscle during a competition, underwent surgery, and was referred to our clinic for rehabilitation. This patient had been a competitive lifter for 10 years. He had

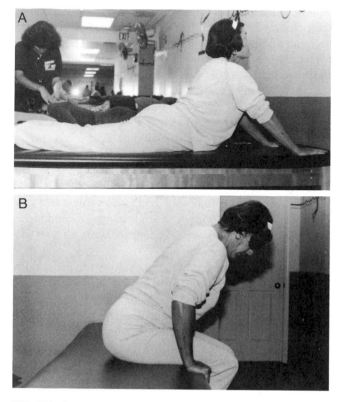

FIG 25–4.
Progression of exercise from prone back extension **(A)** to flexion in sitting **(B)**.

used intramuscular and oral anabolic steroids cyclically for the past 8 years.

Range of motion of the right elbow was from 0 to 75 degrees. The right biceps manual muscle testing grade was F+, and the triceps was F−. The radioulnar joint was restricted in distraction and medial and lateral glides. The radiohumeral joint was not restricted. Wrist and shoulder motions were not restricted.

The patient's goal was to return to competitive power lifting as soon as possible. He stated that he would return to training and lifting regardless of our advice or the advice of his surgeon. We were convinced that he would probably also return to his steroid use.

Treatment consisted of joint mobilization to the humeroulnar joint, passive range of motion, and limited-arc isokinetic exercise at various speeds, progressing from a gravity-minimized to a gravity-resisted position. He began light weight training (bench press, squat, and dead lift) after 4 weeks when his triceps and biceps muscle testing grades were G− to G and his range of elbow motion had increased from 0 to 120 degrees. Shortly after he began weight training, he stopped coming to physical therapy. He was never formally discharged. He subsequently competed successfully in power-lifting competitions.

SUMMARY

Older athletes who are injured present a unique set of circumstances to the rehabilitation professional. In spite of their age, they are athletes, and athletic participation is an important part of their lives. Rehabilitation professionals need to respect this importance and still understand the constraints imposed on athletic participation by injury to musculosketal and cardiovascular systems. This requires knowledge, patience, diplomacy and a healthy respect for the patients' desires to return to activity.

REFERENCES

1. Abraham WM: Exercise induced muscle soreness. *Phys Sportsmed* 1979; 7:57–60.
2. Aloia JF, Cohn SH, Ostuni JA: Prevention of involitional bone loss by exercise. *Ann Intern Med* 1979; 89:356–358.
3. Armstrong RB: Mechanisms of exercise-induced delayed onset muscular soreness: A brief overview. *Med Sci Sports Exerc* 1984; 6:529–538.
4. Clark T: The Master's movement. *Runner's World* 1979; 14:80–83.
5. Costill DF, Miller JM, Fink WJ: Energy metabolism in diabetic distance runners. *Phys Sportsmed* 1980; 8:64–71.
6. Dehn MM, Bruce RA: Longitudinal variations in maximal oxygen uptake with age and activity. *J Appl Physiol* 1972; 33:805–807.
7. Frontera WR, Evans WJ: Exercise performance and endurance training in the elderly. *Top Geriatr Rehabil* 1966; 2:17–31.
8. Gambert SR: Rheumatologic problems in the elderly, in Gambert SR, Benson DM, Gupta KL (eds): *Handbook of Geriatrics*. New York, Plenum Press, 1987, pp 95–120.
9. Grimby G, Danneskiold-Samsoe B, Hvid K: Morphology and enzymatic capacity in arm and leg muscles in 78–81 year old men and women. *Acta Physiol Scand* 1982; 115:125–134.
10. Hagberg JM, Graves JE, Limacher M, et al: Cardiovascular responses of 70–79 year old men and women to exercise training. *J Appl Physiol* 1989; 66:2589–2594.
11. Jette DU: Physiological effects of exercise in the diabetic. *Phys Ther* 1984; 64:339–341.
12. Kasch FW, Wallace JP, Van Camp SP, et al: A longitudinal study of cardiovascular stability in active men aged 45 to 65. *Phys Sportsmed* 1988; 16:117–123.
13. Kendall HO, Kendall FP: Normal flexibility according to age groups. *J Bone Joint Surg* 1948; 30A:690–694.
14. Klein AB, Snyder-Mackler L, Roy SH, et al: Comparison of spinal mobility and isometric trunk extensor forces with electromyographic spectral analysis in identifying low back pain. *Phys Ther* 1991; 71:445–454.
15. Matheson GO, MacIntyre JG, Taunton JE, et al: Musculoskeletal injuries associated with physical activity in older adults. *Med Sci Sports Exerc* 1989; 21:379–385.
16. Nakamura E, Moritani T, Kanetaka A: Biological age versus physical fitness age. *Eur J Appl Physiol* 1983; 58:778–785.
17. Palmer ML, Epler ME: *Clinical Assessment Procedures in Physical Therapy*. Philadelphia, JB Lippincott, 1990.
18. Seals DR, Hagberg JM, Hurley BF, et al: Endurance training in older men and women. 1. Cardiovascular responses to exercise. *J Appl Physiol* 1984; 57:1024–1029.
19. Smith JR, Walker JM: Knee and elbow range of motion in healthy older individuals. *Phys Occup Ther Geriatr* 1983; 2:31–38.
20. Snyder-Mackler L, Ladin Z, Schepsis AA, et al: Electrical stimulation of the thigh muscles after reconstruction of the anterior cruciate ligament. *J Bone Joint Surg* 1991; 73A:1025–1036.
21. Talag TS: Residual muscle soreness as influenced by concentric, eccentric and static contractions. *Res Q* 1973; 44:458–469.
22. Wagner JA, Robinson S, Tzankoff SP, et al: Heat tolerance and acclimatization to work in the heat in relation to age. *J Appl Physiol* 1972; 33:616–622.
23. Walker JM, Sue D, Miles Elkousy N, et al: Active mobility of the extremities in older subjects. *Phys Ther* 1984; 64:919–923.

CHAPTER 26

The Older Adult With Developmental Disability

Jody Delehanty, Ph.D., P.T.

INTRODUCTION

Overview

Professionals with experience in geriatric settings report that they are seeing developmentally disabled elders for the first time in their professional careers. Experts in the treatment and management of cerebral palsy report that they have no experience in dealing with the deformities seen in a 60-year-old individual with spastic diplegia. Who are these people, and where have they been? Individuals with developmental disabilities who are now appearing in Senior Citizen Service centers at the age of 65 have clearly been receiving some degree of assistance in daily living during their adult years. Yet they are an unfamiliar group to other clients at such centers as well as to the staff.

This section will examine the "groups" who are commonly included under the term *developmentally disabled* and the medical and social factors that have influenced their visibility in society. Comparisons with current age cohorts will also be discussed as a general background for the more specific material in the rest of the chapter dealing with the roles physical therapists may play in improving the quality of life for this group of elders.

Diagnostic Groups

The developmentally disabled individual has historically been grouped according to either an associated medical diagnosis or the functional deficit that characterized the individual. When attention turned to the needs of the disabled in the first part of the 20th century, the thrust for programs, money, and attention came mainly from groups of parents organized around diagnostic labels. With the development of the polio vaccine in the late 1950s, there was a public impression that now this talent and money could be converted to curing other diagnoses.

Modeling on the very successful program of the National Foundation for Infantile Paralysis that supported treatment and research in polio, organizations such as the Cerebral Palsy Association, the Association for Retarded Children, and many others came into being as advocacy and fund-raising groups. Most advocacy groups started with the emphasis on children. The Association for Retarded Children did not change its name to the Association for Retarded Citizens until the 1970s.

Attention to many of these disorders revealed that they were not caused by one agent and that the condition did not follow the same course in all clients. The issues that needed to be addressed by the associations in both research for cures and in treatment programs were complex. Furthermore, unlike most of the polio cases, these were chronic disorders and persisted into adulthood. With so many groups competing for both private and governmental funds, pressure was brought on the advocacy groups to come together under one umbrella of need.

At about the same time, in the 1960s, the large social movement of deinstitutionalization emerged and directed attention at the giant residential care facilities that had evolved to serve the needs of individuals who had been judged medically or socially unable to function in society as a result of their mental retardation and/or mental illness (as judged by the standards of that time). Many of the residents of institutions for the "mentally deficient" had been placed there shortly after birth by parents following the strong advice of experts in the medical field that the child would require care and treatment that could be provided only by experts in an institutional environment. Examining these thousands of residents, it quickly became evident that the majority had no "diagnosis" in the usual sense. The most common entry on charts was "congenital encephalopathy, etiology undetermined," giving the reader only the information that the problem had always been there and was probably based in the central nervous system —and no one knew why! The identified needs of many of this group of clients whose supposed problem was mental retardation were stated in terms of therapies and education that seemed very similar to those being described by the advocacy groups. The first major government initiative directed at the care of the mentally retarded reflected this by including the neurologic conditions of autism, cerebral palsy, and epilepsy with mental retardation in the first Developmental Disabilities Act.[1] This specific diagnostic listing excluded many children and families from services. The reaction to these exclusions led to the adoption of functional definitions.

Functional Groups

The amount of segregation by medical diagnosis that existed in pediatrics until the late 1960s is difficult to appreciate today. Children who had deafness in conjunction with athetoid cerebral palsy were often not admitted to speech and audiology programs. Children with Down's syndrome were not admitted for physical therapy, which was not available at centers for the retarded. Traditionally, physical therapists working with children before 1960 worked with children who had polio. Although the impact of this disease on the developing child could continue through growth with many resulting orthopedic complications, the major problems were in the areas of motor control and function. When the caseload in pediatric facilities changed in a short time to being almost entirely composed of children with neurologic dysfunction, the interaction of motor, cognitive, and behavioral deficits on function became immediately apparent. When large numbers of children left the institutions, centers for the mentally retarded suddenly had to deal with individuals who had sensory and motor problems in addition to their "simple" retardation.

The need to establish responsive programs led to compromises between the categorical and functional groups. A *developmental disability,* in the terminology of the 1984 regulations that accompanied the first legislation mentioned earlier, could be attributed to a mental or physical impairment or combination of the two that resulted in substantial functional limitations in three or more areas of life activity: self-care, language, learning, mobility, self-direction, independent living, or economic self-sufficiency. These descriptions meant that many of the old diagnostic groups, such as cerebral palsy, would not mean automatic inclusion for individual clients. Infants and children who had no firm diagnosis but who did have severe lags in early development could receive services.

Medical Management

It is somewhat fashionable for the apparent increase in numbers of developmentally disabled persons in the community to be attributed to medical advances that allow the survival of premature, ill, or injured infants and children. In fact, the less dramatic medical advances in preventive medicine and health maintenance that have increased life expectancy for the entire population in the 20th century have been the greater contributors to increased life expectancy in this part of the population, too. Immunizations, antibiotics, and seizure control measures have been particularly effective for this medically fragile group of children. The willingness and resources to treat the conditions and illnesses that occur in infancy and childhood as complications of many diagnostic groups included within the range of developmental disabilities have steadily increased the number of children who reach a healthy adolescence and adulthood. Old texts still in circulation give life expectancies of 6 to 10 years for individuals with such diagnoses as Down's syndrome and spina bifida. Later in this chapter the importance of ascertaining the knowledge level of clients and care takers in areas such as this will be presented.

Social Management

For the first part of the 20th century, the placement of choice for infants and children with conditions we would now consider as developmental disabilities was residential. Large institutions for those who could not cognitively, behaviorally, and/or physically function within the normal settings of school and work life housed an amazing variety of persons in what was a total community with care from cradle to grave, and indeed, most institutions had a geriatric building. This in itself provides evidence that there has always been a population of aged developmentally disabled and that life expectancy data have always been biased by omitting the data from those who lived in this other community of the institution.

The deinstitutionalization move of the 1960s and 1970s changed residential patterns dramatically. Individuals were rapidly discharged to be placed in community placements that often varied more according to age-group, since this was an easier parameter to identify than any evaluation of function. Twenty years ago, a substantial portion of the community placements were in nursing homes that were seen as age appropriate for a number of former institution residents in mid- or late adulthood. Anecdotally, we know that many of the clients who moved from the crowded and often dirty back wards to the more socially acceptable bright and sunny nursing home did not respond as their advocates and care takers had anticipated. In many cases, they gave every evidence of missing their previous institutional homes, social contacts and sense of personal control and freedom in the same way as their age peers who were coming from "real homes" in the community. Many placements were reversed, and the individual was able to return to the institutional home.

Professionals experienced in this area came to the conclusion that factors other than chronologic age and aging-related characteristics (such as gray hair or lack of teeth) were important for successful community placement of individuals who had lived most of their lives in institutions. We are still trying to identify those factors in the life experiences of the developmentally disabled elder (and in their families) that are important in predicting which programs will be successful for the individual.

In accord with the philosophy of deinstitutionalization, many infants and children born after 1960 and identified as being developmentally disabled have always lived within the community in their family of birth, in foster care, or in community residence programs. Most communities, through social and legal pressures, have established programs that have retained and maintained special needs children in the community. Perhaps because the term *developmentally disabled* has been so linked with infancy and childhood, programs for individuals identified as belonging to this population started with projects addressing the needs of preschoolers. Other age-appropriate programs were initiated as this first generation of children matured.

In most cases, planners have been "surprised" as these individuals have progressed through age-appropriate activities such as school programs and emerged into the post-education adult stage of life. The types of individuals who were made eligible for such programs have steadily increased. For example, initially children with progressive muscular dystrophies were not included, and some of the early programs were not even accessible to those who were not ambulatory. Some of the first plans seemed to have been based on the concept that known interventions properly applied would enable all the children in programs to reach functional independence as adults. The severity of some of the problems and factors such as the interaction of motor and cognitive handicaps were not considered in the earliest interventions. An adolescent might be mainstreamed in the local school system and complete the required number of years of education, but this could not guarantee the ability needed to be employed or to live independently. Issues such as preparation for work, adult leisure, and housing outside the family-parent-child relation have been addressed only in the last 10 years, and models are still being worked out. It is encouraging that appropriate programs and intervention for the aged individual are starting to be considered before large numbers enter this age-group and confront health professionals with problems previously ignored by geriatric practitioners.

The developmentally disabled individual is becoming a part of the community of aging persons as a result of both medical and social evolutions that have caused them to become community members earlier in the life span. *Developmentally disabled,* like *baby boomer,* seems to be a term that is moving along the age continuum successively referring in each decade to an older cohort. At the outset, it is important to remember that the term was coined in the 1960s to describe in functional, rather than diagnostic, terms a group of individuals who had "special needs" and required "special services" to allow them to function in society. The term has always been a description and not a diagnosis. As such, it can and does accommodate a wide variety of individuals and behaviors. Physical therapists may see the term given in a referral as a diagnosis, but it has no more functional meaning than 85-*year-old, spinal cord injury,* or *arthritis* used in such a broad context. The needs of individuals cannot be predicted from labels such as these. They are helpful only in providing some parameters for further evaluation.

DEMOGRAPHICS

The dramatic shifts in demography that we are all experiencing are influencing the life course of all members of society. The growth in the field of geriatrics is one of the more visible results. The developmentally disabled are part of the rapidly growing number of older persons, and as members, they share in both the benefits and the problems of a new population. This section discusses some of these similarities and differences on a group and an individual level.

Similarities to Age Cohort

The developmentally disabled are not exempt from demographic change, and they share the graying of America with their respective age cohorts. From the perspective of health professionals, the view in geriatrics is often bleak. We focus on those elders who have lost function and family, on those who have suffered financial and personal loss from catastrophic illness, and on concern for their increasing numbers. There is, however, a social, financial, and political power in the increasing number of individuals in the senior citizen ranks that is not being ignored by entrepreneurs. This can be seen in the number of marketing efforts at leisure products, retirement homes, travel, and other age-tailored products.

The disabled have shared in some of this benefit. It is now possible to buy a "CP Walker" in an adult size. Seating systems address *all* sizes and do not attempt to maintain normal position to prevent deformity but seek to accommodate function and posture. Program planners and policymakers are considering the numbers of developmentally disabled adolescents and adults in their long-term planning rather than assuming that most of the individuals will be "gone." Family members are empowered by this growth in numbers to ask for, and to expect, responsible agencies to respond to the need for residential care for the older developmentally disabled family member as a viable alternative to the home-care setting.

Differences From Age Cohort

As a group, the developmentally disabled differ from their aging nondisabled peers, as they have differed throughout the life span. There used to be an assumption that the disabled infant varied little from the normal infant and that differences grew through the age span, peaking at full adult status, and then there was a congruence occurring somewhere near retirement age. Today we can question this scenario from the vantage of both the disabled and the nondisabled. Clearly, there is a range and no orderly curve.

One marked difference, by definition inherent in developmental disability, is that of life course. In general, clients who come to the physical therapist have experienced a life course that is somewhat similar for all those who have aged in American society. They have gone to similar schools, attained similar milestones (such as a first date, a driver's license, or leaving the family home), and have had a productive adult role involving a work function either in business, industry, or the home. Experiences such as marriage, divorce, children, home ownership, and the family living constellation vary, but most of these experiences are familiar to all. More than that, these are familiar experiences to most of the health or helping professionals who come in contact with the geriatric client.

This is not the case with the developmentally disabled. Their life courses vary greatly. Adulthood for some may have been spent wholly or partly in an institutional setting; for others in the community, living with their parents or a parent, often without work or leisure out of the home, and eventually in the company of aging or ill parents. Increasingly we will see developmentally disabled senior citizens who have had work experience and an adult family role, but this is not now, and may never be, the majority. Many of their life settings were not by choice and, in a surprising number of cases, simply evolved with no sense of control or ability to choose on the part of the individual or their family who took what was available. The developmentally disabled differ in the quantity and the nature of experiences both from their age peers and from those who will be in a helping relationship with them in their later life phases. This factor alone places a real responsibility on those such as physical therapists who are involved in evaluation of these clients; these individuals must expend considerable time and effort to discover how the person has come to senior citizen status and how this will influence intervention, rather than imposing a diagnostically related management regimen.

Individual Differences

Individuals with developmental disabilities may have unique properties that differentiate them from others with the same label and from their age peers. We learn most about individual variations by long-term observation and documentation. This type of information is just becoming available for the elderly population as a whole and is still lacking for the developmentally disabled.

While most mental health agencies are incorporating life span issues in their programs, both the education and the health care systems continue to be categorized by age. Physical therapists see infants in clinical centers, young children in preschool centers, and adolescents in educational settings. Many programs for young adults do not have physical therapy available or access therapists from pediatric settings. In common with most other health care professionals, very few physical therapists have had longitudinal contact with developmentally disabled clients in either institutional or community programs.

As we acquire this experience, new and challenging questions are arising about the nature of appropriate intervention, long-term outcomes, and the impact of chronicity. An interesting parallel is that of postpolio syndrome, which is emerging years after the initial insult. Many of the developmentally disabled have experienced a similar type of long-term physiologic stress, especially on weight-bearing joints. Lack of intervention, surgical intervention, or long-term "unusual" patterns of movement and weight bearing seem to place direct and indirect pressures on movement and endurance. Joint changes and resulting pain and loss of function may well occur in early adulthood. The issue of pain and that of alternative modes of movement will be addressed later in this chapter.

One area of concern is that of a variety of problems in communication seen among many of the developmentally disabled. This common characteristic may be based on a variety of factors, such as articulation, cognition, language skills, and social experience. A number of geriatric patients suffer a loss in their ability to communicate, but in most cases, this role is assumed by a family member who can relay history and give some sense of preferences that help in both immediate goal setting and long-term planning. Too often the developmentally disabled individual does not have this type of assistance. Proximate care takers, as in the case of elderly parents, may have died, and other family members are not familiar with daily routines. For those living in an institution, attendants and residence staff who know the individuals leave. Written materials and certainly chart records are usually not specific; they may record what is to be done but not how.

Some of the developmentally disabled may experience the physiologic aging process at an earlier chronologic age. This may be actually tissue based, as has been described in chromosomal disorders such as Down's syndrome where graying of hair, cataract formation, and menopause have been reported to occur at earlier ages than would be expected. Exploration in this area is ongoing. Physical therapists working with this population must stay current on work in this area through review of journals in the field and by discussion with colleagues from other fields who are working with this small but growing group. It is important to differentiate functional changes that may be related to physiologic aging and those that may reflect pathology or an inappropriate environment.

Many effects of aging will need special management for the developmentally disabled person. The fitting of reading glasses may be very difficult for some facial malformations, the dexterity to manage a hearing aid may be absent, and partial weight bearing to allow early ambulation after an injury may be a challenge to all those involved. Minor functional changes of aging, especially those in the sensory areas, may come to be major problems in daily life.

PHYSICAL THERAPY CONTACT

The settings where a physical therapist may come into contact with these individuals has expanded far beyond the traditional institution, and the nature of the experience may be determined more by situation than by setting.

Inpatient

An illness, injury, or surgery may bring the older individual into an acute care or rehabilitation center. With age, the frequency of these instances will increase for the developmentally disabled elder as well as for their age peers. Admission to an acute care facility can be disorienting to anyone, and for many adults who are developmentally disabled, it is a terrifying experience. There have been some instances where it has been almost as frightening for the hospital staff. Communication can be difficult or impossible. Three shifts of nursing personnel giving daily care add to the chaos. Motor problems can exacerbate confusion as to function. Imperfect but functional gait is often discouraged, as may be attempts at self-feeding. Concern for safety may require the use of restraints, which may lead to behavior problems and social isolation. Elective procedures may allow preplanning of admissions, as is commonly done in pediatrics. The presence of a familiar care taker, especially for feeding and mobility, may make the experience as calm as possible for all concerned.

In the case of unanticipated admissions, the physical therapist may be the most appropriate professional to evaluate the functional status of the individual to determine what neuromotor problems, such as spasticity, may be present and how these interact with "normal" but immature patterns of function. Staff dealing with adults with long-standing severe spastic hemiplegia will need to know what this means in terms of weight bearing in transfers and in restriction of both active and passive range of motion. These patients may be able to feed themselves independently with the noninvolved arm but, because of their functional level, can effectively use only a spoon. There have been too many instances of trays being placed close to the patient but on the wrong side. When the tray is accessible, the silverware may not include a large-size spoon with a comfortable handle. The practice of sealing silverware and food with plastic covers or packages can present both motor and cognitive frustrations that can easily be avoided. A description of appropriate activities, assistance patterns, and procedures developed with the nursing staff and availability of assistive personnel to carry out these plans may be more helpful than direct treatment.

Home Care

A change in living situation may be precipitated by the disability or death of a care taker. The new situation is usually based on availability, not suitability, and can range from foster care to an emergency room. This situation is very similar to that of an acute admission with the added problem that care taker continuity is often impossible. Recent developments in patterns of care overall give the hope that these particular instances will decrease with more advance planning for transitional residences and with a broader social support network for most clients. In this context, the physical therapist serves a similar function as in the acute care setting. Certainly the information gathered in the functional assessment should be communicated and used in the planning for long-term placements, especially since environmental and architectural changes often cannot be made in the short term.

In the application of normalization principles, individuals with developmental disabilities will change living arrangements in the same, usually age-related, ways that are common in our society. It is socially expected that young adults finishing their education will move out of the family home and that this move is often to group settings, such as college dormitories or shared apartments. More established adults may move on to nuclear family or smaller living groups. Examples of such changes for the developmentally disabled include moves from an institution to a group home, a group home to a supervised apartment, a family home to a group home (when planning averts a crises state), or a supervised apartment to an extended care facility. The greatest difference may be that the developmentally disabled adult may not be making the choice of move (though this is an assumption that is not true in all cases) and may have difficulty anticipating the daily implications of a new setting. A clinical example illustrates this point. Penny was very eager to move from her parent's home to a group home with other adults but had difficulty adjusting to going to bed and getting up on a schedule determined by the times that attendant staff were available. Her reaction was especially negative at 6 A.M. on Saturday and Sunday and became the major motivation in her program directed at independent transfer skills!

Planning

In the best situations, the physical therapist should be involved in the planning on a continuous basis when change can be anticipated. In cases where the change is from parental home to alternative community placements, the physical therapist can often be the effective functional link from one home to another before and after the move is actually made. Long-term planning for these clients, as for others, requires functional evaluation of the client and of the environment resources and barriers. In both group homes and supervised apartments, the developmentally disabled, in contrast to other older individuals, may be moving residence but have a continuing work or recreation program. Besides the usual architectural barriers, it may be important to identify needed transportation services, such as program bus routes and accessibility to loading areas and parking. Since many of the developmentally disabled have long-standing motor problems, distances, textures (hilly or unpaved terrain), and complexity of a neighborhood must be considered.

Some group home settings are designed for those whose cognitive or behavioral problems are paramount but whose motor problems are minimal. If the individual who may be further reducing already limited motor function as a result of aging is placed in such social environments, they may effectively be cut off from participation in internal and external group activities designed for more mobile residents. Some of the more care-oriented homes deal with individuals with severe physical problems. The individual who has some endurance problems and who has spent adult life living with parents and functioning in social activities stressing verbal interaction (visiting and shopping, for example) may lack this type of companionship within the new home and have limited opportunity for these types of activities outside the home. The type and quantity of assistance an individual needs for personal care and life activities must be carefully evaluated, especially at times when the living situation is changing.

Too often, the physical therapist is called in for intervention after the individual has had a change in living situation due to age-related factors in order to "fix" the problem the individual is having in adapting. Examples of these instances have included a referral to teach a 60-year-old to climb stairs because he had been placed where bedrooms were all on the second floor; gait training for a severely handicapped person who was not able to get a wheelchair into the bathroom in a "specialized" apartment (the door was "adapted size," but the hallway was too narrow to permit a large wheelchair to turn into the doorway). In both cases, involvement in planning could have avoided what became insurmountable problems having little to do with aging or developmental disabilities.

EVALUATION

Overview

An evaluation of the elderly developmentally disabled should examine the same factors of strength, endurance, and function as that of any age peer and should be within the context of the living setting. The tools that are used need to be modified for each case, and the observation and analytic skills of the physical therapist will be the most valuable. Range of motion may be determined by choosing the right activity, rather than using a goniometer, and may have meaning when compared with the range necessary to sit at the dining table rather than with the range of flexion

possible in the normal hip. When evaluating the "average" geriatric patient, physical therapists deal with an individual who is experiencing a new and often frightening physical status; when they evaluate the developmentally disabled senior citizen, they see an individual with very long experience with a unique physical status. Sensible physical therapists will tailor their evaluation to take advantage of this experience.

History

In this population, evaluation involves more professional judgment than specific measurement tools. Many assessment procedures are not valid for this population, and their application is difficult if not impossible. This situation is very similar to that experienced in assessing very young children where observation and history as reported by care givers are an important part of valid and reliable measurement. Since motor function is so critical to other decisions that will be made for the individual with a developmental disability, the physical therapist needs to assume the lead in seeking out and integrating material that will aid in this complex process, and this may require creativity in evaluation.

As mentioned earlier, the older individual with developmental disabilities has had lifelong function molded by the presence and management of that disability. This history is an integral part of the individual and therefore an important part of any evaluation. Even in instances where there is a very specific motor handicap of lifelong standing such as spastic diplegia, childhood and adult function will have an important effect on the status of the geriatric client who is developmentally disabled.

Establishing the type of home where the individual lived during most of his life and certainly the most recent living environment will provide some idea of previous functional level. It will also give the therapist a place to start interacting with the patient, especially if the records accompanying the client to an evaluation are either absent or incomplete, as is often the case.

Function

Evaluation is often composed of material gained by observation. While family members are usually excellent reporters of actual behavior, the geriatric client may have outlived parents and siblings before coming into a residential system. The person accompanying the individual to the evaluation may have known that individual for only several days out of a long lifetime. Individuals from workshop or recreational programs as well as long-time neighbors can be the best available sources of longitudinal functional observation. Such data will require professional interpretation to be valid but should not be ignored.

Even in well-recorded cases, the conditions of performance of functional activities are not always maintained in the record as it passes from agency to agency. For example, reports that the disabled individual "used to walk" are a common problem since there is often no indication as to when this actually occurred or if walking terminated when the individual got too tall or too heavy for the parent to assist in ambulation. Many parents working with their child for many years have developed a very sensitive system of weight shift and trunk rotation that enables them to "walk" the developmentally disabled individual within the household. Many therapists have been chagrined when after observing a tiny elderly lady moving a tall, young adult into an erect position, they find that they are unable to duplicate the feat. In one case, a young man who had been managed this way at home all his life spent 2 weeks in a respite care home while his elderly parents had a vacation in Florida. After the family returned home, they were never able to resume this functional pattern, requiring some important changes in daily care. In other cases, the discovery may be made that walking ceased very recently because needed orthoses were left behind in a move.

Independence

A history of functional independence or dependence needs to be carefully explored because of the importance of this measure for successful placement. Some individuals have maintained a level of independence through a life spent with aging parents (astonishing even to the professional). Strategies for assisted function worked out through years of client growth and care-taker decline are sometimes very effective. Conversely, the living environment may have not been one that could allow any risks. It may have been easier for an aging parent to keep a child in a wheelchair or to use a bedpan rather than risk falls or injuries to either. Functional ability in the older years may be more determined by these kinds of social factors than by actual muscle strength or joint range.

Functional settings can be used to stimulate demonstrations of functional activities by the client. This is an instance where the previously gathered history can be very helpful in setting up the appropriate conditions. These functional trials should take place in several settings to observe maximum variation and adaptability. Until the therapist has become acquainted with the client's methods, watchful physical guarding of the client needs to be employed since many of the developmentally disabled have developed methods over their lifetime that are not found in rehabilitation texts and can be fairly dramatic and often very propulsive. This information is important so that the environment can be set up to preserve independence even

if it does mean bolting the bed to the floor. It may be important to know that the client pushes off the arm of the wheelchair to get onto the toilet so that a new wheelchair is ordered with a padded armrest.

Self-care activities need to be evaluated and the conditions of performance noted. In this instance, the developmentally disabled aged differ little from their peers, except that their methods are often homegrown (rather than taught by the therapist and practiced in rehabilitation) and quite novel. Like other geriatric clients, they need the time, the attention, and the interest of care takers to continue at least partial independence in self-care.

Locomotion

The variety in gait patterns mentioned earlier carries over to all types of locomotion. In testing, the therapist should first determine if the individual has a desired place to go, which can serve as a goal for mobility behavior. While it is startling to see a 65-year-old rolling across the floor, this may be functional mobility for many of the severely handicapped, and these age-inappropriate but useful levels of mobility should be considered in the process of an evaluation. In the absence of history in this area, examination of the calluses on arms, legs, and head can provide some clues to innovative methods of progression. While this would be quite inappropriate for the average geriatric patient, these are lifelong functional patterns for some of these clients. If care takers are not aware of the presence of such behaviors, developmentally disabled clients may go on to spend all their time in a condition of restraint that reduces the quality of life.

Many of the elderly developmentally disabled will be in wheelchairs of varying sorts. The methods of progression vary widely. One common pattern is to propel the wheelchair with the feet, often backwards. If the arms are used, clients often use the wheel rather than the rim for propulsion. Recently, severely handicapped individuals have been successfully placed in motorized equipment. This should be particularly valuable to older wheelchair-bound clients as they enter geriatric facilities and to some older persons who have not had a trial at an earlier time.

In some individuals with lifelong gait problems, the use of walkers, canes, and crutches is well established. During the evaluation, the specific size, shape, and style of the assistive device should be noted, since like others with chronic mobility problems, these individuals over their lives have developed strong preferences that they may not be able to articulate. Like wheelchairs, brand-new crutches are often the cause of loss of function. For older individuals who have recently lost functional ambulation, the evaluation may be critical for future functional mobility whether in a wheelchair or with a walker or cane.

In the older population of developmentally disabled,

there are individuals who are household ambulators as long as they have proper support available—the right railing or solid furniture placed strategically—but who have never progressed beyond what could be called "cruising" behavior. This level seems to meet their own needs and should be considered a functional activity for them rather than a transition stage. Other individuals seem to have the ability to ambulate but have chosen not to walk throughout adulthood. For this person, the costs of ambulation in energy, in anxiety, or in cosmetic appearance simply do not match the benefits to them. Whatever the reason, this is usually a lifelong pattern and, again, can be considered a functional state in these elderly.

Communication

The issue of client-therapist communication was mentioned earlier but assumes great importance during the evaluation by the physical therapist. Usual screening should be done for problems in vision or hearing as well as consultation with speech pathology and occupational therapy as to further evaluation and use of aids. Any communication system, such as lipreading, functional signing, or communication boards or devices, should, of course, be used in the evaluation process.

In many clients with developmental disability, language seems to be a particularly difficult area at any age. The individual who has lived to age 70 without a communication language board, however, will not probably adopt one quickly. Fortunately, communication is not limited to words, and this is particularly true in the area of examining motor behavior. Imitation both visual and motoric can be an effective way to elicit desired motor behaviors. Goal-directed activities are usually most effective. For example, having the individual reach for an object (if it is desirable to the individual) is generally more effective as a test of function than isolated elbow extension.

The observation of communication within the evaluation process can be helpful to other evaluators and care takers. How well does the client seem to follow directions? Are verbal or motor prompts more effective in eliciting behavior? How many steps in a procedure can the individual cope with at a time? There are some individuals who can do a safe and independent transfer but require a motor prompt for each step of the task. A toilet transfer for them cannot be done without an individual present to give the motor cues at each stage, but it is a transfer without physical lifting and the attendant risk for both client and care taker.

Medical History

The medical history has been left to last for several reasons. Often this is the best-documented part of the life record, but the information needs to be considered in terms of present status. Past surgery, medication, and intervention regimens will be of interest to the physical therapist as they influence present function. The amount and type of therapy is generally of interest and may provide some clues to past functional level.

At best, there is very little knowledge of the natural history of many of the diagnostic groups included in this population, and prediction is therefore difficult and uncertain. Concern has been voiced about sending elderly developmentally disabled persons on extensive diagnostic tours for either an academic interest on the part of care takers or belief that an exact diagnosis will direct intervention and provide better care and improve function. This elderly individual, along with his cohort, generally requires increased amounts of preventive health care to maintain function, but this is not determined by the diagnostic category.

Routine care in this population is complicated by the lack of ability to report symptoms accurately. The physical therapist's evaluation may contribute to the medical referral by noting symptoms of pain, shortness of breath, unusual fatigue, and so on, that are more easily observed in motor activity. Such findings should initiate referral to the medical staff.

INTERVENTION

Many types of helping persons are involved with programs for geriatric patients. They are professionals, paraprofessionals, and individuals who have had primarily on-the-job training. Formally or informally, most have been indoctrinated with a rehabilitation philosophy that cannot accept that the individual who is not on active therapy is being treated appropriately. Considering the unique behaviors of many of the developmentally disabled, there seems at times to be an attitude in facilities that if they would sit and move more "normally," they would fit in more easily. Often the desire for therapy is based on the erroneous belief that these people have been hidden away and neglected in institutions and now in their later years deserve full access to all available services. Thus, the perceived need for intervention is too often the reason why physical therapists are asked by staff to see an older client with a developmental disability.

Goal Setting

In the great majority of residential settings for the geriatric client and for the adult developmentally disabled, the clients who are able to interact with staff and to participate in the activities of the residence and the community appear to get more attention, to be more content and responsive, and to enjoy what we would term a better quality of life. If, in the judgment of the physical therapist, areas are identified where intervention would aid the client to be more participative in the social setting, then client-related goals should be established. For example, if assistive transfers rather than two-man lifts would allow more and easier participation in recreational activities, then a program directed at such transfers might be a reasonable try. If self-propulsion would mean more participation on community trips, a goal might be to teach wheelchair propulsion or to evaluate the client's ability to use motorized equipment. In some cases, specific exercise programs might be appropriately directed at strengthening or range of motion, but these goals must be considered in light of the fact that many of these older individuals may never have displayed the ability to move against gravity or had "normal" range of motion. Specific environmental demands may indicate goals, for example, the need to do two steps to enter the house.

People within the environment may have different goals, and the therapist may need to involve them in discussion of values. The individual who pushes the wheelchair backwards and will not use foot pedals may be a continuous concern to care takers, but there needs to be a reason to change 70 years of function that is stronger than appearance. An incongruity between the desires of the staff and client desires is often seen in this population, for example, with the client described earlier who seems to choose not to walk as much as he seems able. A projection of the value of walking on the part of staff may lead to labeling the client as unmotivated or uncooperative. The physical therapist may need to spend considerable time with staff to develop the attitude that walking is a goal-directed activity. In some cases, hours of very expensive and scarce therapy time have been directed at forcing an uninterested individual into endurance ambulation. The energy expenditure of the older client must be considered if this is done primarily for staff goals, no matter how well motivated they may be.

Values

The physical therapist has the opportunity to set appropriate goals in this potentially overaggressive atmosphere and must keep in mind both the client and the environment. Based on evaluation, the therapist should make an informed judgment about the client's function, the client's need to change motor behavior, and the client's interest and ability to change behavior. Increasing the range of motion of a knee may not be an appropriate goal unless added range will permit better mobility. Improving quadriceps strength might improve gait, but the treatment program will have value only if the client can understand the concept of resistance and see some value in the repetitive activity as well as have the assistance necessary to engage in the program for the required time to achieve a therapeutic effect. The word *value* is used repeatedly in discussing intervention because programs for this special population must be designed to be congruent with the value systems of the environment, the care takers, the therapists, and ultimately, the client.

Care taker education and monitoring are vital whether or not active physical therapy programs are established. The turnover in staff is generally high, and 24-hour coverage or supervision generally means a number of people are involved in the client's life. For the person who cannot easily communicate or demonstrate his abilities or needs, an organized effort needs to be in place to ensure that opportunities and demands are consistent and follow the established plan. The confusion of changing demands and physical management can produce functional deterioration quite rapidly in many individuals.

Re-evaluation

Regardless of decisions regarding intervention by the physical therapist, re-evaluation should be stated as a part of each evaluation. If physical therapy services are being delivered to the individual, then progress toward goals should be evaluated. Otherwise, programs may simply go on as ends in themselves, wasting client time and health care dollars. Because this is a relatively little known population entering a relatively unknown age period, a recommendation for intervention may be appropriate at one time and not at a later time. Developmentally disabled older people are unlikely to report minor or emerging symptoms or problems, and day-to-day care takers tend to adapt to small changes over time. The physical therapist may be the one who identifies decreases in abilities or function early enough to intervene effectively.

Experience with this population provides what has been called a "sudden onset" problem. A residential program will report a problem in management related to a sudden stiff shoulder. A review of the record may indicate no indication of a problem 2 years earlier, whereas an examination of the client indicates a severe loss of shoulder function. In most cases, there has been a steady decline that becomes suddenly apparent only when it causes a problem in daily care. As in other older persons, deficits of this proportion are often hard to reverse; a routine re-evaluation is the best treatment.

SPECIAL CONCERNS

Appearance

While care takers may become accustomed to a variety of physical manifestations, one of the problems of the developmentally disabled in all age-groups is related to age-appropriate behavior and appearance. This issue continues into the geriatric group and manifests itself in programming and in attempts at intervention. Activities that are enjoyable to the average geriatric client in a day program may be strange and unknown to the developmentally disabled attending the program. Bingo, for example, requires a fairly high level of motor and cognitive behavior. It may distress peers and care takers to see a gray-haired elderly woman playing with a doll or an older man rolling a ball, but efforts to substitute age-appropriate activities should be done carefully and should not be allowed to reduce the developmentally disabled individual to watching television or at least sitting in front of one for a large portion of leisure time. This seemingly simple problem in establishing recreational activities that are age appropriate and enjoyable to the client may need consultation by physical therapy, occupational therapy, recreational specialists, and other professionals.

Long-term Physiologic Stress

As mentioned in an earlier section, the long-term impact of deformities and dysfunctions associated with developmental disabilities is just being seen. Within the older institutional model, gross deformities such as untreated clubfeet and dislocated hips were documented but often blamed on lack of care. The deformities today are not as dramatic, but the best of care is not enough to prevent any deformity in the presence of severe neuromuscular dysfunction or bony abnormalities unless the individual is totally passive and inactive. Arthritic changes in some joints and increasing biomechanical stress on multiple joints are being identified. Some deformities seem to reach a point where a correction that has been effective for years, such as a foot or back orthosis, is no longer tolerated, indicating that a slow progression of the deformity has occurred. Without the external support applied, there is concern that the progression will accelerate in the elder years, impairing general and specific function. In many cases, those concerned with continuing care must keep in mind that they are dealing with structures that have never been "normal," and standards for non–developmentally disabled geriatric clients must be applied with caution.

Pain

The presence of pain and the response of the individual and the environment constitute an emerging and serious problem in this group. Pain may originate from specific physiologic stress and may actually start early in childhood and become a major functional problem fairly early in adulthood. The difficulty of locating the source and treating pain are emerging as major problems for individuals and care takers. The individual in pain is difficult to care

for in any residential setting in both a functional and an interactive sense. The search for a cure often involves "shopping" by the family for a professional who can help and by professional care takers for a technique at considerable energy cost to both. In visible deformity, surgery is often seen as a cure and eagerly sought. In the many cases where medication, surgery, and special equipment have failed to alleviate the pain, the frustrated care takers and family seem to begin to merge the pain and the patient.

Many techniques for managing chronic pain require more cognitive involvement on the part of the patient as well as more predictability of neuromotor responses than currently available for most of the developmentally disabled. Rather than deal with the complaint or risk starting the pain cycle, care takers may start to avoid the client, if possible, and a cycle of social isolation begins. For example, clients do not go on community trips in case the pain might start and their behavioral response would be socially unacceptable and embarrassing for staff and peers.

Less dramatically, the aches and pains of age may be more problematic to those who are dependent on others for movement. In one case, residential staff were experiencing severe behavioral problems with an older man every morning. Bob had never ambulated, had no consistent speech, and had severe cognitive limitations. He did, however, communicate by gesture and demonstrated a sense of humor that had made him a favorite of many of the staff. Behavioral problems had never been a concern. He had always required physical assistance to transfer from bed to chair, but now each morning he struck attendants, cried out, and resisted being transferred. Evaluation conducted during the day revealed no new problems, and no pain could be elicited. The attendant noted almost in passing that the problem was much less severe on weekends. Further exploration revealed that Bob slept in a completely flexed position and rarely changed position during the night. When the staff woke him on weekdays, they did so by straightening him out and quickly transferring him, whereas on the more relaxed weekend schedule, he was allowed to wake on his own and stay in bed until he wished to get up. A minor change in schedule and some assistance in active movement solved the problem and improved everyone's morning. It seems that this problem of pain may increase in frequency and may need more consideration in programs for all aging, especially the chronically disabled.

Stereotypes

There has been considerable concern about stereotyping of the aged and the aging by the rest of society. Nonetheless, most individuals anticipate that they will grow old, and whatever the negative stereotypes, the visible signs of aging are seen by most individuals as something that will happen to them. Throughout life, the developmentally disabled may be especially stereotyped by society since their appearance and/or condition is not something within the expectation of care takers or social contacts—they are and remain different. This difference is often a problem for those whom program planners regard as peers of the developmentally disabled. The problems of mainstreaming developmentally disabled school-age children and youth have been described in the education literature.[2]

In workshop and work-training settings, the physically impaired have, in some cases, objected to being placed in the same program with developmentally disabled, whom they see as reflecting on their own competence. Within extended care facilities, geriatric patients and/or their families have objected to the presence of developmentally disabled age peers in the same room or program since this infers that they share the same limitations, especially in the area of cognition.

In many cases, the joint effect of a cognitive and motor disability has greater functional impact for the individual than would either deficit occurring alone. In the near future, we will discover whether the interaction of age and developmental disability will enhance negative stereotypes for the developmentally disabled or whether the decreasing stereotyping in the area of aging will improve the chances for the developmentally disabled to be considered more as individuals than as a distinct group as they age.

ROLES FOR THE PHYSICAL THERAPIST

This area of practice offers new opportunities for physical therapists to function as consultants and educators in the area of motor and functional behavior. Building on the ability to evaluate across a wide variety of fairly unique diagnostic categories and functional variations, the physical therapist has an important role in disseminating accurate information about and to the developmentally disabled elder.

Educator

In many cases, the physical therapist is the most consistent presence in the program who can read the medical record and has some knowledge of, or knows where to get the knowledge about, the seemingly exotic or rarely seen syndromes that are often attached to the developmentally disabled person. In spite of the earlier comments on increased life expectancy, there are still many care takers who are working with outdated information and mistaken beliefs. One nursing home staff wanted to have a patient admitted to the medical center for a complete diagnostic workup because their client was 50 years old and had Down's syndrome. According to their information, this diagnostic

group died by 10 years of age; so they presumed that the diagnosis of Down's syndrome was incorrect in this case. Persons who have worked exclusively with the geriatric population cannot be expected to be familiar with the characteristics of the diagnostic groups included in developmental disabilities as well as the nature of deformities that are common to chronic disability of lifelong standing.

All professionals, including the physical therapist, should be an educator for the client as well as the care takers. Many of the older developmentally disabled coming from sheltered backgrounds have very little knowledge of their conditions, its functional meaning, or impact on their future. Changes in living situation, however minor, even a change of roommates, can give rise to anxiety, and this needs to be dealt with at the client's level of understanding. One client thought he could not walk because he did not have crutches like a housemate who ambulated; he acted out quite severely until he was assured that this was not a deliberate act on the part of staff to limit his freedom. The example of acute hospital admission is another example where the physical therapist may help other staff in dealing with patient concerns.

Consultant

Many of the care takers who spend the most time with the client in any residential placement do not have formal education in disabilities, and their knowledge ranges from extensive and accurate to very sketchy. Those familiar with common geriatric problems in physical function may be quite unaware of developmental disabilities and the differences in appropriate intervention for a recent v. longstanding motor problem. A specific example is a common desire of nursing home staff to give a new admission with developmental disabilities and hemiplegia the benefit of a one-arm drive wheelchair since these are used by many of their residents with hemiplegia. The complexity of operation of this type of drive and its tendency to mash fingers need to be explained in a tactful way to simultaneously spare the patient and avoid squelching future good suggestions from staff. The physical therapist's role as consultant to the staff may be specific to certain clients in a program and general in the broad area of developmental disabilities as a preparation for the future.

Physical therapists, to date, have not taken the initiative (and this may require some aggressive volunteering) to participate in program planning for community programs for the developmentally disabled. Certainly their input should be valuable in designing programs, choosing sites, and considering the mix of needs that are predicted to increase into the next century. This interaction should be across the range of planning for the aging population from supervised apartments to long-term care. It is important that all the options remain open for the developmentally disabled person since the only sure prediction is that they will vary in their needs in the older ages as much as they do in younger ages in their need for residential settings, work opportunities, and leisure activities.

Traditionally, intervention programs for the developmentally disabled have been termed *habilitation programs* since they are directed at gaining new abilities rather than at recovering lost functions. As this group of individuals age, they may reach a point, as do many adults, where their need or ability to achieve new activities plateaus. Many will come to a point in common with their age peers where they need rehabilitation to regain abilities after injury or illness.

Addressing the needs of the aging person with developmental disabilities offers physical therapists many opportunities to exercise their professional expertise. From evaluation to discharge, the physical therapist has the opportunity to be a detective, an interpreter, a consultant, and an educator to a variety of people. In this problem-solving process, it is important to keep in mind that the evaluation and intervention strategies are the usual ones for the physical therapist, but they are applied to an unusual population.

SUMMARY

This chapter has discussed the social evolution of a group of aging persons who are taking their place as members of the broad community. In many respects, developmentally disabled persons share the changes and risks of aging with other persons their age and display the same variability, but the presence of lifelong functional handicaps presents a special challenge to these individuals and to the helpers who come in contact with them. Physical therapists, applying their professional knowledge and skills in appropriate roles, have the potential to improve the quality of life for the older citizen coping with age and a developmental disability.

REFERENCES

1. Janicki M, Wisniewski H (eds): *Aging and Developmental Disabilities*. Baltimore, Paul H Brookes, 1985.
2. Rostetter D, Kowalski R, Hunter D: Implementing the integration principle of PL 94–142, in Certo N, Haring N, York R (eds): *Public School Integration of Severely Handicapped Students*. Baltimore, Paul H Brookes, 1984.

ADDITIONAL READINGS

Chinn P, Drew C, Logan D: *Mental Retardation: A Life Cycle Approach*. St Louis, CV Mosby, 1979.

Landesman S, Butterfield E: Normalization and deinstitutionalization of mentally retarded individuals: Controversy and facts. *Am Psychol* 1987; 42:809–816.

GENERAL RESOURCES

Since the challenge of providing services to this population is an emerging rather than an established area of service delivery, it may be most helpful to consult current journals in both geriatrics and education/mental health. In the latter area, the periodicals *Mental Retardation, American Journal of Mental Retardation,* and *Journal of the Association for Persons With Severe Handicaps* may be of particular interest. Special issues on aging with a disability and on issues of residential care may be particularly helpful.

Glossary

adherence Consistent behavior that is accomplished through an internalization of learning, enhanced by independent coping and problem-solving skills.

aerobic exercise training Exercise of sufficient intensity, duration, and frequency to improve the efficiency of oxygen consumption during work.

Alzheimer's disease Diagnostic label for a cluster of symptoms including confusion and diminished mental capacity after other diagnoses have been ruled out. Confirmation of the diagnosis can only be made with a brain biopsy, most usually on autopsy.

andragogy Philosophic orientation for adult education.

anticholinergic Any substance that diminishes the effects of acetylcholine in the body.

arteriovenous oxygen difference (a-$\bar{v}o_2$ diff) The difference between the oxygen content of blood in the arterial system and the amount in the mixed venous blood. At rest the normal a-$\bar{v}o_2$ diff averages 4 to 5 mL of oxygen per 100 mL of blood. With vigorous exercise, this value may increase to 15 mL of oxygen per 100 mL of blood.

arthrokinematics The relative rotary and translatory movements that occur between joint surfaces.

arthrokinesiology The study of the structure and function of skeletal joints.

assignment Process through which a provider agrees to accept the amount the insurer pays as payment in full. The only amounts the patient may be billed for are copayments and deductibles.

assisted living settings A type of living situation in which persons live in community housing with attendant care provided for those parts of the day or those activities where assistance is required. One attendant may provide for a number of clients.

automatic postural responses Refers to a set of muscle responses characterized by latencies of approximately 100 to 150 ms, which are longer than monosynaptic reflexes but shorter than voluntary muscle responses. They occur in response to balance disturbance (expected or unexpected) and are important in postural control; there is evidence that these responses become delayed with age.

balance billing Procedure for billing the patient for the balance of amounts not covered by insurance. This can be done only with certain insurers for which the provider does not accept assignment.

blastema Immature substance from which cells and tissues are created.

cardiac output ($\dot{Q}$) The product of heart rate and stroke volume.

chronotropic response Influencing the rate of the heartbeat.

close-packed position The point in a joint's range of motion where maximal stability exists due to the stretch placed on periarticular structures.

cocontraction Simultaneous contraction of agonist and antagonist muscles.

colloid osmotic pressure The pressure exerted by substances capable of influencing osmosis of water across membranes. These substances include serum proteins.

compliance Subservient behavior that implies following orders or directions without self-direction or choice.

creep A measure of the deformation in a material as a result of a constant load applied over a specific time interval.

deinstitutionalization A movement that started in mental health that shifted the location of treatment from hospital to community. This philosophy has extended to current practice in general health care as seen in the move from hospital to home care.

delirium Acute and reversible changes in mental status. Causes include fever, shock, and drug overdose.

dementia Impairment of intellectual functioning, occasionally due to a treatable condition.

depression Affective disorder divided into various separate diagnoses by the third revised edition of the *Diagnostic and Statistical Manual of Mental Disorders* (*DSM III-R*). Two diagnoses of particular interest to physical therapists are major depressive episode (*see* Table 10–1) and adjustment disorder with depressed mood.

developmental disability A physical or mental handicap or combination of the two that becomes evident before age 22 and is likely to continue indefinitely and that results in significant function limitation in major areas of life.

diagnosis-related groups (DRGs) System of categorizing acute care inpatients who are medically related in terms of diagnosis and treatment for the purpose of assigning dollar amounts for reimbursement to hospitals for care of these individuals under the Prospective Payment System.

disability   Defined by the International Classification of Impairments, Disabilities and Handicaps as limitations in functional activities. Refers to inability to fulfill social role obligations in situations of long-term or continued impairments that lead to functional limitations in the model developed by Nagi.

disease   Pathologic condition of the body that presents as a group of characteristic signs and symptoms that indicate the condition is abnormal.

drug half-life   The time required for half the drug remaining in the body to be eliminated.

durable medical equipment (DME)   Equipment covered by the Medicare program for patient use. Equipment must meet specific criteria and may be rented or purchased.

durable power of attorney   Designation by a mentally competent individual of the person who should make decisions for that individual in the event of mental incapacitation. Durable power of attorney may be restricted to certain kinds of decisions, and different individuals may be designated to make different types of decisions.

ejection fraction   The fraction of the end-diastolic volume that is ejected with each heartbeat.

elastic stiffness   The amount of tissue force produced when a tissue is deformed and held at a given length.

elder   *See* older person.

end-diastolic volume   The amount of filling of the ventricles during diastole.

end-systolic volume   The amount of blood remaining in each ventricle after each heartbeat.

extrapyramidal signs   Motor symptoms that mimic Parkinson's disease, dyskinesia, and other lesions in the extrapyramidal tract.

feedback control   Refers to the postural control mechanism of automatic responses that occurs when there is a displacement of one's center of gravity that is not under voluntary control (e.g., a slip or a trip). Automatic postural responses that occur in response to this balance disturbance are critical in the recovery of balance and are not under voluntary control.

feedforward control   Refers to the postural control mechanism of automatic responses that occurs during an intentional displacement of the center of gravity, as during voluntary movement (e.g., lifting arms overhead). Automatic postural responses occur prior to activation of the prime movers, are not under voluntary control, and are

critical to the successful execution of the movement. Persons with impaired balance may have difficulty with the feedforward mechanism of postural control.

FEV$_1$ The percentage of the vital capacity that can be expired in 1 minute.

fibroblast   Chief cell of connective tissue responsible for forming the fibrous tissues of the body such as tendons and ligaments.

Frank-Starling mechanism   The intrinsic ability of the heart to adapt to changing volumes of inflowing blood.

functional limitation   Inability to perform a task or typical daily activities in the normal or anticipated fashion as the result of impairment.

functional reach   A simple clinical measure of functional balance that quantifies one's forward reach. This measure assesses one's ability or willingness to move his center of gravity to the margins of his base support. Reach is known to diminish slightly with age, but markedly restricted reach (less than 6 in.) can be a marker of frailty and signal that a person is at increased risk for falls.

functional reserve   Refers to the excess or redundant function that is present in virtually all physiologic systems. This is diminished in the older adult, lowering the threshold for clinically observable loss of function. For example, sensory loss (vision, proprioception, vestibular function) is common in the older adult. Compensatory capacity then becomes compromised. An older individual with diminished proprioception may have little "visual reserve" with which to compensate for position sense loss.

gyral atrophy   Decreases in the gray or white matter of the brain or both.

handicap   The social disadvantage of a disability.

impairment   Any loss or abnormality of anatomic, physiologic, or psychologic structure or function.

indemnity insurance   Type of insurance based on payments only when an illness or accident has occurred.

individualized habilitation plan (IHP)   A written multidisciplinary plan of care for a developmentally disabled adult that identifies needs, strategies for meeting these needs, and the individuals involved in providing the program. This may be a part of a referral to physical therapy.

informed consent   A process by which a mentally competent individual is given sufficient information to develop adequate comprehension about the risks, benefits, and alternatives to treatment in order to choose a treatment option voluntarily.

intermediate care facility (ICF)   One that provides intermediate care, which is the care most often required in a nursing home. This may include help with activities of daily living. This type of care does not require the constant involvement of licensed professional staff.

kinematics The study of the motion within a joint or between bones, without regard to forces or torques that have caused the motion.

kinetics Describes the joint forces and torques that cause motion at a joint.

learning A change in behavior resulting from an acquisition of knowledge directed toward achieving predetermined goals.

lipofuscin A dark, pigmented lipid found in the cytoplasm of aging neurons.

locus of control An individual's orientation toward internal motivation, autonomy, and control of decisions.

mainstreaming A philosophy of incorporating individuals with special needs into programs in which their age peers participate rather than developing special programs. Has usually been used in relation to educational programs for children but is now being extended to work and leisure.

maximal voluntary ventilation (MVV) The greatest volume of air that can be exhaled in 15 seconds.

microneurography A technique for the recording of action potentials from individual peripheral nerve fibers.

minute ventilation ($\dot{V}E$) The volume of air inspired and exhaled in 1 minute. The highest minute ventilation achieved during exercise is also called the *maximum breathing capacity.*

motor time (MT) In a reaction time (RT) test, the time from onset of electromyographic activity to the initiation of the movement.

motor unit (MU) Single alpha motoneuron and all the muscle fibers it innervates.

muscle fiber types Classification of muscle fibers based on anatomic, physiologic, and functional characteristics.

mutability The muscle fiber's ability to change in response to a new demand.

neuritic plaque A discrete structure found outside the neuron that is composed of degenerating small axons, some dendrites, astrocytes, and amyloid. Neuritic plaque is found in normal aging brains. Also known as *senile plaque.*

neurofibrillary tangle (NFT) A darkly stained, thick, and twisted band of material found in the cytoplasm of aging neurons.

older person Term used to refer to individuals in the later years of the life span. Arbitrarily set between 65 and 70 years old in American society for the purpose of age-related entitlements.

Omnibus Budget Reconciliation Act of 1987 (OBRA '87) Contains a section of the Federal Nursing Home Reform Act, which made sweeping changes in the standards for provision of nursing home care. These mandated changes address areas such as patient care planning, nursing staffing, nurse's aide training, nurse's aide registry, patient's rights, transfers and discharges, and administrator standards.

orthostatic hypotension A sudden decline in blood pressure that occurs on standing. Also known as *postural hypotension.*

oxygen consumption ($\dot{V}O_2$) The difference between the oxygen inspired and the oxygen exhaled is the amount of oxygen used. Maximum oxygen consumption ($\dot{V}O_2max$): The highest amount of oxygen used during exercise. The oxygen consumption will not increase even if the exercise intensity increases. This value is often used to measure maximal exercise capacity.

pacing Accommodating for time in a test or treatment session; the rate at which instruction is given or practice is provided.

pain An unpleasant sensory and emotional experience associated with actual or potential tissue damage, or described in terms of such damage.

pharmacodynamics The study of how drugs affect the body.

pharmacokinetics The study of how the body handles drugs, including the way drugs are absorbed, distributed, and eliminated.

plasticity *Neuroscience:* Adaptive structural or physiologic change in the central nervous system in response to a neuron's disturbed environment. *Biomechanics:* Defined as continued elongation of a tissue without an increase in resistance from within the tissue.

plethysmography Use of a plethysmograph to measure the volume of a body part.

polypharmacy The excessive and unnecessary use of medications.

postural hypotension *See* orthostatic hypotension.

premotor time (PMT) In a reaction time (RT) test, the time between the stimulus onset to the onset of electromyographic activity.

prepaid health plan An insurance plan provided by health maintenance organizations (HMOs) and competitive medical plans. Preventive and wellness services are available in addition to care for illnesses.

presbyastasis Age-related disequilibrium in the absence of known pathology.

presbycusis Age-related decline in auditory function in the absence of known pathology.

Prospective Payment System (PPS) A process under which hospitals are paid fixed amounts based on the principal diagnosis for each hospital stay of Medicare patients.

pseudodementia Term used to describe the misdiagnosis of depression as dementia in the elderly.

pseudoelastin A protein found in aging elastin tissue. The essential constituent of yellow elastic connective tissue.

reaction time (RT) The time required to initiate a movement following stimulus presentation.

resistance exercise training Exercise that applies sufficient force to muscle groups to improve muscle strength. High forces of at least 60% of the maximal voluntary isometric contraction applied over 1 to 15 repetitions and conducted for 6 weeks or longer.

resource-based relative value system (RBRVS) A system of reimbursement being developed by Medicare for outpatient service based on assessing the intensity and complexity of a service and assigning a numerical value and dollar amount related to that value.

respiratory exchange ratio ($\dot{V}co_2/\dot{V}o_2$) The ratio of the volume of carbon dioxide breathed out and the oxygen consumed.

restorative aide A nursing assistant who works in a rehabilitation capacity and assists nursing home residents in carryover of learned functional mobility (ie., ambulation, transfers) and activities of daily living on the patient floors.

senile plaque *See* neuritic plaque.

skilled nursing facility (SNF) Provides care that must by rendered by or under the supervision of professional personnel such as a registered nurse. The care must be required daily and must be a continuation of the care begun in the hospital.

somatosensory evoked potential (SEP) Peripheral nerve stimulation produces potentials that can be recorded from the scalp, over the spine, or in the periphery. The potentials are called SEPs.

strain Refers to the percent change in original length of a deformed tissue.

stress The force developed in a deformed tissue divided by the tissue's cross-sectional area.

stroke volume (SV) The amount of blood ejected from the left ventricle on one beat. *Maximum stroke volume* is the highest volume of blood expelled from the heart during a single beat. This value is usually reached when exercise is only about 40% to 50% of maximum exercise capacity.

synaptogenesis The formation of new synapses.

tensile force Resistive force generated within a tissue in response to elongation or stretch.

tetany A syndrome manifested by sharp flexion of joints, especially the wrist and ankle joints, muscle twitching, cramps, and convulsions, sometimes with attacks of difficult breathing.

transcutaneous electrical nerve stimulation (TENS) Generically, refers to all forms of therapeutic electrical stimulation to intact nerve/muscle done via skin surface electrodes. Most commonly refers to electrical stimulation used specifically for pain management.

ventilatory equivalent (for oxygen) ($\dot{V}e/\dot{V}o_2$) The ratio of minute ventilation to oxygen consumption. The normal ratio is 25:1, meaning that for 25 L of air breathed, 1 L of oxygen has been consumed.

viscosity Describes the extent to which a tissue's resistance to deformation is dependent on the rate of the deforming force.

visual acuity Measure of visual discrimination of fine details of high contrast.

visual evoked response (VER) Presentation of a particular visual stimulus evokes consistent electrocortical activity that can be recorded from electrodes placed on the scalp. The potentials that are recorded are known as VERs.

vital capacity The total volume of air that can be voluntarily moved in one breath from full inspiration to maximum expiration.

$\dot{V}o_2$max The point at which oxygen consumption plateaus and shows no further increase with an additional work load. It is generally assumed that this represents a person's ability to synthesize adenosine triphosphate aerobically.

Wolff's law States that bone is formed in areas of stress and reabsorbed in areas of nonstress.

Index